56.99

Clinical
Surgery
General

RCS Course Manual

Commissioning Editor: Laurence Hunter
Project Development Manager: Janice Urquhart
Project Manager: Frances Affleck
Designer: Erik Bigland
Illustration Manager: Bruce Hogarth
Illustrator: Ethan Danielson

Clinical Surgery in General

RCS Course Manual

Edited by

R. M. Kirk MS FRCS
Honorary Professor of Surgery and Honorary Consultant Surgeon,
The Royal Free Hospital, London, UK

W. J. Ribbans FRCS FRCS Ed Orth
Consultant Orthopaedic Surgeon, Northampton General Hospital,
Northampton, UK

FOURTH EDITION

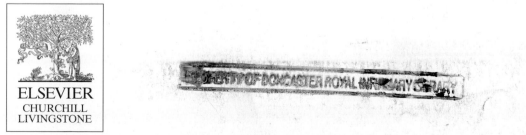

ELSEVIER
CHURCHILL
LIVINGSTONE

EDINBURGH LONDON NEW YORK OXFORD PHILADELPHIA ST LOUIS SYDNEY TORONTO 2004

CHURCHILL LIVINGSTONE
An imprint of Elsevier Limited

© Royal College of Surgeons 1993
© Royal College of Surgeons 1996
© Royal College of Surgeons 1999
© R. M. Kirk, W. J. Ribbans 2004. All rights reserved.

First edition 1993
Second edition 1996
Thrid edition 1999
Fourth edition 2004
    Reprinted 2004, 2006

ISBN 0 443 07262 0

British Library Cataloguing in Publication Data
A catalogue record for this book is available from the British Library

Library of Congress Cataloguing in Publication Data
A catalogue record for this book is available from the Library of Congress

Note
Medical knowledge is constantly changing. Standard safety precautions must be followed, but as new research and clinical experience broaden our knowledge, changes in treatment and drug therapy may become necessary r appropriate. Readers are advised to check the most current product information provided by the manufacturer of each drug to be administered to verify the recommended dose, the method and duration of administration, and contraindications. It is the responsibility of the practitioner, relying on experience and knowledge of the patient, to determine dosages and the best treatment for each individual patient. Neither the Publisher nor the editors assume any liability for any injury and/or damage to persons or property arising from this publication.
The Publisher

The publisher's policy is to use **paper manufactured from sustainable forests**

Printed in China

Preface

What is the book about? Basic science texts deal with anatomy, physiology and pathology. Clinical textbooks deal in a systematic manner with guidance on managing individual patients. We have attempted to create a bridge between the basic sciences and their incorporation into clinical practice. In the past general surgery dominated teaching and postgraduate surgical examinations, but many of the included subjects have successively been separated into specialities. In order to offer the best management to our patients, we may need to know about specialities outside of surgery, such as imaging techniques, radiotherapy, cancer chemotherapy, and terminal care. We have tried to identify and demonstrate some of those subjects.

The chapters fall into three types. Some are intended to be revelatory; not intended to cover the subject in detail but offering a simply presented, comprehensible account, which can be expanded by further reading, for example, *Pathogenesis of cancer*. Some are for reference, because apart from the principles, the specific details cannot be retained in full and need to be looked up, for example *Fluid, electrolyte and acid/base balance*. The third type are intended to emphasize that becoming a surgeon is more than acquiring facts; even more important is the acquisition of professional attitudes of common sense, competence, commitment, and compassion. Books cannot transmit attitude, they can merely set out for young surgeons the high personal and professional standards that are crucial, for example in *Good surgical practice*.

Experts often find it difficult to write 'down' for trainees, and especially for those whose first language is not English and those taught medicine in languages other than English. Teachers often feel, quite reasonably, that aspiring experts should learn the basic specialist terms, but too often the trainees learn the words without fully understanding their clear meaning. Consequently, the contributors have been exhorted to use simple, direct language, define complex terms and acronyms, and, when in doubt, to prefer comprehensibility over comprehensiveness. Most have been very tolerant.

A minority of readers studied Latin or Greek at school and even those who have done so, do not always recognize the words when they encounter them in medical texts. One of us, deprived of such an education, vividly remembers encountering the word 'parotid' in a dictionary; it was a revelation to discover that the parotid gland is simply the 'beside the ear gland' (G *para* = beside + *otis* = ear). In consequence of this the contributors have been encouraged to define interesting or difficult terms. Although it is often frowned upon, the eponymous (G *epi* = upon + *onyma* = a name; a distinguishing name) titles of diseases, instruments, clinical features, incisions and manoeuvres honour those who described or recognized them. They could be inserted as footnotes, or in a glossary at the end of the book. They do not get overlooked within the text and they offer struggling readers moments of relaxation.

Surgery was traditionally taught within the master/apprentice relationship. The master is often not consciously aware of the tacit skills he or she has acquired and passes on to the apprentice by example, rather than by explicit teaching. The trainee is similarly unaware of assimilating it. The transfer of this unrecognized wisdom is often disparaged as mere skill but is described and extolled by Michael Polanyi in his book *Personal knowledge*.[1] Words alone and this book alone, cannot contain the whole of knowledge. In the present day obsession with objectivity, information that defies statistical analysis is often ignored, when in reality it is only our ignorance of it that prevents us from utilizing it. The really important truths defy objective description. Bernard Levin[2] stated, 'Most things that are fundamentally important are not susceptible to logical analysis. I would go so far as to state that that is how we know they are fundamentally important.' Because of the need for trainees to rotate through the sub-specialities, long-term master/apprentice relationships are truncated. As a trainee, assimilate as much as possible by reading but

---

[1]Michael Polanyi. Personal knowledge, Routledge & Keegan Paul, London, 1958
[2]Times, London, 13th February 1989

be receptive to the lessons you can acquire through your contact with experienced senior colleagues. In the longer term, when you become a senior, be receptive to the fresh lessons to be learned from your juniors.

Apology

There is no epicene (G *epi* = upon + *koinos* = common; common to both genders) word for he and she, him and her, his and hers. Most of the older textbooks recognized only male surgeons but this must no longer be so. However, there are times when specifying both sexes several times in a sentence becomes tedious; repeated cutting from singular to plural is clumsy. Some sexually attributable words have acquired special meanings, such as Master, with the connotation of teacher or leader; Mistress has a quite different connotation!

2003   R. M. K.
                                                                             W. J. R

Acknowledgements

We are grateful for the expert and experienced advice of Laurence Hunter, the pleasure of working once again with Janice Urquhart and with a newly encountered and expert copy editor, Rosaline Crum. The contributors have generously agreed to forego any payment in order that the royalties can be donated to the Royal College of Surgeons of England towards funding the very successful Research Fellowships.

Professor Marc Winslet, Head of the Academic Department of Surgery at the Royal Free Hospital, has not only contributed to the book, but he has also generously allowed the organization and editing of the book to be centred within the Department.

Contributors

Tushar Agarwal MB BS MRCS(Ed)
Specialist Registrar, Academic Surgical Unit, St Mary's
Hospital, London, UK

Peter L. Amlot MB BS FRCP
Senior Lecturer, Department of Immunology, Royal Free
and University College Medical School, London, UK

J. L. Atkins MSc FRCS
Registrar in Plastic Surgery, Royal Free Hospital,
London, UK

Wynne Aveling MA MB BChir FRCA
Consultant Anaesthetist, University College London
Hospitals, London, UK

Daryll M. Baker PhD FRCS(Gen)
Consultant Vascular Surgeon, Royal Free Hospital,
London, UK

Tom Bates MB BS MRCS LRCP FRCS
Consultant Surgeon in General Surgery, The William
Harvey Hospital, Ashford, Kent, UK

T. J. Beale FRCS(Eng) FRCR
Consultant Radiologist, Central Middlesex Hospital,
London, UK

Satyajit Bhattacharya MS MPhil FRCS
Consultant Surgeon, Hepatic and Pancreatic Surgery
Unit, The Royal London Hospital, London, UK

Colin Bicknell BM MRCS
Research Fellow, Regional Vascular Unit, St Mary's
Hospital, London, UK

Laura J. Buist MD FRCS
Consultant Transplant Surgeon, Queen Elizabeth
Hospital, Birmingham, UK

Peter E. M. Butler FRCSI FRCS FRCS(Plast)
Consultant Plastic Surgeon, Royal Free Hospital,
London, UK

N. J. W. Cheshire MD FRCS FRCS(gen)
Consultant Vascular Surgeon, Regional Vascular Unit,
St Mary's Hospital, London, UK

John P. S. Cochrane MS FRCS
Consultant Surgeon, Whittington Hospital, London, UK

Richard E. C. Collins FRCS(Eng) FRCS(Ed)
Chairman Intercollegiate Board in General Surgery
1998–2001; Consultant General and Endocrine Surgeon,
Kent and Canterbury Hospital, Canterbury, UK

Carmel Coulter FRCR FRCP
Consultant Clinical Oncologist, St Mary's Hospital,
London, UK

K. Cox MB MS MA FRCS FRACS FACS
Emeritus Professor of Surgery, University of New South
Wales, New South Wales, Australia; Formerly Director
of the World Health Organization Regional Training
Centre for Health Development

M. K. H. Crumplin MB FRCS
Honorary Consultant Surgeon, Maelor Hospital, North
East Wales Trust, UK

Professor Sir Ara Darzi KBE
Professor of Surgery and Head of Department of
Surgical Oncology and Technology, Imperial College of
Science, Technology and Medicine, St Mary's Hospital,
London, UK

Andrew Davenport MA MD FRCP
Director, International Society of Hemodialysis;
Consultant Renal Physician and Honorary Senior
Lecturer, Royal Free Hospital, London, UK

Brian Davidson MB ChB MD FRCS
Professor of Surgery, Royal Free and University College
School of Medicine, London, UK

J. L. Dawson (deceased)

Ahmet Dogan MD PhD MRCPath
Senior Lecturer and Consultant, Department of
Histopathology, Royal Free and University College
Medical School, UCL Hospitals, London, UK

Glenn Douglas BA(Hons) IPFA MIHSM
Chief Executive, Ashford and St Peter's Hospitals NHS
Trust, Eastbourne, UK

Len Doyal BA MSc
Professor of Medical Ethics, Barts and the London
School of Medicine, Queen Mary, University of London,
London, UK

Peter A. Driscoll BSc MD FRCS FFAEM
Consultant in Emergency Medicine, Hope Hospital,
Salford, UK

Roshan Fernando MB ChB FRCA
Consultant Anaesthetist and Honorary Senior Lecturer,
Department of Anaesthesia, Royal Free Hospital,
London, UK

F. Kate Gould MB BS FRCPath
Consultant Microbiologist, Freeman Hospital,
Newcastle upon Tyne, UK

Stuart W. T. Gould FRCS
Senior Lecturer in Surgery, Imperial College of Science,
Technology and Medicine, London, UK

Clair S. Gricks BSc PhD
Post Doctoral Research Fellow, Dana Farber Cancer
Institute, Harvard Medical School, Boston, USA

Pierre J. Guillou BSc MD FRCS FRCPS(Glas) FMedSci
Professor of Surgery, St James's University Hospital,
School of Medicine, Leeds, UK

Amy Guppy MRCP BSc
Specialist Registrar, Mount Vernon Cancer Centre,
Northwood, Middlesex, UK

Mark A. Hamilton BSc MB BS MRCP
Research Fellow, Centre for Anaesthesia, Middlesex
Hospital, London, UK

Chris G. Hargreaves BSc MRCP FRCA
Consultant in Intensive Care Medicine and Anaesthesia,
Whittington Hospital, London, UK

John A. Henry FRCP FFAEM
Honorary Consultant, Head of Academic Department of
Accident and Emergency Medicine, Imperial College
Faculty of Medicine, St Mary's Hospital, London, UK

Barrie Higgs MB BS MSc FRCA
Consultant and Honorary Senior Lecturer, Departments
of Anaesthesia and Physiology, Royal Free Hospital and
Royal Free and University College School of Medicine,
London, UK

Daniel Hochhauser MRCP DPhil
Kathleen Ferrier Reader in Medical Oncology, Royal
Free and University College Medical School, London,
UK

R. W. Hoile MS FRCS(Eng)
Consultant General Surgeon, Medway Maritime
Hospital, Gillingham, Kent, UK; Principal Surgical
Coordinator of National Confidential Enquiry into
Perioperative Deaths (NCEPOD)

Robert A. Huddart MA MB BS MRCP FRCR PhD
Senior Lecturer and Honorary Consultant, Institute of
Cancer Research and Royal Marsden Hospital, Surrey,
UK

Iain A. Hunter BMedSci BM BS FRCS(Eng)
Clinical Research Fellow, St James's University Hospital,
School of Medicine, Leeds, UK

Donald J. Jeffries BSc MB BS FRCP FRCPath
Professor of Virology and Head of Department of
Medical Microbiology, St Bartholomew's and the Royal
London School of Medicine and Dentistry, London, UK

Jennifer Jones BSc MB BS FRCP FRCA
Consultant Anaesthetist, St Mary's Hospital, London,
UK

R. M. Jones MD FRCA
Professor of Anaesthetics, St Mary's Hospital, London,
UK

R. M. Kirk MS FRCS
Honorary Professor of Surgery and Honorary Consultant
Surgeon, The Royal Free Hospital, London, UK

Anna C. Kurowska BSc BA FRCP
Consultant in Palliative Medicine, Whittington Hospital and Edenhall Marie Curie Centre, London, UK

Sunil R. Lakhani BSc MB BS MD FRCPath
Professor of Breast Cancer Pathology, The Breakthrough Toby Robins Breast Cancer Research Centre, Institute of Cancer Research and The Royal Marsden Hospital, London, UK

David Leaper MD ChM FRCS FRCSEd FRCSGlas FACS
Professor of Surgery, University Hospital of North Tees, Stockton-on-Tees, UK

Richard C. Leonard BA MRCP FRCA FANZCA FFICANZCA
Consultant Intensivist, St Mary's Hospital, London, UK

Liang Low FRCSI
Specialist Registrar in Surgery, University Hospital of North Tees, Stockton-on-Tees, UK

Valentine M. Macaulay MD PhD MRCP
Cancer Research UK Senior Clinical Research Fellow and Honorary Consultant in Medical Oncology, Molecular Oncology Laboratories, Weatherall Institute of Molecular Medicine and Oxford Radcliff Trust, Oxford, UK

John W. McClenahan MA MS DiplIndMgt PhD FOR
Fellow in Leadership Development, King's Fund, London, UK

Paul McMaster MA MB ChM FRCS
Professor of Hepatobiliary Surgery and Transplantation, Queen Elizabeth Hospital, University of Birmingham, Birmingham, UK

Caroline A. Marshall MB BS MRCP FRCA
Consultant Anaesthetist, Southampton University Hospitals Trust, Southampton, UK

Atul B. Mehta MA MB BChir MD FRCP FRCPath
Consultant Haematologist, Royal Free Hospital, London, UK

Richard W. Morris BSc MSc PhD
Senior Lecturer in Medical Statistics, Department of Primary Care and Population Sciences, Royal Free and University College London, London, UK

Paul D. Nathan PhD MRCP
Specialist Registrar Medical Oncology, Department of Oncology, Royal Free Hospital, London, UK

Katherine E. Orr MB ChB FRCPath
Consultant Microbiologist and Honorary Senior Lecturer, Freeman Hospital, Newcastle upon Tyne, UK

Jason Payne-James LLM FRCS (Ed & Eng) DFM
Honorary Senior Research Fellow, Central Middlesex Hospital, London; Director, Forensic Healthcare Services, London

Anthony L. G. Peel MA MChir FRCS
Consultant Surgeon, North Tees Hospital, Stockton-on-Tees, UK

Michael W. Platt MB BS FRCA
Consultant and Honorary Senior Lecturer in Anaesthetics and Pain Management, St Mary's Hospital NHS Trust, London, UK

William J. Ribbans FRCS FRCSEdOrth
Consultant Surgeon, Northampton General Hospital, Northampton, UK

Jonathan Robin MRCP
Lecturer in Clinical Pharmacology and Intensive Care Medicine, University College London, London, UK

Gordon J. S. Rustin MD MSc FRCP
Director of Medical Oncology, Mount Vernon Cancer Centre, Northwood, Middlesex, UK

Michael Saleh MB ChB MSc Bioeng FRCSEd FRCSEng
Professor of Orthopaedic and Traumatic Surgery, University of Sheffield; Honorary Consultant, Northern General Hospital, Sheffield; Honorary Consultant, Sheffield Children's Hospital, Sheffield, UK

Hank J. Schneider FRCS
Consultant General and Paediatric Surgeon, The James Paget Hospital, Great Yarmouth, UK

J. A. R. Smith PhD FRCS(Ed) FRCS(Eng)
Consultant Surgeon, Northern General Hospital, Sheffield, UK

Martin Smith MB ChB FRCSEd(A&E) FFAEM
Specialist Registrar in Emergency Medicine, Hope Hospital, Salford UK

Vinnie Sodhi MB BS BSc FRCA
Portex Research Fellow in Obstetric Anaesthesia, Department of Anaesthesia, Royal Free Hospital, London, UK

Jeremy J. T. Tate MS FRCS
Consultant Surgeon, Royal United Hospital, Bath, UK

Clare P. F. Taylor MB BS PhD MRCP MRCPath
Consultant in Haematology and Transfusion Medicine,
Royal Free Hospital and National Blood Service,
London, UK

Adrian Tookman MB BS FRCP
Medical Director, Edenhall Marie Curie Centre, London;
Consultant in Palliative Medicine, Royal Free Hospital,
London, UK

Robin Touquet RD FRCS FFAEM
Consultant in Accident and Emergency Medicine,
St Mary's Hospital, London, UK

Ines Ushiro-Lumb MB BS MSc MRCPath
Consultant Virologist, Department of Virology, Barts
and The London NHS Trust, London, UK

Patricia A. Ward MB BS MRCP FRCSEd(A&E) FFAEM
Director of Resuscitation, Accident and Emergency
Department, St Mary's Hospital, London, UK

Denis Wilkins MB ChB MD FRCS ILT
Consultant General and Vascular Surgeon, Derriford
Hospital, Plymouth; Chairman, Court of Examiners,
Royal College of Surgeons of England; Chairman of the
Specialist Advisory Committee in Training in General
Surgery for Great Britain and Ireland

M. C. Winslet MS FRCS
Professor of Surgery and Head of Department,
University Department of Surgery, Royal Free Hospital,
London, UK

Gillian M. H. Wray MB BS FRCA
Consultant in Anaesthesia and Intensive Care Medicine,
St Bartholomew's Hospital, London, UK

Contents

SECTION 3
PREPARATIONS FOR SURGERY

SECTION 4
OPERATION

SECTION 5
MALIGNANT DISEASE

EMERGENCY

1 Resuscitation

R. Touquet, P. A. Ward, M. W. Platt, J. A. Henry

Objectives

- **Recognize the variety of presentations to an accident and emergency (A & E) department; these are often multidisciplinary, complex, and neither solely medical nor solely surgical.**
- **Understand the rationale for prioritizing resuscitation sequences and basing decisions on the patient's responses to interventions.**
- **Follow protocols to avoid errors of omission.**
- **Understand arterial blood gases, both in terms of acid–base balance and gas exchange.**
- **Understand the difference between oxygen tension (Pao_2, partial pressure) and oxygen saturation (Sao_2).**
- **Recognize that the doctor in A & E may be the last generalist to manage the patient before admission under a specialist team.**

'Scientia vincit timorem'
(Knowledge conquers fear)

INTRODUCTION

Collapse (Latin *col* = together + *lapsare* = to slip; extreme prostration, depression and circulatory failure) or coma (Greek *koma* = deep sleep; unrousable loss of consciousness) are features of diverse life-threatening conditions depressing or injuring the central nervous system. The cause is often unknown when the patient arrives in the resuscitation room. Furthermore, there may be more than one cause, for example a hypoglycaemic patient may fall and sustain a head injury.

When a patient with an altered level of consciousness arrives in the accident and emergency department, apply the resuscitation sequence described in the American College of Surgeons' Advanced Trauma Life Support Course, whether the cause appears medical or surgical. The initial sequence is the primary survey (ABCDE, see below), a systematic assessment that can be performed while undertaking any resuscitative procedures. Institute ongoing monitoring of vital signs while observing their response to any procedure undertaken, such as immediately infusing 2 litres of crystalloid into an adult with hypovolaemic shock.

When the patient is stable, with clinically acceptable vital signs, carry out the secondary survey, a thorough examination from head to toe to avoid missing any pathological condition. You are often the last doctor to carry out a complete examination. If the patient needs to be transferred immediately to the operating theatre, the secondary survey must be carried out later, on the ward, by members of the admitting team.

PART 1: PRIMARY SURVEY WITH INITIAL RESUSCITATION

Greet and talk reassuringly to a conscious patient. Do not treat the patient as an inanimate object. Take notice of the history from the ambulance crew. Involve them in the initial resuscitation and have them immediately available to give any further details of the history. Ensure that the ambulance transfer form is signed by a member of the accident and emergency department staff.

The standard sequence of the initial primary survey is:

Airway, with cervical spine control
Breathing
Circulation
Disability – a brief neurological assessment
Exposure – undress the patient completely, but briefly, to avoid hypothermia.

Key points

- **Apply an appropriately sized cervical collar to steady the head. In-line cervical spine**

immobilization prevents iatrogenic (Greek *iatros* = physician + *gennaein* = produce) spinal cord damage in those with unsuspected neck injury.
- Be particularly careful if you pass an orotracheal tube.

Airway

Assess

Talk to the patient; look for signs of confusion or agitation which may indicate cerebral hypoxia. Listen for stridor or gurgling sounds from a compromised airway. Detect expired warm air with your hand in a patient who is breathing. Check if chest movements are adequate and equal.

If the patient has inhaled smoke, look for carbon deposits in the mouth or nostrils, which raise the possibility of upper airway burns and associated carbon monoxide poisoning. If so, call an anaesthetist to pass an endotracheal tube.

Manage

Keep the airway open and clear it. Remove any foreign bodies, such as sweets; suck out vomit. Lift the chin forwards to bring the tongue off the back of the nasopharynx. If the gag reflex is diminished, insert an oral (Guedel) airway; if this is not tolerated, but obstruction is still present, consider gently inserting a well-lubricated nasopharyngeal airway. Do not insert a nasopharyngeal airway if basal skull fracture is a possibility. Once the airway is secured, deliver 10–15 l min⁻¹ oxygen through a face mask with a reservoir device, which provides about 85% inspired oxygen.

None of these basic airway manoeuvres protects the lungs from aspiration of gastric contents or blood. If the patient has an absent gag reflex, insert a cuffed tracheal tube by the oral or nasal route to facilitate efficient ventilation and protect the lungs.

If you cannot provide an airway in any other way, urgently carry out a needle cricothyroidotomy followed, if necessary, by a surgical cricothyroidotomy.

Breathing

Assess

Assess any cyanosis. If the neck veins are engorged, consider the possibility of a tension pneumothorax, cardiac tamponade, air embolus, pulmonary embolus or myocardial contusion. Check the position of the trachea; if it is deviated to one side, has it been pushed over by a tension pneumothorax on the opposite side? Count the respiratory rate (normally 12–20 per minute) and expose, inspect and palpate the anterior chest wall. Assess breath sounds or their absence by auscultation. A severe asthmatic may present with collapse and have a silent chest because with extreme airway narrowing no air can move in or out of the lungs. If three or more consecutive ribs are fractured in two or more places, with a segment of paradoxical chest wall motion, this is a flail chest. The underlying pulmonary contusion may cause acute respiratory failure. If there is any doubt about the adequacy of the patient's airway or breathing, urgently obtain expert help from physicians and anaesthetists.

Manage

Prevent hypoventilation, hypercapnia (Greek *kapnos* = smoke, vapour – carbon dioxide) and cerebral vasodilatation. They produce increased intracerebral pressure which is extremely dangerous in traumatized patients, especially if they have suffered a head injury. Both adults and children have a normal tidal volume of 7 ml kg⁻¹. A patient with rapid, shallow breathing and signs of fatigue and distress is unable to sustain a normal tidal volume. Hypercapnia is likely, with a resultant increase in cerebral perfusion and oedema. Institute assisted respiration, initially by bag–valve–mask positive pressure ventilation. An arterial blood sample demonstrates a high arterial carbon dioxide tension (Pa_{CO_2}) level if breathing is inadequate. If possible, ventilate and oxygenate the hypoxic or apnoeic patient for at least 3 min before attempting intubation. Do not prolong any attempt for more than 30 s before returning to bag–valve–mask ventilation. An apnoeic patient needs urgent ventilatory support.

With assisted ventilation, aim to keep the arterial blood oxygen above 10 kPa (80 mmHg) and the carbon dioxide below 5.5 kPa (40 mmHg), but above 4 kPa (30 mmHg) to prevent brain ischaemia. In a patient with head injury and decreased consciousness, a reduction of the Pa_{CO_2} to just above 4 kPa (30 mmHg) reduces cerebral oedema and intracerebral acidosis.

 Key points

- Assume that a spontaneously breathing patient who is agitated, aggressive or with a depressed level of consciousness, is hypoxic.
- Remember, though, that restlessness is also caused by, for example, a full bladder or a tight plaster of Paris splint.

Urgently take arterial blood samples from all collapsed patients who are not likely to recover immediately, for measurement of oxygen, carbon dioxide and acid–base balance. Aspirate arterial blood from the radial artery or, failing this, from the femoral artery, into a heparinized syringe (a 2 ml syringe whose dead space has been filled with heparin 1000 units ml^{-1}).

Maintain arterial oxygen tension (PaO_2) above 10 kPa (80 mmHg), with added inspired oxygen, to preserve tissue viability. The exception is the patient with chronic obstructive airways disease (COAD), who depends on hypoxic drive rather than $PaCO_2$ to breathe and will tend to hypoventilate when given added oxygen of more than 35%. Diagnose this from the arterial blood gas, which shows a high $PaCO_2$ with a normal pH. Give all collapsed patients high-flow oxygen initially, as patients whose respiration is dependent on hypoxic drive are uncommonly encountered in A & E.

You may need to administer oxygen to produce a higher than normal PaO_2. In, for example, carbon monoxide poisoning, elevated pulmonary vascular resistance, sickle cell crisis and anaerobic infections the treatment is to produce an elevated PaO_2.

Circulation

Assess

Assess the patient for shock.

Early signs of shock

- **Anxiety, tachycardia of 100–120 min^{-1}, tachypnoea of 20–30 min^{-1}, skin mottling, capillary refill time of more than 2 s, and postural hypotension.**

Initially assume hypovolaemia from occult bleeding if there is postural hypotension with a fall of systolic blood pressure of 20 mmHg, a fall of diastolic blood pressure of 10 mmHg and a rise of pulse of 20 beats per minute (20:10:20 rule). Supine systolic blood pressure does not drop until an adult has lost around 1500–2000 ml of blood, or 30–40% of the blood volume of 70 ml kg^{-1} body-weight; by this time the patient is ashen in colour because of blood-drained extremities.

The level of consciousness is also decreased because of inadequate cerebral circulation, particularly if blood loss was rapid. As a guide, a palpable carotid pulse indicates a systemic blood pressure of at least 60 mmHg.

Key point

- **If the carotid pulse is absent, initiate immediate basic cardiopulmonary resuscitation (CPR, see below).**

Manage

Control haemorrhage from any external bleeding points by direct pressure, with limb elevation where appropriate.

1. *Intravenous access.* The Parisian scientist Jean Poiseuille (1797–1869) calculated that the rate of flow of fluid through a pipe is proportional to the fourth power of the radius, and inversely proportional to the length. In a severely traumatized or hypovolaemic patient, never fail to insert two short, wide-bore cannulae of 14 gauge or larger, sited in peripheral veins, whether introduced percutaneously or by surgical cutdown.

2. *Venous cutdown.* Acquire skill in this safe, simple and quick technique for intravenous access. Prefer the saphenous vein anterior to the medial malleolus or the basilic vein in the elbow crease. Make a transverse, 2 cm incision anterior to the medial malleolus or to the medial epicondyle of the humerus. Delineate, by blunt dissection, the long saphenous or basilic vein. Ligate the vein distally with 2/0 black silk. Control the vein proximally with a similar loose ligature. Make a transverse incision across one-third of the circumference of the vein to enable the insertion of a 14- to 12-gauge cannula. Secure the cannula in place by tightening the proximal suture. This technique is applicable for collapsed infants.

3. *Intraosseous infusion* is an even simpler technique for children under 7 years. In order to avoid the potential risk of osteomyelitis, thoroughly clean the area around the site of insertion, two fingers' breadth distal to the tibial tuberosity, on the anteromedial tibial surface. Insert a specially designed intraosseous trocar and cannula through the cortex of the bone into the marrow cavity. You may slowly infuse crystalloid and colloid solutions into the marrow (20 ml kg^{-1} initially for the collapsed child), together with drugs used in resuscitation, with the exception of sodium bicarbonate and bretylium. The circulation time from here to the heart is only 20 s.

4. *Central venous cannulation*, even in experienced hands, may be dangerous for the trauma patient, who is often restless. Such patients may not survive an iatrogenic pneumothorax or a cervical spinal cord injury caused by turning in the presence of an unsuspected neck injury; as the above routes of access avoid the possibility of these complications, they are to be preferred. Central venous pressure monitoring is useful in the stabilized patient, but these lines are not for resuscitation other than in patients with cardiac arrest, when drugs should be administered centrally. Carry out central vein cannulation after cleaning the area with antiseptic surgical solution.

a. Unless the patient has a head injury, apply a 20° head-down tilt to fill the vein and reduce the risk of air embolus. The easiest route for an anaesthetist is via the right internal jugular vein, which provides the most direct access to the right atrium. Turn the patient's head towards the opposite side and you can feel the vein as the softest part of the neck, usually lateral to the carotid artery in a line from the mastoid process to the suprasternal notch. The easiest route for you, or an accident and emergency clinician, is probably through the right subclavian vein. Pull the right arm caudally, to place the vein in the most convenient relation to the clavicle for cannulation. Unless there is a possibility of spinal injury, to improve access place a sandbag beneath the upper thoracic spine so that the shoulders lie more posteriorly.

b. For jugular vein cannulation, introduce the needle through the skin at approximately the midpoint of a line running from the mastoid process to the suprasternal notch, aiming laterally at 30° to the skin, towards the right big toe or right nipple, or towards the previously palpated jugular vein. For subclavian vein access, introduce the needle through the skin 2 cm inferior to the junction of the lateral and middle thirds of the clavicle. Advance the needle, aspirating continuously and snugging the inferior bony surface of the clavicle, aiming at the superior aspect of the right sternoclavicular joint for not more than 6 cm.

c. Aspirate until blood freely appears; ensure the bevel of the needle is now directed caudally; remove the syringe and immediately insert the Seldinger wire, flexible end first, through the needle. Remove the needle; railroad the plastic cannula over the Seldinger wire, then remove the wire. Check that the cannula is in the central vein by briefly allowing retrograde blood flow into the attached intravenous giving set.

d. Aftercare: secure the line with a suture through the skin and dress the wound with a sterile dressing. Return the patient to the horizontal position and obtain a chest X-ray to check the position of the central venous cannula and to exclude a pneumothorax.

Key point

- **The absence of a pneumothorax on this film does not exclude the possibility of one developing subsequently, possibly under tension.**

If direct venous access is not obtained during CPR, for immediate drug therapy to the heart muscle give drugs via a peripheral venous line, infusing 5% dextrose solution after injecting each drug, to flush it into the central circulation. You may give certain drugs, such as adrenaline (epinephrine), atropine, lidocaine (lignocaine) and naloxone via the tracheal tube route, in double the intravenous dosage.

5. Correct hypovolaemia by rapid intravenous infusion of warmed crystalloid or colloid solutions followed by blood. Rapid loss of more than 40% of a patient's blood volume produces pulseless electrical activity, leading to circulatory standstill unless you carry out immediate resuscitation. You cannot measure the blood volume or blood loss in the resuscitation room. Therefore monitor the vital signs (delineated in Part 2), especially in response to treatment such as fluid replacement, adjusting your treatment accordingly.

6. If the carotid pulse is impalpable, the heart has become an ineffective pump and irreversible brain damage results unless you take immediate action to correct the specific causes of electromechanical dissociation, such as massive blood loss, tension pneumothorax or cardiac tamponade. If there is no improvement or if these conditions are not present, commence cardiac massage for cardiac arrest (Fig. 1.1). Check the heart's electrical rhythm on the monitor. Place the leads in the correct positions as quickly as possible. If no rhythm is visible, turn up the gain knob on the monitor and check for a rhythm in two different ECG leads. Alternatively, monitor through the paddles of a defibrillator, one placed just to the left of the expected position of the apex beat and one inferior to the right clavicle.

7. *External chest compression*. If you cannot feel the carotid pulse after you have controlled ventilation, place one hand over the other on the sternum, the lower border of the hands being two fingers breadth above the xiphisternal–sternal junction. If the hands are lower you risk damaging the liver. Keep your arms straight, with the shoulders in a direct line over the hands so that you do not tire. Depress the sternum smoothly for 4–5 cm, at a rate of 100 per minute, with a ratio of two ventilations to fifteen compressions.

Key point

- **Do not interrupt cardiac massage for ventilations.**

Keep the compression rate regular. In this way the pressure is increased generally in the chest both during compression and by ventilation. In addition, the expanding lungs drive the diaphragm down, leading to compression of the vena cava, further facilitating the driving of blood up the carotid arteries; this is the thoracic pump effect. Feel for the carotid or femoral pulse every 2 min.

8. Diagnose the correct cardiac rhythm quickly. The rhythm is ventricular fibrillation in 70% of patients with non-traumatic cardiac arrest and the chance of successful

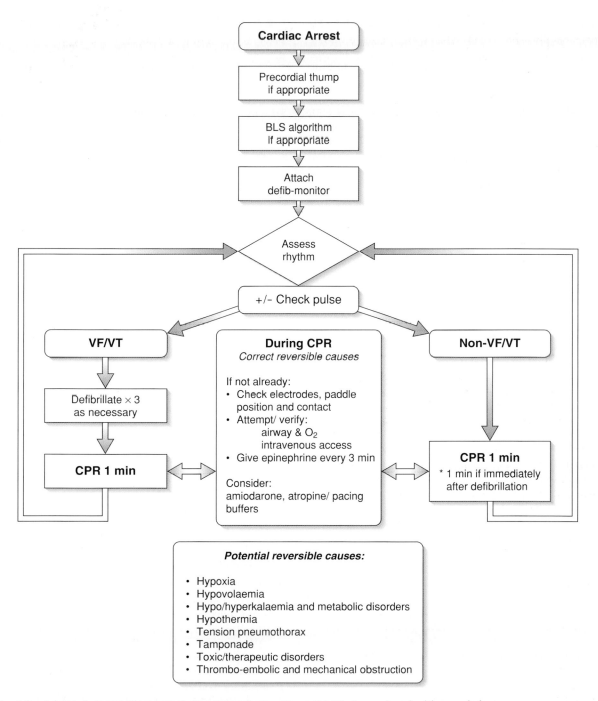

Fig. 1.1 Adult advanced life support. The Resuscitation Council (UK). Reproduced with permission.

resuscitation is directly proportional to the speed of applying a DC shock in the correct manner and sequence (Fig. 1.1). There must be no delay following arrest, and this is why ambulance crews are being trained to use, and are issued with, defibrillators.

9. *Internal cardiac massage.* External chest compression does not effectively resuscitate an empty heart that is in cardiac arrest from hypovolaemic shock; however internal cardiac massage is indicated in the A & E department for direct penetrating trauma only. It is *not* for blunt

trauma, when the patient, at the very least, just has a palpable pulse on arrival. When there is no appropriate response to prompt rapid transfusion, consider internal cardiac massage for penetrating trauma. This is the only indication for an emergency thoracotomy for internal cardiac massage by trained personnel in the A & E department. If you have had appropriate training, it is both safe and haemodynamically superior to external cardiac massage, although the latter can be initiated without delay and performed by non-surgeons. Open-chest cardio-pulmonary resuscitation (CPR) enables you to feel and see the heart, and direct electric defibrillation.

10. Create a left-sided thoracotomy through the fourth or fifth intercostal space once the patient is receiving intermittent positive pressure ventilation through a tracheal tube. Immediately compress the heart using your left hand, without at first opening the pericardial sac, by placing your thumb over the left ventricle posteriorly and fingers anteriorly in front of the heart. Compress the heart at the rate of 100 times per minute, adjusting the force and rate to the filling of the heart. Open the pericardium, avoiding the phrenic and vagus nerves. You may inject adrenaline (epinephrine), atropine and lidocaine (lignocaine), but not sodium bicarbonate, directly into the left ventricle, avoiding the coronary arteries. For internal defibrillation use internal 6 cm paddle electrodes with saline-soaked gauze pads and insulated handles. Place one paddle posteriorly over the left ventricle and one over the anterior surface of the heart (10–20 J).

11. *Drugs.* In a patient with cardiac arrest, if possible give drugs such as adrenaline (epinephrine) centrally, and for this reason become proficient in at least one method of central venous cannulation. Use the approach with which you are most familiar. The infraclavicular approach is often the most convenient and practicable means of access.

Disability

This term signifies a brief neurological assessment you must carry out at this stage of the initial examination. The mnemonic used in the Advanced Trauma Life Support Course is useful:

A = **A**lert
V = responds to **V**erbal stimuli
P = responds to **P**ainful stimuli
U = **U**nresponsive

Now assess the presence or absence of orientation in time (does the patient know the day and month?), space (knows where he or she is?) and person (knows who he or she is?). These perceptions are usually lost in this sequence with lessening of consciousness. Alternatively use the Glasgow coma scale at the outset.

Record the pupil size and response to light (Table 1.1). Bilateral small pupils denote opiate poisoning unless disproved by failure of naloxone to reverse the constriction. If necessary, give up to 2 mg of naloxone (i.e. five vials of 0.4 mg). If there is a response, you may need to give more, because naloxone has a short half-life. You may give it via an endotracheal tube if you do not have intravenous access. The other common cause of bilateral small pupils is a pontine haemorrhage, for which there is no specific treatment.

Expose

In a severely traumatized patient always carry out a complete examination of the entire skin surface. Remove every article of clothing. Carefully protect the spine. Complete examination demands log-rolling by a minimum of four trained people so that you can examine the back. Perform this early if there is a specific indication, such as injury to the posterior chest wall, or at the latest at the end of the secondary survey. Protect all patients, particularly children, from hypothermia.

Consider inserting a nasogastric tube or, if you suspect a cribriform plate fracture, an orogastric tube. Insert a urinary catheter after inspecting the perineum for bruising and bleeding, and carrying out a rectal examination in an injured patient (see Ch. 2).

PART 2: MONITORING

 Key point

- **Throughout the initial assessment, resuscitate, monitor and react to changing clinical and vital measurements (see also Ch. 9).**

- *Pulse.* Remember that in an elderly or even a middle-aged person a rate of more than 140 beats per minute is very unlikely to be sinus tachycardia as this is too fast for someone of that age. Atrial flutter runs at around 300 beats per minute, and therefore if there is 2–1 atrio-ventricular block the ventricular rate is 150 beats per minute. The rate of supraventricular tachycardia is usually 160–220 beats per minute.
- *Respiratory rate* is important. Do not forget it. The normal range is 12–20 breaths per minute. It rises early with blood loss or hypoxia, and, as well as being a very useful indication of the patient's clinical state, it is one of the physiological parameters that is mandatory for the calculation of the revised trauma score.
- *Blood pressure* drops in hypovolaemia when the blood loss is greater than 30–40% of the total blood volume –

Table 1.1	Pupil size and response to light in comatose patients	
	One pupil	Both pupils
Dilated	Atropine in eye 3rd nerve lesion normal consensual light reflex, e.g. posterior communicating artery aneurysm Enlarging mass lesion above the tentorium, causing a pressure cone	Cerebral anoxia Very poor outlook if increasing supratentorial pressure – if dilated pupils preceded by unilateral dilatation or if due to diffuse cerebral damage

	Optic nerve lesion:
	Old: pale disc and afferent pupil
	New: afferent pupil with normal disc, loss of direct light reflex, loss of consensual reflex in other eye – both constrict with light in other eye
		Overdose: e.g. amphetamines (including MDMA "Ecstasy")
		                  carbon monoxide
		                  phenothiazines
		                  cocaine
		                  glutethimide
		                  antidepressants
		Hypothermia

Constricted	Pilocarpine in eye Horner's, e.g. brachial plexus lesion Acute stroke uncommonly (brainstem occlusion or carotid artery ischaemia: small pupil opposite side to weakness)	Pilocarpine in both eyes (glaucoma treatment) Opiates, organophosphate insecticides and trichloroethanol (chloral) Pontine haemorrhage or ischaemia (brisk tendon reflexes, and raised temperature: poor prognostic sign) Alcohol poisoning (dilatation shaking) (Macewan's pupil))
If pupils normal in size, and reacting to light, consider metabolic, systemic non-cerebral causes (N.B. Normal pupils do not exclude a drug overdose)		

about 2000 ml in an adult. Fit young adults, and especially children, maintain their blood pressure resiliently, but then it falls precipitously when compensatory mechanisms are overwhelmed.

- *Pulse pressure* is the difference between systolic and diastolic pressures. Diastolic pressure rises initially following haemorrhage, because of vasoconstriction from circulating catecholamines. Systolic pressure stays constant, therefore the pulse pressure decreases. This is followed by a greater decrease in the pulse pressure as the systolic blood pressure falls once 30% of the patient's blood volume has been lost.
- *Capillary refill time* is the period it takes for blood to return to a compressed nailbed on release of pressure. It may be lengthened by hypothermia, peripheral microvascular disease and collagen diseases, in addition to hypovolaemia. The normal value is 2 s, but this increases early in shock, following a 15% loss of blood volume.
- *Temperature* fall indicates the degree of blood loss in a hypovolaemic patient, quite apart from primary hypothermia. Restore blood volume adequately because simple warming of a hypovolaemic patient produces vasodilatation with resulting further fall in blood pressure. A patient with primary hypothermia is usually also hypovolaemic, so rapid rewarming results in a drop in blood pressure unless blood volume is replaced. Ensure your resuscitation room has a warming device, ideally as part of a rapid transfuser, so that intravenous fluid at 37–38°C can be immediately infused to the hypovolaemic or hypothermic patient.
- *Urinary output.* The minimum normal obligatory output is 30 ml h^{-1}. In a child it is easily remembered as 1 ml kg^{-1} h^{-1}. Suspect renal pathology if you find more than a trace of +protein on stick testing.
- *Central venous pressure (CVP)* is measured in centimetres of water by positioning the manometer on a stand such that the zero point is level with the patient's right atrium. The normal pressure is around 5 cmH$_2$O from the angle of Louis, with the patient at 45° to the horizontal.

The CVP is a measure of the filling pressure (preload) to the right atrium. It reflects the volume of blood in the central veins relative to the venous tone. It is not a measure of left heart function, until right ventricular function is compromised as a result of poor left heart function. It may be low if the patient is hypovolaemic, and rises to normal with correction. If it rises slowly with a fluid challenge, this usually indicates hypovolaemia. Particularly in the young, peripheral vasoconstriction to conserve central blood volume occurs in the presence of hypovolaemic shock, maintaining central venous pressure to a limited degree. It is raised if the circulating volume is too large, as might happen with renal failure or with overtransfusion. Overtransfusion not only precipitates heart failure, due to dilatation of the heart, but in a patient with a head injury the resultant rise in intracranial pressure may cause irreversible damage to the already bruised brain. Therefore assiduously monitor the CVP in these circumstances.

The CVP also rises with malfunctioning of the right side of the heart. It cannot then be used as an indicator of systemic circulatory filling, except as a measure of changing cardiac function. It may be raised for mechanical reasons, such as tension pneumothorax or cardiac tamponade. It is also raised in the presence of pulmonary embolism, or when the heart is failing for lack of muscular power due to contusion or infarction.

Arterial blood gases

pH (normal range 7.35–7.45)

Does the patient have an acidosis, alkalosis or neither (Table 1.2)? The lower the pH, the more acidic is the blood sample, the opposite being the case for alkalosis. Acid (as hydrogen ions) is produced continually from metabolizing cells, mostly as carbon dioxide. More is generated by lactic acid production during conditions of hypoxia, for example in shock, or in cardiac or respiratory arrest. Inadequate tissue perfusion results in acid buildup. Most acid–base abnormalities result from an imbalance between production and removal of H^+ ions (Table 1.3).

Hydrogen is adsorbed by buffers, the largest being proteins, both intra- and extracellularly. In the extracellular fluid, the largest buffer is haemoglobin. However, bicarbonate is a highly dynamic buffer, enabling an exchange to occur between hydrogen and carbon dioxide. This enables hydrogen to be excreted rapidly via the lungs as carbon dioxide:

$$H^+ + HCO_3^- \rightleftharpoons H_2CO_3 \rightleftharpoons CO_2 + H_2O$$

Hydrogen ions are also excreted via the kidneys, but over hours or days, leaving respiratory compensation to be the most rapid method the body has for correction.

The complex proteins of the body are optimally conformed at ideal pH. When the pH of tissues changes, it induces conformational changes in proteins, affecting their function, especially enzymes and cell membrane channels. This is why it is crucial to maintain normal pH. Carbon dioxide is the largest generator of H^+ ions, ten times more than the production of lactic or other metabolic acids (Table 1.3).

P_{CO_2} (normal range 35–45 mmHg, 4.5–5.5 kPa)

- P_{CO_2} is high: suggests a respiratory acidosis (if pH is low); or a compensated metabolic alkalosis (see below).
- P_{CO_2} is low: suggests a respiratory alkalosis (if pH is high); or a compensated metabolic acidosis (see below).

The partial pressure of carbon dioxide is related to the degree of lung ventilation. Hyperventilation reduces P_{CO_2} and vice versa. If the patient is not breathing adequately, carbon dioxide is not adequately excreted and hydrogen ions build up, leading to acidosis caused by inadequate ventilation, that is, a respiratory acidosis. pH falls, indicating acidosis. Anxious patients and those in early hypovolaemic shock have a tachypnoea, resulting in overexcretion of carbon dioxide, with loss of hydrogen and a resulting respiratory alkalosis.

When the patient is ventilated mechanically or manually, an end-tidal carbon dioxide measuring device gives

Table 1.2 Reading of arterial blood gases for acid–base balance	
Acidosis or alkalosis?	pH 7.35–7.45
Respiratory component?	If P_{CO_2} < 4.5 kPa, suggests respiratory alkalosis (pH > 7.45), or attempted compensation of a metabolic acidosis (pH < 7.35 and BE < −3) If P_{CO_2} > 5.5 kPa, suggests respiratory acidosis (pH < 7.35), or attempted compensation of a metabolic alkalosis (pH > 7.45 and BE > +3)
Metabolic component?	Base excess (BE) is always affected by metabolic acid–base changes: Metabolic acidosis causes BE < −3 Metabolic alkalosis causes BE > +3

Table 1.3 Production and elimination of hydrogen ions

Class		Daily production (mol)	Source	Excreted in breath	Metabolic removal possible	Normal organ of elimination
I	CO_2	15	Tissue respiration	+	−	Lungs
II	*Organic acids and urea synthesis*					
	Lactic	1.2	Muscle, brain erythrocytes, skin, etc.	−	+	Liver (50%), kidneys, heart Many tissues (not liver)
	Hydroxybutyric and acetoacetic	0.6*	Liver	−	+	
	Fatty free acids (FFA)	0.7	Adipose tissue	−	+	Most tissues
	H^+ generated during urea synthesis	1.1†	Liver	−	+	Most tissues (see text), small fraction in urine
III	*'Fixed acids'*					
	Sulphuric	} 0.1	Dietary sulphur-containing amino acids	} −	} −	Urinary excretion (partly)
	Phosphoric		Organic phosphate metabolism			

The daily production rates for the organic acids are calculated from results obtained in a resting 70 kg man after an overnight fast, and are proportioned up to 24 h values.
*Because of ingestion of food during daytime and consequent suppression of FFA and ketone body production, the values for these acids may be considerable overestimates.
†On 100 g protein diet.

a good correlation of arterial carbon dioxide, unless there is significant lung disease. End-tidal carbon dioxide partial pressure reflects that in the pulmonary artery, and indicates correct siting of the tracheal tube.

Base excess (or deficit) (normal range −3 to +3)

- High negative value: (e.g. −10) always indicates a metabolic acidosis. pH tends to normalize because of hyperventilation to reduce Pa_{CO_2}, producing a compensatory 'respiratory alkalosis'.
- High positive value: (e.g. +10) always indicates a metabolic alkalosis. Similarly, hypoventilation to increase Pa_{CO_2} tends to compensate and normalizes the pH.

A metabolic acidosis indicates an inability of the kidneys to shift an increased hydrogen load, as occurs in shock, diabetes or renal failure.

Chronic respiratory acidosis with normal pH occurs in chronic lung disease associated with chronic hypercarbia, causing the kidneys to retain bicarbonate ion. This produces an increase in plasma bicarbonate concentration and a normalizing of blood pH, despite the hyper-

carbia (metabolic compensation). These changes take several days to occur but will identify those patients who normally run high Pa_{CO_2} levels, not just those with acute changes. Whenever there is an attempted compensation, the pH never quite reaches completely normal values, which is how you can tell if there has been compensation.

Overenthusiastic treatment with sodium bicarbonate is hazardous (Table 1.4). Do not give bicarbonate during the first 15 min of a cardiac arrest in a previously healthy patient. The principal method of controlling acid–base status during a cardiorespiratory arrest is adequate ventilation to ensure carbon dioxide excretion. If the pH is below 7.1 at 15 min with a normal or low P_{CO_2}, give either 50 ml of 8.4% sodium bicarbonate intravenously (1 ml = 1 mmol) or calculate the amount of bicarbonate needed to correct the metabolic acidosis from the blood gas result. Multiply the base deficit by the estimated extracellular volume (divide the product of the patient's weight in kilograms and the base deficit by 3). Base deficit is defined as the millimoles of alkali required to restore the pH of 1 litre of the patient's blood to normal at P_{CO_2} = 5.33 kPa. In practice, do not normally give more than 1 mmol kg^{-1} initially. Of paramount importance in the traumatized

---

Table 1.4 Hazards of bicarbonate therapy

1. Inactivates simultaneously administered catecholamines
2. Shifts the oxyhaemoglobin dissociation curve to the left, inhibiting the release of oxygen to the tissues
3. Exacerbates central venous acidosis and may, by production of carbon dioxide, produce a paradoxical acidosis
4. Induces hypernatraemia, hyperosmolarity and an extracellular alkalosis; the last causes an acute intracellular shift of potassium and a decreased plasma ionized calcium

---

patient is restoration of blood volume and reperfusion of the tissues.

A lowered pH is desirable, provided that it does not fall below 7.1. Correct it if it falls below this; further acidosis lowers the threshold of the heart to ventricular fibrillation and inhibits normal cell metabolism.

Pao$_2$ and oxygen saturation

The partial pressure of oxygen in the arterial blood (also called the *oxygen tension*) is that pressure which oxygen gas produces if it is in a gaseous phase – if the blood is in a glass vessel with a gaseous phase immediately above it. Gases move down pressure gradients, and so oxygen in the body always moves from an area of higher partial pressure to an area of lower pressure, for example, from lung alveoli to mixed venous blood in the pulmonary artery. The Pao_2 indicates the amount of oxygen reaching the arterial blood from the lungs, or shows if there is some dilution with venous blood by shunting.

Oxygen saturation is the proportion of haemoglobin bound to oxygen, expressed as a percentage. Oxygen carriage depends on haemoglobin, and haemoglobin-bound oxygen is the main supplier of the tissues. The amount of oxygen in solution in the blood is minute, becoming significant only at ambient pressures which are multiples of atmospheric pressure. This is demonstrated in the oxygen flux equation, which gives the amount of oxygen flowing to the tissues per minute:

$$O_2 \text{ flux} = CO\,[(Sao_2 \times Hb \times 1.34) + F]$$

where CO is the cardiac output, Sao_2 is the arterial oxygen saturation, 1.34 is Hoeffner's constant (the amount of oxygen that is capable of combining with Hb) and F is the small amount of oxygen dissolved in the blood. The values are converted to give millilitres per minute: normal oxygen flux is 1000 ml min^{-1}. The minimum flux compatible with life is 400 ml min^{-1}.

Oxygen saturation is now routinely measured non-invasively by shining several infrared wavelengths of light across a finger, earlobe or other piece of skin. A sensor detects those waves not absorbed by haemoglobin. Oxyhaemoglobin and deoxyhaemoglobin have different infrared absorption spectra, so the machine can calculate

the mean oxygen saturation of blood reaching the part with each pulse, compensating for tissue absorption by an algorithm.

The relationship between Pao_2 and Sao_2 is shown in the oxygen dissociation curve (Fig. 1.2). Note how the curve becomes steep below 90% saturation – the situation for many patients with lung disease.

This curve is calculated for HbA, with normal characteristics. Other haemoglobins produce curves in different positions. For example, sickle cell anaemia shows a marked shift to the right, and fetal haemoglobin is shifted to the left.

Acidosis increases ease of unloading oxygen from the blood into tissues; this is the Bohr effect, described by the Danish physiologist Christian Bohr (1855–1911), of pH on the oxygen dissociation curve (Fig. 1.2). Increasing temperature and increasing partial pressure of carbon dioxide have the same effect, the latter not just because of an associated acidosis but also because carbon dioxide combines directly with haemoglobin to form carbamino compounds. Anaemia, heat, raised carbon dioxide, acidosis and increased 2,3-diphosphoglycerate (2,3-DPG) cause a rightward shift to the oxygen dissociation curve, the opposite effects producing a leftward shift.

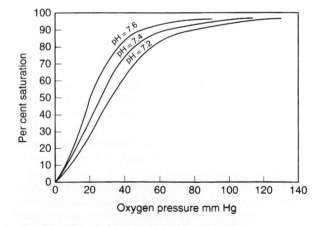

Fig. 1.2 Effect of pH on the oxyhaemoglobin dissociation curve of human blood at 38°C.

Blood sugar (fasting blood glucose normal range 3.6–5.8 mm l⁻¹)

Key point

- **Order an immediate blood glucose estimation, using a reagent strip, on every patient who has an altered level of consciousness, otherwise you will miss hypoglycaemia.**

Follow this with a laboratory estimation. When giving glucose in A & E, be aware of the possibility of precipitating Wernicke's encephalopathy (confusion, ophthalmoplegia, nystagmus, ataxia and peripheral neuritis – described in 1881), and give B vitamins (Pabrinex) intravenously at the same time if there is any evidence of alcohol misuse.

PART 3: THE SECONDARY SURVEY: DETERMINING THE CAUSE OF THE PATIENT'S COLLAPSE

After carrying out the initial assessment (primary survey) and resuscitation of a collapsed patient presenting to the A & E department with no history, a deceptively incomplete history or, worse, an incorrect history, now proceed to make a full head-to-toe examination. This is the secondary survey, during which you aim to gain a clearer picture of the cause of the patient's collapse. Ensure that there is no occult injury. Examine all the skin, including the mouth and throat, the external auditory meati and the perineum. Always consider all the forensic possibilities, noting needle marks, pressure blisters and the presence of any visible soft tissue injuries. Remember that bruising may appear at a distance from the site of injury.

1. Follow a routine to ensure you do not omit any feature. Keep in mind the common causes of collapse (Tables 1.5, 1.6), especially if communication is difficult, because of language, because the patient is unconscious or cannot communicate, or when obvious initial clinical signs deflect you from finding the hidden life-threatening pathology.

2. Strictly adhere to standard guidelines for protection of medical and nursing staff from contamination with body fluids: wear gloves, waterproof gowns and masks with visors. Take special care to avoid needlestick injuries. Ensure all staff are immunized against hepatitis B virus.

3. Leave on the cervical collar in all trauma patients while they are in the resuscitation room. This is mandatory for all patients who have evidence of trauma above the level of the clavicle and have any decrease in level of consciousness, whether it be from the trauma itself or from drugs, especially alcohol.

4. Keep an open mind to all diagnostic possibilities while both collecting the clinical evidence and monitoring the response of the vital signs to treatment. *Beware* a patient found by the police, and smelling of alcohol, who develops an acute intracranial haematoma after a relatively trivial head injury. Involve your anaesthetist early with preparation for the CT scan of brain and possibly cervical spine. Patients with a head injury who misuse alcohol may have a larger subdural space and prolonged clotting times. Patients taking aspirin or warfarin are also at risk.

5. If the conscious level is reduced and the gag reflex is depressed, the patient cannot protect his or her own airway. Call for anaesthetic assistance immediately. Provided he or she is breathing spontaneously, place the patient in the recovery position on the side (ensure first there is no evidence whatever of a spinal injury). Otherwise immediate preparations must be made to intubate the trachea in order to protect the lungs. This also applies if the patient is to receive gastric lavage and cannot protect his or her own airway with complete certainty. If gastric contents are aspirated into the lungs they must be promptly sucked out because they produce a chemical pneumonitis followed by bacterial pneumonia. The clinical picture may well develop into adult respiratory distress syndrome (ARDS).

6. Consider forensic possibilities (Latin *forum* = market place, where courts of law were held; the application of medical science to elucidating appropriate legal questions). Look for needle marks, soft tissue injuries and bruising, which may appear at a distance from the site of injury. Remember the possibility of non-accidental injury in children and in the elderly.

7. Rhabdomyolysis and myoglobinuria may develop in any comatose patient after prolonged tissue pressure and muscle ischaemia, which is then relieved. Local swelling of muscles may be evident and compartment syndromes can develop because of positional obstruction of the circulation. Muscle death starts after 4 h of complete ischaemia. Look for the early symptoms and signs of pain and paraesthesiae in a pallid, cool, weak limb. Passively extend the fingers or flex the foot to test for a developing compartment syndrome (anterior tibial compartment syndrome is the commonest). Losses of distal pulses, numbness, paralysis and development of a flexion contracture are all late signs. With myoglobinuria ensure that the urinary output is maintained at over 100 ml h⁻¹ in an adult, or 2 ml kg⁻¹ h⁻¹ in a child. Alkalinization of the urine in an appropriate high dependency setting with adequate monitoring increases the excretion of myoglobin, and will help prevent renal failure.

Table 1.5 Synopsis of causes of collapse to be considered during secondary survey

System	Diagnosis	Notes
Respiratory	Upper airway obstruction	Inhaled foreign body (try Heimlich manoeuvre) Infection such as epiglottitis (occurs in adults, although commoner in children) Call help urgently Trauma including respiratory burns
	Ventilatory failure	Asthma Chest trauma such as sucking open wound Paralysis such as in Guillain–Barré syndrome
	Failure of alveolar gas exchange	Pneumonia Pulmonary contusions Cardiogenic pulmonary oedema Adult respiratory distress syndrome
	Tension pneumothorax	From trauma (including iatrogenic) Ruptured emphysematous bulla
Cardiac	Ventricular fibrillation Asystole Pulseless electrical activity	Follow Resuscitation Council (UK) guidelines for treatment of cardiac arrest Look for treatable cause: tension pneumothorax, cardiac tamponade, hypoxia or hypovolaemia, drug overdose
	Cardiogenic shock or failure	Acute myocardial infarct Arrhythmia Pulmonary embolism Cardiac contusions after blunt chest trauma Valve rupture
Vascular	Hypovolaemic shock	Revealed or concealed haemorrhage Diarrhoea and vomiting Fistulae Heat exhaustion
	Anaphylactic shock	From stings and bites, drugs or iodine-containing contrast used for radiological investigation
	Dissecting thoracic aorta	Usually in previously hypertensive patients, pain radiates to back
	Leaking abdominal aortic aneurysm	Always check femoral pulses so that you consider aortic pathology (although pulses may not be lost)
	Septic shock	Initially massive peripheral vasodilatation: 'warm shock'. Temperature may be normal
	Neurogenic shock	From loss of sympathetic vascular tone in cervical or high thoracic spinal cord injury
Gastrointestinal	Haemorrhage Perforated peptic ulcer Pancreatitis Mesenteric embolism	 Always check serum amylase Abdominal signs may be absent initially
Gynaecological	Ruptured ectopic pregnancy	Usually at 4–6 weeks gestation. Always think of diagnosis in collapsed young woman
Obstetric	Supine hypotension	The gravid uterus obstructs venous return from the vena cava unless the pregnant woman is turned onto her left side
	Eclampsia Pulmonary embolism Amniotic fluid embolism	

Table 1.5   (cont'd)

System	Diagnosis	Notes
Neurological	Head injury	Isolated head injuries do not cause shock in adults. Look for sites of blood loss elsewhere
	Infection	Meningitis in children (often meningococcal in UK), tetanus, botulism, poliomyelitis, rabies
	Cerebrovascular	Intracranial embolism or haemorrhage Subarachnoid haemorrhage may present solely as a severe headache
	Epilepsy	Including the postictal (following a seizure) state
	Poisoning	See Table 1.6
	Alcohol	
Haematological	Sickle cell crisis	May lead to respiratory failure
	Malaria	Cerebral malaria causes coma
	Coagulopathy	Thrombocytopenia may present with bleeding
Metabolic	Hypoglycaemia	Check blood glucose in *every* patient
	Hyperglycaemia	Coma may be first presentation of diabetes mellitus
	Hyponatraemia	May be addisonian crisis
	Hypocalcaemia	May present with fits
	Hepatic failure	Precipitated by paracetamol overdose in previously fit people, and by intestinal haemorrhage, drugs, or high-protein diet in those with chronic liver disease
	Renal failure	Pre-renal from dehydration Renal, e.g. from crush syndrome and myoglobinuria Post-renal from ureteric obstruction (dangerous hyperkalaemia causes tall tented T waves and widening of the QRS complexes)
	Hypothermia	Resuscitation may include passive or active core rewarming Sepsis and hypovolaemia often coexist
Endocrine	Addisonian crisis	Give 200 mg hydrocortisone i.v. (hypotension, low serum sodium, raised serum potassium)
	Myxoedema	Always consider in hypothermic patients

Table 1.6   Common drugs and poisons

Drug	Symptoms and signs	Treatment
Paracetamol	Liver and renal failure, hypoglycaemia May be asymptomatic initially	Charcoal Acetylcysteine
Salicylates	Tinnitus, abdominal pain Vomiting, hypoglycaemia, hyperthermia, sweating Acid–base disturbances	Lavage and charcoal Rehydration Urinary alkalinization Haemodialysis
Tricyclic antidepressants	Arrhythmias and hypotension Dilated pupils, convulsions Coma	Lavage and charcoal Cardiopulmonary support Sodium bicarbonate
Benzodiazepines	Drowsiness or coma Respiratory depression	Respiratory support (Flumazenil)
Opioids (heroin)	Pinpoint pupils Loss of consciousness Respiratory depression Needle marks	Respiratory support Naloxone

Table 1.6 (cont'd)

Drug	Symptoms and signs	Treatment
Phenothiazines	Dyskinesia, torticollis	Procyclidine
Lidocaine (lignocaine)	Tingling tongue Perioral paraesthesiae Convulsions Ventricular fibrillation	Cardiopulmonary support Diazepam for convulsions
Carbon monoxide	Nausea and vomiting Headache, drowsiness Hallucinations, convulsions	100% or hyperbaric oxygen
Cyanide	Headache, vomiting, weakness Tachypnoea, convulsions Coma	Amyl nitrite inhalation Dicobalt edetate i.v. if diagnosis certain
Iron	Hypotension, vasodilatation Gastric haemorrhage	Lavage Desferrioxamine
Organophosphates (pesticides, nerve gases)	Nausea, vomiting, diarrhoea Salivation, pulmonary oedema Pinpoint pupils, convulsions, coma	Lavage Atropine Pyridostigmine

8. Keep clear, precise medical records of any resuscitation sequence, remembering that, since 1 November 1991, patients or their relatives have had the legal right to see medical records. This record keeping is the responsibility of the senior doctor present. Take appropriate care with forensic evidence, especially from terrorist incidents – anything removed from victims must be removed by a named person and must also be handed to a named person who personally seals the item in a labelled bag.

Key point

- **If there is any clinical deterioration return to the basic initial sequence of the primary survey and recheck AIRWAY, BREATHING, CIRCULATION yet again.**

9. Ensure all patients with a diminished level of consciousness are seen by an anaesthetist before they leave the A & E department. Patients must be in the best possible clinically supported condition for transportation, whether their journey is to the CT scanner, to a ward or to another hospital. If necessary, ensure that the patient is ventilated, depending on the length of journey and the form of transport employed. Order an appropriate trained attendant, such as an anaesthetist.

10. Do not allow the patient to leave the A & E department without stable vital signs, appropriate intravenous lines in place, and having been thoroughly examined, unless there is an acceptable reason. A patient may all too easily deteriorate clinically in the X-ray room or, even more dangerously by reasons of reduced space, in the CT scanner. There must at the very least be a doctor of registrar grade in command of the resuscitation team.

11. For an A & E department to receive patients who need immediate resuscitation from a 'blue-light' ambulance, the hospital must have a minimum of an anaesthetic registrar, a medical registrar and a surgical registrar 'living in' on site 24 hours a day. Even if the patient does not survive, you will be able to tell the relatives truthfully that everything possible was done.

12. Both medical audit and medicolegal considerations dictate the above minimal adequate standards of care. All doctors who are expected to resuscitate the collapsed patient as part of their work practice are expected to be trained in the above. This is your responsibility, but more especially that of the supervising consultant and above all of the employing authority.

Summary

- Do you understand the importance of following routines and protocols when examining and treating collapsed patients?
- Can you perform a competent initial primary survey, and identify and perform appropriate resuscitation procedures?
- Are you capable of setting up monitoring procedures, interpreting the findings and taking the correct actions?
- Do you have a grasp of the basic sciences as regards normal and altered body functions?
- Can you carry out a complete, thorough, secondary survey and interpret the features?
- Are you aware of the forensic aspects of working in the accident and emergency department?

Further reading

Advanced Life Support Course Sub-Committee 2000 Advanced life support course provider manual, 4th edn. Resuscitation Council UK

Advanced Life Support Group 1997 Advanced paediatric life support, 2nd edn. BMJ Publishing Group, London

Advanced Trauma Life Support Course Manual 1997 American College of Surgeons, Chicago IL

Driscoll P, Gwinnutt C, Jimmerson CL, Goodall O 1993 Trauma resuscitation. Macmillan, London

Driscoll P, Brown T, Gwinnutt C, Wardle T 1997 A simple guide to blood gas analysis. BMJ Publishing Group, London

Evans TR 1995 ABC of resuscitation. British Medical Association, London

Henry JA 1997 Poisoning. In: Skinner D, Swain A, Peyton R, Robertson C (eds) Cambridge textbook of accident and emergency. Cambridge University Press, Cambridge

Jones RM 1989 Drug therapy in cardiopulmonary resuscitation. In: Baskett PJF (ed.) Cardiopulmonary resuscitation. Elsevier, Amsterdam, pp 99–101

Royal College of Physicians 1991 Some aspects of the medical management of casualties of the Gulf War. RCP, London

Skinner D, Driscoll P, Earlam R 1996 ABC of major trauma. British Medical Journal, London

Touquet R, Fothergill J, Henry JA, Harris NH (2000) Accident and emergency medicine. In: Powers MJ, Harris NH (eds) Medical negligence, 3rd edn. Butterworths, London

APPENDIX: CHEMICAL WEAPONS

Terrorist or military attacks with chemical weapons may result in pathology and panic. Here we describe the effects of nerve gas and mustard gas.

Nerve gases such as sarin, tabun

These are organophosphorus compounds that act by inhibiting the enzyme acetylcholinesterase and therefore preventing the breakdown of acetylcholine at motor end-plates. The symptoms and signs of poisoning are the same as for organophosphorus insecticide poisoning – overactivity of the parasympathetic system and paralysis of the muscles of respiration.

Initially treat by reversing the effects of acetylcholine at muscarinic receptors, using atropine. Give 2 mg intravenously every 10–15 min in severe poisoning. Support respiration, reactivate inhibited acetylcholinesterase with oximes (pralidoxime mesilate) and suppress convulsions with diazepam. Pretreatment with pyridostigmine (reversible inhibitor of acetylcholinesterase) protects a proportion of the total quantity of enzyme present against a subsequent attack by nerve gas.

Mustard gas (sulphur mustard)

Exposure to the liquid or vapour produces blistering of the skin and damage to the cornea and conjunctiva. Classically there is an asymptomatic latent period of up to 6 h before reddening of the skin develops, leading to blistering. Burns are initially superficial, and blister fluid does not contain free sulphur mustard. Early vigorous scrubbing of the skin with soap and water reduces the severity of the skin burns.

Treat eye exposure with saline irrigations, mydriatics, Vaseline to prevent sticking of the eyelids, dark glasses and antibiotic drops. The damage usually resolves over a number of weeks.

Inhalation produces damage to the upper respiratory tract, with sloughing of the epithelium of the airways and nasal passages. The most severely affected patients need assisted ventilation with oxygen. Absorption of sulphur mustard leads to depression of the bone marrow and a fall in the white count, with a maximum effect at about 2 weeks post-exposure.

In the First World War the death rate from mustard gas was 2% of those exposed, resulting from burns, respiratory damage and bone marrow depression.

2 Trauma

M. Smith, P. A. Driscoll

Objectives

- Describe the biomechanics of injury commonly seen in clinical practice.
- Revise those aspects of human anatomy important in trauma care.
- Discuss the normal and pathophysiological response to trauma.
- Quantify trauma severity by using the anatomical and physiological assessments.

INTRODUCTION

Trauma is a major cause of death in the UK. It is surpassed only by ischaemic heart disease, respiratory disease and carcinoma. Irrespective of gender it is the leading cause of death in the first four decades. Trauma accounts for 8.3% of all potential years lost under age 75. In England and Wales, approximately 10 000 people die each year: just under half of these deaths result from road traffic accidents; a not dissimilar number occur in the home.

There has been a gradual fall in the number of UK deaths and serious injuries following trauma. This is due to primary, secondary and tertiary injury prevention, illustrated for road traffic accidents (RTA) in Table 2.1. Between 1974 and 2000 the number of fatalities fell by 49% to 3409, and the number of seriously injured by 56% to 41 564. In contrast, the number of minor injuries rose by around 35% to 320 283.

It is estimated that for every trauma death 2–3 victims are disabled, a proportion of whom require continuing healthcare facilities for life. The cost to the NHS and social service budgets could exceed £1.2 billion (Department of Health 1998); the cost to the country's economy is considerably greater.

Trimodal distribution of death following trauma

Over a decade ago, Trunkey, an American pioneer in the study of trauma, showed that trauma deaths in San Francisco followed a trimodal distribution over time.

1. The first peak occurs at, or shortly after, the injury; these patients die from major neurological or vascular injury, most being unsalvageable with current technology.

Key point

- **Up to 40% of irrecoverable trauma deaths may be avoided by appropriate prevention programmes.**

2. The second peak occurs several hours after the injury. Patients commonly die from airway, breathing or circulatory problems and many are potentially treatable.

Table 2.1	Initiatives in reducing RTA trauma	
Initiative	Definition	Examples
Primary	Prevents the RTA occurring	Better roads, speed restrictions, better car brakes, drink driving legislation
Secondary	Reduces the effect of the collision	Seat belts, air bags, pedestrian-'friendly' cars
Tertiary	Improvements in medical care	Speedy and effective resuscitation, integrated trauma care, early rehabilitation.

This period is known as the 'golden hour', emphasizing the time following injury when it is critical to resuscitate and stabilize patients.

3. The final peak occurs days or weeks following injury. These victims die from multisystem organ failure (MSOF) or sepsis syndrome. Suboptimal resuscitation in the immediate or early postinjury phase increases the incidence of mortality and morbidity during this phase.

The relative sizes of these peaks are now known to vary depending on the country. In Scotland, the first peak accounts for 76% of all the trauma deaths, the second 7% and the third 17%. This contrasts with San Francisco's figures of 50%, 30% and 20%, respectively. Indeed, recent work questions the existence of the trimodal distribution of death in the UK, suggesting an early peak followed by an exponential decline in mortality over time.

BIOMECHANICS OF INJURY

BLUNT TRAUMA

Over 90% of trauma in the UK is a result of a blunt mechanism. The force is dissipated over a wide area, minimizing the energy transfer at any one spot and so reducing tissue damage. In low energy impacts, the clinical consequences are dependent on the organs involved. In contrast, when high energies are involved, considerable tissue disruption can be produced, irrespective of the underlying organs. There are three types of force:

1. *Shearing* results from two forces acting in opposite directions. Skin lacerations and abrasions produced by shear tend to be irregular, have a higher risk of infection and are associated with more damage to the surrounding tissue and more excessive scarring than follows low energy penetrating trauma. Shearing forces have a maximal effect on abdominal viscera at the points where the organs are tethered. Common examples include the peritoneal attachments at the duodenojejunal flexure, spleen, ileocaecal junction and the vascular attachments of the liver.

2. *Tension* occurs when a force acts on a tissue surface at an angle of less than 90º, causing avulsions and flap formation. Both are associated with more tissue damage and necrosis than are found after a shearing force.

3. *Compression* acts on a tissue surface at 90º and can produce significant damage and necrosis of the underlying structures. The impact site usually shows contusion (Latin *tundere* = to bruise), haematoma if a significant number of blood vessels are damaged, and possibly a breach of the surface tissue. Additionally, compression forces may raise internal pressure sufficiently to rupture the outer layer of closed gas or liquid-filled organs such as the bowel.

A combination of these forces frequently contributes to the pattern of injury seen in victims of blunt trauma. Typically, multiple injuries occur, one system usually being severely affected and one to two others damaged to a lesser degree. Overall, the UK incidence of life-threatening injuries in different systems is: head 50.2%, chest 21.8%, abdomen 23.9% and spine 8.55%. More than 69% of trauma victims also have orthopaedic injuries, but these are not usually life threatening.

Determining how these various forces result in patient injury is complicated. Seek help from the members of the emergency services who have had the opportunity to inspect the scene. For example, a frontal impact with a 'bull's-eye' pattern on the windscreen, a collapsed steering column and indentations on the dashboard indicate that the driver of this vehicle may have sustained a number of injuries (Table 2.2).

Following a frontal impact, the patient is at risk of sustaining a flexion–distraction type injury to the lumbar vertebrae if only a lap seat belt has been worn. This can produce a Chance fracture (vertebral fracture caused by acute flexion, with horizontal splitting of the spinal processes and neural arch), in addition to some or all of the listed injuries. Motorcyclists, pedestrians and victims ejected from a car have a significant risk of multiple injuries, including head, spinal, wrist and lower limb damage.

A completely different pattern of injuries results from rapid deceleration following a fall from a height on to a solid surface, landing on the feet (Table 2.3).

Knowing the mechanism of injury allows you to predict possible life-threatening secondary injuries that may not be immediately apparent (see Ch. 1). It also gives you a clue as to the degree of energy transfer and, consequently, the level of tissue damage.

Table 2.2 Potential driver injuries from a frontal car impact

Facial fractures
Obstructed airway
Cervical injury
Cardiac contusion
Pneumothorax
Flail chest/fractured ribs
Liver and/or splenic injury
Posterior dislocation of the hip
Acetabular fracture
Fractured femur
Patella fracture
Carpometacarpal injuries
Tarsometatarsal injuries

Table 2.3   Potential injuries when landing on the feet from a fall
Tarsometatarsal injuries
Calcaneal compression fractures
Ankle fracture
Tibial plateau fractures
Pelvic vertical shear fracture
Vertebral wedge fracture
Cervical injury
Rupture of the thoracic aorta
Tracheobronchial disruption
Liver avulsion

 Key point

- **Anticipate high energy transfer following road traffic accidents, falls from a height and crush injuries.**

PENETRATING TRAUMA

Around 7% of the annual trauma deaths in the UK are a result of a penetrating mechanism. The clinical consequences of penetrating trauma are dependent on both energy transfer and anatomical factors.

Energy transfer

Energy transferred to tissues surrounding the track of a weapon or missile depend upon:

- The kinetic energy of the weapon or missile (KE = mass/ 2 × velocity^2)
- The mean presenting area of the weapon or missile
- The tendency of the weapon or missile to deform and fragment
- The density of the tissues
- The mechanical characteristics of the tissues.

It follows that if the missile has a high velocity, such as a rifle bullet, then it carries considerable kinetic energy, even though its mass is small. Realize that the crucial speed is the impact velocity, the speed of the missile when it hits the patient, not its initial velocity as it leaves the barrel of the gun. In contrast, a knife has a much lower kinetic energy because it travels at a much slower speed.

Neighbouring tissues may be injured as kinetic energy is transferred to them. If the missile impacts in the tissues and fails to exit, all the kinetic energy is transferred, producing the maximum possible damage. This is more likely if the missile tumbles or fragments within the tissues. High energy pushes away surrounding tissues from the missile track, creating a temporary cavity. Although this lasts but a few milliseconds, it can extend to 30–40 times the diameter of the missile, depending on the amount of energy transferred to the tissues and their elasticity. As the energy waves dissipate, the tissues rapidly retract to a permanent cavity created by the destruction of the tissues in the direct path of the missile. This has three consequences:

1. There is functional and mechanical disruption of the neighbouring tissues, related to energy transfer and the tissue characteristics. Solid organs, such as the liver and spleen sustain severe damage. Lungs and other low density organs such as muscle, skin and blood vessels may escape significant disruption because of their greater elastic properties.

2. A core of any covering clothing is carried deeply into the wound by the missile. The higher the projectile velocity, the finer the shearing of material and the wider its spread. Negative pressure at the exit wound sucks in further material, increasing the chance of wound contamination.

3. If a missile traverses a narrow part of the body the exit wound is usually larger than the entry wound because the temporary cavitation effect extends along the wound track. The temporary cavitation effect finishes if the missile gives up kinetic energy to become a low energy missile before leaving the body. There are, however, no certainties about the size of the entry and exit wounds.

Anatomical factors

An incision with low energy penetrating trauma, such as a stab wound, produces a wound with minimum oedema and inflammation that heals quickly and with minimum scarring (see Ch. 31). Nevertheless it can still be fatal, for example from a stab wound to the heart.

BURNS

There are 16 000 NHS admissions with burns each year in the UK.

Thermal burns are most common, caused by heat from flames, flashes, scalds and contact with hot surfaces. Children and the elderly are the most frequent victims, but scalds are also the most prevalent type of industrial burn.

Electrical burns cause damage depending on voltage, duration, tissue resistance and the direction and path taken by the current (see Ch. 24). Although the entrance and exit wounds are treated as thermal wounds, they do not accurately indicate the extent of the burn. Electric current travels along the path of least resistance; skin is resistant and current travels preferentially along arteries, veins, nerves, bones and tendons, making assessment difficult.

BLAST INJURIES

When a bomb is detonated there is a sudden release of considerable energy. The instantaneous pressure rise in the surrounding air is the shock front or blast wave, which travels at supersonic speed through the surrounding air in all directions. The pressure falls progressively as the wave front travels further from the epicentre. Behind the shock front comes the blast wind, which is movement of the air itself, rapidly spreading out from the epicentre, carrying fragments from the bomb or surrounding debris at high velocity, some of it producing 'high energy transfer' wounds.

Primary effect

This is a result of the shock front, mainly affecting air-containing organs such as lung, bowel and ears. The band of pressure strikes the surface of the body, causing distortion and damage depending on its magnitude and rate of onset. These waves produce most of the damage, at the air–tissue boundary, associated with 'blast' lung, gut and tympanic membrane (Table 2.4). If the pulmonary changes are extensive, a ventilation–perfusion (V/Q) mismatch develops and hypoxia results. High blast pressures may also lead to air emboli; if they obstruct the cerebral or coronary arteries, they may cause sudden death.

Secondary effects

These are the result of the direct impact of fragments carried in the blast wind. In most explosions, the lethal

area for these fragments is much greater than that of the shock front. Furthermore, at distances outside this area, they can still produce considerable damage. The patient usually presents with multiple, extensive wounds of varying depth, which are grossly contaminated. As the distance from the epicentre increases, the wounds become more superficial.

Tertiary effects

These are the result of the dynamic force of the wind itself, which can be so great as to carry all or part of the patient along with it. This results in impact (deceleration) injuries and, in extreme cases, amputations.

Miscellaneous effects

These encompass all other causes of injury, including falling masonry, fires, toxic chemicals, flash burns, together with acute and chronic psychological disturbances. In addition to the primary effects, blasts give rise to penetrating, blunt and burn trauma.

MAIN ANATOMICAL SITES OF TRAUMA

The damage sustained by the patient depends not only on the biomechanics of the trauma but also on the anatomical site of injury.

These are discussed in the order in which they are usually managed clinically.

AIRWAY

The important structures and surface landmarks of the upper airway are shown in Figure 2.1.

THORAX

Chest wall

1. The upper two ribs are extensively protected by the scapula and overlying muscle, requiring considerable force to break them. Consequently, if they do break there is a high risk of concomitant damage to vital structures such as the thoracic aorta, main bronchi, lungs and spinal cord. Therefore, closely assess these vital structures if you discover fractures of the first two ribs. Remember that the neck is mobile and the pleural cavity and lung apex project above the clavicle, so pneumothorax or lung injury may result from penetrating injuries to the lower

Table 2.4 Primary effects of blast on lungs, gut and ears
Haemorrhage into alveolar spaces
Damage to alveolar septae
Stripping of bronchial epithelium
Emphysematous blebs produced on the pleural surface
Contusion of the gut wall
Leakage of blood into the gut lumen
Perforation
Rupture or congestion of the tympanic membrane

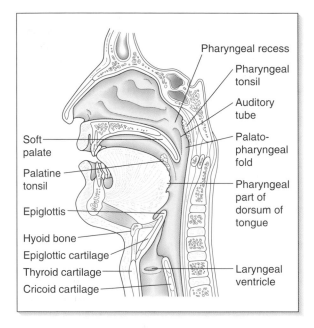

Fig. 2.1 The upper airway.

neck. Similarly, the lower six ribs overlie the abdominal cavity when the diaphragm is elevated during expiration, so both the lung and the upper abdominal viscera may be injured. Trauma to the 'midzone' of the trunk may be associated with both abdominal and chest injuries.

Key point

- **Following stab wounds of the lower chest the incidence of abdominal visceral involvement is 15%. Following penetrating injury to the lower chest from gunshots it rises to 46%.**

2. When two or more adjacent ribs are fractured in two or more places they form a flail segment – a flail (probably from Latin *flagellum*), classically has a loose segment hinged on to the handle. The adjacent doubly fractured clavicle and first rib may also produce a flail segment. On inspiration, when the chest wall rises, the partially detached segment is sucked in – this is paradoxical movement. This may not be visible in the early stages when spasm of the chest wall muscles splint the fractures but becomes apparent when the muscles tire. Flail segment can be life threatening in the presence of underlying pulmonary contusion, which increases the tendency to hypoxia as a result of the impaired ventilation.

3. The neurovascular bundle lying in the subcostal groove may be torn when ribs are fractured. Multiple fractures or significant disruption may cause massive haemothorax. The internal mammary artery may be torn. Large lung lacerations may not stop bleeding when the lung has been re-expanded by insertion of a chest drain.

4. A one-way valve may develop on the lung surface, allowing air to enter the pleural cavity during inspiration but blocking its escape during expiration. This produces a tension pneumothorax unless the intrapleural pressure is relieved.

Mediastinum

The trachea, oesophagus and major blood vessels lie close together, so penetrating injuries of the mediastinum may damage one or more structures. The surface landmarks of the mediastinum are medial to the nipple line anteriorly, or medial to the medial edges of the scapulae posteriorly.

CIRCULATION

1. Tough, inelastic, fibrous pericardium encloses and protects the heart. Even in a healthy person, a small collection of blood within the pericardium creates tamponade (French *tampion* = a plug) occupying space, compromising ventricular filling and hence cardiac output. Intrapericardial haemorrhage usually follows penetrating trauma of the heart.

2. Blunt trauma can cause cardiac contusion, possibly associated with an overlying sternal fracture. A combination of vascular spasm, intimal tearing and neighbouring tissue oedema may lead to coronary artery occlusion. Myocardial damage may cause dysrhythmias, infarction and impaired cardiac performance (see below), with electrocardiographic (ECG) abnormalities. Severe blunt trauma with rupture of the chordae tendinae produces mitral or tricuspid valve incompetence.

3. The distal arch of the aorta is anchored just inferior to the left subclavian artery. During a deceleration injury there is a risk that the mobile aortic arch will shear off the fixed descending aorta, disrupting it. The injury may occur in falls over 9 metres (30 feet) or vehicle crashes at over 50 k.p.h. (30 m.p.h.). In 10% of cases the escaping blood is contained by the outer, adventitial layer of the aorta but eventually this is also breached, rapidly exsanguinating the patient in the absence of surgical intervention.

SKULL

1. The scalp consists of five layers: Skin, subCutaneous layer, Aponeurosis, Loose areolar tissue, Periosteum (SCALP). The vascular subcutaneous layer is divided by

fibrous bands into loculi, while the areolar layer is loose, and this is where scalp haematomas collect. If the aponeurosis is breached, the wound tends to evert.

2. The interior of the neurocranium is divided into two levels by a fibrous structure called the tentorium (tent) cerebelli. The midbrain passes through the opening in the anterior aspect of this layer, partially covered on its anterolateral aspects by the corticospinal tract. The oculomotor (IIIrd) nerve leaves the anterior aspect of the midbrain to run forward, lying between the free and attached edges of the tent. In the intact state, there is free communication above and below the tentorium as well as between the intracranial and spinal subarachnoid spaces.

3. Following head trauma, the development of a mass lesion above the tent, as from haematoma or cerebral oedema, may produce a pressure gradient. If this is unrelieved it can result in one or both medial surfaces of the temporal lobes herniating through the opening in the tent. In so doing, the brain tissue presses on, and damages, structures in this region, namely the oculomotor nerve and motor fibres in the corticospinal tract. This is *tentorial herniation*, resulting in an ipsilateral (same side) fixed dilated pupil and contralateral weakness in the limbs. If the pressure increases further, the medulla and cerebellum are forced downwards into the foramen magnum – *coning*. This is a preterminal condition resulting in compression of the vital centres and disturbance of cardiovascular and respiratory function.

4. The base of the neurocranium is irregular, with the sphenoid wings and petrous processes projecting from its surface. Acceleration and deceleration forces move the brain over the base of the skull so that it collides with these projections, which damage it.

5. The internal surface of the neurocranium is lined with the thick, hard, fibrous *dura mater* (Latin = hard mother, a translation from the Arabic) (Fig. 2.2). Its blood vessels closely adhere to the bone surface, grooving it in places, so they can be torn when forces are applied to the overlying bone. A haematoma collects between the bone and dura – an *extradural haematoma*; 90% of these are associated with a fractured skull. The middle meningeal artery is most at risk and the commonest site is the thin temporoparietal area.

6. The arachnoid (Greek *arachne* = spider; like a spider's web) mater is connected to the pia mater (Latin translation of Arabic *umm raqiqah* = thin mother), across the cerebrospinal fluid (CSF)-filled subarachnoid space, by thin fibrous strands. Running between these strands are bridging veins, carrying blood from the brain to the venous sinuses. With age the brain atrophies, increasing the subarachnoid and subdural spaces, stretching the bridging veins and making them more likely to tear following a head injury. The resulting blood collects in the subdural and subarachnoid spaces.

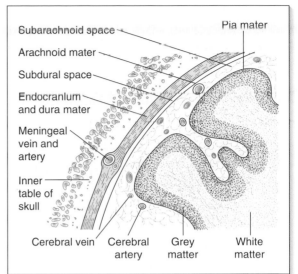

Fig. 2.2 The meninges and their blood supply.

MAXILLOFACIAL SKELETON

 Key point

- **The major acute problem associated with significant facial fractures is the potential for associated airway obstruction secondary to swelling, haemorrhage and structural damage.**

The maxillofacial skeleton consists of a complex series of mainly aerated bones which provide a firm but light foundation to the face (Fig. 2.3). The nasal, frontal and zygomatic–maxillary buttresses provide vertical support, with lateral stability coming from the zygomatic–temporal buttresses. Several of these bones, especially those making up the bony orbits, are closely associated with nerves and blood vessels, which may therefore be damaged when these bones are broken. In addition, the associated bleeding and deformity can lead to obstruction of the patient's airway.

Nasoethmoidal–orbital fractures

These result from trauma to the bridge of the nose or medial orbital wall. In view of their location, they are associated with lacrimal duct (Latin *lacrima*, Greek *dakre* = tear) injury, dural rupture and traumatic telecanthus (Greek *tele* = far + *kanthos* = angle at junction of the eyelids); the medial canthus is tethered to the displaced medial orbital wall, drawing it down and widening the angle.

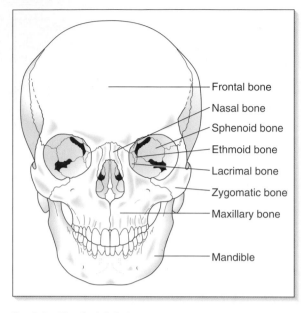

Fig. 2.3 The facial skeleton.

Blow-out fractures

These result from blunt injury to the eyeball, increasing intraorbital pressure, depressing and fracturing the thin floor of the orbit, often with associated fracture of the medial orbital wall. The infraorbital nerve is usually damaged, producing anaesthesia of the cheek, upper lip and upper gum and also diplopia (Greek *diploos* = double + *ops* = eye; double vision), especially to upward gaze. This results from a combination of muscle haematoma, third nerve damage, entrapment of periorbital fat and, in a minority of cases, true entrapment of extraocular muscles. Subcutaneous emphysema (Greek *em* = in + *physaein* = to blow; to inflate) occurs if the fracture extends into a sinus or nasal antrum.

Zygomatic complex fractures

Two types can be caused by blunt trauma. Zygomatic arch fractures are produced by a direct blow and can give rise to limited mouth opening due to impingement of temporalis muscle. The more serious 'tripod' type of fracture involves the displacement of the whole zygoma. This bone can be compared to a four-legged stool, with the 'legs' being the floor and lateral wall of the orbit, the zygomatic arch and the lateral wall of the antrum. The 'seat' of the stool cannot be moved without displacement of at least two of the 'legs'. This is associated with lateral subconjunctival haemorrhage and infraorbital anaesthesia. In addition, the displacement leads to a downward angulation of the lateral canthus and either trismus or an open bite.

Fractures of the middle third of the facial skeleton

It takes approximately 100 times the force of gravity to break the middle third of the face. Consequently, patients with this condition have significant multisystem trauma in addition to the malocclusion, facial anaesthesia and visual symptoms described above. Traditionally, the fractures are classified using the system devised by the French paediatric orthopaedic surgeon, René Le Fort in 1901 (Fig. 2.4). The grade of fracture is often asymmetrical, that is, different on two sides. The Le Fort I fracture runs in a transverse plane above the alveolar ridge to the pterygoid region. Le Fort II extends from the nasal bones into the medial orbital wall and crosses the infraorbital rim. Le Fort III detaches the middle third of the facial skeleton from the cranial base; it is therefore commonly associated with fractures of the base of the skull and bloody CSF rhinorrhoea and otorrhoea (Greek *rhinos* = nose, *otos* = ear + *rhoia* = a flow). A characteristic 'dish face' may be evident due to retropositioning (Greek *retros* = backward) of the midface along the base of the skull.

Mandibular fractures

The mandible, like the pelvis, is a ring structure and therefore rarely fractured in isolation. Usually there are multiple fractures or an injury to the temporomandibular joint. Common fracture sites are the condylar process, through the posterior alveolar margin, and

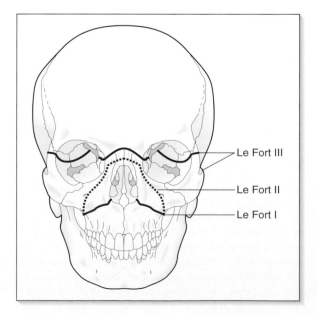

Fig. 2.4 Common sites of fracture of the midface.

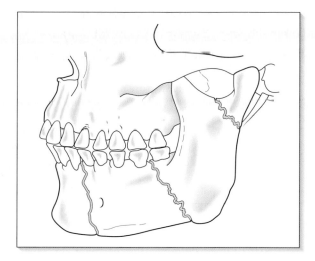

Fig. 2.5 Common sites of fracture of the mandible.

through the alveolar margin anterior to the premolar teeth. In the majority of the latter cases the fracture is open as it extends between the teeth and communicates with the oral cavity (Fig. 2.5). It is common to find numbness of the lower lip on the affected side and malocclusion.

ABDOMEN AND GENITOURINARY SYSTEM

Peritoneal cavity

This can be subdivided into intrathoracic and abdominal regions. Remember, however, that on expiration, the diaphragm rises anteriorly to the level of the fourth intercostal space. As a result, several of the intraperitoneal organs, such as the liver, spleen and stomach, lie within the bony thorax and are therefore at risk if the patient suffers trauma to the lower chest.

1. Diaphragmatic injury is uncommon and rarely occurs in isolation. It may result from both blunt and penetrating injury. The former tends to occur with greater force than the latter and commonly leads to larger tears in the diaphragm, through which abdominal contents may enter the thorax and compromise respiration. Injuries to the diaphragm may be so slight that the patient is asymptomatic and the damage may not be discovered until weeks, months or even years later.

2. The liver and biliary tree are largely covered by the rib cage, affording some protection from injury. Although numerically less common than splenic injury, liver injuries account for more deaths as a result of unsuspected intra-abdominal haemorrhage. Consider the possibility of underlying liver damage when assessing trauma victims.

Because of their location, the gallbladder and extrahepatic biliary tract are usually damaged in association with other viscera. Liver trauma is the most common coexisting pathology (50% of cases), but there is a significant chance of pancreatic damage (17% of cases). Consequently, injury of the gallbladder and biliary tree are usually masked by the features resulting from damage to the surrounding viscera. This condition has an overall mortality of 16% due to coexisting organ injuries. Blunt trauma is the usual cause of gallbladder damage, and rupture is more likely when the gallbladder is distended, as between meals.

3. The spleen is the most commonly injured solid organ in the abdomen following blunt trauma, and is therefore a frequent cause of shock in patients with abdominal injury. Any injury to the left lower chest or upper abdomen may cause splenic damage, ranging from small tears to complete shattering of the organ.

4. Stomach injury is infrequent following blunt trauma but the stomach may be punctured by penetrating wounds; this usually presents as peritonitis.

5. Small bowel damage may result from blunt or penetrating wounds, as well as blast injury. Blunt trauma and blast can cause bowel injury in one of three ways: (1) the force may squeeze the viscus between the anterior abdominal wall and vertebral column; (2) the bowel may rupture as a result of a sudden increase in pressure within the lumen, as when the abdomen is compressed (the closed-loop phenomenon); (3) the bowel may be rendered ischaemic by damage to the mesentery and its vessels. Mesenteric tears often result if the abdomen is subjected to deceleration or shearing forces; it is particularly common at points where the bowel crosses the interface between the intra- and retroperitoneum, including the duodenojejunal flexure and ileocaecal junction. Blast injuries can also lead to multiple intestinal perforations and areas of infarction. Bowel penetration injury usually produces small tears in the wall but may completely transect it. Unlike injuries to the liver and spleen, trauma to the bowel is rarely immediately life threatening. As with the stomach, the major problem is peritonitis, which develops over several hours as a result of leakage of bowel contents into the peritoneum.

Retroperitoneum

1. Injuries to the retroperitoneal organs are more difficult to diagnose than are those in the peritoneal cavity because they are less accessible to physical examination and investigation.

2. Pancreas and duodenum may be injured as a result of both blunt and penetrating trauma, the commonest

mechanism being that of the unrestrained car driver impacting with the steering wheel.

3. Bowel. All of the caecum and ascending colon, as well as between one- and two-thirds of the circumference of the descending colon lie within the retroperitoneal space. The remainder of the colon is located within the peritoneal cavity. Blunt or penetrating trauma can damage any part of the colon, allowing leakage of the bowel contents. However, in cases of retroperitoneal perforation, the symptoms are usually ill-defined and slow to develop, leading to delayed diagnosis and increasing the risk of abscess formation.

4. Vascular. The abdominal aorta is susceptible to damage as a result of penetrating injury. Severe trauma is almost invariably lethal, but lesser injuries manifest as hypotension and/or symptoms of ischaemia. If the haemorrhage is contained within the retroperitoneum, the hypotension may be transient, responding to fluid resuscitation. Later, a retroperitoneal haematoma may become visible as bruising in the flank or back, described by the Newcastle surgeon George Grey Turner in 1920, or around the umbilicus, described in 1919 by Thomas Cullen, gynaecologist of Johns Hopkins Hospital in Baltimore. The inferior vena cava is susceptible to the same types of injury as the aorta, resulting in significant blood loss, although usually less than from an equivalent injury to the aorta. This is because the intravenous pressure is low and the external tissue pressure is relatively higher. However, if this pressure is lost, as occurs in the presence of a large wound, external pressure is diminished, so haemorrhage increases and may be life threatening.

5. Renal system. The kidneys are well protected by soft tissue in front and bone and muscle behind. As a result, isolated injury to the kidneys is uncommon, barring sporting incidents. Significant renal damage following major penetrating or blunt trauma is usually associated with multiple organ injuries. Ureteric injury of either type is uncommon. Assiduously investigate macroscopic haematuria, or microscopic haematuria in the presence of shock.

Pelvis

1. Pelvic injuries mainly involve the bladder and posterior urethra.

2. Urinary system. Although the bladder lies within the pelvis, when full it may extend as high as the umbilicus and be susceptible to injury to the lower abdomen. Compression of the abdomen increases intravesical pressure and may cause 'full-bladder blowout', although more commonly the bladder is punctured by bone fragments generated by fracture of the pelvis. Bladder rupture into the peritoneal cavity produces peritonitis.

Extraperitoneal rupture is usually less dramatic but, if it remains undiagnosed, tissue necrosis follows. The short, female urethra is rarely injured. In males, posterior urethral injury usually occurs above the urogenital diaphragm (which contains the external sphincter urethrae) as a result of pelvic fracture and is therefore often associated with injuries to other body regions. Anterior urethral injury is generally the result of blunt trauma to the perineum, such as falling astride a beam, and is therefore usually an isolated injury. If urethral rupture is complete, the patient is unable to pass urine. In contrast, a lesser injury, such as a submucosal haematoma, makes micturition slow, painful, but possible.

3. The pelvis contains the rectum and the female reproductive organs. In addition to perforation from bony pelvic fragments following trauma, injuries to the rectum are similar to those described for the colon and bowel above. Uterine injuries are uncommon but can result from both blunt and penetrating trauma. The chance of damage from either mechanism is increased during pregnancy because of the greater uterine size.

Abdominal wall

1. In fit, athletic individuals this forms a firm muscular layer, offering considerable protection from blunt trauma. Protection is reduced in children and those with poorly developed muscles. The anterior abdominal muscles can rupture spontaneously, for example following vigorous exercise or coughing. The most common cause of tears is compression from a seat belt in a deceleration injury; if it produces an imprint of the overlying clothes and seat belt on the skin, there is a high probability of significant intra-abdominal injury.

2. Although penetrating trauma can breach the anterior abdominal wall, it may not necessarily cause intra-abdominal injury. The degree of damage sustained depends on the nature of the weapon used: the wound may be either a stab wound or gunshot wound.

Perineum

Blunt or penetrating injury may injure the penis. Fractured penis infrequently results from forceful bending of the erect organ, rupturing one or both corpora cavernosa, causing a large subcutaneous haematoma and detumescence (Latin *de* = reversal + *temure* = to swell). The testes can be damaged by blunt or, more rarely, penetrating trauma. Rupture of the testis following the former is uncommon because of the scrotal position, cremasteric retraction and the frictionless surface of the tunica vaginalis. All these features allow the testis to evade the direct effects of blunt trauma.

BONY PELVIS

The bony pelvis is usually injured as a result of road traffic accidents (60–80%) or falls from a height (10%). These mechanisms give rise to anteroposterior compression, lateral compression or vertical shear acting on the pelvis either singularly or in combination. They are all capable of producing pelvic instability and haemorrhage from the vascular and bony damage. Because of the nature of this high energy transfer, 98% of patients with major pelvic trauma have other injuries (Table 2.5). The mortality rate is therefore high, at 10%, but rises to 30% with an open fracture, and in this case mortality approaches 100% if the open fracture is missed.

The bones of the pelvis can be separated only if the ligaments uniting them are torn. When this occurs, structures running close to the ligaments, such as vessels and nerves, can be damaged. The resulting bleeding is usually venous and extraperitoneal, so it can be life threatening. However, a tamponading (plugging) effect can be achieved if fractures occur while the ligaments remain intact, in which case haemorrhage is less severe, and mortality lower.

Table 2.5 Associations with pelvic fractures	
Major haemorrhage	over 70%
Musculoskeletal injury	over 80%
Intra-abdominal injury	18–35%
Urological injury	12–20%
Lumbosacral plexus injury	8–30%

LIMBS

Bone

The size, shape and consistency of bone varies with age. Old bones require less force to break them than young ones because they are more brittle and often osteoporotic (Greek *poros* = passage; porous or rarefaction). In children, fractures may involve the physis (Greek = nature; growth plate), resulting in deformity if reduction is not accurate.

Bone is a living tissue with a generous blood supply and can bleed profusely after injury. Furthermore, blood loss from adjacent vessels and oedema into the surrounding tissues can be severe enough to cause hypovolaemic shock. The approximate blood loss with some closed fractures is: pelvis 1.0–5.0 litres, femur 1.0–2.5 litres, tibia 0.5–1.5 litres and humerus 0.5–1.5 litres. These volumes can be much higher if there is an open fracture (see below).

Nerves

These tend to lie within neurovascular fascial bundles close to the long bones in the limbs. This close proximity is particularly noticeable around joints, making the nerves prone to damage following fractures and dislocations.

Structure and function of a peripheral nerve

The neuronal processes making up a nerve trunk are grouped into fascicles (Latin *fascis* = bundle). In the more proximal segments there is considerable crossing over and rearrangement between fascicles, but, more distally, below the elbow for example, the fascicular arrangement is constant, predictable and corresponds to the eventual motor and cutaneous branches. Some nerves, such as the ulnar, have small numbers of well-defined fascicles; others, such as the median nerve, have large numbers of smaller ones.

You need to know the connective tissue framework of the nerve in order to understand nerve injuries. The outermost layer is the epineurium (Greek *epi* = upon + *neuron* = nerve), the chief characteristic of which is mechanical strength. It is usually in a state of longitudinal tension, which is why the ends of a cut nerve spring apart. Each fascicle is surrounded by perineurium (Greek *peri* = around); this functions as a blood–nerve barrier and determines the biochemical environment of the nerve tissue. The individual axons are invested in endoneurium (Greek *endo* = within), which forms conduits guiding each axon to the appropriate end organ.

The nerve is nourished by an internal longitudinal plexus of vessels, fed at intervals by perforators from the adventitia. This plexus becomes occluded if the nerve is subjected to undue tension, otherwise it can support the nerve trunk even when it has been lifted from its bed over a distance. The cell body and axonal parts of the neuron communicate with each other chemically by means of the axoplasmic transport system. Under normal conditions this carries transmitter substances centrifugally (Latin *centrum* + *fugare* = to flee); during regeneration after injury, structural proteins are also carried. Signalling molecules from the end organs or from axons which are damaged are conveyed to the centrally sited cell body, thus transmitting peripheral influences proximally to the nucleus, which controls the repair.

Vessels

Following trauma, the intimal layer may be the only part of a limb artery damaged. This can be very difficult to detect clinically, initially because distal pulses and capillary refill are maintained. Subsequently, the intimal tear can become a focus for the formation of an intravascular thrombosis and can also give rise to distal embolization.

More overt acute signs are seen only if a significant area of the lumen is occluded. When all the layers of the artery are transected transversely, the vessel goes into spasm from constriction of the muscle fibres in the media, limiting the degree of blood loss. Conversely, if there is a partial or longitudinal laceration, the muscle spasm tends to keep the hole in the artery open, and blood loss continues.

Veins have less muscle in their walls but the venous pressure is lower than arterial pressure. However, many veins have external attachments, especially in the pelvis and intracranial sinuses, which hold them open. In addition, many venous tears produce side holes rather than transections, prejudicing the sealing effects of annular contraction. Consequently, blood continues to leak from the lumen until direct pressure is applied.

Limb compartments

These are regions in the limbs where skeletal muscle is enclosed by relatively non-compliant fascia. Running through these areas are blood vessels and nerves, the function of which can be affected if intracompartmental pressure rises above capillary pressure. This is most commonly seen in the four compartments around the tibia and fibula. Nevertheless, compartments also occur in the shoulder, forearm, hand, buttocks and thigh, and these can also give rise to the compartment syndrome (see below).

SPINAL COLUMN

The stability of the vertebral column depends mainly on the integrity of a series of ligaments but the vertebral bodies and the intervertebral discs also contribute. These can be considered as three vertical columns. The anterior column comprises the anterior longitudinal ligament and the anterior half of both the vertebral body and intervertebral disc. The middle complex consists of the posterior longitudinal ligament and the posterior half of both the vertebral body and intervertebral disc. The posterior column comprises the remaining posterior ligament complex and the facet joints; it is structurally the most important column. If any two of these columns are disrupted, the vertebral column becomes unstable.

The spinal cord runs down the spinal canal to the level of the second (adult) or third (baby) lumbar vertebra. The size of the space around the cord in the canal varies, depending on the relative diameters of the spinal cord and spinal canal. In the region of the thorax it is very small because the spinal cord is relatively wide. In contrast, there is a large potential space at the level of C2. Consequently, injuries in this area are not automatically fatal because there is a potential space behind the odontoid process or dens (Latin = tooth).

Key point

- **Steel's rule of three states that at the level of the first cervical vertebra one-third of the available space in the vertebral canal is occupied by the odontoid process and one-third by the spinal cord, leaving a free space of one-third.**

Free space in the spinal canal is an important safety factor in adaptation to injury; it can be reduced by spinal stenosis or posterior osteophytes.

Incidents leading to spinal injury are:

- Road traffic accidents   48%
- Falls   21%
- Violent acts   14%
- Sport   14%
- Others   3%

1. Road traffic accidents can result from side, rear or front collision. Ejection from a car increases the chance of a spinal injury to approximately 1 in 14. Rear-end collisions can produce hyperextension of the neck followed by hyperflexion (the 'whiplash phenomenon'). Unprotected victims, such as pedestrians hit by cars or motorcyclists, have a higher chance of sustaining a spinal injury than those within a vehicle.

2. Rugby football, especially following collapse of the scrum, is infamous for producing spinal trauma, but almost all sports have been implicated in spinal injury. Diving into shallow water, particularly by young males following alcohol imbibition, is a common cause of neck injuries during the spring and summer months. The victim usually misjudges the depth of the water or dives from too steep an angle, hitting his head on the underlying solid surface. Because of the mechanism of injury, 50% of patients with spinal trauma have other injuries, 7–20% have head injuries, 15–20% have chest injuries and around 2.5% have abdominal injuries.

3. Injury may result from single or combined forces, including flexion, extension, rotation, lateral flexion, compression and distraction. In the adult, the vertebral column is more likely to be injured at C5/C6/C7 and T12/L1. The more mobile cervical and lumbar regions meet the relatively immobile thoracic segments, focusing stress and increasing the chance of fracture at these points.

SKIN

The principal soft tissue in the body is the skin. Ageing decreases the amount of collagen in both the skin and subcutaneous tissues, as well as weakening the elastic fibres. This process can be accelerated by the administration of long-term steroids. These changes reduce the tensile strength of skin, allowing extensive lacerations to develop with minor trauma.

THE BODY'S RESPONSE TO TRAUMA

Injury initiates many well-developed physiological responses. Consequently, when you treat trauma victims you are presented with a complex combination of pathophysiological changes, some of which are a direct result of the injury and others the body's response to the initial insult. The underlying mechanisms controlling response are a mixture of cardiovascular, paracrine and endocrine reactions. Individual examples of the more important pathophysiological processes are listed in Table 2.6.

METABOLIC RESPONSE TO INJURY

Three phases are recognized: the early, acute *ebb* phase, followed by the *flow* phase if resuscitation and homeostasis

Table 2.6 Pathophysiological effects contributing to the body's response to trauma
Metabolic response to injury
Shock and cardiovascular pathophysiology
Systemic inflammatory response syndrome (SIRS)
Coagulopathy
Multiorgan failure (MOF)
Neuropathophysiology
Spinal injuries
Fractures
Peripheral nerve injury
Compartment syndrome
Crush syndrome
Fat emboli
Wound healing
Burns

are successful, or by *necrobiosis* if treatment fails and death ensues (Fig. 2.6). Following very severe injuries, the ebb phase may be short and necrobiosis may already have started by the time the patient reaches the accident and emergency (A & E) department.

Ebb phase

1. The body anticipates danger and prepares for fight or flight (the defence reaction). Superimposed on this is

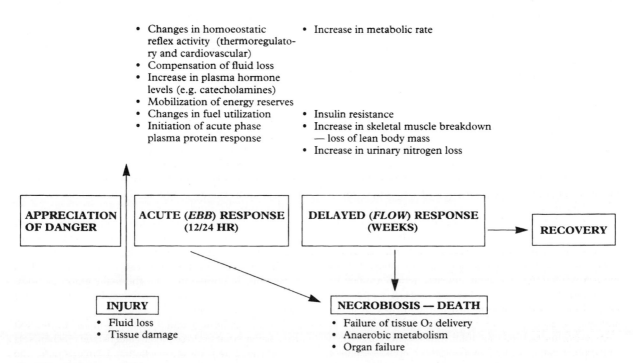

Fig. 2.6 Defence reaction.

the body's response to haemorrhage, tissue injury, pain and hypoxia, the response being related to the severity of the injury. The ebb phase is characterized by mobilization of energy reserves and changes in cardiovascular reflex activity. The latter corresponds to the clinical state commonly referred to as 'shock' (see below). Increased sympathetic nervous activity links these changes and is reflected by rises in plasma catecholamine (derived from catechu an extract of Indian plants), such as adrenaline (epinephrine) and noradrenaline (norepinephrine), with concentrations proportionate to the severity of the injury. Additionally, there is a rapid secretion of hormones from the posterior and anterior pituitary gland as well as the adrenal medulla.

2. Increased sympathetic activity stimulates the breakdown of liver and muscle glycogen, leading to increased levels of plasma glucose. This hyperglycaemia is potentiated by reduced glucose utilization in skeletal muscle because high adrenaline (epinephrine) levels inhibit insulin secretion. A relative intracellular insulin resistance develops, the mechanism of which is unclear, although glucocorticoids may be involved.

3. The changes in carbohydrate metabolism in the ebb phase can be interpreted as defensive. In addition to providing fuel for fight or flight, hyperglycaemia may also play a role in compensating for post-traumatic fluid loss, both by mobilizing water associated with glycogen and through its osmotic effects. The decrease in glucose clearance associated with the development of insulin resistance can be considered as a mechanism for preventing the wasteful use of the mobilized carbohydrate, which is an essential fuel for the brain and the wound, at a time when the supply of nutrients may be limited.

4. Increased sympathetic activity also mobilizes fat from adipose tissue. Plasma concentrations of non-esterified fatty acids (NEFAs) and glycerol are raised following accidental injury in humans, although the relationship with injury severity is complex. Plasma NEFA is lower after severe injuries than after moderate ones, possibly resulting from metabolic effects such as stimulation of re-esterification within adipose tissue by raised plasma lactate levels, or circulatory factors such as poor perfusion of adipose tissue.

5. Increased plasma cortisol, mediated by adrenocorticotrophic hormone (ACTH), occurs rapidly following all forms of injury, although the relationship with severity is again complex. Unexpectedly low cortisol concentrations are found following severe injuries, which cannot be related to a failure of the ACTH response but are possibly caused by impaired adrenocortical blood flow in major trauma.

6. In normal subjects the total consumption of oxygen per minute (V_{O_2}) is constant throughout a wide range of oxygen delivery (D_{O_2}). The normal V_{O_2} for a resting male is 100–160 ml min^{-1} m^{-2} and the normal value of D_{O_2} in the same person is 500–720 ml min^{-1} m^{-2}; therefore, tissues are taking up only 20–25% of the oxygen brought to them. This is known as the oxygen extraction ratio (OER) and demonstrates that normally there is great potential for the tissues of the body to remove more oxygen from the circulating blood.

7. Following trauma, both oxygen delivery and consumption can be affected. In simple haemorrhage, V_{O_2} is maintained in the face of falling D_{O_2} by increasing the oxygen extraction ratio. When tissue injury occurs on the background of haemorrhage, despite the oxygen extraction ratio rising, oxygen consumption falls with oxygen delivery. In other words, V_{O_2} has become supply dependent.

8. Nociceptive (Latin *nocere* = to hurt + *recepere* = to receive) stimulation also complicates the cardiovascular response to fluid loss. The heart rate response to simple haemorrhage is an initial tachycardia, mediated by the baroreflex (Greek *baros* = weight, pressure), followed, as the severity of haemorrhage increases, by a bradycardia (Greek *bradys* = slow) mediated by the 'depressor reflex'. The sensitivity of the baroreflex is reduced by injury, contrary to the increase seen following haemorrhage. Impairment of the baroreflex, which can persist for several weeks following modest injuries, means that vasopressors such as vasopressin (antidiuretic hormone, ADH) released acutely after injury are more effective in maintaining blood pressure than normally, when the baroreflex buffers their pressor effects. The bradycardia caused by the depressor reflex is also markedly attenuated by additional tissue injury. This complex interaction between the cardiovascular responses to haemorrhage and injury may be harmful. Maintenance of blood pressure following haemorrhage and injury can be achieved at the expense of intense vasoconstriction in peripheral vascular beds. Reduced gut blood flow is thought to be pivotal in the production of inflammatory cytokines such as interleukin 6 (IL-6) and tumour necrosis factor α (TNFα). Raised levels of these inflammatory markers, as well as abnormalities in IL-10, an anti-inflammatory cytokine, may lead to further tissue damage and increase the likelihood of developing multiple organ failure.

9. There is clinical evidence for changes in the control of thermoregulation: severely injured patients do not shiver, despite having body temperatures below the normal threshold for the onset of shivering. The selection of the ambient temperature for thermal comfort is modified. This may be centrally mediated, but cytokines are likely to be important.

10. If tissue damage and fluid loss from the circulation are so severe that endogenous homoeostatic mechanisms are overwhelmed and resuscitation is inadequate, the necrobiotic phase begins. This is characterized by a

progressive imbalance between oxygen demand and supply in the tissues, leading to a downward spiral of anaerobic metabolism, with irreversible tissue damage and death.

Key point

- **If the ebb phase is successfully managed and oxygen delivery maintained, the flow phase ensues.**

Flow phase

1. The main features are increased metabolic rate and urinary nitrogen excretion associated with weight loss and muscle wasting, reaching a maximum at 7–10 days following uncomplicated injuries. This response pattern may last many weeks if sepsis and/or multiple organ failure supervene. The increased metabolic rate, which is proportional to the severity of injury, results from neural, hormonal and immunological factors. The wound acts as the 'afferent arc', priming the inflammatory response, while systemically released stress hormones perpetuate the metabolic changes (efferent arc). The complex interaction between the factors is still unclear.

2. The wound, whether a fracture site or a burned surface, can be considered as an extra organ that is metabolically active and has a circulation that is not under neural control. It consumes large amounts of glucose, which is converted to lactate, which in turn is carried to the liver and reconverted to glucose. This is an energy-consuming process, reflected by an increase in hepatic oxygen consumption. Other factors possibly contributing to the hypermetabolism are: increases in cardiac output (needed to sustain a hyperdynamic circulation); the energy cost of the latent heat of evaporation of water from, for example, the surface of the burn; the energy costs of substrate cycling (metabolic processes which involve the expenditure of energy without any change in the amount of either substrate or product); and increased protein turnover.

3. During the flow phase, the metabolic rate seldom exceeds 3000–4000 kcal per day, twice the normal resting metabolic expenditure, with the highest values following major burns. Energy expenditure is often lower than expected and may be close to, or even lower than, values predicted from standard tables. This is because the hypermetabolic stimulus of injury or sepsis is superimposed on a background of inadequate calorie intake, immobility and loss of muscle mass, all of which tend to reduce metabolic rate.

4. Hypermetabolism of the flow phase is fuelled by increases in the rates of turnover of both fat and glucose.

Turnover of NEFAs is raised in relation to their plasma concentration, and the normal suppression of fat oxidation following the administration of exogenous glucose is not seen in these hypermetabolic patients. Both changes have been attributed to increased sympathetic activity, although plasma catecholamine concentrations are not always increased at this time. The rate of hepatic gluconeogenesis is increased from a number of precursors, such as lactate and pyruvate from the wound and muscle, amino acids from muscle protein breakdown, and glycerol from fat mobilization. This increase in hepatic glucose production is not suppressed by infusing large quantities of glucose into burned or septic patients. The apparent resistance to the effects of insulin is mirrored by the failure of peripheral glucose utilization to rise to the extent predicted from the raised plasma glucose and insulin concentrations. This insulin resistance in, for example, uninjured skeletal muscle, seems to be an intracellular, postreceptor change.

5. The balance between whole body protein synthesis and breakdown is obviously disturbed in the flow phase. The observed changes probably represent the interaction between the severity of injury and the nutritional state: increasing severity of injury causes increasing rates of both synthesis and breakdown, while undernutrition depresses synthesis. Thus, increasing nutritional intake should move a patient towards nitrogen balance but, despite technical advances for administering nutrients and modifications to the type and composition of feeding regimens, no amount of nitrogen is sufficient to produce a positive balance following severe injuries. Nevertheless, the use of anabolic agents, such as growth hormone or testosterone derivatives, and manipulations of ambient temperature may be advantageous as the patient moves from the catabolic flow phase into the anabolic convalescent phase.

6. A major site of net protein loss is skeletal muscle, both in the injured area and at a distance. For example, following moderate injury the patient can lose 2 kg of lean body mass, sufficient to compromise mobility, especially in the elderly whose reserves of muscle mass and strength are already reduced. Although the changes in skeletal muscle are very obvious, the liver is another tissue in which changes in protein synthesis are of particular interest after injury; it is the source of the acute-phase reactants such as C-reactive protein, fibrinogen and α_1-antitrypsin, the concentrations of which rise in response to infection, inflammation and trauma.

7. These metabolic changes, not attributable to starvation or immobility, can be mimicked to some extent by the infusion of the counterregulatory hormones glucagon, adrenaline (epinephrine) and cortisol. However, the plasma concentrations required to elicit relatively modest increases in nitrogen excretion, metabolic rate and induce

peripheral insulin resistance are much higher than those found in the flow phase, although they are similar to those noted in the ebb phase.

SHOCK AND CARDIOVASCULAR PATHOPHYSIOLOGY

Shock can be defined as inadequate organ perfusion and tissue oxygenation. Tissue oxidation depends on adequate pulmonary function with satisfactory gas exchange, together with an adequate quantity of functioning haemoglobin able to deliver and release oxygen to the tissues.

When a sufficient cell mass has been damaged, shock becomes irreversible and the patient inevitably dies. Fortunately, the body has several compensatory mechanisms which sustain adequate organ perfusion and lower the risk.

Circulatory control

Pressure receptors in the heart and baroreceptors in the carotid sinus and aortic arch trigger a reflex sympathetic response via control centres in the brainstem in response to hypovolaemia. The sympathetic discharge stimulates many tissues in the body, including the adrenal medulla, which releases increased amounts of systemic catecholamines, so enhancing the effects of direct sympathetic discharge, particularly on the heart. This prevents or limits the fall in cardiac output by positive inotropic (Greek *inos* = muscle, fibre + *trepeein* = to turn, influence) and chronotropic (Greek *chronos* = time + *trepeein*; influencing time or rate) effects on the heart and by increasing venous return as a result of venoconstriction. Furthermore, selective arteriolar and precapillary sphincter constriction supplying non-essential organs, such as skin and gut, maintains perfusion of vital organs, such as brain and heart. Selective perfusion lowers hydrostatic pressure in capillaries serving non-essential organs, also reducing diffusion of fluid across the capillary membrane into the interstitial space, thereby decreasing further loss of intravascular volume. Reduction in renal blood flow is detected by the juxtaglomerular apparatus in the kidney, which releases renin. This leads to the formation of angiotensin II and aldosterone; these, together with ADH released by the pituitary gland, increase renal reabsorption of sodium and water, reducing urine volume, and helping to maintain the circulating volume. Renin, angiotensin II and ADH can also produce generalized vasoconstriction, promoting increase in venous return. In addition, the body attempts to enhance the circulating volume by releasing osmotically active substances from the liver, which increase plasma osmotic pressure, drawing interstitial fluid into the intravascular space.

Oxygen delivery

Although sympathetically induced tachypnoea (Greek *tachys* = rapid + *pnoia* = breathing) occurs, it does not increase oxygen uptake because the blood haemoglobin traversing ventilated alveoli is already fully saturated.

Causes of shock

1. Reduced venous return following haemorrhage is the commonest cause of shock in traumatized patients. Bleeding may be occult, collecting in the large spaces of the thorax, abdomen and pelvis. As well as the potential spaces intrapleurally and within the retroperitoneum, blood may be lost into muscles and tissues around long-bone fractures; in addition, intravascular volume may be reduced as a result of leakage of plasma into the interstitial spaces. This can account for up to 25% of the volume of tissue swelling following blunt trauma. The rate of blood returning to the heart depends on the pressure gradient created by the high hydrostatic pressure in the peripheral veins and low hydrostatic pressure in the cardiac right atrium. Any reduction in this gradient, as from tension pneumothorax, cardiac tamponade or increasing right atrial pressure, reduces venous return to the heart. External compression on the thorax or abdomen can have a similar action in obstructing the venous return.

2. Cardiogenic shock from ischaemic heart disease and cardiac contusions have negative inotropic effects. Nevertheless, it does not occur unless more than 40% of the left ventricular myocardium is dead or severely damaged. In cardiogenic shock the compensatory sympathetic and catecholamine responses only serve to increase the myocardial oxygen demand and further increase ischaemia. Certain dysrhythmias alone, from pre-existing cardiac ischaemia or following cardiac contusion, significantly reduce cardiac performance. Be aware that all antiarrhythmic agents may have negative inotropic effects, impeding the patient's physiological response to the injury. Cardiac tamponade not only prejudices venous return but also restricts ventricular filling.

3. Reduced arterial tone complicates spinal injury above T6 by impairing sympathetic nervous system outflow from the spinal cord below that level. Consequently, both the reflex tachycardia and vasoconstriction responses to hypovolaemia are restricted to a degree proportional to the level of sympathetic block. Generalized vasodilatation, bradycardia and loss of temperature control can follow high level spinal injuries, producing *neurogenic shock*; additional nervous damage may result from the reduced blood supply to the spinal column. Any associated haemorrhage from the injury aggravates this situation, further reducing spinal blood flow. In addition, these patients are very sensitive to any

vagal stimulation. For example, pharyngeal suction can aggravate the bradycardia, leading to cardiac arrest.

4. Septic shock results when circulating endotoxins, commonly from Gram-negative organisms, produce vasodilatation and impair energy utilization at a cellular level. Hypoxia can devlop even with normal or high oxygen delivery rates, because the tissue oxygen demand is extremely high and there is impaired oxygen uptake by the cells. In addition, endotoxin makes the capillary walls leaky at the site of infection; this becomes more generalized, allowing sodium and water to move from the interstitial to the intracellular space. This eventually leads to hypovolaemia, making it indistinguishable from hypovolaemic shock. Further cellular damage by endotoxins causes the release of proteolytic enzymes, which paralyse precapillary sphincters, enhance capillary leakage and increase hypovolaemia. The situation is aggravated by the endotoxin acting as a negative inotrope on the myocardium. It follows that in the late stage of sepsis there are several causes of the shock state.

DISSEMINATED INTRAVASCULAR COAGULOPATHY (DIC)

Trauma, massive blood transfusion, infection, hypothermia, tissue injury and damage to the microvascular endothelium are all common causes of DIC. Procoagulant tissue factors such as IL-6 and TNFα are released, promoting inappropriate intravascular activation of the coagulation, fibrinolytic and complement systems. Both thrombin and plasmin are activated but out of balance; as a result, platelet-fibrin thrombi form in the microvasculature, while fibrin degradation products are raised in the plasma. Platelets are reduced in number and impaired in function; coagulation and fibrinolytic factors are also reduced and coagulation studies show prolongation of clotting time.

Coagulopathy resulting in vascular occlusion can provoke end-organ ischaemia, infarction and failure. At the same time it can lead to haemorrhage and uncontrolled bleeding at many sites, as in surgical wounds, the skin, the pulmonary system, the gastrointestinal tract and the cranium. Haemorrhagic complications usually dominate in acute DIC following trauma.

MULTIPLE ORGAN FAILURE (MOF)

This is defined as the presence of altered function in two or more organs in an acutely ill patient, such that intervention is required to maintain homeostasis (Greek *homoios* = like + *stasis* = standing; tendency to stable state). It represents the final common pathway of many disease processes, of which trauma is one. It is invariably preceded by a condition known as the systemic inflammatory response syndrome (SIRS), characterized by two or more of the following:

- Temperature >38° C or <36° C
- Tachycardia >90 beats per minute
- Respiratory rate >20 breaths per minute or $Pa\text{CO}_2$ <4.3 kPa
- White blood count >12×10^9 l^{-1} or < 4×10^9 l^{-1} or >10% immature (band) forms.

Key point

- **Multiple organ failure is a deadly condition with a mortality rate of about 60%.**

1. The pathophysiology behind MOF has yet to be fully elucidated. A 'one-hit model' accounts for early MOF as a result of massive trauma. The initial insult triggers a severe SIRS, leading to MOF. It was apparent that some traumatized patients who had sustained non-massive trauma developed delayed MOF. The 'two-hit model' was developed to explain the occurrence of MOF in such patients. In this model the initial injury primes the inflammatory machinery to a subclinical level. This gives rise to the exaggerated response seen in MOF only if the patient is subjected to a 'second hit', such as hypoxia, hypotension, infection, operation, anaesthesia or further trauma.

2. Irrespective of the actual cause, it is probable that a stimulus such as injury or infection initiates the release of a number of mediators by macrophages, monocytes and endothelial cells. These include TNF, IL-1β, IL-6 and IL-8. Following 'relook' laparotomies (reoperations to identify and correct any complications that have developed), raised levels of IL-6 were found; this suggests that cytokines may have a role in intensifying and perpetuating the inflammatory state following such a 'second hit'. These changes cause further white cell activation in addition to adhesion of leucocytes to endothelial cells lining blood vessels. This occurs in virtually all organs of the body, but particularly the lungs, liver and intestine. The process leads to the migration of white cells into the interstitial space, the release of proteases and oxygen radicals and the activation of arachidonic acid. Such changes exacerbate existing capillary damage, leading to widespread leakage of fluid into the interstitial space. In addition, arachidonic acid activation gives rise to prostacyclin, thromboxane A_2 and leukotrienes.

3. Tissue damage is simultaneously resulting from vasoconstriction and intravascular thrombosis in the microvascular circulation. In the lungs, this can give rise to right heart failure due to the increases in pulmonary vascular resistance and pulmonary artery pressure.

4. In managing these patients, recognize that the normal relationship between oxygen delivery to tissue (DO_2) and oxygen consumption (VO_2) is altered. In MOF, partly because of the marked increase in VO_2, tissues become flow dependent, that is reliant upon DO_2 (see p. 30). Consequently, any hypovolaemia, pulmonary disease or myocardial dysfunction jeopardizes the delivery of oxygen even further, and so increases the degree of tissue hypoxia and organ dysfunction.

Adult respiratory distress syndrome/acute lung injury

Adult respiratory distress syndrome (ARDS) represents the severe form of acute lung injury (ALI). Although only approximately 2% of trauma patients develop ARDS, they then have a mortality rate of approximately 40–50%.

ALI is a collective term for hypoxaemic respiratory failure, characterized by the American–European consensus as:

- Bilateral pulmonary infiltrates visible on chest X-ray
- Pulmonary capillary wedge pressure <18 mmHg
- PaO_2/FiO_2 <300.

In ARDS:

- PaO_2/FiO_2 <200

Aetiology and pathogenesis

1. Acute lung injury can be caused by local or systemic inflammation. In trauma patients it may result from direct lung injury or, when the injured tissue is more distant, by SIRS (see above).

2. Direct causes include pulmonary contusion, aspiration of gastric contents, near drowning, inhalation of toxic fumes, thermal injury to the respiratory tract, bacterial or viral pneumonia, and radiation injury.

3. Indirect causes include sepsis, massive haemorrhage, multiple transfusions, shock from any cause, DIC, massive burns, major and multiple trauma, pre-eclampsia, amniotic fluid embolism, pancreatitis, head injuries and cardiopulmonary bypass.

4. In addition, it has been suggested that any critical illness that leads to inadequate cellular oxygenation can precipitate the syndrome.

5. Regardless of the cause, pathogenesis follows a common pathway (Fig. 2.7). Neutrophils adhere to the vascular endothelium, then migrate into the interstitium and alveolar airspaces. They release inflammatory mediators that attract and activate other inflammatory cells, stimulate the coagulation cascade and release oxygen free radicals, producing widespread endothelial damage. As a result of the increased capillary permeability, protein-rich fluid occupies the interstitium and alveolar airspaces;

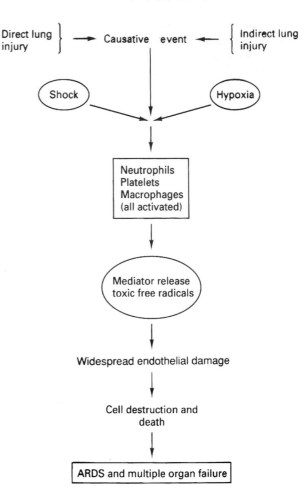

Fig. 2.7 A simplified flow chart illustrating the development of ARDS.

this, coupled with the deactivation of surfactant, causes stiff lungs with decreased compliance. The protein-rich fluid, coupled with increased lung lymph flow, thickens the alveolar capillary membrane, impairing oxygen diffusion. In the later stages of the disease, fibrosis may develop.

NEUROLOGICAL PATHOPHYSIOLOGY

Head injuries are common. In the UK head-injured patients account for 7–10% of all emergency department attendances, of whom 1 in 7 are admitted. Most serious head injuries result from road accidents, falls and assaults. Over 5000 people die from traumatic brain injury in England and Wales every year. It is estimated that a further 1500 patients survive to endure significant lifelong morbidity. Remember that victims have a mean age of 30, so there is a major impact on society. The combination of head injury and extracranial injury is particularly dangerous, as the presence of hypoxia and hypotension is associated with a 75% increase in mortality from severe head injury. This is partly the result of impaired autoregulatory capacity of the injured brain, resulting in the development of secondary brain injury.

Intracranial pressure

1. In the adult the neurocranium is a rigid box and its volume is fixed. The intracranial pressure (ICP) generated inside it depends on the volume of its contents. In the normal state these consist of brain, CSF, blood and blood vessels. Together, these produce an ICP of 5–13 mmHg when the subject lies horizontally.

2. If the ICP is to be kept at normal levels, any increase in the volume of one component must be accompanied by a decrease in the other components. CSF can be displaced into the spinal system and its absorption increased. The volume of cerebral venous blood within the dural sinuses can also decrease. Furthermore, the brain is a compliant organ, so it can mould to accommodate changes. Once the limit of these compensatory mechanisms is reached, the ICP rises.

3. Head trauma results not only in mass lesions but also in increased permeability of the intracerebral microvasculature. This leads to interstitial oedema and cerebral swelling, making the brain relatively 'stiff', so it is less able to adapt to changes in the intracranial contents. This situation deteriorates further if ventilation is impaired, as hypoxia produces additional cerebral swelling. Hypercarbia results in vasodilatation of the blood vessels in the uninjured parts of the brain (see below), thereby increasing intracranial pressure.

4. Alterations in the intracranial contents, including haematoma, not only produce an elevated ICP but also make the brain, CSF and blood less adaptable to any further additions. Even a small rise in volume of the intracranial contents now causes a steep rise in the ICP. Eventually, the brain herniates downwards through the defect between the edges of the tentorium, and this tentorial herniation causes ipsilateral (Greek *ipsos* = same) pupillary dilatation (IIIrd cranial nerve compression) and contralateral (Latin *contra* = opposite) motor weakness (corticospinal tract compression). As ICP rises further, the brainstem is compressed within the foramen magnum, causing coning, leading to ischaemia. This is heralded by Cushing's reflex, described by the great American neurosurgeon (1869–1939), which is usually fatal:

a. Decreased respiratory rate
b. Decreased heart rate
c. Increased systolic blood pressure.

Cerebral perfusion

Adequate ventilation and cerebral perfusion are essential to supply the brain with oxygenated blood. Perfusion depends on a difference between mean arterial pressure (MAP) and the resistance to blood flow due to the ICP: cerebral perfusion pressure (CPP) = MAP – ICP.

In the multiply injured patient, not only is the ICP rising because of the head injury, but the MAP may be falling due to blood loss from an extracranial trauma. The CPP is markedly reduced. If the CPP is 50 mmHg or less, cerebral ischaemia develops; as described above, this leads to additional brain swelling and further rises in ICP as the cycle perpetuates itself. Make every effort to keep CPP at greater than 70 mmHg, as this reduces mortality. A CPP less than 30 mmHg is fatal.

Consciousness

Consciousness depends on an intact ascending reticular activating system, contained within the midbrain and brainstem, and an intact cerebral cortex. Interruption anywhere along this pathway, either structural or metabolic, results in loss of consciousness. There are many possible causes but the mnemonic (Greek *mneme* = memory) 'TIPPS on the vowels' recalls the important ones:

Trauma	**A**lcohol
Infection	**E**pilepsy
Poisons	**I**ncrease in ICP
Psychiatric	**O**piates
Shock	**U**raemia/metabolic

Key point

- **Eliminate hypoxia and hypovolaemia; each can alone induce coma. If they are coupled with head trauma, mortality increases.**

An initial measure of consciousness is the patient's response to stimulation. This is graded on the AVPU scale.

A	Alert
V	Responds to **V**oice
P	Responds to **P**ain
U	No response (**U**nconscious)

The Glasgow Coma Scale is a more complicated but validated assessment based on the patient's best eye, verbal and motor responses to stimulation (Greek *koma* = deep sleep). The scale (Table 2.7) is an objective measure of the condition, used to monitor the patient's progress. The three scores are added; the minimum score is 3 and any score below 8 carries a poor prognosis.

Table 2.7 The Glasgow Coma Scale

Eye opening	Score	Verbal response	Score	Motor response	Score
Spontaneous	4	Orientated	5	Obeys commands	6
To speech	3	Confused	4	Localizes to pain	5
To pain	2	Inappropriate words	3	Withdraws	4
None	1	Inappropriate sounds	2	Flexion to pain	3
		None	1	Extension to pain	2
				None	1

Fractures

Skull fractures usually result from direct trauma and are classified as being linear, depressed or open. The term 'open' implies a direct communication between the brain surface and either the scalp or mucous membrane laceration.

Primary and secondary brain injury

1. Neurological cells may die as a result of energy transferred to them by the injurious event – primary brain injury. Possibly, progressive primary brain damage occurs subsequently because of endogenous neurochemical changes leading to further cellular injury. At present, injury prevention is the only factor that reduces primary brain damage.

2. Secondary brain injury is the neurological damage produced by subsequent insults, such as hypoxia, hypovolaemia and elevation in ICP (remember CPP = MAP – ICP), metabolic imbalance, seizures and later diffuse brain swelling, and infection. Mortality can be reduced by appropriate resuscitation to prevent secondary brain injury.

3. A purely focal injury can follow a contact force. However, there is usually sufficient associated diffuse brain injury to produce an altered level of consciousness from a temporary disruption of the reticular formation (see above). Furthermore, a space-occupying lesion is often accompanied by a swollen brain due to primary and secondary brain damage. This accelerates the rise in intracranial pressure and the development of additional brain damage. Consequently, the trauma patient invariably has diffuse and specific neurological injuries. The clinical features of a focal injury depend on the site injured, as different parts of the brain perform different functions; diffuse brain injuries tend to be bilateral.

4. Selective herniation of the cerebellum through the foramen magnum can be produced by an expanding posterior fossa intracranial haematoma. This is the only cerebral haematoma to produce neurological damage without a preceding deterioration in consciousness level. (See above for tentorial and brainstem herniation.) Among the features, the most common are pupillary dilatation, respiratory abnormalities, bradycardia, head tilt and cranial nerve palsies. Most alarming is sudden respiratory arrest resulting from distal brainstem compression. It is a rare condition but consider it early, especially in patients with an occipital fracture.

Concussion

Concussion (Latin *con* = together + *quatare* = to shake) occurs when the head is subjected to minor inertial forces. The patient is always amnesic of the event and there may also be retro- and antegrade amnesia. A transient loss of consciousness may occur, usually less than 5 min. These patients show no localizing signs but may have nausea, vomiting and headache. It was at first thought that no organic brain damage occurred but this is found not to be the case: microscopic changes occur, and, while the net effect of one episode is minor, the effect of further episodes can be cumulative.

Diffuse axonal injury (DAI) and contra coup injury

1. Diffuse axonal injury results from widespread, mainly microscopic, disruption of the brain, consisting of axonal damage, microscopic haemorrhages, tears in the brain tissue and interstitial oedema. Consequently, it can cause prolonged periods, for days or weeks, of coma and has an overall mortality rate of 33–50%. Autonomic dysfunction is common, giving rise to high fever, hypertension and sweating.

2. The brain that lies beneath the impact point of a contact force is subjected to a series of strains resulting from the inward deformation of bone and the shock waves spreading from the site of impact. The base of the brain can be strained if it impinges on projections on the base of the skull, producing gross neurological damage, with haemorrhages, neuronal death and brain swelling. Consciousness is invariably lost at the time of the incident and neurological signs develop by the time it is regained. Common signs are altered level of consciousness, hemiparesis, ataxia and seizures.

3. The brain is not fixed within the neurocranium but floats in a bath of CSF, tethered by the arachnoid fibres

and blood vessels. As the head moves because of an accelerating or decelerating force, the skull, and then the brain, moves in the direction of the force. Consequently, strains develop in the brain tissue and small blood vessels opposite the impact point, producing the contusional changes previously described. Additionally, the brain continues to move until it impacts against the opposite side of the skull or its base, thus injuring it in two places, most severely at the site furthest from the impact; this is a *contra coup injury* (French = counterblow).

Acute intracranial haematoma

1. Most extradural haematomas (EDHs) develop in the temporoparietal area following a tear in the middle meningeal artery. Much less commonly, they result from torn venous sinuses within the neurocranium. Compared to a venous cause, an arterially produced extradural haematoma develops quickly, producing a rapid rise in intracranial pressure.
2. The 'classic' presentation (Fig. 2.8) occurs in only one-fifth of patients. Some may be unconscious from the time of the impact, others do not lose consciousness at the time but later develop neurological features. Most commonly there is a deterioration of consciousness, pupil-size changes or a focal weakness.

Acute intradural haematoma (IDH)

1. This incorporates both subdural (SDH) and intracerebral (ICH) haematomas, which frequently coexist, and are 3–4 times more common than extradural haematomas. Subdural haematomas usually develop in the temporal lobe and may be bilateral. Following application of an inertial force, some of the bridging veins tear and blood collects in the subdural space. Occasionally, a subdural haematoma develops without an accompanying intracerebral haematoma. Solitary intracerebral haematomas rarely develop in the frontal lobes.
2. Small intracerebral haematomas may result from inertial forces, and increase in volume over time. Depending on their location, they may cause localizing signs or a rise in the intracranial pressure, with deterioration in the patient's clinical state.

3. The forces needed to produce an intracerebral haematoma are greater than those needed to produce an extradural haematoma, so an intracerebral haematoma is usually associated with cerebral contusion and cortical lacerations. Consequently, the patient commonly loses consciousness immediately and may also exhibit focal signs such as contralateral hemiparesis (Greek *parienai* = to relax), unilateral pupil dilatation or focal fits. With a solitary subdural haematoma, an initial lucid period may be followed by deteriorating neurological state. This develops more slowly than following an extradural haematoma because the bleeding is venous rather than arterial. Tears of only a few bridging veins, in the presence of brain atrophy with enlargement of the intracranial space, may delay development of symptoms for several days.

Subarachnoid haemorrhage (SAH)

This occasionally follows a head injury. The patient often develops severe headaches and photophobia, but other signs of meningism can occur. Do not test for neck stiffness until cervical spine injury has been ruled out clinically and radiologically (see Ch. 1).

SPINAL INJURIES

In the UK, 10–15 people per million of the population suffer spinal injuries each year (Table 2.8). The commonest site is the cervical spine (55%), mainly because most people are injured following a road traffic accident (48%).

Table 2.8	Sites of spinal injuries	
Site	Blunt trauma (%)	Penetrating trauma (%)
Cervical	55	24
Thoracic	35	56
Lumbar	10	20
Multiple	10	

- Transient loss of consciousness at the time of the injury from a momentary disruption of the reticular formation.

- Patient then regains consciousness for several hours, the lucid period.

- Localizing signs develop with neurological deficits, headache and eventually unconsciousness from the developing EDH, which causes the ICP to rise.

Fig. 2.8 Classic history of an extradural haematoma (EDH).

Primary neurological damage

1. This results directly from the initial insult, usually from blunt trauma, producing abnormal movement in the vertebral column. Severe trauma may lead to ligamental rupture and vertebral fractures, reducing the space around the spinal canal and allowing bone and soft tissue to impinge directly on the cord. The potential space around the spinal cord may already be small, increasing the chance of neurological damage.

2. Less commonly, penetrating trauma, as by stabbing, causes primary spinal damage. Much more extensive areas of destruction and oedema result when the spinal cord is subjected to a large force such as a gunshot.

Secondary neurological damage

1. The three common causes of damage following the initial injury are mechanical disturbance of the back, hypoxia and poor spinal perfusion. These effects are additive.

2. Hypoxia can result from any of the causes mentioned above, but significant spinal injury alone can cause it (Table 2.9). The underlying problem is usually a lack of respiratory muscle power following a high spinal lesion. Lesions above T12 denervate the intercostal muscles. Injuries above the level of C5 also block the phrenic nerve, paralysing the diaphragm.

3. Inadequate spinal perfusion results either from general hypovolaemia or failure of the spinal cord to regulate its own blood supply following injury. A fall in mean arterial pressure therefore produces a reduced spinal perfusion. Conversely, if the pressure is increased too far it may produce a spinal haemorrhagic infarct. Secondary damage leads to interstitial and intracellular

Table 2.9 Respiratory failure in spinal injury	
Tetraplegic	Paraplegic
Intercostal paralysis Phrenic nerve palsy Inability to expectorate V/Q mismatch	Intercostal paralysis

oedema, further aggravating the deficient spinal perfusion. As this oedema spreads, compressing neurons, it produces an ascending clinical deterioration. In cases of high spinal injury this process can lead to secondary respiratory deterioration.

Partial spinal cord injury

Anterior spinal cord injury results from direct compression or obstruction of the anterior spinal artery. It affects the spinothalamic and corticospinal tracts (Fig. 2.9), resulting in loss of coarse touch, pain and temperature sensation, and flaccid weakness. This type of injury is associated with fractures or dislocations in the vertebral column.

Central spinal cord injury usually occurs in elderly patients with cervical spondylosis. Following a vascular event the corticospinal tracts are damaged, resulting in flaccid weakness. Because of the anatomical arrangement in the centre of the cord, the upper limbs are more affected than the lower.

Sacral fibres in the spinothalamic tract are positioned laterally to corresponding fibres from other regions of the body (Fig. 2.9). It follows that anterior and central injuries, which primarily affect the midline of the spinal

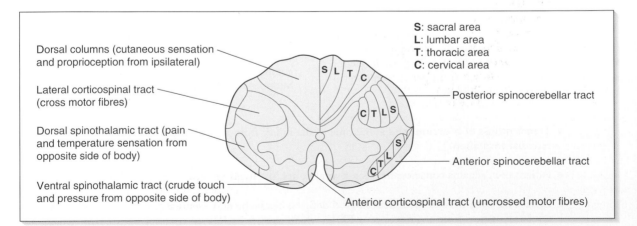

Fig. 2.9 Cross-section of the spinal cord demonstrating the longitudinal tracts. (With permission from Driscoll P, Gwinnutt C, Jimmerson C, Goodall O. In: Trauma resuscitation: the team approach, Macmillan Press Ltd).

cord, may not affect the sacral fibres. This 'sacral sparing' produces sensory loss below a certain level on the trunk, with retention of pinprick appreciation over the sacral and perineal area.

Lateral spinal cord injury (Brown-Séquard syndrome) is the result of penetrating trauma. All sensory and motor function is lost on the side of the wound at the level of the lesion. Below this level there is contralateral loss of pain and temperature sensation with ipsilateral loss of muscle power and tone.

Posterior spinal cord injury is a rare condition, resulting in loss of vibration sensation and proprioception.

Spinal shock

1. This totally functionless condition occasionally occurs following spinal injury. The features are generalized flaccid paralysis, diaphragmatic breathing, priapism, gastric dilatation and autonomic dysfunction associated with neurogenic shock. The English neurologist C.E. Beevor (1854–1908) described movement of the umbilicus when the abdomen is stroked, resulting from paralysis of the lower rectus abdominis muscle.

2. This state can last for days or weeks, but areas of the cord are still capable of a full recovery. Permanent damage results in spasticity once the flaccid state resolves. Upper motor neuron reflexes return below the level of the lesion following complete transection of the cord, producing exaggerated responses to stimuli; however, sensation is lost.

3. During this stage there is risk of pressure sores, deep venous thrombosis, pulmonary emboli and acute peptic ulceration with either haematemesis or, occasionally, perforation.

FRACTURES

1. Fracture occurs in normal bone as a result of trauma. The type of fracture depends on the direction of the violence. A twisting injury causes a spiral or oblique fracture, a direct blow usually causes a transverse fracture, axial compression frequently results in a comminuted (Latin *minuere* = to make small) or burst fracture.

2. Stress fractures occur when the underlying bone is normal. It is the repetitive application of an abnormal load that causes the bone to fracture. The load alone is not sufficient to cause the fracture but rather the cumulative effect of repeated loading. It is most frequently seen in individuals undertaking increased amounts of unaccustomed exercise, such as the 'march' metatarsal fracture in army recruits and dancers.

3. Pathological fractures occur when the underlying bone is weak, perhaps from metastatic cancer or metabolic bone disease; as a result it gives way under minimal trauma.

Fracture repair

1. When a fracture occurs, not only is the bone broken but the encircling tissues are also damaged. The bone ends are surrounded by a haematoma including these injured tissues. Within hours an aseptic inflammatory response develops, comprising polymorphonuclear leucocytes, lymphocytes, macrophages and blood vessels, followed later by fibroblasts. Within this organized fracture haematoma, bone develops either directly or following the formation of cartilage with endochondral ossification. At the same time osteoclasts resorb the necrotic bone ends. The initial bone that is laid down (callus) consists of immature woven bone, which is gradually converted to stable lamellar (Latin *lamina* = a thin plate) bone with consolidation of the fracture. Resorption occurs within the bone trabeculae as recanalizing haversian systems (described by the English physician C. Havers 1650–1702) bridge the bone ends.

2. There are two types of callus. Primary callus results from proliferation of committed osteoprogenitor cells in periosteum and bone marrow. They produce directly membranous bone, a once-only phenomenon limited in duration. The second callus is inductive or external callus, derived from the surrounding tissues, formed by pluripotential cells. A variety of factors, including mechanical and humoral factors, may induce these mesenchymal cells to differentiate to cartilage or bone.

3. The mediators for callus formation are not fully understood. Probably the fracture ends emit osteogenic substances, such as bone morphogenetic protein, into the surrounding haematoma. This is in addition to mediators such as IL-1 and growth factors released from the fracture haematoma. Angiogenic factors probably play an important role in the vascularization of the fracture haematoma.

4. Movement of the fragments increases the fracture exudate. Rigid fixation minimizes the granulation tissue and external callus and may retard the release of morphogens and growth factors from the bone ends. Reaming of the intramedullary canal may cause additional bone damage. Weight bearing stimulates growth factors and prostaglandins, which act as biochemical mediators.

PERIPHERAL NERVE INJURY

1. Blunt trauma to a nerve may produce a temporary block in the conduction of impulses, leaving the axonal transport system intact. The axon distal to the injury survives and complete functional recovery can be expected;

this is *neuropraxia* (Greek *a* = not + *prassein* = to act). More severe trauma will interrupt axonal transport and cause wallerian (Augustus Waller 1816–1870) degeneration: the distal axon dies, the myelin sheath disintegrates and the Schwann cells turn into scavenging macrophages which remove the debris. The cell body then embarks on a pre-programmed regenerative response which is usually known as *chromatolysis*, as it involves the disappearance of the Nissl's granules which are the rough endoplasmic reticulum of the normal cell. An entirely new set of ribosomes appears, dedicated to the task of reconstruction. By their efforts, axon sprouts emerge from the axon proximal to the lesion and grow distally. Injury of this severity is known as *axonotmesis* (Greek *tmesis* = a cutting apart). It eventually produces a good functional result because the endoneurial tubes are intact and the regenerating axons are therefore guaranteed to reach the correct end organs.

2. Laceration or extreme traction producing neurotmesis also leads to wallerian distal degeneration and proximal chromatolysis – loosening of the chromatin of cell nuclei, followed by either cell death or axonal regeneration. In this case, however, the final functional result is bound to be much worse than in any injury that leaves the endoneurial tubes intact. Not only do the axon sprouts have to traverse a gap filled with organizing repair tissue, but each one needs to grow down its original conduit at a rate of approximately 1 mm per day. Axons failing to enter the distal stump may form a tender neuroma, often producing troublesome symptoms. Progress can be monitored clinically using the sign described by the French neurologist Jules Tinel (1879–1952). These are electric feelings in the territory of the nerve produced by light percussion over regenerating axon tips, whether in the distal portion of the nerve or in a neuroma.

3. Motor axons are capable of producing collateral sprouts once they enter muscle, leading to abnormally large motor units with relatively good return of strength. Sensory axons often fail to reinnervate the specialized receptors forming the basis for the sense of touch and this, together with the mismatching of axons with conduits, invariably results in poor sensory recovery except in the very young. The functional result in the hand is poor.

Compartment syndrome

This specific type of neurovascular compromise can occur as part of any extremity injury. Although commonly caused by fractures and soft tissue injuries, the presence of a fracture is not essential. It is a progressive condition in which the elevated tissue pressure within a confined myofascial compartment exceeds capillary pressure, leading to vascular compromise of the muscles and nerves. It can result from a variety of causes, categorized as either expansive or compressive.

External compression of compartment

- Constricting dressing or cast
- Closing fascial defects
- Third degree, full thickness, burns.

Expansion of compartment contents

- Haemorrhage and oedema following fractures or soft tissue injuries
- Haemorrhage following coagulopathy or vascular laceration
- Postischaemic swelling.

The four compartments of the lower leg are the most commonly involved areas, but it can occur in the shoulder, arm, forearm, hand, buttock, thigh or abdomen (following trauma or surgery).

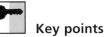

Key points

- **Continuously monitor at-risk sites in order to detect and correct impeding compartment syndrome (Table 2.10).**
- **Increasing pain, exacerbated by passive flexion and extension, is a reliable combination signalling compartment syndrome.**

1. Detect the condition in the early, potentially reversible stage or muscle may infarct, giving rise to rhabdomyolysis, hypovolaemia, hyperkalaemia, hyperphosphataemia, high levels of uric acid, metabolic acidosis, renal failure and death. Locally fibrotic contractures may develop.

2. Detection should be clinical but the intracompartmental pressure can be monitored when clinical assessment is difficult or if you are in doubt about the clinical

Table 2.10   Features of impending or established compartment syndrome
Early   Pain in the limb   Pain on passive movement of the distal joints   Paraesthesia   Loss of distal sensation
Late   Tension or swelling of the compartment   Absent muscle power
Very late   Absent pulse pressure in the distal limb

features. Examples of such cases are when the patient is unresponsive because of neurological injury or sedation, or has a nerve defect from other causes, or has a regional nerve block. Use it as an adjunct to, not a replacement for, clinical monitoring.

3. Absolute pressure values are unreliable because perfusion is dependent upon the difference between the arterial blood pressure and the compartmental pressure. A difference of less than 30 mmHg between diastolic blood pressure and compartment pressure is recommended as a threshold for releasing the tension by carrying out fasciotomy. A fall in the distal pulse pressure is a very late sign and indicates imminent tissue ischaemia. Pulse oximetry is not a reliable help in diagnosing or monitoring impaired perfusion secondary to raised compartment pressure.

CRUSH SYNDROME

1. Crush injuries occur in a variety of ways: for example, in patients becoming trapped under fallen masonry or in a car following a road traffic accident. The patient's own body weight may be sufficient to compress the tissue if the consciousness level is depressed for a considerable time. Severe beatings and epileptic seizures may also be responsible.

2. They present both local and systemic problems. The local injury may be complicated with compartment syndrome. Systemic concerns include intravascular volume depletion, electrolyte imbalance and renal injury from myoglobin. Until the limb is released there is little systemic effect; once reperfusion starts, plasma and blood leak into the previously crushed soft tissues as a result of the increased capillary membrane permeability and vessel damage. The effect depends upon the degree of tissue damage and in severe cases may produce hypovolaemia. Devitalized tissue is at high risk of secondary infection with a further systematic release of toxins.

3. Abnormal systemic blood markers of muscle infarction include rising blood urea nitrogen, raised potassium, phosphate, uric acid and creatine kinase. Metabolic acidosis develops with an increased anion gap. Hypocalcaemia occurs although intracellular calcium is raised. The packed cell volume is raised but there is thrombocytopenia.

Key point

- **The sudden rise in serum potassium concentration may produce cardiac arrhythmias (and arrest) soon after the patient is released.**

4. Myoglobinuria and raised plasma myoglobin result not only from direct myocyte damage but also from polymorphonuclear neutrophil-mediated cell lysis and microvascular coagulation.

Acute renal failure complicates severe crush injury as a result of hypovolaemia leading to prerenal failure, while the released myoglobin from damaged muscle cells precipitates and obstructs flow in the renal tubules. Myoglobin and macrophage-generated cytokines experimentally induce levels of potent vasoconstrictors such as platelet activating factor and endothelins, causing renal arteriole constriction, decreased glomerular filtration and renal ischaemia. A high concentration of myoglobinuria produces a red or smoky brown discoloration of the urine. Look for this when you catheterize the patient and check the urine regularly.

FAT EMBOLISM SYNDROME

1. Ninety per cent of cases result from blunt trauma associated with long bone fractures. It has, however, also been reported following burns, decompression sickness and even liposuction!

2. The classical triad of respiratory failure, neurological dysfunction and petechial rash is not present in all cases; indeed the rash, though pathognomonic, is only present in 50% of cases.

3. As several organs can be affected, there is a wide range of possible clinical presentations, although dyspnoea is the commonest. The onset of symptoms is usually between 24 and 48 h postinjury. Pulmonary changes include ventilation–perfusion (V/Q) mismatch, impaired alveolar surfactant activity and segmental hypoperfusion. Shadowing on chest X-ray is not dissimilar to ARDS. Neurological changes occur as a result of hypoxia and/or the humoral and cellular factors released from the bone. Effects on the heart may result in a fall in mechanical performance and arrhythmias. Renal damage can lead to lipiduria with tubular damage and ischaemic glomerular–tubular dysfunction.

4. Lipid globules are formed mainly from circulating plasma triglycerides, carried by very low density lipoproteins (VLDLs). In trauma, this is commonly a result of the release into the circulation of lipid globules from damaged bone marrow adipocytes; however, it can also occur with increased peripheral mobilization of fatty acids and increased hepatic synthesis of triglycerides or reduced peripheral uptake of plasma VLDLs (Fig. 2.10). It gives rise to thromboembolism of the microvasculature, with lipid globules and fibrin–platelet thrombi. In addition, the local release of free fatty acids can cause a severe inflammatory reaction that initiates the SIRS chemical

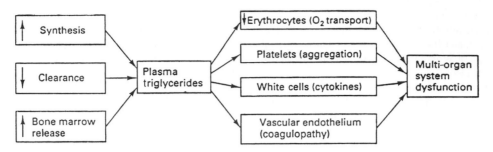

Fig. 2.10   The mechanism of interaction between raised plasma triglycerides and the pathogenesis of multiorgan system dysfunction in fat embolism.

cascade, which is probably responsible for the high association of fat emboli syndrome with both progressive anaemia and pyrexia (> 38.5° C).

Key point

- **Diagnosis of fat embolism rests on identifying fat globules in body fluids, histological recognition, or pulmonary involvement with at least one other organ system dysfunction.**

5. Search for fat globules in body fluids, such as sputum and urine, or lipid emboli in retinal vessels on fundoscopy; histological diagnosis requires demonstration of intracellular and intravascular aggregation of lipid globules with Sudan black stain.

PATHOPHYSIOLOGY OF WOUND HEALING

Soft tissue injuries heal by a complex series of cellular events that lead to connective tissue formation and repair by scar formation. Three fundamental things must happen for wound healing to occur: (1) haemostasis must be achieved; (2) an inflammatory response must be mounted in order to defend against microbial infection as well as attracting and stimulating the cells needed for tissue repair; and (3) many different cells must proliferate and synthesize the proteins necessary for restoring integrity and strength to the damaged tissue. This is covered in more detail in Chapter 33.

Wound healing therefore requires:

- Haemostais
- Inflammation
- Cell proliferation and repair.

Wound contracture

When wounds with tissue loss are left to heal by secondary intention, contraction of granulation tissue reduces the size of the tissue defect. The cell responsible for this process is the myofibroblast, although the exact role of this cell is unresolved. Even though reducing the size of the tissue deficit is of benefit in wound healing, the distortion and scar formation produced by the process inhibit function in certain areas of the body (particularly on the face and around joints).

PATHOPHYSIOLOGY OF BURNS

Three risk factors for death after burn injury have been identified: age more than 60 years; burn surface area of more than 40%; and the presence of inhalational injury.

Increased fluid losses due to uncontrolled evaporation are coupled with fluid shifts for the first 24–48 h after a major burn. Leakage of intravascular water, salt and protein occurs through the porous capillary bed into the interstitial space. This, in turn, results in loss of circulating plasma volume, haemoconcentration and hypovolaemia, the severity of which increases with the severity of the burn. In a burn over 15% of the total body surface area (TBSA), the capillary leak may be systemic, causing generalized oedema and a significant fall in blood volume.

Shock associated with burn injuries

The effect on the circulation is directly related to the size and severity of the burn wound. The body compensates for this loss of plasma with an increase in peripheral vascular resistance, and the patient will appear cool, pale and clammy; however, this compensation will only be effective in maintaining circulation for a period of time, depending on the severity of the burn and the presence of other injuries. Ultimately, the patient will demonstrate signs of hypovolaemic shock as the cardiac output falls. During this time it is rarely possible to keep the circulating volume within normal limits. The end of the shock phase in the adequately resuscitated burn patient is usually marked by a diuresis. This occurs approximately 48 h after the burn and is usually associated with a fluid balance that is more like that of an uninjured individual.

A burn of greater than 15% TBSA almost always requires intravenous fluid administration to expand the depleted vascular volume. However, shock can occur with a burn involving as little as 10% TBSA, as a result of complicating factors such as age, pre-existing disease and other major injuries. In these circumstances, a burn of 25–40% becomes a potentially lethal injury. Numerous fluid regimens have been calculated to assist in burn resuscitation: it is sensible to use the regimen favoured by your local burns department.

Depth of burn and cause of burn

The diagnosis of the depth of burn is not always easy. If doubtful, it should be reassessed at 24 h, using non-adherent dressings between examinations.

Superficial burns

Superficial burns are characterized by erythema, pain and the absence of blisters. Typical examples of superficial burns would be sunburn or simple flashburns. The epithelium remains intact so infection is not usually a problem and they generally do not require fluid replacement. Healing takes place over a few days and, with the exception of some pigmentation changes, no scarring occurs.

Partial thickness burns

Superficial partial thickness and deep partial thickness burns have been described. In the superficial variety the epidermis and the superficial dermis are burnt. They appear pink, moist and have fluid-filled, thin-walled blisters. They are associated with more swelling and are painfully sensitive, even to air current. Healing is by epithelialization from the pilosebaceous and sweat glands, as well as the wound edges. Therefore healing is often prolonged to 3–4 weeks.

In deep partial thickness burns the reticular dermis is involved. The appearance is a mixture of red and white, with blistering also a feature. The capillary refill is often prolonged and two-point discrimination may well be diminished. Healing is from the few remaining epithelial appendages and can take up to 6 weeks. It results in poor quality skin and marked pigmentation change (either hyper- or hypopigmentation). Hypertrophic scar formation may be a problem, as can wound contraction.

Infection may complicate the recovery of any partial thickness burn because the epithelium has been breached. This may take the form of locally delayed wound healing or sytemically-induced multiorgan failure (MOF). Deep dermal burns can result from scalds, contact burns, chemical burns and flame burns.

Full thickness burns

Full thickness burns involve the destruction of both the epidermis and dermis. They appear white, leathery and have no sensation to pinprick. The diagnosis between deep dermal and full thickness burns can be difficult, as they commonly lie adjacent to each other within the same wound. They can only heal naturally by epithelialization from the wound edge, leaving a contracted, poor quality scar. In the acute situation, circumferential full thickness burns around limbs and the chest can act as tourniquets, impeding the distal circulation and respiration, respectively. Urgent escharotomy may be required in these situations so discuss the possibility early with the local burns centre (see Ch. 24).

Simplistically, the depth of a burn is a product of the injurious temperature and the contact time. Thus the arm of an alert individual exposed to a hot flame, and quickly removed, will cause damage similar to that in a comatose patient lying against a warm radiator. The young and elderly are similarly immobile and prone to deep burns from relatively innocuous hazards (e.g. hot bathwater). Patients with peripheral neuropathies (e.g. diabetics) may also present with unexpectedly severe contact burns.

Chemical injury, such as that due to hydrofluoric acid or strong bases, can give rise to full thickness burns requiring specialist treatment. A high index of suspicion is appropriate when dealing with electrical burns because current flows preferentially through the deep structures, and extensive tissue damage may not be evident on early superficial inspection.

Patients with full thickness burns may require blood transfusion, as red cell haemolysis occurs with direct thermal injury; indeed there is generalized fragility of the entire red cell population leading to reduced cell lifespan.

Toxic shock syndrome

Toxin-producing strains of staphylococcal or streptococcal bacteria can colonize wounds. A marked cytokine response is stimulated, leading to a severe systemic illness typified by:

- Pyrexia (usually >39° C)
- Vomiting and/or diarrhoea
- Rash (erythematous, maculopapular)
- Malaise, dizziness, peripheral shutdown or frank shock.

It can occur even with relatively small, superficial burns and is more common in children. Treatment is with oxygen, intravenous fluids and antibiotics.

Response of the respiratory system to inhalational injury

The upper airway may receive thermal burns, and tissue swelling can develop very rapidly in these vascular tissues. Injury to the mouth and oropharynx in particular can cause acute respiratory obstruction. Oedema from these injuries may also involve the vocal cords. Dramatic changes in the patient's ability to maintain the airway have been observed over a short period of time following this type of injury. The lungs themselves are rarely injured from 'burning'. Usually laryngeal spasm occurs from the heat of the inspired gases, thereby protecting the lower airway and lungs from exposure; however, steam, with a heat capacity approximately 4000 times that of dry air, can carry heat to the lower airways, resulting in significant distal thermal injury.

Smoke inhalational injury secondary to confinement in a house fire may be associated with a wide variety of concomitant chemical injuries; for example, plastic furniture and textiles will release hydrogen chloride. Not only does this cause irritation to the eyes and throat but it also causes severe pulmonary oedema. Phosgene, produced from the burning of polyvinyl chloride, is also associated with the development of significant pulmonary oedema. Burning mattresses can produce nitrogen dioxide.

As fires can produce such a wide variety of chemicals, the resultant pulmonary damage may be multifactorial. This may result in necrosis of respiratory epithelium, inactivation of the respiratory cilia, and destruction of type II pneumocytes and alveolar macrophages. This leads to a decrease in lung compliance, which is seen as an increase in the work of breathing and an impairment of diffusion through the alveolar membrane.

In view of the very large surface area of the lung, fluid requirements for resuscitation may increase by as much as 50% of the calculated values if a severe inhalation injury has been sustained. The severity of the injury will not be related to the TBSA burn size, but rather to the length of time and intensity of exposure to the inhalation. Accurate information from the prehospital care providers relative to these conditions is vital in planning the patient's care and anticipating respiratory complications.

Carbon monoxide poisoning

Systemic absorption of inhaled toxins may also occur. Carbon monoxide (CO) is reported to be the leading toxicological cause of death. Burning any carbon-containing material can release CO, a byproduct of incomplete combustion. The mechanisms of CO toxicity are multiple. CO competes with oxygen for binding with haemoglobin, myoglobin and cellular cytochrome oxidase. In addition, off-loading of oxygen to the tissues is impaired by the leftward shift of the oxygen-dissociation curve induced by carboxyhaemoglobinaemia. The result is profound hypoxia both in the intra- and extracellular environments. The areas most affected are those with a high metabolic rate: heart and brain. Fetal tissue is also at significant risk.

Measured carboxyhaemoglobin levels do not necessarily correspond to clinical symptoms. The duration of the patient's exposure to CO is significant, as short exposures to a high concentration may give high carboxyhaemoglobin levels but not cause significant metabolic effects (usually acidosis with bicarbonate deficit). Carboxyhaemoglobin levels greater than 10% are significant and levels greater than 50% are generally lethal. Early treatment with high concentration oxygen is essential.

Carbon monoxide intoxication is the biggest cause of death in people caught in house fires or other types of closed-space fires.

Cyanide poisoning

When the polyurethane foam in modern furniture burns, a thick black smoke is produced. This not only contains CO and the corrosive substances mentioned above but also cyanide gas. The latter is another metabolic poison which binds to mitochondrial cytochrome oxidase. This leads to inhibition of adenosine triphosphate (ATP) production, with rapid onset of profound cellular anoxia and death. Cyanide gas is difficult to measure but should be assumed to be present if the carbon monoxide level is greater than 10%. Severe metabolic acidosis and raised lactate levels found on arterial blood gas analysis provide further clues towards the diagnosis.

TRAUMA SEVERITY SCORING

Essentially two separate types of trauma score have been developed. One type is based on the anatomical injuries sustained by the patient, while the other makes use of physiological data taken from the patient at first contact. They have developed in an attempt to achieve two separate objectives: firstly, to predict the probability of survival of an individual patient; and, secondly, to compare outcomes between different hospitals, or the same hospital over time.

The Injury Severity Score (ISS) is an anatomical scoring system that gives an overall score for patients with multiple injuries. The body is divided into six regions. Within each region every injury is given an Abreviated Injury Scale (AIS) score. This is a predetermined score from 1 (minor) to 6 (unsurvivable). The three highest grading scores, which are found in separate regions, are squared and then added together to make the final score. An obvious deficiency in this model is that it does not take account of multiple injuries within one body region. More recent scores such as the New Injury Severity Score (NISS) have been developed in an attempt to take account of such inaccuracies.

The Revised Trauma Score (RTS) is a physiological scoring system which attempts to predict outcome based on the first set of data obtained on the patient. The timing of first data recording and the effect of any treatment previously instigated will have a variable effect. None the less, it has been shown to correlate well with the probability of survival. It is calculated by combining three separately weighted scores based on the observed GCS, respiratory rate and systolic blood pressure.

TRISS determines the probability of survival of a patient by combining the ISS and RTS along with weightings to take account of the patient's age and the mechanism of injury (i.e. blunt or penetrating). The weightings have been calculated from a large database of trauma victims and allow comparative audit to be carried out.

ACKNOWLEDGEMENTS

Thanks are due to Geraldine McMahon, Richard Cowie, Charles Galasko, Roop Kishen, Roderick Little, David Marsh, Mohamed Rady, Stewart Watson and David Whitby.

Summary

- Trauma is an important clinical and economic problem because it is a major cause of mortality and morbidity in all countries of the world.
- In order to be effective in trauma care, the clinician needs a good understanding of the biomechanics of injury and how they relate to specific anatomical regions of the body.
- The clinician also needs to be aware of both the physiological and pathophysiological response to trauma, as this has direct implications for optimum patient resuscitation.
- These anatomical and physiological assessments can be used to quantify the severity of the trauma so that comparisons between treatment methods can be made.

References

Department of Health 1998 Our healthier nation – a contract for health. DoH, London

Further reading

Beal AL, Cerra FB 1994 Multiple organ failure syndrome in the 1990s. JAMA 271:226–233

Burgess AR, Eastridge BJ, Young JW et al 1990 Pelvic ring disruptions: effective classification system and treatment protocols. Journal of Trauma 30: 848–856

Colucciello S 1995 The treacherous and complex spectrum of maxillofacial trauma: etiologies, evaluation and emergency stabilisation. Emergency Medicine Reports 16: 59–70

Committee on Trauma 1997 Head trauma. In: Advanced trauma life support manual. American College of Surgeons, Chicago, pp 181–206

Committee on Trauma 1997 Biomechanics of injury. In: Advanced trauma life support manual. American College of Surgeons, Chicago, pp 345–366

Demling RH, Seigne P 2000 Metabolic management of patients with severe burns. World Journal of Surgery 24: 673–680

Foex BA 1999 Systemic responses to trauma. British Medical Bulletin 55: 726–743

Greenberg C, Sane D 1990 Coagulation problems in critical care medicine. Critical Care: State of the Art 11: 187–194

Grundy D, Swain A 1997 ABC of spinal cord injury, 3rd edn. British Medical Journal, London

Irving M, Stoner H 1987 Metabolism and nutrition in trauma. In: Carter D, Polk H (eds) Butterworths international medical reviews: trauma surgery 1. Butterworths, Oxford, pp 302–314

Lee CC, Marill KA, Carter WA, Crupi RS 2001 A current concept of trauma-induced multi-organ failure. Annals of Emergency Medicine 38: 170–176

Little R, Kirkman E, Driscoll P, Hanson J, Mackway-Jones K 1995 Preventable deaths after injury: why are traditional 'vital' signs poor indicators of blood loss? Journal of Accident and Emergency Medicine 12: 1–14

Mellor A, Soni N 2001 Fat embolism. Anaesthesia 56: 145–154

Moore J, Moore E, Thompson J 1980 Abdominal injuries associated with penetrating trauma in the lower chest. American Journal of Surgery 140: 724–730

Nathan AT, Singer M 1999 The oxygen trail: tissue oxygenation. British Medical Bulletin 55: 96–108

Nicholl JP 1999 Optimal use of resources for the treatment and prevention of injuries. British Medical Bulletin 55: 713–725

Proctor J, Wright S 1995 Abdominal trauma: keys to rapid treatment. In: Bosker G (ed). Catastrophic emergencies. Diagnosis and management. American Health Consultants, Atlanta, GA, pp 65–74

Skinner D, Driscoll P, Earlam R 1996 ABC of major trauma. British Medical Journal, London

Slater MS, Mullins RJ 1998 Rhabdomyolysis and myoglobinuric renal failure in trauma and surgical patients: a review. Journal of the American College of Surgeons 186: 693–716

Tiwari A, Haq AI, Myint F, Hamilton G 2002 Acute compartment syndromes. British Journal of Surgery 89: 397–412

Ware LB, Matthay MA 2000 The acute respiratory distress syndrome. New England Journal of Medicine 342: 1334–1349

Wyatt J, Beard D, Gray A, Busuttil A, Robertson C 1995 The time of death after trauma. BMJ 310: 1502

Useful links

www.doh.gov.uk/HPSSS Department of Health 2002 Indicators of the nation's health

PATIENT ASSESSMENT

SECTION 2

3 Clinical diagnosis

R. M. Kirk

Objectives

- **Clinical diagnostic skills are the basic requirements for successful surgical practice.**
- **For success you need to know the range of normality against which to measure abnormalities.**
- **Try to be positive in your opinions. Do not hide behind vagueness.**

Should you read this chapter? Are you already too experienced to need further instruction? If you think so, you are lacking in self-knowledge. None of us is completely competent in the complex, and still not yet fully understood, process by which we seek out a diagnosis of our patients' clinical problems.

INTRODUCTION

Much has been spoken and written about clinical diagnosis. Although Sir Peter Medawar, the Nobel Prize-winning immunologist, was not a clinician, he described the process of making a diagnosis as similar to the process of scientific research – hypothetico-deductive (Medawar 1969). A hypothesis (Greek *hypo* = under + *thesis* = a placing) is a supposition or idea; deduction (Latin *de* = from + *ducere* = to lead) is the application of critical testing to the idea. The great scientific philosopher, Sir Karl Popper, uses the parallel terms, 'conjectures (Latin *con* = with + *jacere* = to throw) and refutations' (Latin *refutare* = to drive back), suggesting that we should rigorously attempt to destroy our hypotheses. If they withstand the critical testing, we may accept them for practical purposes. If we refute them, we are free to develop further, perhaps more successful ideas (Popper 1959).

It has been said that an experienced clinician makes a provisional diagnosis within a few seconds of seeing most patients. Analyse your thought processes as you take a history and examine patients. You will recognize that you

repeatedly think, 'I wonder if this is condition X?' – a hypothesis, followed by the intention to ask a further question or carry out a specific test to see if the idea survives it or is refuted – the deductive process.

Why do we not employ computers, into which patients may enter information directly, for diagnosis? Computers are often used to harvest preliminary information as they can hold much more information than we usually have easily accessible. But they are valuable only when critically assessed information is entered. They are mere repositories, hence the pithy American acronym 'GIGO' (garbage in, garbage out).

Key point

- **All facts are not of equal importance. Identify, register and rely on the significant ones.**

Computers lack intuition – the power of perceiving truth without reasoning or analysis. As we communicate with our patients, we take in, partly consciously and partly unconsciously, details that weigh in the balance alongside the words. A quiet response to the question, 'How severe is the pain?' of, 'Chronic,' by a grey-faced London dock-worker may signal greater suffering to you than the vehement retort of, 'Excruciating,' by someone with a more volatile personality. Yet the first person may enter a score of 6 out of 10 and the second 10 out of 10 in response to a computer questionnaire in which 10 signals the highest pain level. You have interpreted the Cockney slang word 'chronic,' (Greek *chronos* = time, hence longstanding), to mean its opposite, 'acute'. Someone in excruciating pain (Latin *crucifigere crux* = cross + *figere* = to fix, hence to crucify; agonizing, anguished), often finds it difficult forcefully to express their suffering.

HISTORY

1. We have traditionally prided ourselves as surgeons on our ability to elicit physical signs and make accurate 'spot'

diagnoses. We have not always sufficiently developed our communication and history-taking skills. An effective history directs your attention to the cause of the surgical problem. You can apply the famous statement of Louis Pasteur about scientific discovery to the diagnosis of surgical disease, which may be translated as, 'Chance favours the prepared mind.' The history directs you towards the correct area of examination and investigation.

2. There are two, usually separate, parts of the history. Initially you should concentrate on the presenting complaint. Having clarified this, you need to investigate the general physical and mental health of your patient and identify coexisting or alternative disease.

3. Taking a history requires great tact. You must control the direction it takes, otherwise you may be led away from the line of pursuit of the diagnosis. When you ask a question and hear the response, the timing and phrasing of your next question is important. Too soon, too sharp, a sudden change of topic, and you may prevent the patient from adding a vital clue. Too late and the patient may have led you on a false track.

4. As you take a history you are establishing a relationship with the patient. For this reason prefer to speak together in a quiet, relaxed atmosphere. You cannot take an accurate history unless you and the patient can communicate verbally. Make sure you understand the meaning of the patient's statements – and the patient understands yours. If you do not have a common language, try to recruit an interpreter.

5. Ask 'open' questions whenever possible, for example, 'Where is your pain?' rather than 'Is your pain here?'

6. Avoid appearing judgemental; patients often withhold information if you seem to disapprove. Equally, they may give an incorrect answer, thinking that it may elicit your approval.

Presenting complaint

1. As you encounter each patient take in every detail of gender, age, expression, speech, gait, dress and attitude. This prejudices your interpretation of everything you are told and subsequently find. Do not misinterpret 'prejudice'; it means prejudging; although it is usually used disparagingly, it is reprehensible only if it is rigidly maintained against the evidence. Treat your interpretations as working hypotheses, to be tested and abandoned if the evidence refutes it. By sensibly incorporating your impressions of the patient with the history you are more likely to reach a balanced judgement (Fig. 3.1).

2. Do you think that the complaint made by the patient is the one that is the cause of anxiety? Sometimes patients find a reason to see a doctor, worried about a condition, yet are unable to express it, from diffidence, embarrassment or fear of the consequences.

3. The next time you sit before a patient, try to follow the sequence of your questions. What is your motivation for asking each one? Each one should elicit a clue to the diagnosis, clarify the answer to the previous question or elicit fresh information.

4. If you can identify the exact site of the symptoms, you may be able to identify the likely system. If so, ask about the effect of system function on the symptoms and the effect of symptoms on the system function. In this way you can sometimes recognize a pattern of features that form a syndrome (Greek *syn* = together + *dromos* = a course; hence, a concurrence of features).

5. If you think you have identified the cause of the presenting features, do not relax. While you are questioning the patient the answers you receive should trigger other possible diagnoses and you need to ask questions that will substantiate or exclude them. Thus, you are running several lines of thought in parallel.

6. Your targeted history is incomplete until you have sought out evidence of the severity of the cause of symptoms, its extent and rate of progression.

General assessment

1. There are well-established questions to check the function and health of the main body systems. Employ them to identify or exclude coexisting problems. For example, the answer to, 'Can you climb stairs?' may reveal preliminary information about the function of the

• Young child	• Appendicitis
• Young woman	• Gynaecological
• Young man	• Hernia, appendicitis
• Middle-aged woman	• Gynaecological, diverticulosis coli
• Middle-aged man	• Diverticulosis coli or colon cancer
• Elderly woman	• Gynaecological; cancer or diverticular disease of the colon
• Elderly man	• Colon cancer

Fig. 3.1 Your intuitive diagnosis for lower abdominal pain depends upon the patient before you. These are some preliminary diagnoses – but do not consider them to be a final judgement.

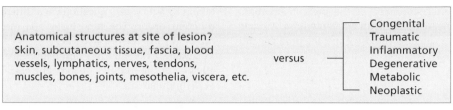

Fig. 3.2 Mentally test each of the likely tissues in the detected lesion against the pathological grid. You hope to identify the combination that fits the information that you have acquired.

cardiorespiratory, haematological, musculoskeletal and neuromuscular systems.

2. While taking the history, carefully assess the personality and attitude of your patient. Try to identify any anxieties or misapprehensions that need to be discussed.

EXAMINATION

1. You cannot carry out a thorough examination in an atmosphere of hysteria, noisy distraction or pressure of time. Relax and reassure the patient, and also make an effort to relax yourself.

2. When you took the history, you should have identified the important clinical signs you need to seek, but seek to identify further ones as you proceed through the examination.

3. Do not rush. Take each examination in turn and do not proceed until you have decided confidently, 'Is the sign present, or not?'

Key points

- **You can confidently reassure your patient that all is well only if you know the range of normality.**
- **You learn the range of normality only by assiduously building up your experience every time you have the opportunity.**

4. If you find a suspicious lesion, identify exactly where it lies both 'geographically' and in depth, including its attachments. You may then apply the anatomico-pathological grid (Fig. 3.2).

5. If you find an enlarged lymph node, examine the whole of its potential drainage area – and remember that when lymphatics are blocked, the flow may become retrograde (Latin *retro* = backward + *gressus* = to go).

6. If you find an abnormality in one part of a system, examine the whole system, such as the reticuloendothelial, vascular, neurological, joint, bone, muscles, skin systems.

7. If you need to curtail the full examination in an emergency, or in order to start treatment, determine to complete it as soon as possible.

8. Even though you may be certain of the clinical signs, be prepared to repeat the examination before you take action. Especially in emergency circumstances, such as an acute abdomen, physical signs often change rapidly.

9. Record your findings in full. If you do not record negative findings it may be assumed you did not seek them. Write legibly and do not use abbreviations or jargon. Write the time and date, and then sign the record.

10. Your hope is that you will reach a likely clinical diagnosis, excluding other possibilities so that you may plan the investigations (Fig. 3.3).

Key points

- **The commonest condition is the most likely.**
- **Remember, though, the 'pay-off' diagnosis – the one that may be less common but has important consequences if you miss it.** (Warning expressed by Hugh Dudley, formerly Professor of Surgery, St Mary's Hospital, London.)

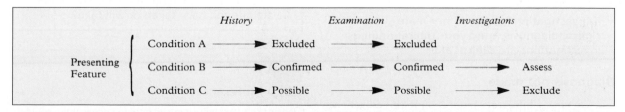

Fig. 3.3 As you proceed, you often accumulate further possible diagnoses. You run with all of them in parallel, hoping to exclude some. Some you confirm but need to assess the extent of disease. Others you keep in mind, hoping to confirm or exclude them by means of carefully chosen investigations (see Ch. 4).

11. Write a brief summary of the present situation: what will be done, why, and with what intention. Anyone reading the notes can now rapidly grasp the problem and the intended management of the patient.

DIAGNOSIS

1. As you discover symptoms and signs, decide if they are significant and reliable. Sometimes you find features that are contradictory and must decide which ones, if any, to trust.

2. Pattern recognition contributes powerfully to diagnosis. The almost subconscious recognition of a type of patient, a particular symptom and the discovery of a significant feature produce a pattern. Try asking yourself to describe someone close to you; remarkably, you may not be able to articulate many observations, yet you instantly recognize the person in a crowd. Overreliance on pattern recognition is dangerous. As you become experienced, having become acquainted with a large number of syndromes, you risk accepting them without further corroboration. Remember Karl Popper's admonition to test your hypothetical diagnosis. The extra effort often discloses a feature that throws doubt on the initially recognized likely diagnosis.

3. Perhaps the most daunting declaration to your patient is to state that there is no disease. This demands confidence in your findings and your diagnosis. It is also one of the most satisfying acts – at least comparable with pulling off a dramatic life-saving action. If you can look the patient in the eye and say, 'It is all right,' imagine the relief and joy your declaration brings. In many cases you can send the patient away, feeling relieved and happy, or order carefully selected investigations to confirm your diagnosis.

4. Not every patient's clinical features correspond to textbook descriptions. Be alert to the exceptions. Sometimes an apparently capricious finding warns you that you are misinterpreting the evidence; sometimes you are able to discover a previously undiscovered feature.

Key point

- If investigation results do not match your clinical diagnosis, trust your clinical findings; investigations are clinical aids.

Diagnosis not made

1. Do not rush to order more complex investigations. One of the most productive methods is to put aside the previous notes and start afresh. This is particularly so if someone else previously saw the patient. A fresh person taking a history asks questions in a different manner and different order. The new history is often surprisingly different from the original one.

2. Repeat the clinical examination. Do not automatically accept the findings of someone else, however senior or distinguished.

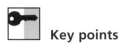

Key points

- **Did you ignore or dismiss information that clashed with your preconceptions?**
- **Never fail to respond to changed circumstances or 'uncomfortable' new information.**

3. Did you order the correct investigations? Remember that many investigations are operator dependent. If the investigation does not confirm your clinical judgement, consider repeating it after discussion with the person carrying out the procedure, rather than ordering another one that is perhaps more complex, expensive and potentially dangerous.

4. It is not always necessary to make a diagnosis before taking action. In an emergency you may need to act without knowing the exact cause of cardiorespiratory failure, calamitous bleeding or acute abdominal symptoms.

Summary

- Do you appreciate the immense and crucial value of history taking?
- Do you recognize that to diagnose a lesion, or confidently reassure your patients that all is normal, you must be thoroughly familiar with the range of normality?
- Will you remember that clinical diagnosis is not an end in itself? It offers a valuable opportunity to assess the character of the patient and establish a relationship.
- Will you assiduously record what you asked, what you were told, what you examined, what you found, what it means and what actions you have taken or will take?

References

Medawar PB 1969 Induction and intuition in scientific thought. Methuen, London, pp 42–45
Popper K 1959 The logic of scientific discovery. Routledge, London

4 Investigations

N. J. W. Cheshire, C. Bicknell

Objectives

- Define the aims of investigation used in surgical practice.
- Understand the principles underlying selection of appropriate investigations.
- Determine the limitations of commonly used investigations.
- Consider appropriate sequences and timing of multiple investigations.
- Highlight important principles of investigations most commonly used in clinical practice.

INTRODUCTION

The use of investigations in surgical practice is no substitute for clinical skill. An investigation is only worthwhile when it is requested in order to answer a specific question, or to confirm a clinical impression prior to intervention. There is an ever-expanding range of investigative modalities available and unwary surgeons who are clinically uncertain can easily find themselves overwhelmed with information if too many poorly considered investigations are requested. Furthermore, many modern tests are expensive and the costs of any investigation must always be considered in today's financially conscious health service. Other important issues that govern the effective use of special investigations include their selection, timing and interpretation. This chapter outlines some of the principles that should be applied before investigations are requested in surgical practice, highlights the limitations and discusses the practical use of common investigations.

AIMS

Investigations are performed for different reasons but all should share the common feature of directing management. The most common reasons for ordering investigations in surgical practice are outlined below.

Confirm the diagnosis

Use investigations to confirm a suspected clinical diagnosis, if clinical features are equivocal. Do not assume that tests are essential to diagnose, however, as there remain conditions for which clinical diagnostic acumen matches or exceeds the accuracy of any investigative tool (acute appendicitis), as well as conditions whose treatment uncontroversially confirms the diagnosis (ischiorectal abscess). Nonetheless, even in these instances confirmation of the clinical diagnosis is useful, usually histologically, to avoid missing an underlying condition, such as carcinoid as a cause of appendicitis or Crohn's disease leading to ischiorectal abscess formation.

 Key point

- **Remember that investigations are only worthwhile when they direct management.**

Exclude alternative diagnoses

Perform specific investigations in order to exclude an important alternative or additional diagnosis (frequently malignancy). Many examples of this practice exist. An older patient with new per-rectal bleeding presenting to the colorectal clinic may well have piles easily visible on examination, but must undergo further examination to exclude colonic cancer. Remember resource and financial implications when planning investigations in this manner; inappropriate investigations need to be avoided in all the surgical specialities, especially when pursuing ill-defined abdominal pain (in general surgery), vague back pain (in orthopaedic surgery), 'cystitis' in young women (in gynaecology and urology), chronic rhinitis (in ear, nose and throat (ENT) surgery), ill-defined and longstanding headaches (in neurosurgery). Never ignore these symptoms, but take a full history and examination to form a clinical impression of the likely cause and think carefully of the diagnoses that cannot be missed or may occur concurrently. A combination of clinical and risk assessment for each individual patient should guide the investigations performed.

Key point

• Treat all patients on an individual basis when considering tests to exclude alternative diagnoses.

Confirm the need to intervene in the absence of a diagnosis

In an emergency you may need to act after investigations confirm a need for emergency treatment without knowing the specific cause.

Determine the extent of disease and staging

It is considered best practice to map out the extent of the disease before surgery, especially in the elective setting. In fact when treating patients with neoplasia, staging is essential. Although the diagnosis of oesophageal cancer has been made, it is necessary to map out the extent of the disease, as the presence of an advanced tumour stage negates the need for operation and the physician may concentrate on palliative or chemotherapy treatment. You should also determine the extent of disease to optimize the use of operating theatre time and equipment, plan the operation carefully, avoiding having to make hasty decisions in the operating theatre, and minimize the chances of the surgical team being presented with any unpleasant surprises during the operation.

Evaluate comorbidity

Assess fitness for anaesthesia using a well thought out plan of investigations. A patient with an asymptomatic aortic aneurysm typically presents with a history of smoking and widespread cardiovascular disease; he or she requires particularly careful evaluation of cardiac, pulmonary and renal function if the risks of surgery are to be balanced against the risk of conservative treatment, and informed advice about mortality and outcome are to be given to the patient when consenting for operation. While in many cases a combination of the use of cardiac, renal and lung function tests can appropriately assess fitness for anaesthesia, expensive and time-consuming tests cannot be undertaken on all patients. If the clinical history is not straightforward, seek a cardiological or respiratory opinion instead of indis-

criminately investigating in the domain of another speciality. Consult the anaesthetist ahead of planned surgery to reduce avoidable cancellations on the day of surgery.

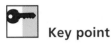

Key point

• You cannot undertake a full and informed discussion of the diagnosis, treatment options and likely outcomes with the patient and family prior to surgery until these necessary investigations have been performed.

Risk to others

Consider all patients to be at high risk for blood-borne infectious disease so that the risk of needlestick injury is minimized. However, in some circumstances hepatitis B, C and human immunodeficiency virus (HIV) serology (with consent) may be appropriate in patients being prepared for surgery in order to determine risk to others. In all patients the methicillin-resistant *Staphylococcus aureus* (MRSA) status should be determined and appropriate isolation procedures activated where necessary. This is particularly true of patients who have been transferred from another hospital and those with leg ulcers, who may have colonization of the wound site with MRSA.

Medicolegal considerations

Although you may be certain in your own mind about the diagnosis and appropriate management, you may need to protect yourself against future claims of incompetence against you, or the patient may wish to have objective evidence available in claims against a third party following, most commonly, an accident. When in doubt take advice from a senior colleague or from a medicolegal expert.

SELECTION

There is often more than one modality that may be used to answer the clinical question the surgeon is faced with, in which case you need to consider the selection of the most appropriate investigation, which varies on an individual basis. Various factors influence this choice.

Sensitivity and specificity

If one test is known to be more sensitive than the alternative, this is obviously a good reason to choose it. Colonoscopy is more sensitive than barium enema for the detection of small polyps and is the investigation of choice with lower gastrointestinal tract bleeding. The investigation must be specific for the disease when alternate diagnoses are to be excluded. [123]I scintigraphy for investigation of thyroid nodules is hard to justify as only 10% of low-uptake nodules are subsequently shown to be malignant. Sometimes the combination of tests can raise the sensitivity and specificity to the acceptable standards, such as triple assessment of a breast mass, which combines radiological, cytological and clinical assessment to improve the sensitivity and specificity of the assessment.

Definitions

Sensitivity: number of cases of the condition detected by the test/total number of cases in population studied.
Specificity: number of truly negative results/total number of negative results.

Simplicity

A simple investigation may be the first line of investigation and may be all that is needed. If a plain radiograph confirms the clinical diagnosis of osteomyelitis in a diabetic foot and the management plan is clear, it is not necessary to order a bone scan or magnetic resonance imaging (MRI). Free air seen on an erect chest X-ray confirms the diagnosis of bowel perforation and no further investigation is necessary. A simple investigation that proves to be undiagnostic, however, will require more detailed studies to be performed.

Safety

Think carefully about the complications of an investigation. Endoscopy may provide useful information as to the cause of bowel perforation but it is not safe in this situation, nor is the use of barium-based contrast. While a Tru-cut biopsy may confirm a diagnosis, it may also result in tumour seeding – ask the cyto/histopathologist whether a fine needle aspirate (FNA) may give sufficient information for management decisions to be made. For example, parotid tumours are at high risk from wound tumour seeding if investigated in this way and histological confirmation of the diagnosis often must wait until the mass is resected.

Cost

If an ultrasound can show liver metastases and this is the only information you require to decide on appropriate management, then why order a computed tomography (CT) scan that may be up to ten times more expensive?

Remember that resources are limited. Reassurance and certainty are purchased at a price. Moving from a position of 95% to 100% certainty is often very expensive. When using investigations it is vital to understand the need to manage risk while at the same time remaining accountable to the patient and to society for the way in which money is spent.

Acceptability

In general the less invasive the investigation the more acceptable it is to the patient. This is especially true in paediatric practice, where the acceptability of the investigation to the child is essential if meaningful results are to be gained from investigations. Consider carefully the acceptability of the test when patients are being screened for asymptomatic disease. One of the limitations of the use of faecal occult blood testing as a screening investigation for colorectal cancer has been the relative unacceptability of this investigation to patients. Unacceptable tests suffer from poor compliance and a screening programme may achieve poor results in this situation.

Availability

The gold standard may be the ideal choice of investigation for a patient but may not be possible. For example, an MRI scan may provide more information about the brain after injury or prior to neurovascular or neurosurgical intervention, but if the institution you are working in does not have an MR scanner and you need information rapidly you must make do with a CT scan.

Routine

Surgical departments may have their own series of investigations set out within a protocol. You should discuss with your consultant and the anaesthetic staff the circumstances in which investigations that do not conform to the categories outlined under 'Aims' should be performed.

LIMITATIONS

Remember that all investigations have limitations that need to be considered when ordering tests and interpreting results.

Incorrect result

Do not discard your clinical impression, if the result of any investigation conflicts with your clinical judgement, without considering the possibility that the test may be misleading. Check that the correct procedure was performed and the procedure was performed correctly.

Take into account any problems encountered with the procedure when interpreting results.

Gaining sufficient confidence in your clinical ability to question the opinion of others is difficult but also essential if a safe and rewarding clinical practice is to be developed. Remember that in many circumstances you, as the surgeon, may be the only individual who has actually spoken to and examined the patient and therefore you are in a unique position to judge the likely accuracy of the investigation result you are presented with.

Key point

- **Do not blindly read a test result without considering the clinical picture.**

The investigation may also be misleading as a result of the limited sensitivity of an investigation. For example, a technically adequate breast fine needle aspiration may have been taken and correctly interpreted but may miss a carcinoma because of a sampling error of the lump assessed. Remember also that an investigation may yield a false-positive as well as false-negative result.

Consider repeating or choosing another test to answer the same question if an investigation does not support a firm clinical diagnosis. Discuss the test with the person who performed it to ensure that as much clinical information as possible has been passed on to the individual who is trying to give you a result. An inadequate report may have been based on inadequate information given on the request form. Combined clinical meetings between the surgical team and specialized radiologists, histopathologists, etc. are often the ideal forum for the presentation of clinical information and review of investigations. In this situation interpretation of radiological images or histological diagnoses may be revised and fit with your clinical impression. If a test is thought to be misleading it is often useful to repeat it, consulting the most clinically reliable investigator.

Key points

- **Many investigations are operator dependent – subjective opinions, not objective proofs.**
- **If an investigation does not conform with your firm clinical impression, first discuss it with the investigator before embarking on more complex tests, and consider repeating the test.**

Complications

An investigation may be associated with a significant complication rate, an issue that may not only influence one's choice of its use, but also may have medicolegal implications if it has not been discussed at the time of consent. Is a selective carotid arteriogram really worth the 1% stroke rate when a duplex scan may give all the necessary information? Think whether this complication rate could be reduced or should be avoided altogether. Hydrate the patient intravenously and consider pretreatment with N-acetylcysteine in a patient with a raised creatinine before giving contrast to perform CT or an angiogram. Give the older patient Klean-Prep rather than Picolax before a colonoscopy.

SEQUENCE AND TIMING OF INVESTIGATIONS

Organization

Do not collect data indiscriminately when you are investigating a patient prior to surgery or during follow-up. Always organize the flow of information you require so that it follows a logical sequence that will culminate in you being able to discuss the patient's condition and management, with any attendant risks, in a fully informed manner and from a position of strength. During the preoperative process of diagnostic confirmation, determination of the extent of disease and exclusion of specific alternative diagnoses, you will frequently need more than one special investigation. In these circumstances thought must be given to determining the appropriate order of such investigations. Avoid the temptation to arrange all investigations at one sitting to prevent the patient having to come back repeatedly to the clinic. It is obviously inappropriate to arrange cardiology and pulmonary function tests to assess fitness for surgery at the same time as determining the primary disease and any spread. If the surgical problem turns out to be inoperable, then the other investigations undertaken have usually been a waste of time and resources as well as putting the patient at potential risk. Patients often understand the need for a logical sequence of investigations and the time this may require.

Urgency

Consider the urgency of each individual investigation and request appropriately. For the patient with a potentially curable carcinoma, investigations must be carried out quickly and efficiently. Conversely, there is no sense in flooding the radiology department with urgent requests that are to determine the cause of problems that have dragged on for many years.

The purpose of investigations is to reduce the management options and to seek to obtain crucial information once, not repeatedly. Sometimes an impasse is reached.

Reflect, reconsider and perhaps postpone a decision for a while, using time as a diagnostic tool. If you rush to make a decision where there is no indication for urgency you will make mistakes. A high negative laparotomy rate in a surgeon usually indicates an unwillingness to use time in this way, perhaps because of organizational constraints. Avoid the temptation to do a laparotomy in the middle of the night just because of the difficulties you might encounter if the need for surgery emerges the next day.

Protocols

Often the sequence and choice of investigations is presented in the form of protocols, where guidelines are set out enabling all staff to follow the preferred investigative methods of a department. These are useful in common conditions, both as a diagnostic tool (such as the investigation of rectal bleeding) and as a preoperative work-up regimen (in the case of complex surgical procedures, such as complex aneurysm surgery or cardiac surgery, where a number of preoperative investigations must be performed). A well-written protocol allows the surgeon who is unfamiliar with the working practices of the hospital to be able to investigate a particular condition appropriately. They may also form guidelines for specialist nurses or nurse consultants to work from, making services more efficient and decreasing waiting times. Protocols are invaluable in the procedure of audit as all staff must work to a standard, which they are expected to maintain. They also prevent unnecessary and costly investigations being performed. A rigid protocol has a number of advantages but you must remember that they are no substitute for clinical acumen and all cases must be dealt with on an individual basis, with investigations directed to a particular patient.

PRACTICAL USE

Blood tests

Most laboratories use automated analysers that give all the common haematological and biochemical indices. You only need ask for a full blood count to receive a full set of haematological parameters. Interpret the results in the light of the patient's general condition. For example, dehydrated patients have a high haemoglobin and packed cell volume (PCV, haematocrit) because of haemoconcentration; a normal haemoglobin in such patients may mask anaemia.

Levels of substances may be affected by the timing of blood sampling. The creatinine kinase is only transiently raised in the plasma after myocardial infarction; other enzymes are increased later. There is a diurnal rhythm with hormones such as cortisol that may produce misleading results. Binding proteins and plasma proteins affect hormone, enzyme and drug levels, so allow for this when interpreting results.

Remember the biochemical picture is obtained from just a sample of plasma. You are only indirectly discovering what is going on inside cells. Potassium levels, for instance, reflect poorly the intracellular potassium. In diabetic ketoacidosis the plasma potassium level is high but the patient is intracellularly depleted of potassium as insulin levels are low and potassium is not taken into cells.

Discuss unusual cases with an expert. Examination of a blood film by an experienced haematologist can prove diagnostic in the case of a raised white cell count (WCC) where the cause is in doubt. Further investigation of the patient may also be influenced by an opinion from an expert. It may be that if the peripheral blood picture shows involvement (as in chronic lymphatic leukaemia), peripheral blood marker studies will lessen the need for lymph node biopsy. This will avoid the need for a general anaesthetic, and a bone marrow sample can be taken under local anaesthetic instead.

Microbiology (see also Ch. 19)

A pus swab only briefly contains a representative sample of organisms from an infected source. Organisms die because they are anaerobic (e.g. *Bacteroides*), because they are delicate (e.g. *Neisseria*) or because the other organisms in the sample proliferate faster and overwhelm them. Therefore lose no time between taking the swab and transferring it to an appropriate medium for culture. If pus is available, collect a quantity and send that, rather than a swab, to the microbiologist. Store pus swabs (in appropriate transport medium) at 4°C when taken at night and ensure that they are sent to the laboratory the next day. Remember that prior consultation with a microbiologist may increase the yield of relevant positive cultures obtained.

Taking many swabs for culture without clinically assessing the patient or careful thought may cause you to miss the diagnosis. Make sure you ask the correct question in order to select the best method of answering it. The detection of amoebic dysentery is not accomplished by taking a swab for culture but by examining a fresh specimen immediately under the microscope. The positive identification of bacteria responsible for late vascular graft infections often requires special techniques (e.g. sonication) to separate the bacteria prior to culture and this requires all the clinical information to be passed on to the microbiologist before the arrival of the specimen.

Inform the laboratory of all relevant clinical information and antibiotic treatment so that the microbiologist can read the results sensibly. For instance Gram-positive cocci within a blood culture may indicate a skin contaminant, such as *Staph. epidermidis*, or an MRSA septicaemia.

In the patient with no sign of sepsis, it is sensible to wait for the full report from the bacteriologist.

Always seek the help of the microbiologist whenever you deal with superadded infection, especially in transplant patients and in the immunocompromised (as in HIV infections or in patients on chemotherapy). *Pneumocystis carinii* is the commonest opportunistic infection here. The picture can, however, become quite complicated, partly because several infective agents can become involved (bacterial, viral or fungal) and partly because the picture may change from day to day.

Radiological investigations (see also Ch. 5)

X-ray examinations are one of the simplest and cheapest radiological investigations to perform. Use these as a first-line investigation in cases of suspected perforation and obstruction before more expensive and complicated tests. Think whether introduction of a contrast agent into a cavity or lumen would improve the diagnostic accuracy of the test if initial plain films are inconclusive. For most patients the radiation experienced from X-rays will not cause problems but the dose is cumulative, so when possible avoid repeated tests that use radiation, especially in the case of long-term screening.

Histopathology

A biopsy is a representative sample of tissue that may be examined by a histopathologist. The tissue may be obtained in a variety of ways and biopsies are classified according to how they are obtained. Excision biopsies remove the entire lesion and undoubtedly provide the best tissue for histopathological examination. Wedge biopsies provide a section of tissue from a lesion, while a core biopsy is performed with a Tru-cut biopsy needle to take a small core of the lesion. Discuss with an expert the best type of biopsy to get an accurate answer and consider radiological methods of obtaining tissue to avoid open biopsy and obtain an accurate sample. Be careful when taking a biopsy to include a representative sample of the lesion. From the histologist you want to know what the lesion is, whether the lesion is malignant and the prognostic indicators. When taking a biopsy, therefore, be careful to take tissue and not only the necrotic centre; when obtaining samples from polyps sample the stalk, so that you may find out the degree of invasion; and when sending resected specimens orientate them appropriately. Talk to the pathologist, relay important clinical information and find out about resection margins, the grade and stage of disease.

Fine needle aspiration does not give the same architectural detail as histology but is quick, relatively painless, requires no anaesthetic, the complications of biopsy are avoided and it can provide cells from the entire lesion, as many passes through the lesion can be made while aspirating. For all cytological examinations there are errors that may occur in the sampling stage, where the lesion may be missed or an inadequate sample taken, or in the pathological examination. You need to know from the cytologist whether the sample was adequate and whether normal or malignant cells were seen. If the sample is inadequate the test will usually need repeating. Cytological specimens can also be obtained from spun down samples of fluid from a patient. Urine, pleural aspirate and sputum can all be examined for malignant cells. Think of these simple ways of obtaining cytological evidence of malignancy.

Invasive diagnostic procedures

The use of endoscopy provides a direct method of visualization of pathology and also allows biopsy or definitive treatment of lesions. A negative endoscopy is usually more reliable than a negative contrast study, but remember that it is operator dependent and that subtle lesions may have been missed (ask about the seniority and experience of the operator if you did not perform the investigation yourself). It may need repeating in cases of doubt.

Diagnostic laparotomy, and more commonly laparoscopy, is used as a diagnostic tool in specific circumstances such as preoperative staging of certain cancers. The need for diagnostic procedures of this kind has fallen with the advent of high-resolution scans such as CT and MR.

Physiological assessment

Use this type of assessment when you require information on the physiological workings of an organ or part of an organ. Motility disorders may be investigated effectively by oesophageal or rectal manometry, which will supplement anatomical and pathological information that has been gained. Manometry will quantify the problem, as well as facilitate the selection of operative therapy.

Summary
- Do you understand the purpose of each investigation ordered in common conditions?
- How do you decide which investigation is the most appropriate?
- Can you name investigations with a limited reliability?
- Which tests have serious complications?
- Can you formulate sensible investigation plans for complex diagnostic problems?

5 Imaging techniques

S. W. T. Gould, T. Agarwal, T. J. Beale

Objectives

- Become familiar with the basic techniques and principles of radiological investigation.
- Be able to enumerate the different types of radiological modalities, together with their advantages and limitations.
- Understand the principles of selection of the most appropriate radiological technique for a given clinical problem.
- Identify the key roles of radiology in the diagnosis and management of surgical disorders.

INTRODUCTION

Radiology is one of the most rapidly expanding specialties. This is due to continuing advances in both computer and machine technology. New imaging techniques, dramatically affecting patient assessment, are constantly being introduced. It is thus becoming increasingly difficult for surgeons to keep up to date with them. There must therefore be close communication between surgeons and radiologists to ensure that the most appropriate imaging technique is utilized for specific surgical problems. This is best achieved by regular interdepartmental meetings and individual case discussions of the more problematic patients.

The correct imaging technique can be chosen only if you make all the facts available to the radiologist. To this end, include the appropriate clinical details on the imaging request form.

Bear in mind the high cost and limited availability of some of the more sophisticated imaging techniques when deciding on the radiological investigation. Do not forget that the required information can often be obtained from plain X-rays and simple contrast studies.

No radiological technique replaces clinical skills. Do not base clinical decision making on imaging findings alone.

Key point

- Remember the maxim, 'treat the patient and not the X-ray'.

TYPES OF RADIOLOGICAL INVESTIGATION

The wide range of imaging techniques available includes plain film radiographs (X-rays), fluoroscopic screening, ultrasound, computed tomography (CT), magnetic resonance imaging (MRI) and nuclear medicine. Each of these will be described briefly.

Plain radiographs (X-rays)

1. X-rays were first demonstrated by the German physicist W. K. Roentgen, in 1895. He discovered, fortuitously, that X-rays not only expose photographic plates, they are also absorbed to varying degrees by intervening structures, which are then projected onto the photographic plate as negative images. The clinical relevance of this discovery was immediately apparent as, for the first time, imaging of the living skeleton was possible, enabling deformities, fractures and dislocations to be seen. To this day the indications for plain radiology have not changed, although X-ray imaging has now been used in every other system of the body. This has come about mainly due to the use of contrast agents. Plain radiographs are used to demonstrate contrast between tissues of different densities and, as such, obviously show the skeletal system well. However, they also demonstrate differences between gas and fluid and are therefore the most sensitive imaging technique for the detection of free intraperitoneal air after gastrointestinal perforation. The use of radio-opaque contrast agents increases the diagnostic yield of plain radiography. For example, iodine-containing agents are excreted rapidly by the renal route and so clearly outline the kidneys, ureters and bladder. The same agents also delineate the internal characteristics of blood vessels in angiography.

2. Plain radiography is the most frequently requested examination. It is relatively cheap and simple to perform. These images can, however, be difficult to interpret, particularly soft tissue images, and of course ionizing radiation can be hazardous to health and to the developing fetus. The actual radiation dose to the patient varies greatly and depends on the density of the tissue through which the X-ray beam must pass. The greater the density of tissue, the more X-rays are absorbed in the patient and fewer reach the film. Table 5.1 shows the relative dose of common surgical requests compared to the radiation dose of a chest X-ray. The radiation dose of a chest X-ray is equivalent to 3 days of natural background radiation.

Ultrasound

1. Ultrasound waves are created in a transducer (Latin *trans* = across + *ducere* = to lead; a device that transfers power from one system to another) by applying a momentary electric field to a piezoelectric crystal which vibrates like a cymbal, producing sound waves. The transmitted waves interact with soft tissue interfaces and are reflected back, deflected or absorbed. The sound waves that are reflected are alone used to make the image. The greater the difference in density between two adjacent tissue planes, the greater the amount of reflected sound waves. For example when the sound waves reach a solid gallstone, most of it is reflected back, resulting in a bright collection of echoes and an acoustic 'shadow' beyond the stone. Ultrasound waves, however, are transmitted through the surrounding biliary fluid, which appears black.

2. Ultrasound examinations are useful for visualizing soft tissues. They easily demonstrate fluid collections in the subcutaneous tissues, such as breast cysts, and within the body cavities, as in the chest and abdomen. Ultrasound has become the first line of investigation in many conditions, such as gallstone disease. Its use is limited by structures that obscure the passage of the ultra-sound waves, so it cannot give images of, for example, the brain. Large amounts of bowel gas may prevent adequate examination of the abdominal cavity, and the retroperitoneum is often poorly visualized. It is highly operator dependent. It does, however, give dynamic, real time images and is safe to use in any patient, including those who are pregnant. It is relatively cheap and is mobile. It is also useful for guiding diagnostic procedures such as aspiration cytology or needle biopsy (see below).

3. Intracavitary ultrasound has been used for transvaginal assessment of the pelvic organs in females and transrectal evaluation of the prostate gland. More recently endoscopic ultrasound (EUS) has been developed, combining the benefits of high frequency ultrasound and endoscopy. A small ultrasonic transducer is incorporated into the tip of an endoscope. It is particularly useful in assessing the extent and especially the 'T' (tumour) staging of oesophageal, gastric, pancreatic and pulmonary tumours.

4. Focused abdominal sonography in trauma (FAST) is gaining wide acceptance for assessing the abdomen in haemodynamically stable patients suspected of having abdominal injuries.

Fluoroscopic imaging

Many common requests to the radiology department involve the use of X-ray screening. These include all barium examinations, most interventional procedures (except those under ultrasound, CT or MRI guidance) and sinograms, cholangiograms, nephrostograms, etc. Each screening room has an image intensifier that converts the X-ray image into a light image, then to an electron image and finally back to a light image of increased brightness. Fluorescence (hence the term fluoroscopy) is the ability of crystals of certain organic salts (called phosphors) to emit light when excited by X-rays. This process is used both in film cassettes for plain radiographs and in an image intensifier.

Barium salts are used to delineate the mucosa of the gastrointestinal tract and are also used in dynamic studies to help define the function of this system (e.g. in barium swallow examinations). Gastrografin is a thin, water soluble contrast medium which has the added advantage of not being a peritoneal irritant like barium. It is used for the evaluation of intestinal obstruction (both small bowel and colonic) and for confirming the presence of a suspected anastomotic leak.

Computed tomography (CT)

1. Some of the major advances in radiology in recent years have been in the field of cross-sectional imaging. Computed tomography (Greek *tomos* = slice + *graphein* = to write: abbreviated to CT) and magnetic resonance

Table 5.1 Relative dose of common surgical requests	
Radiograph	Equivalent number of chest X-rays (approx.)
Chest PA	1
Abdomen AP	50
Pelvis AP	35
Lumbar spine AP and Lat	65
Barium meal	150
Barium enema	250
IVU	125
CT head	115
CT chest or abdomen	400

imaging (MRI) have revolutionized the investigation of the central nervous system and other soft tissues.

2. The CT image is derived from computer integration of multiple exposures as an X-ray tube travels in a circle around a patient. The circular track is called the gantry. A fan-shaped beam is produced by the X-ray tube(s) and is picked up by a row of sensitive detectors aligned directly opposite. The computer constructs the image by dividing the gantry into a grid. Each box in the grid is called a voxel and has a length, width and depth – slice thickness. Each voxel is given a value representing the average density of the tissue in the box; the value is measured in Hounsfield units (HU) after Sir Godfrey Hounsfield who invented the CT scanner in 1972. Water has an HU of 0, air –1000, fat –80 to 100, abdominal organs 30–80 and compact bone >250. Each voxel is assigned a shade of grey according to its HU. The window level (WL) is the HU number in the middle of the grey scale; the window width (WW) is the range of HUs over which the grey scale is spread. Both the WL and the WW can be adjusted to emphasize differences in soft tissue, lung or bony detail on the stored data. These figures are always seen on the printed film.

3. Modern three-dimensional spiral CT scanners have not only drastically cut down the time taken for the imaging but multiplanar reconstruction is now possible. This is particularly useful for the head, neck and face but has found important applications in general surgical conditions, a prime example being CT pneumocolon.

Magnetic resonance imaging (MRI)

1. Each body proton can be thought of as a very small magnet. When the body is placed in a magnetic field, these protons line up along the direction of that field. The images in MR are generated by the energy released from the protons when they realign within the magnetic field after the application of radiofrequency energy pulses. This electromagnetic energy is received by a 'coil' and converted to images by a computer. Scanning methods in MR are referred to as 'pulse sequences' and the images generated are often classified as T1-weighted or T2-weighted. In simple terms, in a T1-weighted image, fat appears as a bright signal and water appears dark, and in a T2-weighted image, water appears as the brightest signal with fat appearing dark. There is therefore much scope for image manipulation by employing different pulse sequences during a single examination.

2. MR images give unparalleled soft tissue resolution but are generally less useful than other imaging methods for bony structures. MR has inherent advantages over CT and other imaging techniques, the most important being the lack of ionizing radiation. It has multiplanar capabilities, allowing imaging in any arbitrary plane, not just the orthogonal planes (the standard projections) permitted

by CT. It has great sensitivity to flow phenomena and unique sensitivity for temperature changes.

3. Its disadvantages include expense and availability. It is safe in the majority of patients but those with implanted magnetic devices or metallic objects, such as certain intracranial aneurysm clips, indwelling pacemakers, cochlear implants or metallic intraocular foreign bodies, cannot be safely scanned. Most orthopaedic implants, however, are safe. Due to the physical constraints of the machine, obese or claustrophobic patients may be unsuitable for imaging by this technique.

Nuclear medicine

1. A radionuclide is administered into the body and subsequently undergoes radioactive decay. The commonest radionuclide used in medicine is technetium-99m (^{99m}Tc). The 'm' is placed after the mass number to indicate a metastable state, i.e. an intermediate species with a measurable half-life. ^{99m}Tc has a half-life of 6 h and is a pure gamma emitter. This results in a relatively low dose of ionizing radiation being delivered to the patient. The radionuclide is labelled so that it can be targeted to the tissue that needs to be imaged. For example, it may be labelled by attaching it to red or white blood cells or a variety of chelates. In the decay process gamma rays are given off. These are detected by a gamma scintillation camera and from them the images are formed.

2. The latest addition to the armamentarium is PET (positron emission tomography), which has been useful in the staging of various gastrointestinal malignancies. It is particularly useful in preoperative assessment of nodal involvement and detection of recurrence and metastases. It is reserved for the assessment of equivocal cases, not as a first choice procedure.

3. Tomographic techniques, commonly used in X-ray and CT, have also been developed in nuclear medicine. Tomography refers to the technique of 'cutting' the body into the required imaging planes. An example is SPECT (single photon emission computed tomography) and involves gamma camera(s) rotating around a gantry, as in X-ray CT. A volume of data can then be collected and transaxial images reconstructed.

HOW ARE RADIOLOGICAL TECHNIQUES USED IN SURGERY?

Radiological techniques are used in the management of surgical diseases in one of three main ways:

1. To aid in the diagnosis of a surgical disorder
2. As an interventional technique to treat a surgical disorder or one of its complications
3. To guide a surgical procedure.

Each of these main areas will be considered in turn, with a few specific examples.

Aid to diagnosis

1. This is of course the simplest and best known application. Examples include the use of an erect chest X-ray to detect free intraperitoneal gas, and CT scan of the brain to detect intracranial bleeding following trauma.

2. Radiology is a valuable screening aid, as in population screening such as mammography, and also as part of protocol-based preoperative imaging such as a chest X-ray when preparing patients for major surgery. Always prefer the simple, hence cheaper, investigation before the complex, hence costlier, one if the simpler investigation has a good chance of providing the diagnosis.

3. If possible, avoid those with a significant associated complication rate or inherent danger; for example, in pregnant women ultrasound techniques are safer than those using X-rays.

4. All investigations, no matter how complex or invasive, have a given sensitivity and specificity and therefore there will always be a false-negative and a false-positive rate.

Key point

- **Prefer safer, and non-invasive tests, to potentially dangerous and invasive ones.**

Interventional techniques

1. Interventional radiology has developed into a speciality in its own right. There can be very few radiology departments that do not perform at least some interventional techniques. Interventional radiology may be defined as the performance of a procedure on some part of the anatomy while using a radiological modality to guide that procedure. Perhaps the simplest example is image-guided biopsy. This is commonly performed using ultrasound or CT guidance, although it is now possible to perform biopsies using the added advantage of MRI. In places this has replaced the need for an open surgical biopsy. A good example is stereotactic (Greek *stereos* = solid + *tassein* = to arrange; location within three dimensions) core biopsy of the breast, guided by digital mammography. The placement of drainage catheters using ultrasound or CT has revolutionized the management of postoperative complications such as subphrenic abscess. Vascular surgery has been completely changed by the advent of interventional radiology. The techniques include angioplasty, catheter thrombolysis and stenting of aneurysmal or occlusive diseases, and novel techniques that replace the need for high-risk surgery, for example transjugular portosystemic shunting in portal hypertension.

2. This is a field that is likely to improve further, given the rapid development and integration of computer technology into imaging methods and the availability of new imaging systems, such as interventional MRI, and tissue destruction techniques, such as focused ultrasound and radiofrequency ablation systems.

Image-guided surgery

1. Image-guided surgery is the use of a radiological modality during a surgical procedure to give more information than is available by direct inspection of the surgical field. The information so gained is used to influence or guide the performance of the operation. There are many examples in everyday surgical practice (Table 5.2). The best known are fracture manipulation using image intensification, and intraoperative cholangiography during cholecystectomy to determine the presence or absence of gallstones within the main bile ducts.

2. More advanced techniques include stereotactic CT-guided neurosurgery and the use of intraoperative ultrasound in hepatic and pancreatic surgery, to determine resectability and to determine the anatomical location of vital structures as resection proceeds. This technique may be used in both open and laparoscopic procedures. It has recently become possible to perform surgical operations within interventional MRI units, harnessing the soft tissue and image manipulation power of MR to guide the procedure. There have been recent reports demonstrating the use of intraoperative MR to guide complete tumour resection in the brain (Moriarty et al 1996), breast (Gould et al 1998), and soft tissues (Gould et al 2001). It has been shown to be a useful guide when

Table 5.2	Examples of image-guided surgery
Modality	Procedure
X-ray	Fracture reduction
X-ray	Removal of foreign bodies
X-ray	Intraoperative cholangiography
X-ray	ERCP
X-ray	Retrograde ureterography
X-ray	Intraoperative arteriography
Ultrasound	Laparoscopic staging of pancreatic cancer
Ultrasound	Hepatic resection
Ultrasound	Complex anal fistula surgery
CT	Stereotactic neurosurgery
MRI	Neurosurgery
MRI	Breast surgery

operating on complex anal fistulae (Gould et al 2002). MR-guided interstitial laser thermotherapy is being carried out for ablation of irresectable and metastatic tumours. It has the added advantage of intraprocedural monitoring and can be performed under local anaesthesia. Some survival benefit has already been described for this technique for ablation of colorectal metastases in the liver.

3. Finally, radiological data obtained preoperatively can be used to plan or guide surgical procedures. The best examples are three-dimensional CT reconstructions of the face or skull for surgical planning prior to major maxillo-facial reconstructive surgery. This technique is now used to plan the best approach for major hepatic surgery for trauma or tumours. An extremely exciting area of current investigation is the combination of information obtained from a number of radiological techniques, such as CT, and conventional and functional MRI to make a comprehensive three-dimensional preoperative model of lesions and surrounding anatomical structures. Work is underway to 'register' this image to the patient during surgery, so that it may truly be used as an intraoperative guide.

Summary

- Do you appreciate the wide variety of radiological imaging methods that are currently available?
- Are you aware of the value of consulting your radiologist in order to select the most relevant investigation?
- Do you recognize that selecting an appropriate investigation demands balancing the aim of the investigation, effectiveness, cost and safety?
- Are you aware that radiological images should not be used in isolation but must be used in conjunction with the rest of the available clinical information?
- Do you recognize the three key areas of diagnostic radiology, interventional radiology and image guidance of surgical procedures?
- Can you foresee the likely future applications of interventional radiology and image-guided surgery?

References

Gould S, Lamb G, Lomax D, Gedroyc W, Darzi A 1998 Interventional MR-guided excisional biopsy of breast lesions. Journal of Magnetic Resonance Imaging 8: 26–30

Gould SWT, Agarwal T, Benoist S, Patel B, Gedroyc W, Darzi A 2001 Resection of soft tissue sarcomas with intra-operative magnetic resonance guidance. Journal of Magnetic Resonance Imaging 15(1): 114–119.

Gould SWT, Agarwal T, Martin S, Gedroyc W, Darzi A 2002 Image guided surgery for anal fistula in a 0.5T interventional MRI unit. Journal of Magnetic Resonance Imaging 16: 267–276

Moriarty T, Kikinis R, Jolesz F, Alexander III E 1996 Magnetic resonance imaging therapy. Neurosurgical Clinics of North America 7: 323–330

Further reading

Royal College of Radiologists 1998 Making the best use of a department of clinical radiology, 4th edn. Royal College of Radiologists, London

6 Influence of coexisting disease

R. M. Jones, C. A. Marshall

Objectives

- Recognize which coexisting disease processes are associated with increased morbidity.
- Understand which features of the patient's condition can be improved.
- Realize that a simple operation does not always mean an equally simple or risk-free anaesthetic.
- Understand that sick patients are best managed in daylight hours with fully trained staff.
- Recognize that in some circumstances it may be better to transfer patients to another hospital preoperatively if there are inadequate facilities for their postoperative care.

INTRODUCTION

About half of adult patients presenting to you have a coexisting disease unrelated to the pathological process necessitating surgery. The proportion is increased in the elderly and patients presenting for emergency surgery. The morbidity and mortality associated with surgery and anaesthesia are increased in patients with coexisting disease, and the more significant the coexisting disease the greater the risk (Buck et al 1987, Campling et al 1993). The medical diagnoses most commonly associated with increased surgical morbidity and mortality are:

- Ischaemic heart disease
- Congestive cardiac failure
- Arterial hypertension
- Chronic respiratory disease
- Diabetes mellitus (Greek *dia* = through + *bainein* = to go + *mellitus* = honeyed)
- Cardiac arrhythmias

- Anaemia
- Obesity.

You can see that pre-existing cardiac-related problems account for the most significant increase in operative risk.

The National Confidential Enquiry into Perioperative Deaths (NCEPOD) for 1990 (Campling et al 1992) emphasized the importance of discussion between surgeon and anaesthetist before a decision to proceed in a particular patient. All patients presenting for surgery should have a full clinical history and examination performed, including details of concurrent drug therapy, previous medical history and history of allergy. Depending on the nature of the coexisting medical disease and that of the planned surgery, additional specialized investigations may subsequently be needed. Young (< 45 years), fit patients undergoing minor elective surgery do not need routine blood haematology or chemistry, a chest X-ray or an electrocardiogram ECG).

The NCEPOD report for 1992–1993 (Campling et al 1995) identified a substantial shortfall in critical care services, and a failure to anticipate the need for these services. Furthermore, it emphasized that the skills of the surgeon and the anaesthetist should be appropriate for the medical condition of the patient. These professionals would not always be doctors of the same grade.

Who Operates When (Campling et al 1997), an NCEPOD report into timing of operations, found that the patients who died were for the most part elderly and in poor preoperative health (82% suffered from at least one coexisting disease, of which cardiorespiratory disease was the most common, followed by malignancy). Preoperative management was criticized as sometimes poor, and the rush to operate before adequate resuscitation contributed significantly to morbidity and mortality. Particular attention was drawn to the low use of intravenous fluids, infrequent use of objective cardiac assessment, and patchy application of thromboembolic prophylaxis.

The 2001 NCEPOD report *Changing the Way We Operate* noted that 95% of patients had coexisting medical problems at the time of the operation.

Aims of management

- To diagnose and determine the extent of pre-existing medical disease.
- To optimize the patient's medical condition before surgery.
- To ensure that specialized postoperative care facilities are available if required.

CARDIOVASCULAR DISEASE

Coronary artery disease

1. Coronary atherosclerosis is the commonest type of cardiovascular disease; NCEPOD has not previously been able separately to identify patients with either a previous myocardial infarction or ischaemic heart disease; for the first time, however, in 2001, NCEPOD identified that 60% of the patients had known ischaemic heart disease at the time of their final operation; an incidence higher than previously identified by national statistics.

2. Established major risk factors for coronary artery disease include: (1) age (male > 45 years, female > 55 years); (2) family history of early myocardial infarction; (3) current or treated hypertension; (4) smoking; (5) diabetes mellitus; and (6) low levels of high density lipoprotein (HDL) cholesterol.

3. High risk procedures (risk of perioperative cardiac morbidity and mortality > 5%) include major emergency operations, especially in the elderly, major vascular procedures including peripheral vascular, and prolonged surgery (> 3 h) with major fluid shifts.

4. In 1996, the American College of Cardiology and the American Heart Association issued joint guidelines for cardiovascular assessment for non-cardiac surgery (ACC/AHA Task Force Report 1996). These utilize a preliminary screening step followed by further investigation where necessary.

5. Assess the degree of activity that precipitates symptoms of myocardial ischaemia and note the presence or absence of congestive heart failure (does the patient also become breathless on exertion?). Enquire about a history of arrhythmias (palpitations) and presence of a pacemaker. Determine blood pressure, height of jugular venous pressure (JVP), cardiac murmurs, lung crepitations, dyspnoea and evidence of peripheral vascular disease.

6. The most important routine test is the electrocardiogram (ECG). Remember that the preoperative ECG is normal in 20–50% of patients with proven ischaemia. The ECG is a poor predictor of perioperative cardiac morbidity. However, features shown to be associated with increased risk include: rhythm other than sinus, atrial fibrillation, Q waves or left ventricular hypertrophy (LVH), and ventricular premature beats, all detectable on electrocardiography.

Key points

You should now be able to identify three broad groups of patients:

- **High risk patients such as those with unstable coronary syndromes, or decompensated congestive cardiac failure (CCF): delay elective surgery, consult a cardiologist.**
- **Intermediate risk patients: proceed with non-vascular surgery, possibly with the addition of a beta blocker. Further evaluate for vascular surgery.**
- **Low risk patients: proceed with surgery.**

7. The basis of management depends on the fact that myocardial ischaemia will occur whenever the balance between myocardial oxygen supply and demand is disturbed, such that demand exceeds supply. The major determinants of myocardial oxygen supply are the coronary perfusion pressure (the aortic diastolic pressure minus the left ventricular end-diastolic pressure) and diastolic time.

8. The major determinants of myocardial oxygen demand are increasing heart rate, increasing inotropic state, afterload, which is the impedance to left ventricular ejection (the systemic arterial pressure is an approximate determinant of afterload), and preload, which is the left ventricular end-diastolic pressure.

9. In the perioperative period avoid factors that decrease supply and/or increase demand. Encourage smokers to stop for at least 12 h before surgery. Almost without exception, continue concurrent drug therapy until the time of surgery. Short term beta blockade may improve survival after discharge from hospital, although, in the study by Mangano et al (1996), atenolol was given under close monitoring and it may not be appropriate simply to adapt this as an oral premedication to be given on the ward. It can be seen that an increase in heart rate and an increase in preload is especially deleterious as they increase myocardial oxygen demand and decrease myocardial oxygen supply. During the perioperative period do not allow a decrease in systemic arterial pressure to a significant degree (a decrease in diastolic pressure greater than 20% of the patient's normal resting diastolic pressure is a useful guide) because this decreases coronary perfusion pressure, which is very poorly tolerated in patients with multiple sites of coronary artery narrowing. Ensure that pain management is effective

postoperatively, as the presence of pain leads to hypertension and tachycardia. If necessary, refer the patient to the hospital's acute pain team. In addition, after major surgery, especially intra-abdominal or intrathoracic, administer supplemental oxygen for 24 h. Consider providing supplemental oxygen overnight for the first four postoperative days.

10.   While myocardial ischaemia is commonest over the first three postoperative days, myocardial infarction tends to occur on the day of surgery or on the first postoperative day; therefore, institute invasive monitoring for the first 24–36 h postoperatively.

Key points

- **Coronary artery disease is the commonest cardiac disease; it is associated with the majority of perioperative mortality and morbidity.**
- **Early postoperative ischaemia is a much stronger predictor of morbidity and mortality than any identifiable preoperative factors.**
- **Acute cardiac failure and unstable angina pose unacceptably high perioperative risks; treat it prior to elective non-cardiac surgery.**

Arterial hypertension

1.   Moderate or marked, longstanding, untreated hypertension increases perioperative morbidity and mortality, and is a significant risk factor for the production of coronary atherosclerosis. Stabilize patients with sustained systemic arterial hypertension (systolic > 160 mmHg, diastolic > 110 mmHg) on antihypertensive therapy before proceeding with long duration elective surgery.

2.   Untreated or inadequately treated hypertensives respond in an exaggerated manner to the stress of surgery, with a resultant increase in operative morbidity and mortality. Assume that patients with longstanding moderate to marked hypertension have coronary atherosclerosis and manage them appropriately, even in the absence of overt signs and/or symptoms of ischaemic heart disease.

3.   Antihypertensive therapy is associated with its own unique considerations for anaesthetic and surgical management, the specific issues depending upon the medication the patient is taking (see Concurrent drug therapy, p. 80).

Heart failure

1.   This implies an inadequacy of heart muscle secondary to intrinsic disease or overloading. The latter may

be due to an increase in volume (an increase in intravascular volume or valve incompetence), or pressure (systemic arterial hypertension or aortic stenosis). It is usual for one ventricle to fail before the other, but disorders that damage or overload the left ventricle are more common (e.g. ischaemic heart disease and systemic arterial hypertension), and hence symptoms attributable to pulmonary congestion are usually the presenting ones.

2.   Left ventricular failure is the most common cause of right ventricular failure and, if this supervenes, dyspnoea may actually decrease as right ventricular output decreases, leading to a reduction in pulmonary congestion. Conventionally, congestive heart failure refers to the combination of left and right ventricular failure with evidence of (and symptoms relating to) systemic and pulmonary venous hypertension. Physiologically, heart failure may be thought of as the failure of the heart to match its output in order to meet the body's metabolic needs. Treatment is aimed at normalizing this imbalance. Thus, cardiac output can be improved or metabolic needs decreased. Traditionally, digitalis glycosides have been thought of as mediating their beneficial effects by improving cardiac output. Their use is now superseded by angiotensin converting enzyme (ACE) inhibitors, often combined with diuretics. Vasodilators can also be used to decrease peripheral demand. Digitalization is indicated in patients with atrial fibrillation or flutter.

Key points

- **Manage symptomatic heart failure by optimum medical therapy preoperatively in all but the direst of surgical emergencies.**
- **Surgery in the presence of decompensated heart failure is associated with a high mortality.**

3. The operative mortality and morbidity of patients with well-compensated heart failure is small. After operation admit the patient to a high dependency unit or an intensive care facility with the ability to measure and adjust preload, afterload and cardiac output. A principal recommendation of the 2001 NCEPOD report was that nurses and doctors on the wards need to improve their proficiency in interpreting and managing central venous pressure (CVP). Ward equipment must include facilities for transducer pressure monitoring, to allow accurate and continuous CVP monitoring.

Congenital heart disease

1.   Congenital anomalies of the heart and cardiovascular system occur in 7–10 per 1000 live births (0.7–1%). It is

the commonest form of congenital disease and accounts for approximately 30% of the total burden of congenital disease. In affected children 10–15% have associated anomalies of the skeletal, genitourinary or gastrointestinal system. Nine lesions comprise more than 80% of congenital heart disease; of these, ventricular septal defect is by far the most frequent at 35%. Approximately 10–15% of patients with congenital heart disease may survive untreated to adulthood but the majority require some form of cardiac surgery as children.

2. A large cohort of patients with treated congenital heart disease is now surviving into adult life. Although these patients have traditionally returned to paediatric cardiac surgery centres for non-cardiac surgery as adults, this is not always possible. If the patient has been lost to cardiac follow-up, request a new cardiological opinion.

Key points

- **Adults with congenital heart disease form a very high risk group, often with multiple anatomical and pathophysiological abnormalities.**
- **Fully assess them preoperatively and request perioperative care from experts familiar with these problems.**

3. It is not possible to review the subject comprehensively here; read the article by Findlow et al (see Further reading). In summary, the problems fall into four groups: arrhythmias, shunts (volume and direction), pulmonary disease and hypertension, and ventricular dysfunction. Patients with Eisenmenger's syndrome (right-to-left shunt due to pulmonary hypertension) are very high risk patients. As well as circulatory failure, they run the risk of air embolism during surgery, postoperative deep vein thrombosis (DVT) and infective endocarditis. Give antibiotic prophylaxis to all patients with congenital heart disease, and take care to avoid air in the tubing during the siting of intravenous lines.

Acquired valvular heart disease

Mitral stenosis

This is nearly always of rheumatic origin, but symptoms do not appear until the valve area is reduced to less than 2.5 cm², i.e. half the normal valve area. This may take 20 years following the episode of rheumatic fever. As valve area decreases below 2 cm², an increase in left atrial pressure is required at rest to maintain cardiac output. A valve area below 1 cm² is classified as severe mitral stenosis and is associated with a left atrial pressure in excess of

20 mmHg, and even at rest cardiac output may be barely adequate; there is pulmonary hypertension. Eventually right ventricular failure supervenes and atrial fibrillation is common. Patients with mild to moderate mitral stenosis and sinus rhythm tolerate surgery well. All patients should receive antibiotic prophylaxis. Fluid balance should be carefully monitored, as overtransfusion may precipitate pulmonary oedema, whereas undertransfusion will compromise left ventricular filling. Similarly, changes in heart rate are poorly tolerated, and during surgery the anaesthetist will use a technique which minimizes changes in cardiac parameters. If major surgery is to be undertaken, with the possibility of large blood loss, consideration should be given to monitoring pulmonary capillary wedge pressure by means of a balloon-tipped flow-directed catheter. Unless the patient is taking oral anticoagulants, a local anaesthetic technique may be used for surgery, but a high spinal or epidural block may be associated with adverse cardiovascular effects (systemic arterial hypotension) and should be employed with caution.

Patients who are dyspnoeic at rest and have a fixed and reduced cardiac output present a significant risk during surgery. Digoxin should be continued up until the time of operation and plasma electrolytes checked, as hypokalaemia will increase the incidence of cardiac rhythm disturbances. These patients may have to be ventilated electively postoperatively.

Aortic stenosis

Valvular aortic stenosis is commonest in elderly males, although it may occur at any time of life. The presence of any of the following significantly increases the likelihood of aortic stenosis: effort syncope, slow rise of the carotid pulse, late systolic murmur with radiation to the right carotid and absent second heart sound. The aetiology is diverse and includes congenital, rheumatic, senile and mixed forms. It must be remembered that it is most common in patients in whom the incidence of ischaemic heart disease is also high. Severe aortic stenosis is associated with an increased perioperative morbidity and mortality. These patients may be asymptomatic even with a large (> 80 mmHg) gradient across the valve, if the left ventricle has not failed. A preoperative echo and cardiac assessment is essential to determine the gradient, as the risk of surgery can be predicted from this. The 1994–1995 NCEPOD report made the specific recommendation that any patient with an ejection systolic murmur in association with evidence of left ventricular hypertrophy or myocardial ischaemia requires referral to a cardiologist preoperatively for assessment of the aortic valve (Gallimore et al 1997). Systemic arterial hypotension must be avoided at all times because it will compromise coronary perfusion. Thus, peripheral vasodilatation, hypovolaemia and myocardial depression are all poorly tolerated. A change in cardiac rhythm is also poorly tolerated, as the atrial component to ventricular filling is essential to maintain normal cardiac output. For major procedures it is advisable to monitor left ventricular filling pressure, as higher than normal filling pressures are needed to maintain cardiac output.

Cardiomyopathies

Using echocardiography, three principal forms of cardiomyopathy are described.

1. Congestive or dilated cardiomyopathy: this may be associated with toxic, metabolic, neurological and inflammatory diseases. There is decrease in contractile force of the left or right ventricle, resulting in heart failure.

2. Hypertrophic or obstructive cardiomyopathy: this is an autosomal dominantly inherited condition in which there is hypertrophy and fibrosis; it mainly affects the interventricular septum but may involve the whole of the left ventricle.

3. Restrictive cardiomyopathy: this is a rare form of cardiomyopathy and the main feature is the loss of ventricular distensibility due to endocardial or myocardial disease. Restrictive cardiomyopathy in many ways resembles constrictive pericarditis, and the endocardial disease may produce thromboembolic problems.

Table 6.1 summarizes the treatment and management of these patients.

Disturbances of cardiac rhythm

Atrial fibrillation

This is the most commonly encountered disturbance of cardiac rhythm and it is important to define the disease processes causing the fibrillation. These are: ischaemic heart disease, rheumatic heart disease (especially mitral stenosis), pulmonary embolism, bronchial carcinoma, thyrotoxicosis, thoracotomy, alcoholism.

If there appears to be no underlying cause, the rhythm disturbance is usually termed 'lone atrial fibrillation'. The atrial discharge rate is usually between 400 and 600 impulses per minute, but the atrioventricular (AV) node cannot conduct all these impulses, so that some fail to reach the ventricle or only partially penetrate the node, and this results in a block or delay to succeeding impulses. Ventricular response is therefore irregular, but seldom more than 200 impulses per minute; the use of drugs or the presence of disease of the AV node often causes the response rate to be lower than this. The medical management of patients with atrial fibrillation must include the management of the underlying cause of the rhythm disturbance. It is important to ensure that the fibrillation is well controlled, i.e. that the response rate of the ventricle is not too rapid. Digitalis alkaloids remain the primary method of slowing AV nodal conduction, but if these fail to control the response rate, amiodarone is usually effective. Occasionally, cardioversion will restore sinus rhythm if the atrial fibrillation is of recent onset. Anticoagulate the patient prior to this.

Atrial flutter

The causes of this disturbance of cardiac rhythm are similar to those of atrial fibrillation, and the perioperative considerations are principally those of the underlying disease process. Atrial flutter is less commonly seen than atrial fibrillation. Although control of ventricular rate is more difficult in flutter, unlike fibrillation cardioversion is often successful. Anticoagulate the patient with warfarin prior to cardioversion. Second line therapy includes flecainide or digoxin. A bolus of adenosine may be used to aid in the differential diagnosis of atrial flutter versus paroxysmal supraventricular tachycardia (SVT).

Table 6.1 Cardiomyopathies: diagnosis and treatment			
	Congestive (dilated)	Hypertrophic (obstructive)	Restrictive
Presenting signs/symptoms	Heart failure Rhythm disturbance Systemic emboli	Syncope Dyspnoea Angina Rhythm disturbance Systolic murmur appearing during longstanding hypertension	Heart failure Eosinophilia
Treatment	Diuretics Vasodilators Antiarrhythmics Anticoagulants	Antiarrhythmics β-Adrenergic antagonists Anticoagulants	Steroids Cytotoxic agents

Heart block

There are two basic types of heart block: atrioventricular heart block and intraventricular conduction defects.

Atrioventricular heart block. This may be incomplete (first- or second-degree AV block) or complete (third-degree AV block). In first-degree heart block the PR interval of the ECG exceeds 0.21 s, but there are no dropped beats and the QRS complex is normal. It does not always imply significant underlying heart disease, but is seen in patients on digitalis therapy. Do not expose the patient to any drug in the perioperative period which will further decrease AV nodal conduction (e.g. halothane anaesthesia, β-adrenergic antagonists or verapamil).

There are two types of second-degree heart block: Mobitz types 1 and 2. Mobitz type 1 block is also known as the 'Wenckebach phenomenon' and this is usually associated with ischaemia of the AV node or the effects of digitalis. There is progressive increase in the length of the PR interval until the impulse fails to excite the ventricle and a beat is dropped. As a generalization, patients with this type of heart block do not require a pacemaker prior to surgery, and should it be necessary the administration of atropine will often establish normal AV conduction. Mobitz type 2 block is less common than type 1; it is a more serious form of conduction defect and may be a forerunner to complete AV block. The atrial rate is normal and the ventricular rate depends on the number of dropped beats, but it is commonly 35–50 beats per minute. The net result is that of an irregular pulse. The ECG indicates that there are more P waves than QRS complexes, but the PR interval, if present, is normal. It is probably acceptable to undertake minor surgery in patients with Mobitz type 2 block without the need for the insertion of a prophylactic pacemaker. However, in these circumstances ensure that you have immediately available drugs such as atropine and isoprenaline, and also the means for temporary pacing. Prophylactic pacemaker insertion is indicated for major surgery, especially if this is likely to result in significant blood loss and associated haemodynamic instability.

Third-degree heart block is also termed 'complete heart block'. It may result from conduction defects located within the AV node, bundle of His, or the bundle branch and Purkinje fibres. An escape pacemaker emerges at a site distal to the block (e.g. if the impulses are blocked within the AV node, the bundle of His usually emerges as the subsidiary pacemaker). In general, the more distal the site of the escape pacemaker, the more likely is the patient to suffer symptoms such as dyspnoea, syncope or congestive heart failure and to need permanent ventricular pacemaker therapy. Pacemaker therapy is always indicated before surgery, although in emergency situations (such as complete heart block appearing intraoperatively) various drugs may be tried to increase the heart rate. Atropine may be of value if the escape pacemaker is junctional. Isoprenaline may be of value if the escape pacemaker is more distal. A pacing Swann–Ganz catheter or a transoesophageal pacemaker can be inserted in an emergency and may be easier to place than a temporary wire.

Intraventricular conduction defects. Left bundle branch block is always associated with heart disease. The QRS complex is wide (>0.12 s). A hemiblock occurs if only one of the two major subdivisions (anterior and posterior) of the left bundle is blocked. The QRS complex is not prolonged in left hemiblocks. Left anterior or posterior hemiblock may occur with right bundle branch block and it is generally considered that left anterior plus right bundle branch block is not an indication for temporary pacemaker therapy before surgery, but that left posterior plus right bundle branch block is an indication for a pacemaker. The latter patients are at risk of developing complete heart block. Right bundle branch block is not invariably associated with underlying heart disease. The principal significance lies in its association with a left posterior hemiblock, as there is then a risk of complete heart block; in these patients a temporary pacemaker is indicated before surgery and anaesthesia.

Pacemakers

The patient with a pacemaker can safely undergo surgery and anaesthesia, but review the medical condition that gave rise to the need for pacemaker therapy. The usual indications for a pacemaker are congenital or acquired complete heart block, sick sinus syndrome and bradycardia, associated with syncope and/or hypotension.

Acquired complete heart block is probably the commonest indication, the underlying cause for this usually being ischaemic heart disease. Specifically ask the patient about the return of symptoms such as syncope, which may indicate that the pacemaker is failing to capture the ventricle (or atria if an atrial pacemaker is present). The heart rate should be within a couple of beats per minute of the pacemaker's original setting. It is important to determine the type of pacemaker that has been implanted and the time when it was put in.

All patients with pacemakers are normally reviewed regularly in a pacemaker clinic.

 Key points

- **Whenever a pacemaker is in situ, have atropine, adrenaline (epinephrine) and isoprenaline available for use in the event of pacemaker failure.**

- During surgery, diathermy is usually safe, but place the indifferent electrode as far from the pacemaker as possible, on the side of operation, in 1–2 s bursts more than 10 s apart (Simon 1977).
- Have the anaesthetist ensure that diathermy has not inhibited the pacemaker function, by checking the pulse (Aitkenhead & Barnett 1989)

RESPIRATORY DISEASE

Asthma

Patients with asthma have bronchospasm, mucus plugging of airways and air trapping. These result in a mismatch of ventilation and perfusion and total effective ventilation may be severely impaired. A number of exogenous and endogenous stimuli may produce reversible airway obstruction. The most active chemical mediators are histamine and the leukotrienes. Expiration is prolonged, functional residual capacity and residual volumes are increased and vital capacity is decreased. Bronchospasm may be aggravated by anxiety, by instrumentation of the upper airway, by foreign material or irritants in the upper airway, by pain, and by drugs. The latter include morphine, papaveretum, unselective β-adrenergic antagonists, and various anaesthetic drugs including tubocurarine and anticholinesterases. In taking the clinical history, pay special attention to factors which precipitate an attack, and review the patient's normal drug therapy. If possible, arrange the timing of surgery to coincide with a period of remission of symptoms. Continue the patient's normal bronchodilator therapy up until the time of surgery, and consider ordering preoperative chest physiotherapy. Allay preoperative anxiety, and prescribe suitable premedication – diazepam, pethidine, promethazine and atropine are free from bronchospastic activity. If the patient is taking steroid therapy, you may need to give additional doses during the perioperative period (see Concurrent drug therapy, p. 80). In the postoperative period, pay careful attention to pain management and give nebulized or intravenous bronchodilators if necessary. In appropriate cases consider using local anaesthetic techniques in severe asthmatics. Postoperative analgesia can be achieved with, if necessary, epidural blocks.

 Indications for intermittent positive pressure ventilation in asthmatics

- If the patient is distressed and exhausted.
- In the presence of systemic arterial hypotension or significant disturbance of cardiac rhythm.

- If the arterial oxygen tension is less than 6.7 kPa or arterial carbon dioxide tension is greater than 6.7 kPa, associated with an increasing metabolic acidosis in the face of maximum medical therapy.

Chronic bronchitis and emphysema

1. Patients who have a cough with sputum production on most days for 3 months of the year for at least 2 years have chronic bronchitis. They are often smokers (see below), and have irritable airways leading to coughing and some degree of reversible airways obstruction in response to minimal stimulation.

2. Patients with destruction of alveoli distal to the terminal bronchioles and loss of pulmonary elastic tissue have emphysema. They experience airway closure with air trapping and, therefore, inefficient gaseous exchange.

3. Chronic bronchitis and emphysema commonly coexist in the same patient. Many of the considerations in the perioperative period that apply to the asthmatic patient also apply to patients with chronic bronchitis and emphysema; there are, however, some additional points to note. These diseases are usually slowly progressive and may eventually result in a respiratory reserve which is so low that the patient is immobile and dyspnoeic at rest, and even speaking and eating may be difficult. Arrange elective surgery during the months in which symptoms are least noticeable – usually during the summer. Make every effort to persuade smokers to quit their habit. If the patient requires major surgery, and if the disease is severe, consider performing elective tracheostomy and arranging postoperative ventilation. These will facilitate the clearing of secretions, and thus gaseous exchange, during the postoperative period when diaphragmatic splinting and pain or respiratory depression may cause acute respiratory insufficiency.

4. Smokers have about six times the incidence of postoperative respiratory complications compared with nonsmokers. Cigarette smoking has wide-ranging effects on the cardiorespiratory and immune systems and on haemostasis (Jones 1985). They may have arterial carbon monoxide concentrations in excess of 5%; the resultant carboxyhaemoglobin decreases the amount of haemoglobin available for combination with oxygen, and inhibits the ability of haemoglobin to give up oxygen (i.e. the oxygen dissociation curve is shifted to the left). Carbon monoxide also has a negative inotropic effect. Nicotine increases heart rate and systemic arterial blood pressure. Thus, carbon monoxide decreases oxygen supply, while nicotine increases oxygen demand, and this is of particular significance in patients with ischaemic heart disease. It is especially important that these patients stop smoking for 12–24 h before surgery; this results in a significant

improvement in cardiovascular function (the elimination half-lives of carbon monoxide and nicotine are a few hours).

However, the respiratory effect of smoking, especially mucus hypersecretion, impairment of tracheobronchial clearance and small airway narrowing take at least 6 weeks before there is any improvement in function after smoking cessation. Similarly, the effects of smoking on immune function (smokers are more susceptible to post-operative infections) require at least 6 weeks before improvement occurs. Many smokers complain that they find it difficult to clear their mucus if they stop smoking, and use this as an excuse not to stop smoking before surgery; there may be some substance to this claim, but it does not outweigh the benefits of stopping. Emphasize the risks of smoking to smokers, and encourage them to stop smoking for as long as possible before elective surgery.

Key points

- **Arrange elective surgery on patients with chronic bronchitis and emphysema at times of the year when symptoms are minimal.**
- **In an emergency, encourage smokers to stop smoking for 12–24 h preoperatively, especially if they also have ischaemic heart disease.**
- **Before elective surgery encourage smokers to stop for as long as possible before operation.**

ENDOCRINE DYSFUNCTION

Thyroid gland

Excluding diabetes, disorders involving the thyroid gland account for about 80% of endocrine disease. There are two practical issues for you and the anaesthetist:

1. Firstly, there are problems related to the local effects of a mass in the neck. These include airway problems and the potential for difficult tracheal intubation.

2. Secondly, there are problems associated with the generalized effects of an excess or deficiency of hormone. Before surgery, prepare and render euthyroid patients with hyperthyroidism, to avoid problems. Propylthiouracil (average daily dose 300 mg) inhibits hormone synthesis and blocks the peripheral conversion of thyroxine to tri-iodothyronine. As a generalization, the larger the gland the longer it takes to achieve the euthyroid state. The vascularity of the gland can be con-siderably decreased by 7 days treatment with potassium iodide solution. Propranolol is an alternative treatment to thiouracil: 60–120 mg daily for 2 weeks may be the

only treatment required, and is now routinely used at many centres.

3. Avoid, if possible, an emergency operation in a poorly or non-prepared patient because it carries signifi-cant risk. Cardiovascular complications are potentially life-threatening so consider giving intravenous esmolol before induction of anaesthesia (using increments every 5 min to decrease the resting heart rate by 10 beats per minute). Disturbances of cardiac rhythm, hypoxia and hyperthermia may all occur. If appropriate, choose a local anaesthetic technique.

4. Hypothyroidism is not uncommon, especially in elderly patients. Cardiac output is low and blood loss is poorly tolerated; however, you must give blood transfu-sion with caution to avoid overloading the circulation. It has been said that in hypothyroidism the respiratory centre is less responsive to hypoxia and hypercarbia, so that it may be necessary to ventilate patients electively in the postoperative period. These patients are especially sensitive to opioid analgesics so use them with caution in the perioperative period. Monitor the patient's tempera-ture and prevent hypothermia, as this will aggravate the circulatory and respiratory depression.

Key point

- **Beware the potential complications of missing, and therefore failing to anticipate, complications of hyperthyroidism and hypothyroidism.**

Pituitary gland

1. In hypopituitarism, the varying involvement of the several hormones which the anterior pituitary produces leads to a variety of clinical presentations: amenorrhoea in females and impotence in males are common present-ing features. If hypopituitarism is unrecognized, there is a greatly increased perioperative risk of hypoglycaemia, hypothermia, water intoxication and respiratory failure. If the diagnosis is known, planned substitution therapy is indicated before surgery. Oral hydrocortisone (15 mg twice daily) is administered. This is increased during the operative period; thyroxine is also given and the dose slowly increased to about 0.15 mg daily and the plasma thyroxine level is measured.

2. Acromegaly is caused by excessive production of pituitary growth hormone. This results in overgrowth of bone, leading to an enlarged jaw and kyphoscoliosis, as well as connective tissue and viscera. There is cardiomegaly, early atherosclerosis and systemic arterial hypertension, and diabetes mellitus is common.

Management should include consideration of all associated conditions and the anaesthetist will carefully assess the patient, as tracheal intubation may be difficult.

3. Diabetes insipidus (Latin *in* = not + *sapere* = to taste; hence tasteless as opposed to diabetes mellitus = honeyed) is the result of deficiency of antidiuretic hormone. A water deprivation test is used to differentiate diabetes insipidus from compulsive water drinking, and measurements are made of urine and plasma osmolality. When the plasma osmolality reaches about 295 mOsmol kg^{-1} normal patients will concentrate their urine, but patients with diabetes insipidus cannot do so. If the syndrome is differentiated from compulsive water drinking, the operative management of these patients is usually uncomplicated. The patient should receive a bolus of 100 milliunits of vasopressin intravenously before surgery, and during the operation 100 milliunit h^{-1} are administered by continuous infusion. Isotonic solutions, such as 0.9% sodium chloride, may then be administered with minimal risk of water depletion or hypernatraemia. Plasma osmolality should be monitored perioperatively (the normal range is 283–285 mOsmol kg^{-1}).

Adrenal gland

Adrenocorticol insufficiency is known as Addison's disease. It may present in acute and chronic forms and may be due to disease of the gland itself or to disorders of the anterior pituitary or hypothalamus. A patient with adrenocortical insufficiency undergoing surgery presents a major problem. The cardiovascular status of the patient and the blood glucose and electrolytes must be measured. The patient is prepared by infusing isotonic sodium chloride and glucose solutions in order to correct hypernatraemia and hypoglycaemia. The day before surgery, an intramuscular injection of 40 mg methylprednisolone is administered. Before induction of anaesthesia a further 100 mg hydrocortisone is administered, and for major surgery an infusion of hydrocortisone should be given during the operation. Hydrocortisone has approximately equal glucocorticoid and mineralocorticoid effects. Postoperatively, the dose of hydrocortisone is decreased from 100 mg twice daily to a replacement dose of about 50 mg daily.

Adrenocortical hyperfunction is commonly iatrogenic. Whatever the aetiology, these patients will have glucose intolerance manifest as hyperglycaemia or frank diabetes mellitus, systemic arterial hypertension (possibly associated with heart failure) and electrolyte disturbances, especially hypokalaemia and hypernatraemia. Protein breakdown leads to muscle weakness and osteoporosis. Muscle weakness will be aggravated by obesity, and respiratory function should be carefully assessed before surgery, as well as postoperatively. Osteoporosis may lead to vertebral compression fractures and patients should be positioned with great care during surgery. Prolonged immobilization after surgery will lead to further demineralization of bone, and hypercalcaemia may lead to the formation of renal calculi. Vitamin D therapy may therefore be needed in the postoperative period.

Aldosteronism may be primary (an adrenocortical adenoma – Conn's syndrome), or secondary, in which the condition is associated with an increase of plasma renin secretion (e.g. the nephrotic syndrome and cardiac failure). Patients will have hypokalaemia and hypernatraemia, which may be associated with systemic arterial hypertension. If the diagnosis is made before surgery, the administration of spironolactone (up to 300 mg daily) will reverse hypertension and hypokalaemia.

Phaeochromocytoma

These catecholamine-secreting tumours may produce sustained or intermittent arterial hypertension. During surgery, arterial hypertension and disturbances of cardiac rhythm are common, due to the release of adrenaline (epinephrine) and noradrenaline (norepinephrine) into the circulation. Prolonged secretion of these produces not only arterial hypertension but also a contracted blood volume; α- and β-adrenergic blockade will help to reverse both these effects.

Preoperative α-adrenergic blockade must not be complete because:

- It may cause preoperative postural syncope.
- It may cause difficulties in controlling the profound hypotension that sometimes occurs after tumour removal.
- A rise in systemic blood pressure on tumour palpation is a useful sign in searching for small tumours or metastases.

Phenoxybenzamine is the agent usually used to induce partial α-adrenergic blockade. Careful preoperative preparation using α- and β-adrenergic blockade, as well as the introduction of anaesthetic techniques that promote cardiovascular stability, have greatly decreased the mortality of patients undergoing surgery for removal of a phaeochromocytoma, from 30–45% in the early 1950s to less than 5% recently.

Pancreas
Diabetes mellitus

Diabetes mellitus is a syndrome characterized by hyperglycaemia due to insulin deficiency, impaired insulin action or a combination of both. It may be primary (most cases) or secondary diabetes associated with other medical problems, such as pancreatitis or steroid treatment. Primary diabetes mellitus is subdivided into type 1 diabetes, characterized by absolute insulin deficiency (formerly insulin-dependent diabetes mellitus, IDDM) and type 2 characterized by insulin resistance and relative insulin deficiency (formerly non-insulin-dependent diabetes mellitus, NIDDM). Type 1, which is due to autoimmune destruction of pancreatic islet β cells, is treated with insulin, whereas type 2 diabetes (whose pathogenesis is less well understood) may be managed by diet and oral agents, although many patients will eventually require insulin for optimal management. Most insulin now used is bioengineered human sequence insulin. Recently the first two artificial insulin analogues, lispro and insulin aspart, have been introduced to clinical practice. These have been developed by amino acid substitution in the insulin sequence in order to create an insulin which is absorbed more rapidly after subcutaneous administration, giving a faster onset and shorter duration of action.

Sulphonylureas and metformin remain the main oral hypoglycaemic drugs used in the UK and are safe and effective. Two other types of oral agent have recently become available for the treatment of type 2 diabetes. Acarbose reduces the breakdown of complex carbohydrates in the gut and reduces postprandial blood glucose levels; however, many patients experience excess flatulence, which limits its acceptability. The thiazolinediones are a new group of drugs that improve insulin sensitivity. Troglitazone was withdrawn after reports of severe hepatic toxicity but two further drugs, rosiglitazone and pioglitazone, have since been introduced. These appear to be effective when used in combination with either a sulphonylurea or metformin.

The chronic complications of diabetes include large vessel disease, microvascular disease, coronary heart disease and neuropathy. Despite advances in management, diabetes is the single greatest cause of end-stage renal failure requiring replacement therapy. In addition to coronary heart disease there is a high incidence of asymptomatic myocardial ischaemia. Clinically significant silent coronary artery disease has been found in 20% of middle-aged men with type 2 diabetes screened by exercise testing. The prognosis of myocardial infarction is considerably worse in diabetic patients, with higher early and late mortality and a greater incidence of left ventricular failure after infarction. Abnormalities of peripheral or autonomic nerve function can be found in most patients with diabetes of long duration. The most common is a classical symmetrical sensory neuropathy which affects the feet and legs and can predispose the patient to the risks of pressure ulceration. Autonomic dysfunction is relatively rare and symptoms usually relate to postural hypotension. Before surgery, the cardiovascular status of the patient should be carefully reviewed and the blood pressure taken both supine and erect to test for the possibility of autonomic neuropathy. An association between sleep apnoea and autonomic neuropathy has been documented and respiratory arrests have been observed following surgery and the use of sedative drugs. Patients with symptomatic autonomic neuropathy should therefore be considered to be at increased risk following anaesthesia, and appropriate steps taken to monitor respiratory function.

Table 6.2 summarizes the regimens suitable for minor and more major surgery in diabetics patients who are either controlled by diet alone, by oral hypoglycaemic agents, or with insulin.

Chlorpropamide is a sulphonylurea with a very long duration of action, and hypoglycaemia is a particular concern in patients taking this agent; it should be stopped 48 h before planned surgery and the blood sugar measured regularly after the patient becomes nil by mouth.

Table 6.2 Severity of diabetes		
	Type of surgery	
	Minor	Intermediate/major
Controlled by diet	No specific precautions	Measure blood glucose 4-hourly: if >12 mmol l^{-1} start glucose-potassium-insulin sliding scale regimen
Controlled by oral agents	Omit medication on morning of operation and start when eating normally postoperatively	Omit medication and monitor blood glucose 1–2 hourly; if >12 mmol l^{-1} start glucose–potassium–insulin sliding scale regimen
Controlled by insulin	Unless very minor procedure (omit insulin when nil by mouth) give glucose–potassium–insulin sliding scale regimen during surgery and until eating normally postoperatively	

Patients taking long-acting insulin preparations should be converted to Actrapid insulin, and surgery should be scheduled for the early morning if possible. A number of regimens for blood sugar control have been described, but the following is easy to use.

Infuse 10% glucose 500 ml + 10 mmol potassium chloride (KCl) at 100 ml h^{-1}. Prepare a 50 ml syringe containing 50 units of Actrapid (short-acting) insulin in 50 ml normal saline (= 1 unit ml^{-1}) and connect via a 3-way tap to a glucose infusion. Adjust the rate of the syringe driver according to the following sliding scale:

Blood glucose (mmol l^{-1})	Rate of syringe driver (ml h^{-1})
<5	Switch off
5–7	1
7–10	2
10–20	3
>20	4

If two successive blood glucose values are > 20 mmol l^{-1}, leave instructions to consult the duty doctor.

The blood sugar is measured at least 2-hourly during surgery and the amount of insulin adjusted to maintain the blood sugar between 6 and 12 mmol l^{-1}. Following surgery, blood sugar and plasma potassium are measured at least 4-hourly. Sepsis and high dose corticosteroid treatment markedly increase insulin requirements.

Postoperatively, as soon as the patient starts eating, those who are normally treated with oral hypoglycaemics may need subcutaneous insulin for a few days before oral therapy is recommended. Patients normally treated with insulin can be converted to Actrapid insulin to a total equal to the normal preoperative dose. After 3 days the original regimen can usually be restarted (i.e. using long-acting insulins). In the perioperative period lactate-containing fluids (e.g. Hartmann's solution) should be avoided in diabetics. If oral feeding has not started within 72 h of surgery, consideration should be given to the institution of parenteral nutrition.

Obesity

Life expectancy is decreased by obesity, and operative morbidity and mortality increase with increasing weight. In moderate obesity, the individual presenting for surgery should be instructed to decrease weight and be given dietary advice appropriate to the patient's social and economic circumstances. They should also be examined carefully for the presence of conditions with which obesity is commonly associated; these include diabetes mellitus and systemic arterial hypertension. Patients who are double or more their ideal weight are usually termed 'morbidly obese'. These patients present a number of problems to both surgeon and anaesthetist. Their preoperative cardiorespiratory status should be assessed carefully and, as

these patients are at an increased risk of inhalation of gastric contents, all should receive appropriate antacid therapy before surgery. Obesity is one of a number of conditions that will lead to an increase in postoperative deep vein thrombosis and associated thromboembolic phenomena; obese patients should receive appropriate preoperative prophylaxis for this. Transport and positioning of morbidly obese patients may cause difficulties, and occasionally two standard operating tables used side by side may be needed. Intravenous access may be difficult and non-invasive methods of monitoring arterial blood pressure may be inaccurate; therefore, an intra-arterial line is indicated for all but the most minor procedures. This will also enable arterial blood gases to be monitored in the intraoperative and postoperative periods. Patients may need continued ventilatory support after surgery.

BLOOD DISORDERS

Primary blood disorders produce a wide range of clinical manifestations, which may affect any organ in the body. Conversely, there are nearly always some changes in the blood accompanying general medical and surgical disorders. Thus, haematological investigations form an important part of the assessment and subsequent monitoring of most disease processes.

Anaemia

This is defined clinically as a reduction in haemoglobin level below the normal range for the individual's age and sex. It becomes clinically apparent when the oxygen demand of the tissues cannot be met without the use of compensatory mechanisms. The level of haemoglobin at which elective surgery should be postponed has been under review and many guidelines have been revised downwards. This is due to concern over the dangers of transmissible agents in blood which may not, as yet, be detectable. An acceptable level will depend on factors such as whether there is a known cause for the anaemia, the nature of surgery planned, and the physical fitness of the patient. A haemoglobin concentration of 8–10 g dl^{-1} may be adequate for minor surgery. It is important to realize that blood transfusion to raise the haematocrit should be carried out at least 48 h before the operative procedure, as this period of time will allow full recovery of the stored erythrocytes' oxygen-carrying capacity. In order to minimize the risk of transmitting the human immunodeficiency virus (HIV), blood transfusion should be undertaken only if the urgency of surgery necessitates this. Tissue oxygenation appears to be maximal at around a haemoglobin concentration of 11 g dl^{-1} (tissue oxygenation depends upon cardiac output, peripheral vascular resistance, blood viscosity and blood oxygen-carrying capacity). Patients with ischaemic heart disease are likely to suffer more from the consequences of decreased oxygen-carrying capacity from untreated anaemia, and it is especially important to treat preoperative anaemia in these patients.

Haemoglobinopathies

This term encompasses a range of different genetic conditions, which can be broadly divided into two groups: the structural variants and the thalassaemia syndromes. The thalassaemia syndromes are due to the abnormal production of one or more globin chain; there are several hundred variants, but they have no implications for anaesthetic or surgical practice. The main structural mutation with clinical significance is sickle haemoglobin. Haemoglobin S is an abnormality in the amino acid sequence of the haemoglobin. When a deoxygenated haemoglobin molecule becomes distorted, this may lead to capillary occlusion and tissue hypoxia. The disease is inherited and it may be in the heterozygous or homozygous form. The former (HbAS) does not usually cause problems during surgery, as the molecular distortion, known as 'sickling', only occurs at very low oxygen saturations. However, in the homozygous state (HbSS) there is a real risk of sickling during surgery and this may cause tissue infarction. Screening tests are available for the presence of haemoglobin S, and electrophoresis is used to determine the exact nature of the abnormality. During surgery it is important to avoid low oxygen tensions and thus an elevated inspired oxygen concentration is used, and the patient is kept warm and well hydrated in order to maintain cardiac output and avoid circulatory stasis. These patients are prone to dehydration because of renal papillary damage and the resultant passage of large volumes of dilute urine. If very major surgery is planned, where there is the possibility of perioperative hypoxia, for example pulmonary surgery, an exchange transfusion should be considered in an attempt to reduce the level of haemoglobin S to below 25%. Patients with haemoglobin C and haemoglobin SC should be managed in a similar way to those with haemoglobin SS.

Bleeding and coagulation disorders

As a generalization, purpura, epistaxis and prolonged bleeding from superficial cuts are suggestive of a platelet abnormality, and bleeding into joints or muscle is suggestive of a coagulation defect. Both forms may be congenital or acquired and it may be possible to differentiate these from the patient's history, a recent onset being indicative of an acquired disorder. A family history should be sought but it must be remembered that the absence of other relatives with a positive history does not exclude a hereditary bleeding diathesis (one-third of haemophilia patients show no family history). Many systemic diseases may be complicated by bleeding, as may treatment with a number of drugs which can cause bone marrow depression leading to thrombocytopenia.

Platelet disorders

Thrombocytopenia arises from a number of causes:

- Failure of megakaryocyte maturation
- Excessive platelet consumption
- Hypersplenism.

Bone marrow disorders leading to failure of maturation may be due to hypoplasia or infiltration. Increased consumption occurs in disseminated intravascular coagulation, idiopathic thrombocytopenic purpura and certain viral infections. Sequestration in an enlarged spleen occurs in lymphomas and liver disease. Spontaneous bleeding does not usually occur until the platelet count has decreased to $30 \times 10^9 \, l^{-1}$. Treatment has to be directed at the underlying disease, but thrombocytopenia resulting in clinically important bleeding necessitates a platelet transfusion. Ideally, the count should be increased to $100 \times 10^9 \, l^{-1}$, but transfusing platelets until a clinically acceptable effect is attained is often performed. Routine major surgery should not be undertaken in the presence of an abnormal platelet count until the result is confirmed and the cause identified.

Haemophilia

Before surgery in patients with haemophilia A or B, the concentration of the coagulation factors should be increased to a level that will minimize bleeding, and this concentration should be maintained until healing has occurred. It is important to seek specialist advice in determining the dosage of factors required. Cryoprecipitate and fresh frozen plasma or factor IX fraction are used to manage bleeding episodes, but the patients should be tested for antibodies to the products. If these are present, only life-saving operations should be contemplated. If cryoprecipitate or freeze-dried factor IX concentrate are administered, complications, including viral hepatitis and possibly prior transmission, may occur. Recombinant (genetically engineered) factor VIII and IX are now available and are the treatment of choice.

RENAL DISEASE

Chronic renal failure

This is said to be present when chronic renal impairment, from whatever cause, results in abnormalities of plasma biochemistry. Usually, this happens when the glomerular filtration rate (GFR) has fallen to less than 30 ml min^{-1}. Fluid balance is precarious in these patients; they may have a very limited ability to excrete water and/or sodium. Management before surgery depends on the severity of the renal failure. Moreover, in a situation of renal insufficiency, anaesthesia and surgery may precipitate acute renal failure. Patients in late and terminal degrees of chronic renal failure (GFR < 10 ml min^{-1}) may already have commenced on dialysis. If not, dialysis should be performed before surgery if at all possible. Dialysis does not reverse all the adverse effects of chronic renal failure; for example, systemic arterial hypertension and pericarditis may still be present. In addition, patients who are dialysed very soon before surgery may have cardiovascular lability during anaesthesia and surgery because they may have a relatively contracted blood volume. These patients are also vulnerable to infection, anaemia, blood coagulation defects, electrolyte disturbances and psychological problems. Systemic hypertension is a constant feature of chronic renal failure and arteriovenous shunts may cause a hyperdynamic circulation with a low systemic vascular resistance, predisposing the patient to myocardial ischaemia. These patients may depend on an increased minute ventilation to maintain respiratory compensation for their metabolic acidosis, and respiratory compromise postoperatively may exacerbate their poor metabolic condition. It is important to define the degree of renal failure present before surgery, and review the dialysis regimen. Blood biochemistry, coagulation and haemoglobin must be checked. Care should be taken when prescribing potentially nephrotoxic drugs and consideration given to pathways of drug elimination (see Concurrent drug therapy, p. 80). A careful search should be made for the presence of occult infection and all patients should have a preoperative chest X-ray. The susceptibility to infection is compounded in transplant patients by the administration of immunosuppressive drugs, and prophylactic antibiotics may be necessary preoperatively and postoperatively. Chest physiotherapy may also be needed. Procedures such as arterial or central venous cannulation must be carried out under strict aseptic conditions. Before, during and after surgery, fluid and electrolyte balance must be very carefully monitored.

Nephrotic syndrome

The clinical association of heavy proteinuria, hypoalbuminaemia and generalized oedema is usually referred to as the 'nephrotic syndrome'. The hypoalbuminaemia is the result of urinary albumin loss and the syndrome becomes apparent if more than 5 g of protein are lost per day, and the plasma albumin concentration falls to less than 30 g l^{-1}. It is important to define the underlying cause of the nephrotic syndrome. Before surgery, the plasma protein and electrolyte levels must be estimated and corrected as indicated. An albumin infusion (up to 50 g) will restore circulating blood volume and may in itself initiate a diuresis. An alteration in plasma proteins will cause changes in drug effect due to an alteration in drug binding. The anaesthetist may use more conservative doses of some drugs. Central venous cannulation is advisable for all but the most minor surgery.

LIVER DISEASE

Chronic liver disease is a continuum of pathophysiology, from the patient with an abnormality of liver function tests with no adverse physiological consequences to the patient with severe end-stage liver disease who represents an extreme surgical risk. Patients with liver disease were classified for general surgical risk by Child and Turcotte in 1964 (Table 6.3) and this is still valid today. The only important addition is the observation that prothrombin time is the most significant preoperative predictor of mortality in patients undergoing surgery for variceal bleeding.

A patient with moderate to severe cirrhosis has numerous pathophysiological changes affecting various organ systems and should always be managed by experienced personnel, both anaesthetic and surgical. Child and Turcotte grade C (even in the absence of coma) carries a very high perioperative mortality, even for elective surgery. Although it is impossible to review the pathophysiology of end-stage liver disease in this text, concise reviews are available (see Further reading).

Table 6.3 Child's classification for hepatic functional reserve			
	A (Minimal)	B (Moderate)	C (Advanced)
Serum bilirubin (mg dl^{-1})	<2.0	2.0–3.0	>3.0
Serum albumin (g dl^{-1})	>3.5	3.0–3.5	<3.0
Ascites controlled	None	Easily controlled	Poorly controlled
Neurological disorder	None	Minimal	Advanced 'coma'
Nutrition	Excellent	Good	Poor 'wasting'

Organ systems affected by cirrhosis

- **Cardiovascular system**
- **Lungs**
- **Kidneys**
- **Brain**
- **Gut**
- **Coagulation**
- **Immunocompetence.**

Prior to surgery the patient's condition must be optimized. All patients should be screened routinely for hepatitis B viral infection. They must be kept adequately hydrated to preserve renal function (although paradoxically they may be on diuretics to control ascites). Respiratory function may be poor due to basal atelectasis and/or intrapulmonary shunts. Ascitic drainage may improve the situation. If renal function deteriorates in the face of adequate filling, a low dose dopamine infusion should be started. These patients are prone to sepsis and spontaneous bacterial peritonitis so body fluids should be cultured and strict aseptic precautions adhered to. Finally their coagulation will be deranged. In patients with predominantly cholestatic disease this may improve with vitamin K injection. Patients with hepatocellular disease are likely to have a combination of clotting factor deficiencies, chronic fibrinolysis and a low platelet count. The situation is best assessed and treated using a dynamic measure of clotting – thromboelastography (Mallett & Cox 1992).

These patients often lose large amounts of blood at operation due to a combination of surgical (varices) and medical (coagulopathy) causes; in addition they have a very high cardiac output and low systemic vascular resistance circulation, which is often unresponsive to noradrenaline (norepinephrine). It cannot be overemphasized that these are very high risk patients to operate on.

NEUROLOGICAL DISEASE

Multiple sclerosis

The aetiology of this disease of temperate climates has become clearer in recent years. It appears that in genetically susceptible individuals activated T cells and macrophages responding to environmental triggers interact with type 1 astrocytes, causing a disruption of the blood–brain barrier and a leak of immune mediators into the nervous system. This causes demyelination. Patients may present for incidental surgery or surgery associated with alleviation of the complications, e.g. implantation of extradural stimulating electrodes. In order to decrease

perioperative morbidity, careful preoperative examination is needed. Patients may have a labile autonomic nervous system associated with postural hypotension. Muscle atrophy may lead to significant kyphoscoliosis and this may result in a restrictive form of pulmonary disease. Urinary tract infections commonly occur, but the patient must be carefully examined to identify other infective foci. An elevation in temperature is the one definite factor known to precipitate an exacerbation of the disease, so all but the most urgent surgery should be postponed until the patient is free from infection. Epilepsy is not uncommon in patients with multiple sclerosis.

Epilepsy

This term refers to a variety of types of recurrent seizure produced by paroxysmal neuronal discharge from various parts of the brain. Seizures may have a cerebral cause (e.g. tumour) or be due to a systemic disorder (e.g. uraemia or hypercalcaemia). The symptomatology is variable and seizures may cause total loss of consciousness or only a minimal alteration in awareness. The disease occurs in all age groups, with an incidence of about 1%. About 75% of patients have no recognizable underlying cause. If there is an underlying cause, the surgical management should take this into account. Otherwise management is usually uncomplicated; it is important that the patient's usual anticonvulsant medication be continued until the time of surgery and restarted as soon as possible postoperatively, if necessary using parenteral drug administration (see Concurrent drug therapy, p. 80). Anticonvulsant drugs such as phenytoin lead to induction of liver microsomal enzymes, and thus the patient's response to a variety of drugs that may be given during the perioperative period may be altered.

Myasthenia gravis

This is an autoimmune disease of the neuromuscular junction, involving the postjunctional acetylcholine receptors. Specific autoantibodies have been identified and microscopic changes in the membrane demonstrated. The disease is characterized by muscle weakness of fluctuating severity, most commonly affecting the ocular muscles. Facial and pharyngeal muscle weakness also occurs, leading to dysarthria and dysphagia. It can occur at any age in life but is most frequently seen in the fourth decade. There is an association with thymic enlargement and thymomas, both benign and malignant. About two-thirds of patients without a thymic tumour will improve after thymectomy, although the outlook is less good for patients with tumour, whether this is excised or not. Inhibitors of the enzyme cholinesterase (e.g. edrophonium, neostigmine and pyridostigmine) are used in the treatment of myasthenia gravis, as are drugs which suppress the immunological response and eliminate circulating antibodies. The latter have now become the first line of treatment, and 90% of patients will benefit from the use of azathioprine or steroids.

Patients may present for thymectomy or incidental surgery, and the surgical management depends upon the nature of the operation and severity of the disease. As usual, the patient's normal medication must be continued up until the time of surgery. If the disease is severe, or major thoracic or upper abdominal surgery is planned, elective postoperative ventilation is advisable and, occasionally, a tracheostomy will be required, but this should only be needed if ventilation is prolonged and excess secretions are a problem. Respiratory failure in myasthenic patients may be secondary to either a myasthenic or a cholinergic crisis. Assisted ventilation should be instituted and anticholinesterase drug therapy stopped, and then cautiously reintroduced after testing with small doses of intravenous edrophonium (2–5 mg). Elective postoperative ventilation may also be advisable for lesser forms of surgery, including thymectomy, if the patient's preoperative vital capacity is less than 2 litres or there is a history of intercurrent respiratory problems. Following surgery, the requirements for anticholinesterase and other drug therapy may be changed and it is important to titrate drug dosage against clinical response. It should be remembered that overtreatment can cause weakness, just as can undertreatment. Postoperatively, the adequacy of ventilation can best be assessed by repeated blood gas measurement and, therefore, before surgery there are advantages to the placement of an intraarterial line. This will also facilitate accurate cardiovascular monitoring during surgery.

ALCOHOLISM AND DRUG ABUSE

Addiction is characterized by psychological dependence, change in tolerance and a specific withdrawal syndrome. Drugs, including alcohol, are used by susceptible individuals in order to obtain oblivion or excitement. Aetiological factors include psychiatric illness, personality disorders and social pressures. It should be remembered that many addicts abuse more than one drug. In general, it is advisable to maintain normal doses of the addict's usual drug in the immediate pre- and postoperative periods. The perioperative period is not the best time to attempt to wean a patient from an addiction and it may only serve to precipitate an acute withdrawal reaction. Addicts may not admit to their addiction and the first sign that there is a problem may be the appearance of a withdrawal syndrome.

Specific organ damage may result from drug addiction. Alcohol gives rise to liver damage and can progress to cirrhosis, and thus a change in protein synthesis, altered glycogen storage and susceptibility to hypoglycaemia. In addition, alcoholics are prone to bleeding, especially from the gastrointestinal tract, and there may be hypomagnesaemia. They may also have cardiomyopathy, and careful assessment of cardiovascular status is necessary in the alcoholic patient. Solvent or glue sniffers may have hepatic or renal damage and bone marrow suppression. Addicts to opioids will often have used contaminated needles and syringes, and there is a high incidence of hepatitis and liver damage and also of infection with the HIV virus (see below). If sudden hypotension occurs in the operative or postoperative period in a narcotic addict, and if other obvious causes are excluded, this may respond to the administration of intravenous morphine.

PSYCHIATRIC DISEASE

Anxiety and concern are a normal reaction of patients to forthcoming surgery and anaesthesia. A significant proportion of the population will suffer from an affective disorder at some time in their lives. A depressive illness is the commonest affective disorder and treatment may involve psychotherapy, antidepressant drug therapy or, if the disorder is severe, electroconvulsive therapy. It is important that the patient's preoperative drug therapy is continued, although both tricyclic antidepressants and monoaminoxidase inhibitors significantly interact with the drugs used during anaesthesia (see Concurrent drug therapy, p. 80). Before surgery both a psychiatrist and an anaesthetist should be consulted. Many anaesthetists would prefer that the drugs be continued up until the time of surgery, and their anaesthetic technique modified to take account of the potential for drug interactions. It should not be forgotten that severe affective disorders are accompanied by a very significant mortality rate in terms of suicide, and supportive drug therapy should not automatically be withdrawn before planned surgery unless there is a very good reason to do so. The postoperative course in patients with a depressive illness may be more prolonged and these patients should be treated with appropriate forbearance.

ACQUIRED IMMUNE DEFICIENCY SYNDROME (AIDS)

This is caused by infection with a retrovirus, the human immunodeficiency virus (HIV). Acquired immunodeficiency syndrome is now a worldwide epidemic with an estimated 33×10^6 persons infected. The recent decline in death rates from HIV in developed countries has been due to the expanding use of antiviral drugs; however, resistance to the new drugs has developed in as many as 20% of patients and, although life expectancy has increased, these drugs do not represent a cure. HIV infection may also be seen in patients who have received infected blood products (e.g. haemophiliacs). The disease is not very infectious and is transmitted primarily in blood, and there is little evidence to support transmission via saliva or airborne transmission. The risk of occupationally acquired HIV is low (compared for example to hepatitis B) and it is estimated that the risk of developing HIV after percutaneous exposure to HIV infected blood is 0.3%. The risk after comparable exposure to hepatitis B virus (HBV) is greater than 30%, and HCV 1.9%. Occupational health departments all have their regimen of postexposure prophylaxis and should be contacted immediately in the event of a needlestick injury from a high risk patient.

THE PATIENT WITH A TRANSPLANTED ORGAN FOR NON-TRANSPLANT SURGERY

The era of transplant surgery dawned in the 1950s with the first kidney transplant (see Ch. 25). It is therefore not uncommon now to be faced with a patient with a transplanted organ presenting for non-transplant surgery.

Some aspects of management are common to all patients. It is essential to continue with their immunosuppressant regimen but consideration should be given to whether they are exhibiting signs of toxicity from the medication. These patients are all immunosuppressed. Apply strict aseptic precautions. Are they suffering from an infectious complication that may be due to an unusual pathogen such as a fungus? Have they developed a tumour as a consequence of the immunosuppression? The incidence of lymphomas is increased in these patients. Finally, are they displaying signs of rejection? This may be difficult to differentiate from infection in, for example, a lung graft.

Some specific considerations in a cardiac transplant recipient are as follows. The heart is denervated; it will be preload dependent to achieve an adequate cardiac output. There will be a delayed heart rate response (e.g. to hypoxia), which will be generated by catecholamine secretion. These patients have accelerated coronary atherosclerosis but may not develop angina in response to myocardial ischaemia. The heart will have unusual responses to vasoactive drugs due to the denervation. Finally, arrhythmias and a low cardiac output may be signs of rejection.

SURGERY IN THE ELDERLY

Although patients over the age of 65 years comprise only 22% of the surgical caseload, they are reported to account for 79% of perioperative deaths (Buck et al 1987). The mortality of surgery in elderly patients is significantly higher in those suffering from serious coexisting medical conditions. In a study of 100 000 surgical operations, the relative risk of dying within 7 days, comparing patients over 80 with those under 60 years, was 3, but the risk factor comparing patients having symptomatic medical disease with those having none was over 10 (Cohen et al 1988). Not only do elderly patients have an increased likelihood of coexisting disease, but physiological function in general decreases with age. As a generalization, many physiological functions (e.g. cardiac output, glomerular filtration rate and renal blood flow) decrease by about 1% per annum after the age of 30 years. Respiratory function also declines with age (maximum breathing capacity decreases from about 100 l min^{-1} at 20 years to 30 l min^{-1} at 80 years). The elderly are also more sensitive to the majority of drugs that might be used in the perioperative period (e.g. diazepam has a half-life measured in hours that is approximately equal to subject age in years). As in all other situations where a patient presents for surgery with a significant coexisting disease, the morbidity and mortality associated with surgery can be reduced to a minimum after careful preoperative evaluation and by optimizing the patient's condition.

If the decision is made to operate on an elderly patient then that must include a decision to provide appropriate postoperative care, which may include high dependency or intensive care support. Hypotension and hypovolaemia are common and should be corrected before surgery whenever possible. Fluid imbalance can contribute to serious postoperative morbidity and mortality and is more likely in the elderly, who may have renal impairment or other comorbidity. Accurate monitoring, early recognition and appropriate treatment of fluid balance are essential. Non-steroidal anti-inflammatory drugs should be prescribed with particular caution in elderly patients in the postoperative period.

Finally, the NCEPOD report *Extremes of Age* (1999) found that, in the elderly, unsuspected gastrointestinal complications are commonly found at post mortem to be the cause, or contribute to the cause, of death following surgery.

 Key points

- **Fluid management in the elderly is often poor; it should be accorded the same status as drug prescription.**

- **Elderly patients have a high incidence of coexisting disorders and a high risk of early postoperative death.**

CONCURRENT DRUG THERAPY

It is a general rule that any patients stabilized on long-term drug therapy should continue to take their normal medication until the time of surgery, and that this should be recommenced as soon as possible after surgery. If the patient is unable to take drugs by mouth, appropriate parenteral administration is required. This is especially important for patients taking drugs such as antiepileptics, antiarrhythmics or antihypertensives. A thorough knowledge of the pharmacokinetic and pharmacodynamic profile of the individual drugs is needed in order that the appropriate doses and interval between doses is arrived at for parenteral administration. A number of drugs (e.g. propranolol) undergo extensive first-pass liver metabolism after oral administration, and drugs such as this need much lower doses administered parenterally than they do orally.

Admission to hospital for surgery gives the opportunity to review the appropriateness of long-term drug therapy and dosage; this may be especially important in elderly patients as they are more likely to suffer from toxic symptoms. The nature of some operations may mean that the need for continued drug therapy has to be reviewed postoperatively, or the dosage of the drugs may need to be altered. An example of this would be a myasthenic patient undergoing thymectomy. Although the majority of patients stabilized on long-term therapy should continue their normal drugs up until the time of surgery, there are a number of drugs whose administration or dosage will need to be modified before surgery (see Table 6.4 for the more important examples of these).

Summary

- If there is a reversible feature to the patient's coexisting medical disease, elective surgery should be postponed until the patient is optimally treated.
- It may be appropriate to delay even emergency surgery until the patient's condition is stabilized or improved.
- A patient presenting for a minor surgical procedure may none the less require a high degree of anaesthetic expertise.

 References

ACC/AHA Task Force Report 1996 Guidelines for perioperative cardiovascular evaluation for non-cardiac surgery. Journal of the American College of Cardiology 27: 910–948

Buck N, Devlin HB, Lunn JN 1987 The report of a confidential enquiry into perioperative deaths. Nuffield Provincial Hospitals Trust, London

Burke M, Callum KG, Gray AJG et al 2001 Changing the way we operate. NCEPOD, London

Callum KG, Gray AJG, Hoile RW 1999 Extremes of age. NCEPOD, London

Table 6.4 Some important drugs, the administration or dosage of which needs to be modified before surgery	
Oral contraceptives	Maintain for minor or peripheral procedures and institute prophylaxis against deep vein thrombosis before surgery. Stop one complete monthly cycle before abdominal (especially pelvic) surgery
Anticoagulants	Stop oral agents several days before surgery and substitute heparin if continued anticoagulant is necessary. The action of heparin can be rapidly reversed with protamine
Agents used in diabetes	See section on diabetic management
Levodopa	Omit dose before surgery
Monamine oxidase inhibitors	Significant potential for drug interactions, causing severe physiological disturbance. Discuss with psychiatrist and anaesthetist and treat each case on its merits
Steroids	Supplement with hydrocortisone 100 mg i.v. 30 min before surgery, repeated 3-hourly during surgery, reducing slowly postoperatively to the patient's preoperative dose. Treat similarly if taking large dose regularly any time during 3 months before surgery

Campling EA, Devlin HB, Hoile RW, Lunn JN 1992 The report of the national confidential enquiry into perioperative deaths, 1990. King's Fund Publishing, London

Campling EA, Devlin HB, Hoile RW, Lunn JN 1993 The report of the national confidential enquiry into perioperative deaths, 1991/1992. King's Fund Publishing, London

Campling EA, Devlin HB, Hoile RW, Lunn JN 1995 The report of the national confidential enquiry into perioperative deaths 1992/1993. King's Fund Publishing, London

Campling ER et al 1997 Who operates when? NCEPOD, London

Child CG III, Turcotte J 1965 Surgery and portal hypertension. In: Child CG III (ed) The liver and portal hypertension. Saunders, Philadelphia

Cohen MM, Duncan PG, Tate RB 1988 Does anaesthesia contribute to operative mortality? JAMA 260: 2859–2863

Gallimore SC, Hoile RW, Ingram GS, Sherry KM 1997 The report of the national confidential enquiry into perioperative deaths 1994/1995. NCEPOD, London

Jones R M 1985 Smoking before surgery: the case for stopping. BMJ 290: 1763–1764

Mallett SV, Cox D 1992 Thromboelastoplasty. British Journal of Anaesthesia 69: 307–313

Mangano DT, Layug EL, Wallace A et al 1996 Effect of atenolol on mortality and cardio-vascular morbidity after non cardiac surgery. New England Journal of Medicine 335: 1713–1720

Simon A 1977 Perioperative management of the pacemaker patient. Anesthesiology 16: 127–131

Further reading

Findlaw D, Doyle E 1997 Congenital heart disease in adults. British Journal of Anaesthesia 78: 416–430

McIntyre N, Benhamon JP, Bircher J et al 1991 Oxford textbook of clinical hepatology. Oxford University Press, Oxford *See especially section 31: Surgery, anaesthesia and the liver*

7 Immunity in surgery

P. L. Amlot, C. S. Gricks

Objectives

- **Appreciate the functions and components of the immune system.**
- **Recognize that most disease processes are prevented by *innate immunity*.**
- **Recognize that specific disease processes are prevented by *adaptive immunity*.**
- **Understand the implications of immune processes in surgery.**

INTRODUCTION

The immune system evolved to protect the body from infection. Innate (inborn) immunity provides common effector mechanisms that protect against a wide range of pathogens. As pathogens evolved to escape control by the innate immune system, co-evolution of adaptive immune mechanisms developed, providing specific and variable receptors that can recruit effector mechanisms already provided by innate immunity that has been evaded by the pathogen.

INNATE IMMUNITY

Innate (Latin *natus* = to be born) immunity needs no prior contact with a pathogen to be activated and there is no 'learning' phase. The innate immune mechanisms are maximally effective the first time a pathogen is met and the response does not change with repeated exposure to pathogens. Clinically pathogenic organisms are broadly defined by their ability to cross epithelial surfaces and to evade other innate immune mechanisms; for example, mycobacterial cell walls are resistant to acid, and cholera has a specific receptor to bind to the gut wall.

Physical barriers

A large part of innate immunity is mechanical and applies to pathogens that have no selective method of crossing intact epithelial surfaces. Damage to skin by penetrating wounds and burns, or to mucosal surfaces by perforation, allow normally non-pathogenic organisms to cause disease. Epithelial cells do not function purely as a mechanical barrier but they produce intracellular chemical messengers known as *cytokines* and molecules that enhance the adaptive immune system's response. These physical barriers are reinforced by secretions.

Secretory system

Lysozyme in saliva and tears digests peptidoglycan in bacterial cell walls. Bacteria with susceptible cell walls are rendered non-pathogenic. *Gastric acid* inhibits bacterial growth and *mucus* inhibits bacterial motility.

The complement system consists of many proteins that can self-assemble to cause lysis of cells to which they are attached. Complement may be activated by two pathways:

- Alternative pathway – initiated directly by xenogeneic molecules, such as sugars forming part of microbial cell walls
- Classical pathway – initiated by antibody and requires adaptive immunity.

Complement, C-reactive protein and mannose-binding protein can all coat foreign particles, making them more easily digestible by phagocytes in a process called '*opsonization*.' Opsonization (G opsonein = to prepare food for; hence, make more digestible by phagocytes), by complement and antibody makes phagocytosis by granulocytes 1000 fold more efficient.

Cellular system

Phagocytes – neutrophils, monocytes or tissue macrophages – possess a wide variety of receptors, capable of increasing in quantity but not in quality. The receptors recognize xenogeneic (Greek *xenos* = foreign) molecules not present on human tissues, such as mannose, for which receptors are expressed on macrophages. Other, non-phagocytic cells may facilitate the immune response. For example, stimulated mast cells release factors that increase vascular permeability, allowing more rapid access of leucocytes to sites of infection. Many of the receptors expressed by leucocytes enable their movement through blood vessels and include selectins, adhesion molecules and chemokines.

Natural killer (NK) lymphocytes are unlike other lymphocytes and lack specific receptors capable of qualitative change. NK cells are involved in the surveillance of altered cells, particularly against tumours and viruses. Activated NK cells are capable of killing nucleated target cells, unless they are inhibited. On the membranes of NK cells are killer inhibitory receptors (KIRs) which bind to self-MHC (major histocompatibility complex) class I molecules of target cells, protecting them from being killed. Both viruses and tumour cells interfere with, or eliminate, MHC class I on the surface of their transformed cells. Although this allows the cells to escape surveillance by the adaptive immune system, it makes them susceptible to NK cells, since KIR now has nothing with which to bind and inhibition of killing does not occur.

Dendritic cells within the epithelium, especially the epidermis where they are known as Langerhans cells, play an important role in carrying antigens from the skin to local lymph nodes, where an adaptive immune response can be generated.

The response of the innate system is amplified in an integrated manner. For example, complement breakdown products are chemotactic (Greek *taxis* = arrangement; power to attract) for neutrophils, encouraging phagocytic removal of complement-coated bacteria.

Deficiencies of innate immunity

Primary immunodeficiencies affecting the innate system are very rare and carry the same consequences as *acquired* or *iatrogenic deficiency*, which is common. Operative surgery is naturally a major violator of epithelial barriers and secretions through incisions, intravascular lines, catheters, anaesthesia and drug use, including anaesthesia. Widespread desquamation, as with burns, severely compromises innate immunity. There is no known deficiency of lysozyme, but achlorhydria is associated with infection and malignancy. Deficiency of complement leads to susceptibility to infection by encapsulated bacteria or, surprisingly, to autoimmunity (Greek *autos* = self). Low neutrophil counts reflect the status of an important component of innate immunity and lead rapidly to severe consequences because of the wide range of infectious processes that require this final common phagocytic pathway. Neutropenia following administration of cytotoxic drugs can lead to severe infection within a few days. It is a key feature of deficiencies in innate immunity that they lead rapidly to infectious complications because most, if not all, infection is ultimately controlled by it. The

chances of meeting any of a wide range of infectious organisms is high and the time to a chance encounter, including organisms in our own digestive system, is therefore short.

ADAPTIVE IMMUNITY

In the adaptive response, exposure to infection leads to qualitative changes of specific receptors. The cells that bear these receptors compete in a darwinian fashion for binding to pathogens. The molecular structure that stimulates an adaptive, specific receptor is known as an *antigen*. Adaptive immunity has two collaborative branches, antibody- and cell-mediated immunity.

ANTIBODY-MEDIATED IMMUNITY

Antibodies belong to a class of proteins known as *immunoglobulin*. In humans, antibody-producing B lymphocytes originate in the bone marrow and the B cell receptor is the membrane-bound form of antibody secreted into body fluids. Pathogens coated with antibody can fix complement by the classical pathway and are phagocytosed (Greek *phagein* = to eat) far more rapidly than uncoated pathogens. It is estimated that our B cell system can create more than 10^{11} unique antibody molecules but each B cell can produce antibody of only a single specificity. There is not enough DNA to encode all the possibilities and the mechanism of shuffling and mixing discrete genes coding for immunoglobulin is known as *gene rearrangement*. This occurs randomly and allows B cells to create antibodies with diverse specificities and includes the possibility of creating antibodies that react with 'self', which can lead to *autoimmunity*.

Antibody-binding region

Antibody in the B cell membrane acts as a receptor for antigen on its surface. The B cell may be stimulated by the binding of an antigen to undergo proliferation, become a memory B cell or differentiate into a plasma cell. B cell stimulation by antigen occurs mainly within lymphoid follicles (structures in which B cells aggregate) and generates germinal centres, where a process known as *somatic hypermutation* takes place. This occurs in 0.1% of cell divisions and allows a few B cells to develop antibodies that bind to antigen with greater affinity. Normally, within 2 weeks the affinity of the antibody increases by 10- to 100-fold in the mutated B cells and allows them to compete successfully against other B cells for antigen, leading to their preferential proliferation – a process known as *clonal expansion*.

Antibodies: structure and synthesis

One part of the antibody, the variable or V region, binds to the antigen. The other part, the constant or C region, interacts with the invariable receptors of the innate immune system. An antibody is composed of at least two heavy and two light chains of immunoglobulin linked together so that there is a minimum of two antigen-binding sites per molecule (Fig. 7.1). This explains why antibodies can cross-link antigens and cause agglutination, for example, during the testing for blood group in transfusion or in the immobilization of flagellated microorganisms.

The constant domain is the major part of the antibody and is so named because it is largely invariable, which endows the antibody with different functional properties. There are five heavy chain genes giving rise to immunoglobulin: IgM, IgD, IgG, IgE and IgA. Immature B cells usually express IgM but they can switch the constant region when stimulated by antigen. The switch is influenced by the environment and T helper cells. This is called *isotype switching*.

IgM is so named because in its secreted form it is a macroglobulin composed of five immunoglobulin molecules bound together. Because of its large size it is largely retained within the vascular system, where it is effective at complement fixation and in protection against blood-borne infections. IgD is a largely membrane-bound immunoglobulin of unknown function. IgG is the most abundant isotype (Greek *isos* = equal; of the same type) in the blood and tissues. It is small enough to diffuse readily in the tissues and contains most of the high affinity antibody. There are several subclasses, each with different functional properties. Apart from coating pathogens for phagocytosis, they are also able to induce antibody-dependent cellular cytotoxicity (ADCC), which may play a part in transplantation and tumour immunity. Because it can cross the placental barrier it provides the fetus with antibody protection. IgG and IgA are also provided in breast milk. IgA can be transported across mucosal epithelium, resists gastrointestinal digestion and is the principal isotype in respiratory and gastrointestinal secretions. It is thought to prevent adherence of microorganisms and toxins to receptors and so is sometimes termed 'antiseptic paint'. IgE is bound to receptors on blood basophils and mast cells, in skin, mucosa, connective tissues and along blood vessels. Antigen binding causes degranulation of mast cells, which release mediators invoking coughing, sneezing, vomiting and diarrhoea. IgE protects against infestation with worms but causes allergies such as hay fever, urticaria, asthma and anaphylaxis.

Monoclonal antibodies and flow cytometry

In a normal immune response many B cells produce many different types of antibodies – a *polyclonal* response. A single B cell can produce only a single antibody; when a B cell proliferates, each daughter cell produces the same antibody – a *monoclonal* antibody – unless somatic mutation occurs during division. Monoclonality is characteristic of B cell malignancy and high levels of monoclonal antibody are recognized as paraprotein in multiple myeloma. These paraproteins can be detected by electrophoresis or immunofixation. Kohler and Milstein in 1975 fused a single B cell from a mouse spleen to a myeloma cell line, allowing infinite production of monoclonal antibodies with defined antigen specificity. Monoclonal antibodies of mouse or rat origin have revolutionized diagnostic processes and have enabled the identification of many cellular molecules. As monoclonal antibodies to lymphocyte receptors and antigens were being generated, a prototype fluorescein activated cell sorter (FACS) was being built. These flowcytometers are able to detect and count cell-

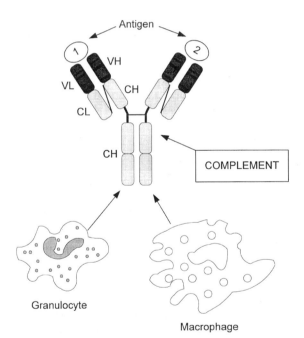

Fig. 7.1 Antibody structure and effector relationships. VL, variable region of the light chain; VH, variable region of the heavy chain; CL, constant region of the light chain; CH, constant region of the heavy chain that consists of three domains. Note that there are two binding sites to the antibody molecule, each binding an identical antigen (1 and 2). Granulocytes and macrophages bind to antibody molecules via their Fc receptors (known as Fc because it is an old term for the constant region of the heavy chain of the antibody molecule). The complement system interacts with the constant region of the heavy chain and leads to lysis of cells.

bound fluorochromes, allowing rapid counting of cells expressing specific antigens. Furthermore, up to four different fluorochromes on the same cell can be detected. This has enormously increased the scope for measuring minor cell populations within blood and other fluids. FACS machines are used to count CD4 and CD8 subsets of patients with human immunodeficiency virus (HIV), identify leukaemic, lymphomatous or other malignant cells and assess the activation status of lymphoid cells, simply by counting fluorochrome labels bound to monoclonal antibodies of the appropriate specificity.

Deficiency of antibody-mediated immunity and bacterial infections

Antibody deficiency predisposes predominantly to bacterial infection. Immunodeficiency of B cells is relatively uncommon but should be excluded in patients suffering repeated infections, especially infections recurring after an adequate course of antibiotic therapy. The slow tempo of infection due to antibody deficiencies means that the diagnosis is often delayed by several years. Antibody deficiency occurs at birth in primary agammaglobulinaemia (Bruton's disease) but more frequently later on in life as common variable immunodeficiency (CVID). Acquired immunodeficiency is often iatrogenic (Greek *iatros* = physician, hence resulting from medical treatment), and as a result of diseases affecting B cells, such as lymphoma. Corticosteroid therapy is the most common iatrogenic cause of poor antibody production. It is yet to be seen what effect the widespread use of the recently licensed anti-B cell monoclonal antibody, rituximab, will have upon iatrogenic immunodeficiency. Bacterial infection can be treated in patients with hypogammaglobulinaemia by replacement immunoglobulin therapy every 2–4 weeks.

- Specific operations may have an effect on bacterial infection from a combination of reduced innate immunity and antibody deficiency. Splenectomy in children, particularly infants, increases their susceptibility to infection and children should be given long-term oral penicillin. There is a lesser risk in older children and adults. Overwhelming postsplenectomy infection, usually with encapsulated bacteria such as *Pneumococcus, Haemophilus* or *Meningococcus* spp, occurs in 1–20% of splenectomized individuals; it is fatal in 50% of cases.

Key point

- **Give polyvalent pneumococcal vaccine, haemophilus (HIB) and meningococcal vaccine to boost antibody levels before elective splenectomy.**

- The small bowel is richly supplied with T, B and plasma cells and secretes the immunoglobulin IgA into the lumen. If it is diseased, it becomes susceptible to infection with, for example, *Giardia lamblia*. Remarkably, extensive bowel resection does not appear to have major immunological effects.

T CELLS AND CELL-MEDIATED IMMUNITY

T lymphocytes have specialized membrane-bound T cell receptors (TCR) that are not secreted and remain cell bound. T cells arise in the bone marrow but migrate to the thymus, a primary lymphoid organ, in order to differentiate. The thymus is a site of enormous cellular proliferation, like the germinal centres in B cell follicles; it is most active early in life and atrophies with age.

The T cell receptor, like immunoglobulin, is made up of two chains. It shows remarkable similarity to the heavy and light chains of immunoglobulin in that they undergo the same process of gene rearrangement, producing a unique antigen-binding variable region and a conserved constant region which is largely anchored in the T cell membrane.

T cell recognition of antigen

T cells can recognize only protein antigens that have been broken down or 'processed' by antigen-presenting cells (APCs). Peptide fragments from proteins are incorporated into specialized cell surface molecules that have been misnamed the major histocompatibility complex (MHC) because of the complications this region causes in transplanting tissues. The MHC is also known as HLA (human leucocyte antigens). T cell receptors recognize the combination of the MHC and the peptide antigen that it 'presents'. T cells cannot recognize free antigen or antigen outside the context of the MHC.

There are two major classes of MHC molecules, structurally related but differing in their tissue expression, the subcellular compartment in which they process peptides and the presentation to separate T cell populations.

MHC class I molecules are present on most nucleated cells and bind endogenous (Greek *endon* = within + *gennan* = to produce; formed within the cell) peptides that originate in the cell's cytoplasm. Cells degrade cytoplasmic proteins and transport peptides to the cell surface in MHC class I molecules where they are recognized by cytotoxic T cells, identified by the CD8 molecule (a surface antigen that can be detected with a specific monoclonal antibody – CD = cluster designation). Cytotoxic T cells that recognize an MHC class I viral peptide complex on the surface of a virally infected cell will kill the cell.

MHC class II molecules are located on B lymphocytes, macrophages and dendritic cells, collectively known as antigen-presenting cells. These cells can assimilate exogenous antigen from outside the cell by phagocytosis or receptor-mediated endocytosis into vesicles within the cell. During the process of MHC class II synthesis it incorporates the peptides from the vesicles and transports it to the cell surface. The T cell receptor of T helper cells, identified by the CD4 molecule, is capable of binding to the antigen bound to the MHC class II molecule. T helper and cytotoxic T cells are selected in the thymus (Fig. 7.2).

In both types of MHC a molecular groove exists into which peptides can fit, facilitating interaction with the T cell receptor. Pathogens with peptide sequences that cannot bind to specific MHC molecules are ignored. To counter this, the MHC gene cluster on chromosome 6 accommodates highly polymorphic (Greek *polys* = much + *morphe* = form; many formed) genes; this benefits the population at the expense of the individual and explains why some individuals are more susceptible to specific infections than others.

T cell function

The T cell receptor detects MHC 'signatures' of non-self and in turn is linked to intracellular enzymatic pathways that activate the T cell via a complex of molecules known as CD3. The activated T cell produces intercellular messengers known as *cytokines*, of which more than 50 have been identified, with many different effects. Most of them transmit between leucocytes and are therefore termed *interleukins* (IL), and the different types and actions are designated by a number, e.g. IL-1, IL-2 to IL-n. Inhibition of cytokines is the basis of selective immunosuppressive drugs such as ciclosporin and tacrolimus which inhibit the secretion of IL-2.

The T cell response, directed by T helper cells, is modified by the antigenic context (microenvironment) and may in some situations cause cellular destruction, including suicide of the target cell – apoptosis (Greek *apo* = away + *ptosis* = a falling), or in other situations enhance antibody production in order to clear or inhibit antigens (see Fig. 7.3). The T cell recognition of 'self' is largely due to ignorance, in that most self-reactive T cells are eliminated in the thymus.

Deficiency of cell-mediated immunity and infections by viral and other intracellular pathogens

The rare failure to develop a thymus, resulting in severe deficiency of T cells, is known as DiGeorge's syndrome

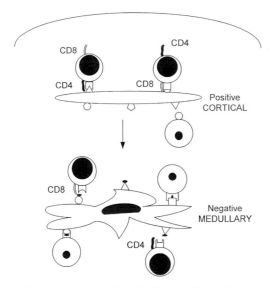

Fig. 7.2 Thymic 'education' in T cell differentiation. CD4 = T helper cells; CD8 = cytotoxic T cells. During 'positive' selection T cells express both CD4 and CD8. Those cells capable of binding to MHC molecules on cortical epithelial cells are destined to survive. During 'negative' selection, T cells express either CD4 or CD8, selected on the ability of the T cell receptor (TCR) to bind to MHC class II or class I, respectively. During 'negative' selection, avid binding of TCR to MHC expressing self-antigens on medullary dendritic cells leads to the apoptotic death of such T cells, thus minimizing autoimmunity. Cells depicted with small nuclei represent apoptotic cells destined for elimination in the thymus. Binding ability of the TCR for MHC is depicted by the degree of 'fit' between the two molecules.

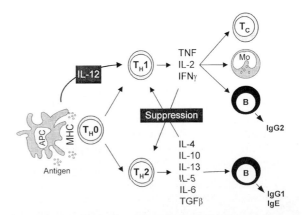

Fig. 7.3 T helper cell (CD4) functions. APC, antigen presenting cell; MHC, major histocompatibility complex; IL, interleukin; T_H0, T_H1, T_H2, T helper cell subsets (CD4+); TNF, tumour necrosis factor; IFN, interferon; TGF, T cell growth factor; T_c, cytotoxic T cell (CD8+); Mo, monocyte/macrophage series; B, B cell.

(after the American paediatrician who described it). Much more common are acquired T cell deficiencies, of which acquired immune deficiency syndrome (AIDS) is the best known. The human immunodeficiency virus (HIV) selectively infects T helper cells, resulting in susceptibility to intracellular infections and virally mediated malignancies such as lymphomas (human herpes virus 4–HHV-4) and Kaposi's sarcoma (HHV-8). Remarkably, thymectomy carried out for the treatment of myasthenia gravis or during cardiac surgery does not appear to have severe effects on immunity. Among the acquired forms of predominantly T cell deficiency are:

1. Malignant disease.
2. Surgical operations, including the response to trauma as well as anaesthetic drugs such as halothane.
3. Infection, particularly viral effects on lymphoid cells.
4. AIDS, which results from infection with HIV. It initially affected male homosexuals, intravenous drug users and haemophiliacs given factor VIII derived from pooled plasma from the USA. More recently in Europe and the USA and elsewhere in the world, most notably Africa, it has become primarily a heterosexual disease. The virus attaches itself to the CD4 molecule on the helper T cell, while cytotoxic T cells are initially unaffected. It is particularly associated with susceptibility to opportunistic infections such as *Pneumocystis carinii*, cytomegalovirus, *Aspergillus* and in certain circumstances the development of Kaposi's sarcoma.
5. Deficiency caused by radiotherapy for malignant disease, which produces lymphopenia, neutropenia and thrombocytopenia and largely depresses cellular immunity; however, the dose and rate of irradiation is such that marked cytopenias are rare and infection is not as common as with cytotoxic drugs.
6. Deficiency resulting from the use of immunosuppressant drugs such as azathioprine, ciclosporin A or tacrolimus used in transplantation.

Deficiency of both T and B cell immunity

The rare failure of lymphocyte differentiation leads to an absence of both B and T cells and a condition known as severe combined immune deficiency (SCID). This immunodeficiency of the adaptive immune system is the most likely to present rapidly but even then takes several months from birth to be diagnosed, after repeated infections, failure to thrive and diarrhoea. As in each form of defects in adaptive immunity, the tempo is much slower than that seen with deficiency of innate immunity. Acquired forms of combined immunodeficiency are the result of:

1. Poor nutrition, which affects both cell-mediated immunity and antibody production.

Key point

- **Postoperative infection rates are likely to be higher in countries where starvation is common.**

2. Chemotherapy to treat malignant disease, which is cytotoxic to neutrophils, leucocytes and lymphocytes. It is associated with increased bacterial and opportunistic infections, of which the effects on innate immunity predominate.
3. The administration of glucocorticoid steroids, which are used in transplantation and in treatment of autoimmune diseases, with potent effects on both arms of adaptive immunity as well as some on innate immune mechanisms.

AUTOIMMUNITY

Random generation of antigen-binding sites in antibodies risks the development of autoimmune disease. One safeguard against autoantibodies is that immature B cells emerging from the bone marrow are sensitive when their antibody receptor binds to self proteins, leading to tolerance or death by apoptosis. Another safeguard is that B cells require a number of growth factors (cytokines) derived from T cells, and in their absence B cell differentiation and antibody production may fail. Autoimmunity arises in genetically predisposed individuals, affecting both B and T cells. Autoantibody may mediate disease by a number of immune mechanisms:

- Binding to and blocking important physiological receptors, such as the acetylcholine receptor in myasthenia gravis
- Damaging cells and tissues by complement fixation or antibody-dependent cellular cytotoxicity (ADCC)
- Forming immune complexes that are deposited on the intimal surface of blood vessels and causing vasculitis.

Immune deficiency is closely associated with autoimmunity; for example, Crohn's disease, which may have an autoimmune component and is often treated with immunosuppressive drugs, coeliac disease and atrophic gastritis are all associated with immune deficiency.

TRANSPLANTATION

Autotransplantation (Greek *autos* = self) of tissue, such as a skin graft, has no immunological consequences; nor does grafting between identical twins (isograft: Greek *isos* = equal). Non-vascularized allografts (Greek *allos* = other), such as corneal grafts, do not normally evoke a cellular rejection. On the other hand, kidney, liver, heart, lung, pancreas, small bowel and bone marrow grafts induce rejection (see Ch. 25). Allografts are mainly cadaveric organs but there is increasing use of live related donors. Bone marrow allografts are from live donors and may be related or unrelated. Rejection of allografts is predominantly acute and cell-mediated early in the course of transplantation, unless the recipient has had prior contact with the donor tissues or is of a different blood group, in which case hyperacute rejection occurs. A slower onset of chronic 'vascular' rejection, causing graft dysfunction and progressive graft loss, is due to a variety of mechanisms, including cell- and antibody-mediated responses, physical effects, accelerated vasculopathy and immunosuppressive drug-induced effects. Tubular structures, such as blood vessels and biliary ducts, are affected by this process.

Avoiding rejection

1. Except when transplanting the cornea, the donor and recipient tissues are matched for ABO blood groups and as closely as possible for human leucocyte antigens (HLA). In addition, the recipient's serum is cross-matched with the donor lymphoid cells to exclude preformed cytotoxic antibodies.

2. Except when transplanting between identical twins, the recipient is immunosuppressed, with agents selected from a variety of drugs, including corticosteroids, azathioprine, mycophenolate mofetil, ciclosporin, tacrolimus and sirolimus. The anchors of current therapy are still ciclosporin and tacrolimus, whose action prevents the development of cytotoxic T cells; however, both are nephrotoxic. Antilymphocytic globulin (ALG) or antithymocyte globulin (ATG) are polyclonal antibodies preferably raised in rabbits, and may be used to increase immunosuppression early in transplantation. Monoclonal antibodies such as OKT3 (CD3) or Campath 1 (CDw52) have been used to reverse acute rejection. Newer monoclonal antibodies reacting with the IL-2 receptor (CD25) are effective at prophylactically reducing acute rejection episodes.

3. Graft versus host disease (GVHD) may develop if the graft contains competent T cells which react against the host cells that are incapable of rejecting them. This is most likely to develop following bone marrow transplantation. GVHD predominantly affects the skin, liver and gut.

CANCER IMMUNOLOGY

- The occasional but well documented spontaneous regression of tumours suggests that immunity may develop against cancers.

- Immunosuppressed patients have a higher than normal risk of malignancy, especially skin cancers and lymphoid tumours.
- Cancers are often infiltrated with lymphocytes and macrophages – this may be associated with an improved prognosis.
- Latent cancers, especially of the thyroid and prostate glands, are often disclosed at postmortem examination, suggesting that the tumours develop but lie dormant for many years without clinical disease. This has been attributed to immune mechanisms.

Tumour antigens

Specific antigens can be found on the surface of tumour cells, especially those that are virally induced, without being present on normal cells of this type. Some tumour cells express antigens normally found only in fetal tissue, such as α-fetoprotein (AFP) and carcinoembryonic antigen (CEA). These may be used as markers for some cancers or to monitor progress by measuring serum levels, but there is little evidence that they act as targets for the immune system. Radiolabelled monoclonal antibody to CEA may be used to localize residual bowel tumour. Malignant cells can overexpress proto-oncogenes on their surface, which contribute to malignant behaviour; these were identified by antibodies developed for the recognition of specific tumour types.

Monoclonal antibodies that attach to receptors highly expressed in tumours can be labelled with isotopes such as ^{111}In and ^{99m}Tc. These can be identified by external scintigraphy. This is especially valuable in identifying residual tumour following treatment.

Immunotherapy

The identification of immune aspects of cancer has led to the search for therapeutic uses, especially for disseminated tumour cells beyond the scope of conventional treatment, or residual tumour following treatment. Antibodies alone are rarely cytotoxic to tumour cells and are largely restricted to haemopoietic malignancy. Monoclonal antibodies can be conjugated to radioisotopes, immunotoxins or enzymes. Radiolabelled antibodies can target highly expressed epidermal growth factor receptors (GFRs) in lung and brain tumours and there is hope that monoclonal antibodies to GFRs will be effective in treating tumours. Monoclonal antibody to Her-Neu has proven effective in a minority of breast cancers expressing this on the tumour.

Summary

- Do you understand that the immune system is composed of humoral and cellular elements and is made up of innate and adaptive mechanisms?
- Are you aware that normally the immune system distinguishes self from non-self but autoimmunity may develop in predisposed individuals?
- Do you recognize that immune deficiency arises from many causes, including operation, which predisposes to postoperative complications?
- Are you aware that, except in specific circumstances, organ transplants must be protected from rejection by immunosuppressive drugs and other techniques?
- Can you foresee the immunological aspects of cancer becoming increasingly valuable in identifying, monitoring and treating malignancy?

References

Kohler G, Milstein C 1975 Continuous cultures of fused cells secreting antibody of predefined specificity. Nature 256(5517): 495–497

Further reading

Goldsby RA, Kindt TJ, Osborne BA, Kuby J 2003 Immunology, 3rd edn. W H Freeman, New York

Janeway CA, Travers P, Walport M, Shlomchik M (eds) 2001 The adaptive immune response. In: Immunobiology, 5th edn. Churchill Livingstone, Edinburgh

Medzhitov R, Janeway CA 2000 Innate immune recognition: mechanisms and pathways. Annual Review of Immunology 173: 89–97

Norman D, Turka L 2001 Primer on transplantation, 2nd edn. Blackwell Science, Oxford

Stites DP, Terr AI, Parslow TG 1997 Medical immunology. Appleton & Lange, Stamford CT

8 Haematological assessment and blood component therapy

C. P. F. Taylor, A. B. Mehta

Objectives

- Understand the need for preoperative detection of blood abnormalities which may affect the outcome of surgery and anaesthesia.
- Be aware of the range of blood components available for clinical use.
- Understand how to use blood components appropriately and the hazards associated with their use.
- Be aware of alternatives to allogeneic blood transfusion and know when they are appropriate.
- Understand the underlying mechanisms and management of excessive intra- or postoperative blood loss.

INTRODUCTION

This chapter outlines the investigation and management of patients undergoing surgery. It includes patients who have a prior abnormality of their blood count or blood plasma constituents and also discusses appropriate use of blood components in patients with no prior haematological problems.

Anaemia and excessive bleeding are symptoms and not diagnoses. An accurate diagnosis is an essential step in the formulation of a management plan. In the majority of hospitals, a clinical haematologist will be available to advise you on optimum use of laboratory diagnostic facilities, interpretation of results and appropriate therapy. Make sure you discuss problems early, and take advice on the appropriate specimens to send and tests to order. If a result is puzzling, go and discuss it with the haematologist.

PREOPERATIVE ASSESSMENT

Growing pressure on hospital beds and increasing use of day surgery means that the preoperative assessment should, wherever possible, be performed prior to admission. This allows for efficient use of hospital resources and limits the number of cancelled operations. The key aims are to assess a patient's fitness to undergo surgery and anaesthesia, anticipate complications, arrange for supportive therapy to be available perioperatively and to liaise with the appropriate specialists regarding non-surgical management. This assessment needs to take place at a presurgical clinic at least 1 month prior to the planned date of surgery.

Preoperative planning

Arrange for the patient to attend a preoperative clinic at least 4–6 weeks prior to operation, to:

- Take a full history and examination, including previous surgical episodes and bleeding history
- Arrange full blood count, group and antibody screen, routine chemistry, coagulation screen (if indicated) and tube for haematinics assessment (ferritin level for iron stores, vitamin B_{12} and folic acid), which can be put on hold pending full blood count (FBC) results
- Consider autologous predeposit if the patient is fit enough and there is a greater than 50% likelihood of significant blood loss requiring transfusion
- Consider using erythropoietin (Greek *erythros* = red + *poiesis* = making), even with normal haemoglobin, at a dose of 600 units/kg weekly for 4 weeks preoperatively
- Prescribe iron and folic acid supplement if there is any suspicion of iron deficiency
- Establish whether the patient is taking regular aspirin, non-steroidal anti-inflammatory drugs (NSAIDs) or warfarin and make necessary arrangements to stop this drug preoperatively
- Consider a staged surgical approach in major surgery.

After the clinic, ensure that all the results of the above tests are seen within a few days so that you can take necessary action. In addition, discuss with the anaesthetists whether acute normovolaemic haemodilution (ANH) or intraoperative cell salvage may be appropriate.

Anaemia

1. Anaemia is defined as a reduction in haemoglobin concentration below the normal range after correction for age and sex (approximately 13–16 g dl^{-1} in males, 11.5–15 g dl^{-1} in females). The most common causes of anaemia in surgical patients are iron deficiency (from chronic blood loss) or anaemia of chronic disease. Both may be due to the underlying condition for which operation is required.

2. Every anaemic patient, that is those whose haemoglobin level is below their laboratory normal range, should have iron studies and ferritin levels performed sufficiently in advance of operation to allow for corrective measures to take effect. A subnormal ferritin indicates iron deficiency and the patient should be treated preoperatively with iron supplements orally or intravenously. Defer elective surgery until the maximum haemoglobin is attained. One should not use allogeneic blood unless there are no reasonable alternatives (Table 8.1).

Key point

- **Anaemia in elective surgical patients should be assessed and appropriately treated preoperatively.**

3. A normal or high ferritin level does not exclude iron deficiency (although it is less likely), as ferritin is an acute phase protein. Anaemia of chronic disease (ACD) may be present in many presurgical patients, including those with malignancy or joint disease requiring orthopaedic surgery. ACD is usually normochromic and normocytic, although it is sometimes slightly microcytic. Iron levels are normal but iron-binding capacity is reduced (in contrast to iron deficiency where iron-binding capacity is raised). Ferritin (an intermediary in the absorption of iron from the gut) may be normal or raised. ACD may respond to erythropoietin therapy preoperatively. Although iron stores may be adequate, supplemental iron and folic acid may be required. Anaemia accompanied by thrombocytopenia or neutropenia may indicate a bone marrow disorder, a complex autoimmune condition or systemic disease, so seek the advice of a haematologist, and other specialists, without delay.

A classification of anaemia is given below:

- *Decreased red cell production*
  - Haematinic deficiency:
    Iron, vitamin B$_{12}$, folic acid
  - Marrow failure:
    Aplastic anaemia, leukaemia, pure red cell aplasia.
- *Abnormal red cell maturation*
  - Myelodysplasia
  - Sideroblastic (Greek *sideros* = iron) anaemia
- *Increased red cell destruction*
  - Inherited haemolytic anaemia, such as sickle cell anaemia or thalassaemia (Greek *thalassa* = sea)
  - Acquired haemolytic anaemia:
    Immune (e.g. autoimmune)
    Non-immune (e.g. microangiopathic haemolytic anaemia, disseminated intravascular coagulation)
- *Effects of disease in other organs*
  Anaemia of chronic disorder; renal, endocrine, liver disease.

Examination of red cell indices provides important clues to the cause of anaemia. The following alterations in red cell indices offer a clue to the cause of anaemia.

- *Lowered mean cell volume (MCV), mean cell haemoglobin (MCH)*
  - Iron deficiency
  - Thalassaemia trait
  - Homozygous thalassaemia
  - Hyperthyroidism
- *Raised MCV*
  - Megaloblastic (Greek *megalo* = large) anaemia
  - Hypothyroidism
  - Liver disease
  - Reticulocytosis
  - Myelodysplasia
  - Aplastic anaemia
  - Paraproteinaemia
  - Alcohol abuse
- *Normochromic normocytic*
  - Anaemia of chronic disease
  - Renal failure
  - Bone marrow infiltration
  - Haemorrhage.

Table 8.1 Reasons to reduce blood exposure

- Immunological complications
  - Red cell alloantibodies: HTR
  - HLA antibodies: refractoriness
  - TRALI, PTP, TA-GvHD, etc.
- Errors and 'wrong blood' episodes
- Infections – bacterial, viral, ? prion
- Immunomodulation – infection, malignancy
- Litigation
- Resource

HTR, haemolytic transfusion reaction; PTP, post-transfusion purpura; TRALI, transfusion-related acute lung injury; TA-GVHD, transfusion-associated graft versus host disease.

A reduction in MCV and MCH (microcytic hypochromic picture) is highly suggestive of iron deficiency. Nutritional deficiency or very slow chronic blood loss leads to a well-compensated anaemia of gradual onset. A raised MCV is highly suggestive of megaloblastic anaemia and malabsorption (due to pernicious anaemia, coeliac disease, or after gastrectomy) or poor dietary intake are the commonest causes. The underlying cause of the anaemia should be specifically treated as far as possible and elective surgery delayed until this is achieved.

Haemoglobinopathies

These are a group of inherited disorders (autosomal recessive) of haemoglobin synthesis in which affected individuals (homozygotes) suffer a lifelong haemolytic anaemia. They are the commonest human inherited disorders.

The carriers (heterozygotes) have a small degree of protection against malaria; haemoglobinopathies are therefore common in all parts of the world where malaria is (or was) prevalent – southern Europe, Asia, the Far East, Africa, South America and immigrant populations in northern Europe and North America. Carriers are asymptomatic and have a normal life expectancy, but may have a mild degree of anaemia. Haemoglobinopathies are divided into two types: disorders affecting haemoglobin structure and disorders of haemoglobin synthesis. In the structural haemoglobin variants, a single deoxyribonucleic acid (DNA) base mutation leads to an amino acid substitution in haemoglobin to give rise to a variant haemoglobin, e.g. haemoglobin S (sickle haemoglobin, which leads to sickle cell anaemia). The variant haemoglobin may be functionally abnormal; thus, haemoglobin S tends to crystallize under conditions of low oxygen tension and this distorts red cell shape to cause 'sickling'. The second type of haemoglobinopathy is thalassaemia, where there is no change in the amino acid composition of the haemoglobin molecule but there is deficient synthesis of one of the globin chains (α or β), leading to imbalanced chain synthesis and anaemia. Thalassa (Greek = sea) recognizes that the disease was discovered in countries bordering the Mediterranean sea.

It is important to detect carriers of some haemoglobinopathies (e.g. sickle cell) prior to operation because anaesthesia and hypoxia can precipitate sickling. All patients of non-northern European origin should be screened prior to operation, for example in the preadmission clinic, by haemoglobin electrophoresis and/or a sickle solubility test. Affected individuals (homozygotes) usually present in childhood but occasionally patients present incidentally. Patients with sickle cell disease (HbSS) should be managed jointly with a clinical haematologist. The consultant anaesthetist performing the case needs to know in advance of the sickle status of the patient because special anaesthetic precautions and practices are required, including exchange transfusion prior to major surgery such as hip replacement. This involves venesection of the patient together with transfusion of donor blood (6–8 units) resulting in a postexchange haemoglobin S level of less than 30%. It can be performed manually or using a cell separator. Minor surgery such as dental procedures can be safely carried out without transfusion in the majority of patients. Intermediate procedures such as cholecystectomy can be performed following transfusion with 2–3 units of packed red cells to a haemoglobin level of 10 g l^{-1} (Vichinsky et al 1995). Pay particular attention to the hydration of the patient, at least 3 litres per day, and to oxygenation during anaesthesia. Patients with some haemoglobinopathies, especially HbSC disease, are at increased risk of postoperative thrombosis, and appropriate prophylaxis with low molecular weight heparin is desirable unless there are contraindications.

Other inherited red cell disorders

Deficiency of the red cell enzyme glucose-6-phosphate dehydrogenase (G6PD) is a sex-linked disorder affecting more than 400 million people worldwide. It results in a reduced capacity of the red cell to withstand an oxidative stress. Patients are asymptomatic in the steady state and have a near normal FBC, but may suffer haemolysis of red cells in response to an oxidative challenge. Common precipitants are infection and drugs, principally antimalarials such as primaquine, pamaquine and pentaquine but not usually chloroquine or mefloquine, and sulphonamide antibiotics (Mehta 1994).

Excessive bleeding

1. Preoperative assessment should allow us to anticipate problems. Many patients with an inherited or acquired defect of coagulation (Table 8.2) leading to peri- and postoperative complications cannot be detected preoperatively. However, take a careful history, which may reveal features such as excessive bleeding at times of previous surgery, bleeding while brushing teeth, nose bleeds, a family of history of bleeding disorders, spontaneous bruising, a history of renal or liver disease and a relevant drug history.

2. Request a coagulation screen, prothrombin time (PT), activated partial thromboplastin time (APTT) and thrombin time (TT) and platelet count, in any patient with a suspected bleeding disorder, although disordered platelet function can be difficult to detect. A bleeding time is the best in vivo test of platelet function and involves a standard skin incision and timing of clot formation, provided the tester is expert and performs it regularly. Laboratory platelet function analyses may also be necessary.

Table 8.2 Bleeding disorders associated with excessive bleeding which may cause peri- or postoperative complications

Disorder type	Cause
Congenital	
Clotting factors	Haemophilia A, B
	von Willebrand's syndrome
Platelets	Congenital platelet disorders
Vessel wall	Hereditary haemorrhagic telangiectasia
Acquired	
Clotting factors	Drugs (anticoagulants, antibiotics)
	Liver disease
	DIC (in sepsis)
Platelets – function	Drugs (aspirin, NSAIDs)
	Liver disease, renal disease, myeloproliferative disorders, paraproteinaemic disorders
Platelets – number	Autoimmune thrombocytopenia
	Hypersplenism
	Aplastic anaemia, myelodysplasia
Vessel wall	Drugs (steroids)
	Vasculitis
	Malnutrition

DIC, disseminated intravascular coagulation; NSAIDs, non-steroidal anti-inflammatory drugs.

3. Ask advice from a haematologist specialising in haemostasis before elective operation on patients with coagulation and platelet abnormalities, since their pre-operative management may be complex. A very common cause of excessive intra-operative bleeding due to platelet dysfunction is pre-operative ingestion of aspirin, clopi dogrel, NSAIDS, or warfarin. The need for these drugs must be assessed at the pre-operative clinic and low dose aspirin should be stopped 10 days prior to surgery, unless this is contraindicated. Platelets may be required to achieve haemostasis in bleeding patients, even with satisfactory platelet counts, if they have been taking aspirin within one week of surgery.

Anticoagulation therapy

1. The dose of oral anticoagulants such as warfarin (named for *Winconsin Alumni Research Foundation* + couma*rin*) is adjusted to maintain the international normalized ratio (INR, which is a measure of the patient's PT to that of a control plasma) within a therapeutic range.

The therapeutic range varies depending upon the indication for which the patient was warfarinized.

2. Heparin is a parenteral anticoagulant and may be given in either low molecular weight or unfractionated forms. Low molecular weight heparin (LMWH) is not usually monitored at prophylactic doses, but at therapeutic doses an anti-Xa assay is required for monitoring. Unfractionated heparin is monitored by measurement of the ratio of the patient's APPT compared to that of control plasma. The short half-life of unfractionated heparin allows safer management during the perioperative period.

Key point

- **Always check the platelet count before starting heparin and every second day on treatment to detect heparin-induced thrombocytopenia (HIT).**

3. For elective surgery in patients on oral anticoagulants, you must balance the risk of haemorrhage if the INR is not reduced against the risk of thrombosis if the INR is reduced for too long or by too great an amount. For minor surgery (e.g. dental extraction) it is normally sufficient to stop the oral anticoagulant for 2 days prior to the procedure and restart with the usual maintenance dose immediately afterwards. For high risk patients such as those with prosthetic heart valves, or for patients undergoing more extensive procedures, you must stop warfarin and substitute heparin, either subcutaneously or by continuous intravenous infusion, under close haematological supervision to provide thrombosis prophylaxis. Patients on warfarin who present for emergency surgery or who have bled as a result of anticoagulant therapy may need reversal of the anticoagulant. This can be done using vitamin K with either a concentrate of factors II, VII, IX and X or, if this is unavailable, fresh frozen plasma (FFP).

ARRANGING INTRAOPERATIVE BLOOD COMPONENT SUPPORT

Elective surgery

1. The standard red cell product is SAG-M blood, that is, red cells suspended in an optimal additive solution of saline, adenine, glucose and mannitol, with a citrate anticoagulant. Whole blood is not used in the UK, although it is available in some other countries in Europe, and plasma-reduced blood is available for specific multitransfused patients. All cellular products, such as platelets and red cells, are leucodepleted at the blood

centres in the UK, and have been so since November 1999. There is therefore no role for an in-line white cell filter in these products. Special products, such as blood with extended red cell phenotyping or rare blood from the frozen blood bank, are available after discussion with laboratory staff and haematology consultants at the blood service.

2. Give the laboratory time to perform a 'group' and antibody screen on every patient before elective surgery. Although in most patients crossmatched blood can be provided, after the group and screen (G & S) in 1 hour, the 1–4% of patients with atypical red cell alloantibodies require extra laboratory time for antibody identification and to obtain compatible units of blood from the blood centre. For this reason, grouping and saving of blood is best performed at a preoperative clinic, even if this is several weeks in advance, and even though a new sample may then be required for crossmatching a day or two before operation, depending on local hospital policy.

3. If no atypical antibodies are present, many procedures can now be performed after grouping and saving alone, blood being provided only if it is required during or after operation. If the antibody screen has been performed already and is negative, blood can be issued on an immediate spin test taking 10 min. In some hospitals a so-called 'electronic' crossmatch allows blood to be issued without any further wet testing.

4. Most hospitals operate a standard, or maximum, blood order schedule (SBOS/MBOS) (British Committee for Standards in Haematology 1990). This agreed schedule for blood ordering improves efficiency within the blood bank and can also simplify the ordering process for junior doctors. An order can be placed prior to major vascular or hepatic operation, where there is a strong likelihood that FFP or platelets may be required, but the components are not usually issued until they are required; this avoids wastage. Discuss these arrangements preoperatively with a clinical haematologist and agree the procedures for regularly recurring events.

Key point

- **Blood component therapy should be given after reviewing recent laboratory results, not on an empirical basis.**

5. Elective surgery should be undertaken on patients with thrombocytopenia, or congenital and acquired disorders of coagulation, only after careful preoperative assessment, and under the direction of a haematologist.

6. Many patients can avoid allogeneic transfusion by normalization of haemoglobin preoperatively, using erythropoietin and iron therapy as appropriate, minimization

of intra- and postoperative blood loss, and acceptance of a lower postoperative haemoglobin, such as 7–8 g dl^{-1}. A blood loss of 1.5 litres is well tolerated by most patients who have a normal initial blood haemoglobin, without the need for red cell transfusion of any sort, provided they are given adequate volume support with crystalloid and colloids.

Preoperative autologous transfusion

There are three kinds of autologous (derived from the same individual) blood transfusion that are practised to varying degrees at hospitals in the UK.

1. Intra- and postoperative cell salvage
2. Acute normovolaemic haemodilution
3. Preoperative autologous deposit (PAD).

Intra- and postoperative cell salvage

A number of companies manufacture equipment that can be used to collect shed blood from intraoperative wounds and drains, and also postoperative drainage containers. Some of these return the blood as collected or they may be used to wash and process the blood to remove plasma constituents. If large volumes of shed blood are returned without processing, the patient may experience coagulation problems that can cause further bleeding. These cell salvage procedures have been evaluated by clinical trials in cardiac and orthopaedic surgery. There is definite evidence that salvage can reduce the proportion of patients who receive allogeneic red cell transfusion in orthopaedic surgery. In cardiac surgery, trials show only a slight reduction in transfusion of allogeneic red cells. The systems have also been used in liver surgery and liver transplantation and are increasingly used in other major vascular surgical procedures. Many clinicians believe from clinical experience that patients with major surgical blood losses do better if they are managed by reinfusing salvaged blood. These systems should not be used for 'dirty' wounds where there is risk of infection from bowel contents or abscesses. Great caution is also exercised over the use of this equipment in patients with malignancy.

Acute normovolaemic haemodilution

There is some controversy over the value of this procedure, in which the anaesthetist withdraws several packs of the patient's blood in the anaesthetic room immediately before surgery, replacing the volume straight away with crystalloid or colloid. The collected blood is then reinfused during or immediately after the operation. The blood must be taken into a clearly labelled blood pack containing standard anticoagulant and should remain with the patient until it is reinfused to avoid problems of transfusion to an inappropriate patient. Reinfusion must be completed before the patient leaves the responsibility of the anaesthetist. This procedure is most likely to be of benefit where the anticipated blood loss is greater than one litre and where the patient's haematocrit is relatively high. The degree to which the haematocrit can be lowered preoperatively depends on the status of the patient but patients who can tolerate a low haematocrit are likely to benefit most from this procedure.

Preoperative autologous deposit (PAD)

1. It may be possible for the patient to make a preoperative donation of 2–4 units of red cells – typically 1 unit per week – for autologous transfusion at or after operation. This is suitable for patients undergoing major surgery likely to require transfusion, especially if there are red cell phenotypying problems or refusal to receive donated blood. Directed donations from family or friends are not recommended in the UK, primarily because of confidence in the general safety of donor blood and concern that coercion may inhibit voluntary withdrawal of unsuitable donors.

2. Autologous donations may not be given by patients with active infections, unstable angina, aortic stenosis or severe hypertension. A haemoglobin level of > 10 g dl^{-1} is maintained with oral iron supplements. Trials have failed to demonstrate a consistent advantage from using recombinant human erythropoietin (rhEPO) to accelerate haemopoiesis. Elective orthopaedic and gynaecological surgery are two areas where up to 20% of patients may be suitable for autologous donation.

3. A number of issues mitigate against the wider applicability of this procedure:

a. Late cancellation of surgery can lead to waste.

b. Relatively few patients are suitable for PAD because of age, drug therapy or comorbidity.

c. Criteria for transfusion of donated units should be identical to those for ordinary units and not be relaxed simply because it is available.

d. Many patients become more anaemic following PAD and the likelihood of receiving a transfusion increases, whether autologous or allogeneic.

e. Current UK guidelines (British Committee for Standards in Haematology, Blood Transfusion Task Force 1993) stipulate that autologous units be tested for the same range of markers of transmissible disease as homologous donations, which increases costs and leads to ethical dilemmas if the results prove positive.

f. Although some risks of transfusion are reduced by using autologous predeposit, errors in patient identification may still occur. It is possible that bacterial contamination is more likely than with standard donor blood.

g. Hospitals need to operate secure laboratory and clinical protocols to ensure proper identification of autologous units and separation from homologous donation.

h. The practice is likely to be associated with increased cost, and benefits are difficult to quantify.

Emergency surgery

1. Patients who are clinically shocked, as from sepsis or haemorrhage, or actively bleeding, require preoperative clinical and laboratory assessment. If possible, stabilize the patient prior to operation unless there is immediate access to the operating theatre to stop the bleeding. Maintain blood pressure, circulating volume and colloid osmotic pressure. First priorities in treating acute blood volume depletion are to maintain blood pressure, circulating volume and colloid osmotic pressure and then to restore the haemoglobin level. The appropriate initial therapy is to give a synthetic plasma substitute and crystalloid.

2. Replace massive blood loss with red cells, FFP, platelets and cryoprecipitate, as indicated by results of testing for PT, APTT, TT, fibrinogen levels and platelet count. The thromboelastogram (TEG), which gives a global assessment of clotting efficiency, is used routinely in some hospitals. Maintain normothermia by transfusing all blood and fluids through a warming device. Even mild hypothermia can contribute to coagulopathy.

3. In an extreme emergency you may give uncrossmatched group O RhD negative blood, 'flying squad blood', immediately. As soon as a sample from the patient reaches the laboratory, group-compatible uncrossmatched blood may be issued within approximately 10 min. It requires 45–60 min for a full crossmatch. A retrospective crossmatch will always be performed on any uncrossmatched units transfused in an emergency.

BLOOD COMPONENTS

1. The supply of blood components in the UK is based on unpaid volunteer donors. Over 99% of donor blood is separated into components, predominantly red cells in additive solution, fresh frozen plasma (FFP), platelets and cryoprecipitate. Cryosupernatant and buffy coats are also produced (Table 8.3). The collection, testing and processing of blood products is organised within the UK by the National Blood Service under the aegis of the National Blood Authority (NBA). Fractionated plasma products, produced by the Bio Products Laboratory (BPL) section of the NBA, are now produced entirely from imported USA plasma. This is because of fears about potential transmission of variant Creutzfeldt–Jakob disease (vCJD) through the British blood supply. The fractionation process is used to produce intravenous immunglobulin (IVIg), albumin, specific immunglobulins and other products.

Table 8.3 Blood constituents available for clinical use		
Whole blood*		
Blood components*	Red cells	– plasma reduced
		– leucocyte poor
		– frozen
		– phenotyped
	Platelets	
	White cells (buffy coat)	
	Fresh frozen plasma	
	Cryoprecipitate	
Plasma products	Human albumin solution	
	Coagulation factor concentrate	
	Immunoglobulin	
	– specific	
	– standard human	

*These products are not heat treated, and all may transmit microbial infection.

2. The hospital transfusion laboratory is concerned with grouping and antibody screening of patient samples, compatibility testing and issuing of appropriate components, together with running an appropriate and accurate documentation system. Remember that, unlike the rest of pathology, the transfusion laboratory, under the direction of its consultant haematologist, is offering a therapy for patients, not merely a testing service. Seek advice regarding the appropriate use of therapeutic components from the haematologist in change.

3. All the functions of the hospital transfusion laboratory require regulation and monitoring and both internal and external quality assurance schemes are performed regularly. Hospital laboratories have standard operating procedures for all the laboratory work carried out within them. Hospitals are also required by the Department of Health, via the Better Blood Transfusion initiative, to have a set of protocols and guidelines in place which are issued to all medical staff, detailing the range of components available together with procedures and indications for their use. The standard blood-ordering schedule is one of these, as mentioned above. The Hospital Transfusion Committee (HTC) provides a forum whereby the clinical users of blood components can meet with the laboratory staff, the haematologist in charge of transfusion and the local transfusion specialists from the blood centre. The responsibilities of such a committee are to organize audit so that activity can be assessed against protocols, to provide information on use of resources, to monitor inappropriate use and adverse effects of transfusion and to provide a mechanism whereby the audit loop can be completed. Plans for education and training in blood transfusion may be drawn up by the HTC

along with new protocols and initiatives to improve blood transfusion practice within the hospital. The HTC is directly accountable to the Chief Executive and once again this pattern of responsibility is now formally expected and monitored by the Department of Health. Serious adverse events in transfusion are reported to SHOT (Serious Hazards of Transfusion), which is a national reporting body that collates anonymized data nationwide on serious adverse events. An annual report is brought out and actions are drawn up to try and improve transfusion practice in hospitals nationwide. In the 5 years since this scheme began, nearly 70% of reports to SHOT have been in the category of 'incorrect blood component transfused'.

Blood grouping and compatibility testing

Red cells carry antigens, which are typically glycoproteins or glycolipids attached to the red cell membrane. Antibodies to the ABO antigens are naturally occurring. Antibodies to other red cell antigens, such as the Rh group (CDEce), Kell, Duffy and Kidd, appear only after sensitization by transfusion or pregnancy and may cause haemolytic transfusion reactions and haemolytic disease of the fetus and newborn.

1. Naturally occurring antibodies are usually IgM antibodies but may be IgG and are found in individuals who have never been transfused with red cells or who have not been pregnant with a fetus carrying the relevant red cell antigen. They are believed to be produced in response to exposure to substances that are found within the environment, including the diet, which have similar structure to red cell antigens. Naturally occurring anti-A anti-B and anti-AB antibodies are reactive at 37°C and are complement fixing antibodies which cause intravascular lysis of ABO incompatible red cells.

2. Immune red cell antibodies are principally IgG, but can contain an IgM and/or an IGA component and these are formed as a result of exposure to foreign red cell antigens during transfusion or pregnancy. Frequency of these immune red cell alloantibodies is determined by the frequency of the antigen in the population and its immunogenicity. Of these D is by far the most immunogenic, followed by Kell (K) and c. The concentration of the antibodies decreases over time if the individual is not exposed to further antigenic stimulus and they may become undetectable in the laboratory.

 Key point

- **Report to the clinical haematologists and transfusion laboratory staff any patient with a history of a previous red cell alloantibody.**

3. In the blood transfusion laboratory all samples sent for 'group and screen' or 'group and save' have the ABO and RhD group determined using monoclonal antibodies, which cause direct agglutination of red cells at room temperature if the relevant antigen is present on those red cells. A screen for atypical red cell alloantibodies is performed in which the patient's serum is incubated with reagent red cells, usually three different ones, which between them carry all the commonest red cell antigens. Any antibodies present in the serum will coat the reagent red cells during the incubation period. The red cells are then washed to remove free antibody, and antihuman globulin (AHG) is added to cause visual agglutination of any red cells that are coated with antibody. This is known as the indirect antiglobulin test (IAT) or Coombs' test. If antibodies are detected using this test, a more extended red cell panel is used to identify which alloantibodies are present. These techniques may be carried out in glass tubes, in microtitre plates or in solid phase (Diamed) columns.

ABO, Rh compatible blood may then be crossmatched, or a G & S sample can be held until blood is required. A lower threshold for crossmatching is necessary if a patient has alloantibodies as this may cause delay in finding compatible blood at short notice.

Red cell transfusion

Major indications for transfusion of red cells are bleeding, anaemia (if severe, and the cause has been established and cannot be treated with alternatives) and bone marrow failure.

1. The majority of red cells issued in the UK are resuspended in optimum additive solution, most commonly SAG-M (sodium chloride, adenine, glucose and mannitol). The blood is anticoagulated with a citrate anticoagulant. The approximate volume of an SAG-M unit of red cells is 270 ml $\pm$ 50 ml. The haematocrit is between 0.5 and 0.7. All cellular components are leucodepleted in the UK and the white cell count per unit is less than 5×10^6. There is therefore no indication for the use of a bedside in-line filter in the UK.

2. The blood has a shelf life of 35 days when stored between 2°C and 6°C. It can be out of controlled storage temperature for up to a maximum of 5 h before transfusion is completed.

3. During storage the concentration of the red cell 2,3-diphosphoglycerate (2,3-DPG) gradually falls, which increases the oxygen affinity and reduces the amount of oxygen the cells can deliver to tissues. Red cells in SAG-M are not usually used for exchange transfusion or large volume transfusion in neonates. An alternative product using citrate phosphate dextrose and adenine (CPDA) is used.

4. There is almost no whole blood issued to any hospital in the UK at present (less than 1% of units are issued as whole blood), but alternative plasma-reduced products are sometimes available for multitransfused problem patients.

5. Red cells matched for extended phenotype are issued for patients who are transfusion dependent and at risk of producing multiple red cell alloantibodies.

6. There is a bank of frozen red cells available through the National Blood Service stored at Birmingham. These include rare units negative for specific common antigens, for use in patients with multiple red cell antibodies. These are made available for particular patients after discussion with the consultant haematologists in the National Blood Service.

Indications

1. For the majority of patients undergoing elective or emergency surgery a transfusion trigger of 8 g dl^{-1} is appropriate. Patients with known cardiovascular disease, previous myocardial infarction and the very elderly or infirm may require a higher haemoglobin perioperatively. A patient undergoing operation with a normal haemoglobin of approximately 14 g dl^{-1} can afford to lose 1.5 litres of blood before red cell transfusion becomes necessary. Clearly the patient should not be allowed to become hypovolaemic or hypotensive and the volume lost must be replaced with colloids and crystalloid as appropriate. Except in an emergency, patients should not undergo operation if they are anaemic. At preoperative clerking clinics, iron deficiency anaemia or anaemia of chronic disease can be corrected using iron therapy or erythropoietin as appropriate. This reduces unnecessary use of a limited resource and exposure of patients to potentially risky blood products.

2. A recent large randomised clinical trial in critically ill patients demonstrated that a restrictive transfusion policy aimed at maintaining Hb in the range 7–9 g dl^{-1} was at least equivalent, and possibly superior, to a liberal policy maintaining Hb at 10–12 g dl^{-1}. A trigger haemoglobin of 7–8 g dl^{-1} is therefore appropriate even in the critically ill, except perhaps for those with unstable angina or acute myocardial infarction (MI). This leaves some margin of safety over the critical level of 4–5 g dl^{-1}. At this level, oxygen consumption begins to be limited by the amount that the circulation can supply.

3. In those patients with abnormal bone marrow function from bone marrow failure resulting from drugs or marrow infiltration, it may be less appropriate to allow the haemoglobin to become so low; a maintenance trough level of 9 g dl^{-1} may be appropriate. There is now some evidence that patients receiving radiotherapy for malignancy have better outcomes if the haemoglobin is maintained at

a normal level, 12 g dl⁻¹ or more, throughout the period of radiotherapy. It relates to the effects of hypoxia on tumour growth and therefore on the efficacy of radiotherapy. Remember though, that this is a small group; the vast majority of elective surgical patients do not fall into this category.

4. As a rule of thumb, in an average-sized adult, one unit of red cells raises the haemoglobin by 1 g dl⁻¹. There is only 200 mg of bioavailable iron in a unit of red cells, so remember that this is not an appropriate treatment for iron deficiency anaemia. Transfusion may correct a severely low haemoglobin in those who are symtomatically anaemic, but it will not correct iron deficiency. Oral iron replacement therapy is required for 4–6 months. Alternatively, give a total dose infusion of iron.

Platelet transfusion

Platelet concentrates may be produced by the pooling of platelets from four standard whole blood donations or may be from donors who give platelets alone via an apheresis (Greek *apo* = from + *haireein* = to take; to separate) machine, in which case only one donor's platelets are present in each adult dose. A standard adult dose in either case is 2.4×10^{11} platelets, suspended in 150–200 ml of plasma. This product has a shelf life of 5 days and is stored at 22°C on a platelet agitator. Platelets express ABO antigens but not Rh antigens and therefore they should be ABO matched as far as possible. There are a small number of red cells present in platelet concentrate and therefore women of child-bearing age should receive RhD matched platelets. If a RhD-negative women has to be given RhD-positive platelets she should be given anti-D cover as appropriate. A standard adult dose of platelets normally raises the count by $10 \times 10^9 \text{ l}^{-1}$ at 1 h posttransfusion.

Indications

1. They are most commonly used to support patients with acute bone marrow failure, for instance after chemotherapy or stem cell transplant. If patients requiring platelet support are undergoing invasive procedures, a count of $50 \times 10^9 \text{ l}^{-1}$ may be required for line insertion and minor procedures, and a count of $80–100 \times 10^9 \text{ l}^{-1}$ for major surgery.

2. Patients with platelet function disorders, whether inherited or acquired, may have normal platelet counts but abnormal platelet function. They may require platelet support during or after surgery. The most common acquired platelet function disorder results from the ingestion of aspirin in the 7–10 days before operation. Platelet transfusion may be indicated for patients who have ingested aspirin within this period and who suffer from prolonged intra- or postoperative oozing.

3. Platelets, together with FFP and cryoprecipitate, may need to be given for consumptive coagulopathy such as disseminated intravascular coagulation (DIC). The transfused blood components should be given on the basis of laboratory coagulation parameters and platelet counts.

4. Massive red cell transfusion may eventually produce dilutional thrombocytopenia and require platelet transfusion, controlled as far as possible from the laboratory results.

5. Patients may require platelet support when on extracorporeal bypass, undergoing for example open heart surgery, even though the platelet count is normal or near normal, because the platelets are activated while in the extracorporeal circuit and therefore may be ineffective in haemostasis.

Platelets are not indicated for:

- Chronic thrombocytopenia, unless there are bleeding problems
- Prophylatically for patients undergoing bypass
- Immune thrombocytopenic purpura, except in the case of critical bleeding.

Platelet transfusion is contraindicated because it may aggravate the underlying conditions in:

- Heparin-induced thrombocytopenia, which is an autoimmune-mediated condition resulting in arterial blood clotting
- Thrombocytic thrombocytopenic purpura.

All patients receiving prophylatic or therapeutic heparin using unfractionated or low molecular weight heparin should have a platelet count performed prior to commencement of heparin, on the day following and every 2 days thereafter.

 Key point

- **Suspect heparin-induced thrombocytopenia if there is a drop in platelet count below $100 \times 10^9 \text{ l}^{-1}$ and urgently seek advice from a haematologist. Amputation results in 30% of cases. Stop heparin, use an alternative anticoagulant.**

Fresh frozen plasma (FFP)

1. FFP is prepared by centrifugation of donor whole blood within 8 h of collection, and frozen at –30°C. It may be stored for up to 12 months and is thawed prior to administration, 300 ml taking approximately 20 min to thaw. Once thawed it should be used within 2 h as there

is exponential degradation of the clotting factors at room temperature.

2. Compatibility testing is not required, but group compatible units are used. FFP contains coagulation factors, including the labile factors V and VIII and the vitamin K-dependent factors II, VII, IX and X.

3. In clinical practice FFP is frequently given unnecessarily, and, when it is indicated, not enough is given. To correct abnormal coagulation a dose of 15 ml kg^{-1} is required. In a 70 kg adult this is almost 1 litre of FFP; corrected to the nearest whole bag this is three bags.

4. Standard FFP carries the same risks as red cells for transmitting viral, bacterial and prion disease. Some virally inactivated plasmas are now available. Solvent detergent-treated plasma is created from pools of up to 1000 donors, which are available as Octaplas™, and non-pooled methylene blue-treated plasma is now available for paediatric use via the National Blood Service. Both of these products are safer in terms of viral transmission than standard FFP, although they are still not completely safe and some viruses may not be inactivated. Viral inactivation procedures have no effect on possible prion transmission. Clotting factor levels are slightly diminished in both products, possibility resulting in the need to use a greater number of units per patient.

Indications

The indications for FFP transfusion are:

1. Coagulation factor replacement where there is no concentrate available. In hospitals with an interest in haemophilia and haemostasis the vast majority of inherited clotting factor deficiencies are treated with specific concentrates, with the exception of factor V deficiency for which there is no concentrate available. In hospitals without a specialist unit, FFP may be used more widely for clotting factor deficiencies.
2. To correct abnormal clotting in patients with DIC or those who have undergone massive transfusion or cardiopulmonary bypass. In all these give FFP guided by the coagulation results obtained from near-patient testing, or from the central laboratory.
3. To correct abnormal coagulation in patients with liver disease and poor synthetic function. Administration of vitamin K may also help in this situation.
4. To reverse oral anticoagulation as from, for example, over warfarinization, if there are no concentrates available.
5. Specifically indicated for plasma exchange in the management of thrombotic thrombocytopenic purpura (TTP) and haemolytic uraemic syndrome (HUS). Cryo-poor FFP may be a superior product in this setting.

FFP should not be used:

1. To treat hypovolaemia which can adequately be managed using colloid and crystalloid solutions.
2. For plasma exchange except in the specific circumstances stated above.
3. As a 'formula' replacement; for example, there is no need to administer two bags of FFP for every 4 or 6 units of red cells transfused. Give replacement with FFP on the basis of clotting results, or, if necessary, for clinical indication.
4. In the management of nutritional or immunodeficiency states.
5. In bleeding due to thrombocytopenia or hypofibrinogenaemia, for which platelet concentrates and cryoprecipitate, respectively, are indicated.

Cryoprecipitate

1. This is prepared from FFP by freezing and thawing plasma and then separating the white precipitate from the supernatant plasma. Cryoprecipitate (Greek *kryos* = frost) contains half of the factor VIII, fibrinogen and fibronectin from the donation and also the majority of the von Willebrand factor. In common with FFP, it is stored at −30°C for up to 12 months. As the volume of each pack is only 10–20 ml, the product thaws very quickly and can be ordered when it is about to be given. Also, like FFP, the effectiveness of the product decreases rapidly once it has been thawed. A standard adult dose is 10 units, which should be ABO compatible but not crossmatched.

2. Cryoprecipiate is indicated when replacement of fibrinogen is required in those with congenital or acquired hypofibrinogenaemic states. In DIC, if the fibrinogen drops below 0.8 g l^{-1}, give cryoprecipitate. Remember to request a fibrinogen level in patients with massive bleeding or DIC as this is not automatically performed with a clotting screen in most laboratories. Cryoprecipitate was formerly the mainstay of management of patients with von Willebrand's disease but a concentrate is now available for this condition at many centres.

Plasma products

These are produced by a fractionation process and are derived from pooled human plasma. The product is concentrated and sterilized and the risk of infection is markedly reduced. However, there is still a theoretical risk that they could transmit prion proteins, which are implicated as a transmissible cause of new variant Creutzfeldt–Jakob disease (nvCJD). For this reason all plasma for fractionation in the UK is now imported from the United States, where it is taken from accredited donors. The processing still takes place in the UK.

Albumin solution

This is usually available as 20 g albumin in 400 ml, as a 5% solution, or 100 ml of 20% solution. Each unit also contains sodium 130–150 mmol l^{-1} plus other plasma proteins and stabilizer. The main indications for albumin are hypoproteinaemia with nephrotic syndrome (20%) and chronic liver disease (20%) and acute volume replacement (5%), for example, for plasma exchange. It may also be used in hypoproteinaemia following burns after the first 24 h. There is no evidence that albumin solutions are necessary to restore circulatory volume following haemorrhage, shock or multiple organ failure; colloid and crystalloid solutions are equally efficacious, cheaper and probably safer.

Coagulation factor concentrates

1. These are largely used in patients with congenital bleeding disorders, and recombinant factor VIII and factor IX are now widely used. Concentrates are also available, manufactured from pooled fractionated human plasma, sourced from outside the UK.

2. Prothrombin complex concentrate contains factors IX, X and II and is used to treat bleeding complications in inherited deficiencies of these factors. When given with vitamin K, it is also used to treat oral anticoagulant overdose, and in severe liver failure. Its use carries a risk of provoking thrombosis and DIC.

3. Other concentrates include the naturally occurring anticoagulant factors protein C, antithrombin (see below) and factors VII, XI and XIII; they are used in corresponding congenital deficiencies. FEIBA (factor VIII bypassing activity concentrate) is used in patients with inhibitors to factor VIII, as is recombinant factor VIIa in some circumstances. Recombinant factor VIIa has also recently been used experimentally for management of massive bleeding that is not responding to other clotting concentrates and platelet infusions. There is now a substantial body of anecdotal evidence that this may be effective and life saving in some cases. Recombinant factor VIIa has significant prothrombotic effects; it is extremely expensive and should only be used under the guidance of a haematologist experienced in its use. A fibrinogen concentrate is now available for severe forms of hypofibrinogenaemia, both congenital and acquired, and fibrin sealants are also available.

Immunoglobulins

These are prepared from pooled donor plasma by fractionation and sterile filtration. Specific immunoglobulins include hepatitis B and herpes zoster and can provide passive immune protection. Standard human immunoglobulin for intramuscular injection is used for prophylaxis against hepatitis A, rubella and measles, whereas hyperimmune globulin is prepared from donors with high titres of the relevant antibodies for prophylaxis of tetanus, hepatitis A, diphtheria, rabies, mumps, measles, rubella, cytomegalovirus and *Pseudomonas* infections. Intravenous immunoglobulin is used as replacement therapy in patients with congenital or acquired immune deficiency and in autoimmune disorders (e.g. idiopathic thrombocytopenic purpura).

Plasma substitutes

These include products based on hydroxyethyl starch (HES), dextran (a branch-chained polysaccharide composed of glucose units) and modified gelatin. Such components remain in the circulation longer than crystalloid solutions – up to 6 h for modified gelatin and up to 24 h for some high molecular weight starch-based products. Other advantages are that they are relatively non-toxic, inexpensive, can be stored at room temperature, do not require compatibility testing and do not transmit infection. Adverse effects include anaphylaxis, fever and rash, such effects being more frequent with starch-based products. Dextran can also impair coagulation and platelet function and can interfere with compatibility testing.

 Key point

- **Take a blood sample for crossmatching before administering dextran.**

The maximum dose of synthetic plasma expanders is approximately 20–30 ml kg^{-1}. Patients receiving larger volumes or with significant evidence of other organ failure, such as pulmonary or renal disease, or a bleeding diathesis, may be given albumin.

ADVERSE CONSEQUENCES OF BLOOD TRANSFUSION

In general, transfusion of blood and products is a safe and effective mode of treatment.

1. The safe administration of blood components is a deceptively complex process involving phlebotomists, clerical staff, junior doctors, porters and nurses as well as transfusion laboratory staff. A survey in the UK (McClelland & Phillips 1994) suggests that a 'wrong blood in patient' incident occurs approximately once per 30 000 units of red cells transfused. By far the commonest cause is a failure at the bedside of pretransfusion identity checking procedures, either at the time of phlebotomy or while setting up the actual transfusion.

Key point

- **Pay rigorous attention to all administrative and clerical aspects of blood component therapy; they are overwhelmingly the commonest cause of fatal errors.**

2. In the UK all hospitals participate in the SHOT (Serious Hazards of Transfusion) reporting scheme which allows for anonymized reporting of serious transfusion events to a centralized data collecting body. Cumulative data from the past 5 years has shown that 'Incorrect blood component transfused' is by far the commonest reported event, with nearly 70% of all reports coming into this category. Conversely, the most feared and well-publicized complication, that of infectious disease transmission, is one of the very least common categories, with only 1–2% of cases. It is now mandatory for all hospitals to participate in the SHOT scheme as set out in the Department of Health circular *Better Blood Transfusion*, published in July 2002 (Table 8.4).

Immune complications

ABO-incompatible red cell transfusions lead to life-threatening intravascular haemolysis of transfused cells, manifesting as fever, rigors, haemoglobinuria, hypotension and renal failure (immediate haemolytic transfusion reaction (HTR)). In the anaesthetized patient, the only signs may be persistent hypotension and unexplained oozing from the wound.

Atypical antibodies arising from previous transfusions or pregnancy may cause intravascular haemolysis but more commonly lead to extravascular haemolysis in liver and spleen and may be delayed for 1–3 weeks (delayed HTR). Typical manifestations are jaundice, progressive anaemia, fever, arthralgia and myalgia. Diagnosis is easily established by a positive direct antiglobulin test (DAT) and a positive antibody screen. Non-haemolytic febrile transfusion reaction (NHFTR) usually occurs within hours of transfusion in multitransfused patients with antibodies against HLA antigens or granulocyte-specific antibodies. The reaction is due to pyrogens released from granulocytes damaged by complement in an antigen–antibody reaction. It presents as a rise in temperature, with flushing, palpitations and tachycardia, followed by headache and rigors. Hypersensitivity reactions to plasma components may cause urticaria, wheezing, facial oedema and pyrexia, but can cause anaphylactic shock, for example, in patients with congenital IgA deficiency who have anti-IgA antibodies following previous sensitization.

Treatment

Stop the transfusion immediately in all cases except for the appearance of a mild pyrexia in a multiply transfused patient. Check clerical details and send samples from the donor unit and recipient for analysis for compatibility and haemolysis. Have the recipient serum analysed for the presence of atypical red cell leucocyte HLA and plasma protein antibodies. Treat severe haemolytic transfusion reactions with support care to maintain blood pressure and renal function, to promote diuresis and treat shock. Intravenous steroids and antihistamines may be needed, with the use of adrenaline (epinephrine) in severe cases. Manage NHFTR by administering antipyretics.

Table 8.4 Hazards of transfusion

	Non-immune complications	Immune complications
Acute	Hypothermia Hyperkalaemia ($\uparrow K^+$) Hypocalcaemia ($\downarrow Ca^{2+}$) Air embolism Bacterial (endotoxic) shock	Febrile non-haemolytic transfusion reaction Acute haemolytic reaction (ABO incompatibility) Allergic reactions (urticarial or anaphylactic) TRALI (transfusion-related acute lung injury)
Delayed	HIV Hepatitis C Hepatitis B CMV Parvovirus B19 **Others**: e.g.: hepatitis A, malaria, brucellosis, syphilis, trypanosomiasis, vCJD?	Delayed haemolytic transfusion reaction (due to red cell alloantibodies) Post-transfusion purpura Transfusion-associated graft versus host disease Immune modulation

Transmission of infection

1. Blood transfusion is an important mode of transmission of a range of viral, bacterial and protozoal infections. There is also a theoretical risk of transmitting infections mediated by prion proteins such as new variant CJD (Flanagan & Barbara 1996, 1998), although no proven or even probable instances of such transmissions have ever been identified. However, concern has been raised by a study in which one (of 19) asymptomatic sheep, 318 days after being given 5 g of brain infected with bovine spongiform encephalopathy (BSE) in the feed, appeared to transmit BSE to a second sheep via a 400 ml venous transfusion (Brown 2000, Houston et al 2000). A recent update on this study suggests that up to four sheep may now be suffering from transfusion transmitted prion disease. Therefore, until definitive evidence becomes available, steps have been taken to reduce the risk of transfusion as a possible secondary route of transmission of vCJD (Brown et al 2001):

- In UK from November 1999:
  - ban on using UK plasma for manufacture of fractionated products (e.g. albumin, clotting factors, IVIg)
  - leucodepletion of all blood, platelets, FFP, cryoprecipitate (as leucocytes believed to play key role in vCJD pathogenesis)
- In other countries (e.g. USA, Canada, New Zealand etc.):
  - exclusion as blood donors of people who have lived in the UK for >6 months between 1980 and 1996.

2. It should be emphasized that the safety of blood components and fractionated plasma products has improved greatly in recent years. Bacterial infections can occur through failure of sterile technique at the time of collection, commonly by organisms such as *Staphylococcus aureus* or *Staph. epidermidis*, or bacteraemia in the donor – especially if organisms such as *Yersinia*, which can survive at 4°C, are incriminated.

3. There are more fatalities per annum from bacterial or endotoxic complications, usually relating to platelets, than from viral transmissions. Donors at risk of malaria are not eligible to donate, but a malarial antibody test is likely to be available for screening at-risk donors in the near future. Transmission of syphilis is now very rare.

Viral infection

Transmission of viruses may occur in spite of mandatory screening because: serological tests may not have had time to become positive in a potentially infectious individual; the virus may not have been identified; or the most sensitive serological tests may not be routinely performed. The risk of transmission is much lower, although still present, for those blood products that have undergone a manufacturing and sterilization process (Table 8.5).

Key point

- **The perceived risk of viral transmission is high: the actual risk in the UK is very low – less than 1 in 4 million for HIV and 1 in 3 million for hepatitis C (Williamson et al 1996).**

Table 8.5 Risk of virus transmission

Risk factor	Estimated frequency per unit transfused	Deaths per million units
Acute haemolytic reactions	1 in 250 000 to 1 in 1 000 000	0.67
Hepatitis B	1 in 100 000 to 1 in 400 000*	<0.5
Hepatitis C	1 in 3 000 000†	<0.5
HIV	1 in 4 000 000	<0.5
Bacterial contamination of red cell concentrates	1 in 500 000	<0.25

*Data on viral markers from Kate Soldan, National Blood Service/CPHL.
†Data on hepatitis C markers from Dr Pat Hewitt and Dr John Barbara, National Blood Service.

Adapted from British Committee for Standards in Haematology, Blood Transfusion Task Force 2001 Guidelines for the Clinical Use of Red Cell Transfusions. British Journal of Haematology 113: 24–31

Other complications

1. There is increasing evidence that transfusion of blood components can cause immunosuppression in the recipient. This may lead to earlier relapse or recurrence of malignant disease after surgical removal of malignant tumours (shortened disease-free interval), as well as an increased incidence of postoperative infection. These effects are probably due to defective cell-mediated immunity and are reduced by giving leucocyte-depleted components.

2. Circulatory overload may result from the infusion of large volumes in patients with incipient heart failure. Iron overload occurs in patients who have received repeated red cell transfusions and these patients require iron chelation therapy (Greek *chele* = claw; attaching the iron to an agent that renders it harmless).

3. Graft versus host disease may be caused by transfusion of T lymphocytes into severely immunosuppressed hosts, and cellular components should be irradiated prior to transfusion to severely immunodeficient patients.

INTRAOPERATIVE ASSESSMENT

1. Rapid bleeding confined to one site is almost always a technical problem. Suspect haemostatic failure in a high risk patient with multiple sites of bleeding, or if the pattern of bleeding is unusual; confirm it with appropriate laboratory tests.

2. The following tests are useful in assessing the degree of blood loss and should serve as a guide for determining the need for replacement therapy:

- *Oxygen-carrying capacity of blood*
  - haemoglobin concentration
  - pulse oximetry
- *Haemostatic function*
  - coagulation screen:
    prothrombin time (PT)
    activated partial thromboplastin time (APTT)
    thrombin time (TT)
  - platelet count
  - fibrinogen level
  - thromboelastography.

3. Quantification of intraoperative blood loss is imprecise. Confirm clinical evaluation with laboratory tests (Table 8.6), many of which cannot be performed outside the main laboratory. Thromboelastography is a useful and rapid test, producing a graphical record of in vitro blood clot formation and dissolution; it provides a global test of coagulation and fibrinolysis which can be performed rapidly within the operating suite in high risk patients.

4. There has been a recent resurgence in other forms of near-patient testing, in particular in coagulometers, which are becoming available at the bedside in intensive care units, operating theatres, high dependency units and obstetric units, and also in accident and emergency units. These provide a 5 min turnaround time for PT and APPT, instead of over an hour when samples are sent to the central laboratory. The availability of a Hemacue for rapid haemoglobin results has also improved management of the bleeding patient in these sites.

Intraoperative autologous transfusion

1. Acute normovolaemic haemodilution (ANH) involves removal of 1–2 units of whole blood during induction of anaesthesia, with replacement by crystalloid, reducing the haematocrit to 25–30%. Operation is usually well tolerated, the collected blood can be returned later during the operation, and there is no need to undertake virological testing of the unit (Williamson 1994).

2. Salvage of blood lost during an operation (British Committee for Standards in Haematology, Blood Transfusion Task Force 1997) is accomplished using a simple device such as Solcotrans, or a cell saver such as Haemonetics, Dideco or Fresenius.

Table 8.6   Results of laboratory tests as an aid in differential diagnosis of excessive bleeding

Cause of bleeding	Laboratory test				
	PT	APTT	TT without protamine	TT with protamine	Platelet count
Loss of platelets	N	N	N	N	↓↓
Lack of coagulation factors	↑↑	↑↑	N	N	N or ↓
Excess of heparin	↑	↑↑	↑	N	N or ↓
Hyperfibrinolysis	↑	↑	↑↑	↑↑	N or ↓
DIC	↑↑	↑↑	↑↑	↑↑	↓↓
Massive blood transfusion	↑	↑	N	N	↓
Vitamin K deficiency	↑↑	↑	N	N	N

N, normal; ↑↑, markedly raised; ↑, mildly raised; ↓↓, markedly decreased; ↓, mildly decreased.

3. Blood shed into the thoracic or abdominal cavity is aspirated and mixed with anticoagulant. It can then be returned to the patient (Solcotrans), or the red cells can be washed, suspended in saline and transfused to the patient (cell savers). The use of a cell saver may considerably reduce the number of units required for transfusion. Contraindications to using the blood salvage procedure are exposure of blood to a site of infection or the possibility of contamination with malignant cells. Postoperative blood lost into drains can also be salvaged using the cell saver.

Methods of reducing intraoperative blood loss

Meticulous surgical technique clearly plays a major role, but there is increasing interest in the use of pharmacological agents to improve haemostasis. Desmopressin (DDAVP) improves platelet function by increasing plasma concentrations of von Willebrand factor, but has not been convincingly shown to reduce blood loss in cardiac surgery. Aprotinin is a serine protease inhibitor which inhibits fibrinolysis and has been shown to reduce blood loss and operative morbidity in cardiac surgery (particularly in repeat procedures) and major hepatic surgery such as liver transplantation (Hunt 1991).

Special situations

Massive blood transfusion

This is defined as transfusion of a volume greater than the recipient's blood volume in less than 24 h. Standard red cell concentrates in SAG-M can be transfused rapidly using a pressure infuser or a pump, and a blood warmer prevents the patient developing hypothermia. FFP, cryoprecipitate and platelet concentrates of the same blood group as the red cells may also be required. They should be given on the basis of clotting screens, fibrinogen levels and platelet counts as far as possible.

Complications include:

1. Cardiac abnormalities such as ventricular extrasystoles, ventricular fibrillation (rarely) and cardiac arrest from the combined effects of low temperature, high potassium concentration and excess citrate with low calcium concentration. They can be prevented by using a blood warmer and a slower rate of transfusion, particularly in patients with hepatic or renal failure. Routine administration of calcium gluconate is unnecessary and may even be dangerous unless the ionized calcium concentration in the plasma can be monitored.

2. Acidosis in the patient with severe renal or liver disease may be aggravated by the low pH of stored blood.

3. Failure of haemostasis manifests as local oozing and, infrequently, as a generalized bleeding tendency due to the lack of coagulation factors and platelets in stored blood. Laboratory assessment is essential (see above). FFP (15 ml kg^{-1}) corrects the abnormalities of coagulation and may need to be given without the benefit of laboratory results in an emergency if 10 units or more of red cells have been given. Platelet transfusion may be required when the platelet count is lower than 50×10^9 l^{-1} or to maintain a count at 80×10^9 l^{-1} if the patient is bleeding.

4. Hypothermia contributes to failure of haemostasis, as the enzymatic clotting cascade functions best at 37°C. Patients receiving large quantities of red cells, colloids and crystalloids become hypothermic and their clotting is suboptimal. Anticipate this problem, as clotting tests from the laboratory may be normalized by being performed at 37°C in vitro.

 Key point

- **Avoid hypothermia by using a blood warmer and fluid warmer, and keeping the patient as warm as possible.**

5. Adult respiratory distress syndrome (ARDS), also called non-cardiogenic pulmonary oedema, occurs in severely ill patients after major trauma and/or surgery. Clinical features include progressive respiratory distress, decreased lung compliance, acute hypoxaemia and diffuse radiographic opacification of the lungs. The mortality is high; post-mortem studies show widespread macroscopic and microscopic thrombosis in the pulmonary arteries. Local DIC, microvascular fluid leakage and embolization of leucocyte aggregates and microaggregates from stored blood all contribute to pathogenesis. Management consists of stopping the transfusion, administering corticosteroids and providing supportive treatment to combat pulmonary oedema and hypoxia, by administering oxygen and giving positive pressure ventilation.

Transfusion in open heart surgery

This requires cardiopulmonary bypass (CPB) for maintaining the circulation with oxygentated blood. In adults, blood is not required for priming of the heart–lung machine, but it is needed in neonates and small children. Usually 4 units of blood, ideally less than 5 days old, are initially crossmatched, or 6–8 units for repeat procedures.

It is unnecessary to use albumin solutions, either for priming the heart–lung machine or postoperatively.

Bleeding associated with CPB results from activation and loss of platelets and coagulation factors in the extra-corporeal circulation, failure of heparin neutralization by the first dose of protamine, activation of fibrinolysis in the oxygenator and pump and/or DIC in patients with poor cardiac output and long perfusion times.

Management requires:

- Administration of 1–2 pools of platelet concentrate when the platelet count is less than 30×10^9 l^{-1}
- Transfusion of 15 ml kg^{-1} of FFP to correct the loss of coagulation factors
- Neutralization of excess heparin by protamine (1 mg of protamine neutralizes approximately 100 units of heparin)
- Administration of tranexamic acid, or a similar anti-fibrinolytic agent, when hyperfibrinolysis is confirmed by laboratory testing
- Treatment of DIC, in the first instance by correcting the underlying cause, such as poor perfusion, oligaemic shock, acidosis or infection, and then by transfusing FFP and platelet concentrate, as required.

Prostatic surgery

This may be followed by excessive urinary bleeding, the result of local fibrinolysis related to the release of high concentrations of urokinase. Antifibrinolytic agents, which include ε-aminocaproic acid (EACA) and tranex-amic acid, are often helpful in reducing clot dissolution, but use them cautiously, as fibrinolytic inhibition can lead to ureteric obstruction, caused by clot formation, in patients with upper urinary tract bleeding. Patients undergoing prostatic surgery are frequently the same patients who are taking low dose aspirin prophylactically to reduce the risks of coronary artery disease and stroke; determine preoperatively if it can safely be stopped. Following prostate surgery, bleeding can be extreme if aspirin intake has resulted in platelet dysfunction.

Liver disease

This warrants special mention as the liver is an important site of manufacture of the components as well as the regu-latory factors of the coagulation and fibrinolytic pathways (Mehta & McIntyre 1998). Vitamin K is required for hepatic synthesis of the coagulation factors II, VII, IX and X, as well as the coagulation inhibitors protein C and S. Impaired vitamin K absorption can occur in biliary obstruction, so give 10 mg vitamin K by intramuscular injection preoperatively. The liver is also the site of manu-facture of factor V and fibrinogen (factor I), the regulatory factors antithrombin and α_2-antiplasmin. In addition, defects of both platelet function and number, such as thrombocytopenia due to complicating hypersplenism, can occur. These patients are at increased risk of DIC and renal failure, and require assessment by a gastroenterologist/ hepatologist as well as a haematologist (see Chs 6, 15).

POST-OPERATIVE ASSESSMENT

1. Anaemia, coagulopathy and excessive bleeding in the immediate postoperative period are often the result of the operation or its complications. Continue blood com-ponent therapy that was commenced intraoperatively for the management of special situations, adhering to the same transfusion triggers for all components that were used intraoperatively (see above).

2. Patients with excessive bleeding and clinical evi-dence of haemostatic failure require laboratory assess-ment (Table 8.6). The trauma of operation triggers both the coagulation and fibrinolytic pathways and places patients at increased risk of DIC. Do not routinely use red cell transfusions to correct postoperative anaemia, unless the haemoglobin falls to below 8 g dl^{-1} or is excessively symptomatic, as this practice has not been shown to improve wound healing or aid surgical recovery. Recovery of haemoglobin to normal levels may result from routinely giving iron and folic acid supplements after operation. Thromboprophylaxis is an important aspect of postoperative care (see Ch. 34).

FUTURE DIRECTIONS

The field of transfusion medicine is rapidly developing and there is increasing awareness of the risks of hom-ologous blood (Greek *homos* = the same; from the same species. Not autologous, Greek *autos* = self.). The advent of recombinant DNA technology has already led to use of recombinant erythropoietin, but granulocyte and granulocyte-monocyte colony stimulating factors are in routine use to elevate the white cell count in leucopenic patients. Synthetic oxygen carriers ('artificial blood') have been under development for many years (Ogden & MacDonald 1995). Perfluorocarbons dissolve oxygen but function only in high concentrations of ambient oxygen and are useful only for short-term perfusion in intensive care unit situations, such as following coronary angio-plasty. Recombinant haemoglobin solutions and liposo-mal haemoglobin are under active development.

Summary

- Do you recognize the need for preoperative haematological assessment to identify those who are already anaemic, requiring investigation and treatment before operation? You may also detect inherited or acquired factors, such as anaemia, haemoglobinopathy, excessive bleeding tendency, affecting outcome of surgery and anaesthesia.
- Are you aware of the available range of blood components and plasma products for intra- and postoperative use, their specific indications and associated risks?
- What are the benefits of the increasingly used intraoperative cell salvage and autologous transfusion?
- Do you accept that administrative and clerical failures dwarf the perceived risks of transmitting infection?
- Do you appreciate the need to seek early advice from the clinical and scientific haematology staff on perioperative care of patients with inherited or acquired haematological conditions, and also in special situations, such as massive transfusion?
- Are you aware of written policies and procedures in your institution governing the ordering, prescription, administration and documentation of blood components and plasma product therapy?

References

British Committee for Standards in Haematology 1990 Guidelines for implementation of a maximum surgical blood order schedule. Clinical and Laboratory Haematology 12: 321–327

British Committee for Standards in Haematology, Blood Transfusion Task Force 1993 Guidelines for autologous transfusion. 1. Pre-operative autologous donation. Transfusion Medicine 3: 307–316

British Committee for Standards in Haematology, Blood Transfusion Task Force 1997 Guidelines for autologous transfusion. II. Peri-operative haemodilution and cell salvage. British Journal of Anaesthesia 78: 768–771

Brown P 2000 BSE and transmission through blood. Lancet 356: 955–956

Brown P, Will RG, Bradley R, Asher DM, Detwiler L 2001 Bovine spongiform encephalopathy and variant Creutzfeldt–Jakob disease: background, evolution and current concerns. Emerging Infectious Diseases 7: 6–16

Flanagan P, Barbara J 1996 Prion disease and blood transfusion. Transfusion Medicine 6: 213–215

Flanagan P, Barbara J 1998 Blood transfusion the risk: protecting against the unknown. BMJ 316: 717–718

Houston F, Foster JD, Chong A, Hunter N, Bostock CJ 2000 Transmission of BSE by blood transfusion in a sheep. Lancet 356: 999–1000

Hunt BJ 1991 Modifying peri-operative blood loss. Blood Reviews 5: 168–176

McClelland DBL, Phillips P 1994 Errors in blood transfusion in Britain: survey of hospital haematology departments. BMJ 308: 1205–1206

Mehta AB 1994 Glucose-6-phosphate dehydrogenase deficiency. Prescribers Journal 34: 178–182

Mehta AB, McIntyre N 1998 Haematological changes in liver disease. Trends in Experimental and Clinical Medicine 8: 8–25

Ogden JE, MacDonald SL 1995 Haemoglobin based red cell substitutes: current status. Vox Sanguinis 69: 302–308

Vichinsky EP, Haberkern CM, Neumayr L et al 1995 A comparison of conservative and aggressive transfusion regimens in the peri-operative management of sickle cell disease. New England Journal of Medicine 333: 206–213

Williamson L 1994 Homologous blood transfusion: the risks and alternatives. British Journal of Haematology 88: 451–458

Williamson LM, Heptonstall J, Soldan K 1996 A SHOT in the arm for safer blood transfusion. BMJ 313: 1221–1222

Further reading

Asher D, Atterbury CLJ, Chapman C et al 2002 SHOT Report 2000–2001. Serious Hazards of Transfusion Steering Group, London

Contreras M (ed.) 1998 ABC of transfusion, 3rd edn. British Medical Journal, London

McClelland DBL (ed.) 1995 Clinical Resources and Audit Group: optimal use of donor blood. Scottish Office, Edinburgh

McClelland DBL (ed.) 2001 Handbook of transfusion medicine, 3rd edn. HMSO, London

Mintz P (ed.) 1999 Transfusion therapy: clinical principles and practice. American Association of Blood Banks, Virginia

Regan F, Taylor C (2002) Recent developments in transfusion medicine. BMJ 325: 143–147

Useful link

www.doh.gov.uk/publications/coinh.html   Better blood transfusion: HSC 2002/009

9 Fluid, electrolyte and acid–base balance

W. Aveling, M. A. Hamilton

Objectives

To understand:

- **The physiology of fluid distribution throughout the body**
- **Methods of detecting hypovolaemia**
- **Managing fluid balance**
- **Principles of acid–base balance**
- **Interpretation of arterial blood gas results.**

INTRODUCTION

To be able to manage the surgical patient optimally you must ensure that all tissues are perfused with oxygenated blood throughout the course of the operation and the postoperative recovery period. To do this well you need to understand the basics of fluid balance in the healthy person and then be able to apply this knowledge, along with that of basic physiology, to your patient. Understand the results provided by both arterial blood gas analysis and modern monitoring systems, including their limitations, in order to achieve optimal tissue perfusion. This has been shown to result in reduced mortality, morbidity and length of hospital stay.

FLUID COMPARTMENTS

Every medical student knows that humans are mostly water. For you, the key to fluid and electrolyte balance is a knowledge of the various fluid compartments. An adult male is 60% water; a female, having more fat, is 55% water; newborn infants are 75% water. The most important compartments are the intracellular fluid (ICF) – 55% of body water – and the extracellular fluid (ECF) – 45%. Extracellular fluid is further subdivided into the plasma (part of the intravascular space), the interstitial (Latin *inter* = between + *sistere* = to stand; the fluid between the cells) fluid, the transcellular water (e.g. fluid in the gastrointestinal tract, the cerebrospinal fluid (CSF) and aqueous humour). Water associated with bone and dense connective tissue, which is less readily exchangeable, is of much less importance. The partitioning of the total body water (TBW) with average values for a 70 kg male, who would contain 42 litres of water, is shown in Figure 9.1 (Edelman & Leibman 1959).

To understand fluid balance you need to know from which compartment or compartments fluid is being lost in various situations, and in which compartments fluids will end up when administered to the patient. For practical purposes you need only consider the plasma, the interstitial space, the intracellular space and the barriers between them.

The capillary membrane

1. The barrier between the plasma and interstitium (Latin *inter* = between + *sistere* = to stand; hence intercellular spaces) is the capillary endothelium, which allows the free passage of water and electrolytes (small particles) but restricts the passage of larger molecules such as proteins (the colloids – Greek *kolla* = glue + *eidos* = form). Although no one has demonstrated holes in the membrane, capillaries behave as if they had pores of 4–5 nm (Greek *nanos* = dwarf; 10^{-9}) in most tissues. Kidney and liver capillaries have larger pores but brain capillaries are relatively impermeable.

2. The osmotic (Greek *otheein* = to push) pressure generated by the presence of colloids on one side of a membrane which is impermeable to them is known as the colloid osmotic pressure (COP). Only a small quantity of albumin (mol. wt 69 000) crosses the membrane and it is mainly responsible for the difference in COP between the plasma and the interstitium. In fact any particle, electrolyte or protein, can exert an osmotic pressure, but the free diffusion of electrolytes across the capillary wall negates their osmotic effect. Passage of proteins across the capillary wall is impeded in the normal state. For this reason they exert an osmotic effect within the capillary, commonly referred to as the colloid osmotic pressure or oncotic (Greek *onkos* = mass; referring to the

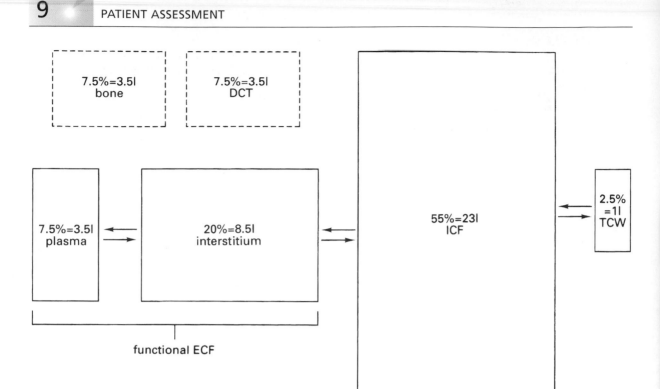

Fig. 9.1 Distribution of total body water in a 70 kg man. DCT, dense connective tissue; ECF, extracellular fluid; ICF, intracellular fluid; TCW, transcellular water.

larger particle size) pressure. The osmotic effect of these proteins is about 50% greater than would be expected for the proteins alone. The reason for this is that most proteins are negatively charged, attracting positively charged ions such as sodium – the Gibbs–Donnan effect. These positively charged ions are osmotically active and therefore increase the effective osmotic pressure.

3. The COP is normally about 25 mmHg and tends to draw fluid into the capillary, while the hydrostatic pressure difference between capillary and interstitium tends to push fluid out. This balance was first described by the physiologist Henry Starling at University College, London, in 1896.

4. Staverman (1952) introduced the concept that different molecules are 'reflected' to a different extent by the membrane. This term, the reflection coefficient, varies between zero (all molecules passing through the membrane) and +1 (all molecules reflected). In disease states when the capillary membrane becomes leaky, such as sepsis and the systemic inflammatory response syndrome (SIRS), the reflection coefficient falls. Flow across the membrane is represented by the equation:

$$V = K_f S[P_c - P_{IF}) - \sigma\ (\pi p - \pi_{IF})]$$

where V is the rate of movement of water, K_f is the capillary filtration coefficient, S is the surface area; P_c and P_{IF} are the capillary and interstitial hydrostatic pressures, πp

and π_{IF} are the plasma and interstitial oncotic pressures, and σ is the reflection coefficient.

The cell membrane

The barrier between the extracellular and intracellular space is the cell membrane. This is freely permeable to water but not to sodium ions, which are actively pumped out of cells. Sodium is therefore mainly an extracellular cation, while potassium is the main intracellular cation. Water moves across the cell membrane in either direction if there is any difference in osmolality between the two sides. Osmolality expresses the osmotic pressure across a selectively permeable membrane and depends on the number of particles in the solution, not their size. Normal osmolality of ECF is 280–295 mOsm kg^{-1}. Since each cation is balanced by an anion, an estimate of plasma or ECF osmolality can be obtained from the formula:[1]

Osmolality (mOsm kg^{-1})
= 2 (Na$^+$ + K$^+$) + glucose + urea (mmol l^{-1})

---

[1]Osmolality is expressed per kilogram of solvent (usually water), whereas osmolarity is expressed per litre of solution. The presence of significant amounts of protein in the solution, as in plasma, means that the osmolality and osmolarity will not be the same.

Note that the colloids contribute very little to total osmolality as the number of particles is small, although, as we saw above, they play an important role in fluid movement across the capillaries.

Movement of water between compartments

1. Consider what happens when a patient takes in water, either by drinking or in the form of a 5% glucose infusion, the glucose in which is soon metabolized. It is rapidly distributed throughout the ECF, with a resultant fall in ECF osmolality. Since osmolality must be the same inside and outside cells, water moves from ECF to ICF until the osmolalities are the same. Thus 1 litre of water or 5% glucose given to a patient distributes itself throughout the body water. In spite of being infused into the intravascular compartment (3.5 litres) it will be distributed throughout the body water space (42 litres) of which only 3.5/42, approximately 7.5%, is intravascular. For this reason approximately 13 litres of 5% glucose need to be infused to increase the plasma volume by 1 litre. By a converse argument we can see that someone marooned on a life raft with no water will lose water from all compartments.

2. Normal saline (0.9%) contains Na+ and Cl− at concentrations of 150 mmol l−1. If this is infused into a patient it stays in the ECF because the water tends to follow the sodium ion and osmolality matches that inside the cells, thus there is no net movement of water into the cells. Therefore a volume of normal saline given intravascularly tends to distribute throughout the extracellular space. The extracellular fluid makes up approximately 45% of the body water, with the plasma volume being approximately 7.5%, and therefore 1/6 remains intravascular and 6 litres need to be given to increase the plasma volume by 1 litre. Equally, a patient losing electrolytes and water together, as in severe diarrhoea, loses the fluid from the ECF and not the ICF.

Key point

- Only 1/6 of 0.9% saline fluid given intravenously remains in the vascular compartment, the remainder enters the interstitium.

3. Finally, consider the infusion of colloid solutions (e.g. albumin, starch solutions and gelatins). The capillary membrane is impermeable to colloid and thus the solution stays in the plasma compartment (there are, of course, circumstances in which it can leak out). A burned patient losing plasma loses it from the vascular compartment and initially there is no shift of fluid from the interstitial space. As blood pressure falls, hydrostatic pressure in the capillary falls, and if colloid osmotic pressure is maintained, the Starling forces draw water and electrolytes into the vascular compartment from the interstitium. Because there are only 3.5 litres of plasma, losses from this compartment lead to hypoperfusion and reduced oxygen transport to tissues and are potentially life-threatening. The use of hypertonic saline as a resuscitation fluid has become topical lately with reports of improved survival (Mattox et al 1991). The theoretical advantage of these solutions is that a small volume of administered fluid provides a significant plasma volume expansion. The high osmolarity of these solutions draws tissue fluid into the intravascular space and thus should minimize tissue oedema for a given plasma volume increment, leading to better tissue perfusion. They are limited at present to single dose administrations and clinical data are still relatively sparse.

4. Since the plasma is part of the ECF, any loss of ECF results in a corresponding decrease in circulating volume and is potentially much more serious than loss of an equivalent volume from the total body water. For example, compare a man losing 1 litre a day of water because he is marooned on a life raft with a man losing 1 litre a day of water and electrolytes due to a bowel obstruction. The man on the life raft will lose 7 litres in a week from his total of 42 litres body water, i.e. a 17% loss. The plasma volume will fall by 17%, which is survivable. The man with a bowel obstruction, on the other hand, loses his 7 litres from the functional ECF of 12 litres, i.e. a 58% loss. Losing more than half of the plasma volume is not compatible with life.

NORMAL WATER AND ELECTROLYTE BALANCE

1. We take in water as food and drink and also make about 350 ml per day as a result of the oxidization of carbohydrates to water and carbon dioxide, known as the metabolic water. This has to balance the output. Water is lost through the skin and from the lungs; these insensible losses amount to about 1 litre a day. Urine and faeces account for the rest. A typical balance is shown in Table 9.1.

2. The precise water requirements of a particular patient depend on size, age and temperature. Surface area (1.5 litres H_2O m−2 daily) is the most accurate guide, but it is more practical to use weight, giving adults 30–40 ml kg−1. Children require relatively more water than adults, as set out in Table 9.2. Add requirements for the first 10 kg to the requirements for the next 10 kg and

Table 9.1 Average daily water balance for a sedentary adult in temperate conditions

Input (ml)		Output (ml)	
Drink	1500	Urine	1500
Food	750	Faeces	100
Metabolic	350	Lungs	400
		Skin	600
Total	2600	Total	2600

Table 9.2 Daily water requirements by body weight in children

Weight (kg)	Water requirements
0–10	4 ml kg^{-1} h^{-1}
10–20	40 ml h^{-1} + 2 ml kg^{-1} h^{-1} for each kg >10 kg
>20	60 ml h^{-1} + 1 ml kg^{-1} h^{-1} for each kg >20 kg

likewise add to subsequent weight. Therefore, for a 25 kg child the basal requirements per hour should be:

$$(10 \times 4) + (10 \times 2) + (5 \times 1) = 65 \text{ ml h}^{-1}$$

3. The average requirements of sodium and potassium are 1 mmol kg^{-1} day^{-1} of each. Humans are very efficient at conserving sodium and can tolerate much lower sodium intakes, but they are less good at conserving potassium. There is an obligatory loss of potassium in urine and faeces and patients who are not given potassium becomes hypokalaemic. As potassium is mainly an intracellular cation, there may be a considerable fall in total body potassium before the plasma potassium falls.

PRESCRIBING FLUID REGIMENS

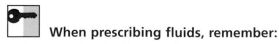

When prescribing fluids, remember:

- **Basal requirements**
- **Pre-existing dehydration and electrolyte loss**
- **Continuing abnormal losses over and above basal requirements.**

Give special consideration to intraoperative fluid balance, as all three of the above apply. Normally nourished patients taking nothing orally for a few days during surgery unusually require intravenous feeding, although some reports have shown that early feeding improves postoperative recovery. Only in special circumstances is intravenous feeding required; this topic is outside the scope of this chapter.

Basal requirements

We have seen above the daily requirements of water and electrolytes. From the various crystalloid solutions that are available (Table 9.3), we can design fluid regimens for basal requirements. Normal (0.9%) saline, Hartmann's Ringer-lactate solution, 5% dextrose, and dextrose 4%-saline 0.18% are the most commonly used. Note that their osmolalities are similar to that of ECF, that is, they are isotonic with plasma. The purpose of the glucose is to make the solution isotonic, not to provide calories, although a small amount of glucose does have a protein-sparing effect during the catabolism that follows a major operation and trauma. Our standard 70 kg patient can be provided with the 24 h basal requirements of 30–40 ml kg^{-1} of water and 1 mmol kg^{-1} of sodium in any of the ways shown in Table 9.4.

Potassium

None of these regimens supply significant amounts of potassium. Potassium chloride can be added to the bags and is supplied as ampoules of 20 mmol in 10 ml or 1 g (=13.5 mmol) in 5 ml. Bags of crystalloid are available with potassium already added and this is safer than adding ampoules.

Key points

- **Be aware that potassium can be dangerous; hyperkalaemia and acute change in potassium levels may cause cardiac arrhythmias and asystole.**
- **Never inject it as a bolus.**

Tragedies have been reported to the medical defence societies in which potassium chloride ampoules are mistaken for sodium chloride and used as 'flush', with fatal consequences. Hyperkalaemia may also occur if potassium supplements are given to anuric patients. Usually wait until you are certain of reasonable urine output before adding potassium to the regimen postoperatively.

Safe rules for giving potassium are:

- **Urine output at least 40 ml h^{-1}**
- **Not more than 40 mmol added to 1 litre**
- **No faster than 40 mmol h^{-1}.**

Table 9.3 Content of crystalloid solutions

Name	Known as	Na$^+$	Cl$^-$	K$^+$ (mmol l^{-1})	HCO$_3^-$	Ca^{2+}	Calculated (mOsm l^{-1})
Sodium chloride 0.9%	Normal saline	150	150				300
Sodium chloride 0.9%, potassium chloride 0.3%	Normal saline + KCl	150	190	40			380
Sodium chloride 0.9%, potassium chloride 0.15%	Normal saline + KCl	150	170	20			340
Ringer's lactate	Hartmann's	131	111	5	29 (as lactate)		280
Glucose 5%	5% dextrose						280
Glucose 5%, potassium chloride 0.3%	5% dextrose + KCl			40	40		360
Glucose 5%, potassium chloride 0.15%	5% dextrose + KCl			20	20		320
Glucose 4%, sodium chloride 0.18%	Dextrose saline	30	30				286
Glucose 4%, sodium chloride 0.18% potassium chloride 0.3%	Dextrose saline + KCl	30	70	40			366
Glucose 4%, sodium chloride 0.18%, potassium chloride 0.15%	Dextrose saline + KCl	30	50	20			326
Sodium chloride 0.45%	Half normal saline	75	75				150
Sodium chloride 1.8%	Twice normal saline	300	300				600
Sodium bicarbonate 8.4%	–	1000			1000		2000
Sodium bicarbonate 1.4%	–	167			167		334

Continuing loss

Patients with continuing losses above the basal requirements need extra fluid. The commonest example in anaesthetic and surgical practice is the patient with bowel obstruction. Fluid can be aspirated by a nasogastric tube to assess both volume and electrolyte content. Give saline with added potassium to replace it. Dextrose saline is not an appropriate fluid for this purpose because it contains only Na 30 mmol l^{-1}, and 5% glucose is even worse. Hyponatraemia results if these solutions are used to replace bowel loss.

Table 9.4 Basal water and sodium regimens for a 70 kg patient on intravenous fluids

Solution	Volume (ml)	Na$^+$ (mmol)	K$^+$ (mmol)
5% glucose	2000	–	
0.9% saline	500	75	
5% glucose	2000	–	–
Hartmann's	500	65.5	2.5
4% glucose 0.18% saline	2500	75	–

To keep track of the fluids, keep a fluid balance chart. Record all fluid in (oral and intravenous) and all fluid out (urine, drainage, vomit, etc.). Every 24 h total them, allow for insensible losses and record the balance, positive or negative. Any patient on intravenous fluids should have a daily balance, daily electrolyte measurements and a new regimen calculated every day. Never use the instruction 'and repeat' in fluid management; it has led to disasters in the past.

Correction of pre-existing dehydration

Patients who arrive in a dehydrated state clearly need to be resuscitated with fluid over and above their basal requirements. Usually this will be done intravenously.

 Key points

- **Identify from which compartment or compartments the fluid has been lost.**
- **Assess the extent of the dehydration.**

Resuscitate the patient with fluid similar in composition and volume to that which has been lost. From what you know about the movement of fluid between compartments (see above) and the patient's history, you can usually decide from where the losses are coming. As we have seen, bowel losses come from the ECF, while pure water losses are from the total body water. Protein-containing fluid is lost from the plasma, and there may sometimes be a combination of all three types of loss.

Assessment of deficit

Key point

- **Occult untreated intraoperative hypovolaemia may lead to organ failure and death long after the operative period.**

1. Assessment of deficit is, by its very nature, retrospective and reactive. It is still far better to predict loss, such as that experienced by patients who have received bowel preparation for surgery, and replace fluid prospectively. In estimating the extent of the losses, take into account the patient's history, clinical examination, measurement and laboratory tests. A dehydrated patient may be thirsty, have dry mucous membranes, sunken eyes (and in infants fontanelles), cheeks, loss of skin elasticity and weight loss. They feel weak and, in severe cases, are mentally confused, all of which are soft endpoints for adequate resuscitation; do not rely upon them in isolation. The cardiovascular system provides harder endpoints for resuscitation, with tachycardia and peripheral vasoconstriction as the body responds with an endogenous sympathetic drive, so that the patient feels cold. Prior to the fall in blood pressure seen in continuing haemorrhage, there is evidence that other organs, such as the gut, can suffer from occult hypoperfusion. A study by Hamilton-Davies et al (1997) showed that, in progressive haemorrhage, gastrointestinal tonometry demonstrated gut mucosal hypoperfusion greatly in advance of blood pressure, heart rate or arterial blood gas changes.

The famous American surgeon, Alfred Blalock (1899–1964), commented in 1943 after his experiences of war, 'It is well known by those that are interested in this subject that the blood volume and cardiac output are usually diminished in traumatic shock before the arterial blood pressure declines significantly.'

2. Next follow decreases in stroke volume, which up until this point have been maintained by a decrease in the capacitance of the vascular system. Cardiac output falls, causing a compensatory rise in heart rate and, eventually, a fall in blood pressure. At this point the protective autoregulation of blood flow to the brain, heart and kidneys may fail and severe dehydration produces clouding of consciousness and oliguria. Carry out the simple, essential measurements of weight, pulse, blood pressure

and urine output, to assess and treat fluid loss – although sympathetic drive from the nervous system may misleadingly maintain blood pressure until very late.

3. Measure central venous pressure (CVP). Insert an intravenous catheter into a central vein. The catheter tip should lie within the thorax, usually in the superior vena cava. In this position, blood can be aspirated freely and there is a swing in pressure with respiration. Measure the pressure, usually with an electronic transducer, although it can be done quite simply by connecting the patient to an open-ended column of fluid and measuring the height above zero with a ruler. The zero point for measuring CVP is the fifth rib in the midaxillary line with the patient supine, corresponding to the position of the left atrium. The normal range for CVP is 3–8 cmH$_2$O (1 mmHg = 1.36 cmH$_2$O). A low reading, particularly a negative value, confirms dehydration, but the converse is not true. A high or normal CVP does not indicate an adequately filled vascular system. For example, a patient on a noradrenaline (epinephrine) infusion or with a high intrinsic sympathetic tone may have a high CVP in spite of a low volume, high resistance vascular system. CVP measurements are of more use as a guide to the adequacy of treatment.

Key point

- **The response of the CVP to a fluid challenge of 200 ml colloid tells you more about the state of the circulation than a single reading.**

4. A dehydrated patient's CVP rises in response to the challenge but then falls to the original value as the circulation vasodilates to accommodate the fluid. If the response to the challenge is a sustained rise (5 min after the challenge) of 2–4 cmH$_2$O, this indicates a well-filled patient. If the CVP rises by more than 4 cmH$_2$O and does not fall again, this indicates overfilling or a failing myocardium. A fluid challenge is the only logical way of attempting acutely to restore the intravascular volume.

5. The CVP reflects the function of the right ventricle, which usually parallels left ventricular function. In cardiac disease, either primary or secondary to systemic illness, there may be disparity between the function of the two ventricles. The left ventricular function can be assessed by inserting a balloon-tipped catheter (Swan–Ganz) into a branch of the pulmonary artery. When the balloon is blown up to occlude the vessel, the pressure measured distally gives a good guide to the left atrial pressure. This is called the pulmonary capillary wedge pressure (PCWP) and is normally 5–12 mmHg. In certain circumstances the CVP may be high when the PCWP is low, which then indicates that, although the right atrium may be well filled, the

filling state of the systemic circulation is low. Here, as with the fluid challenge of the CVP, manage the filling status of the patient by means of fluid challenging the PCWP. Similar changes in level apply.

6. Both intraoperatively and on the intensive care unit there are many ways to monitor flow-based values such as stroke volume and cardiac output. Measurement is easy and with minimal morbidity, using simple and effective systems such as the oesophageal Doppler monitor. Slightly more invasive systems, such as pulse contour analysis or pulmonary artery flotation catheters, also provide useful flow-based information but do cause a slightly higher morbidity. Whatever method you choose, and it is most likely that variants will be used on the general wards in the near future, they all allow you to challenge a haemodynamic variable with fluid to bring about an improvement in flow. Pressure is of secondary importance; it is easy to generate pressure in an occluded vessel but impossible to generate flow which brings with it oxygen and all the means by which a cell survives.

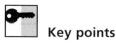

Key points

- **Elderly patients have poor cardiovascular system compliance.**
- **Consider frequent small volume fluid challenges.**
- **Left ventricular failure does not equate to hypervolaemia.**

7. Work performed by Shoemaker et al (1988) demonstrated that the Swan–Ganz catheter can be used to treat patients to oxygen delivery/consumption goals when undergoing high risk surgery. They found that an improved outcome followed in those who achieved goals of:

- Oxygen delivery[2] > 600 ml min^{-1} m^{-2}
- Oxygen consumption[3] > 170 ml min^{-1} m^{-2}
- Cardiac index > 4.5 l min^{-1} m^{-2}

However, one argument is that these patients are self-selecting and that they would have had a good outcome anyway as they are able to achieve these goals, thus demonstrating better cardiovascular function. Boyd et al (1993) also demonstrated an improvement in outcome in

patients treated with the inotropic sympathomimetic dopexamine to achieve these goals. Again, the same arguments apply. There are now many studies based around boosting oxygen delivery with a combination of fluids and inotropes in an attempt to decrease surgical morbidity and mortality. These have recently been analysed in a formal Cochrane meta-analysis by Grocott et al (2003), which proves that high risk surgical patients undergoing a process of optimization are not only significantly less likely to die as a result of surgery but may also suffer less morbidity as well. This is not true of an intensive care population where it has been shown that, if critically ill patients are subjected to a similar style of management by driving their cardiovascular systems to achieve these goals with fluid and inotropes, this group fare worse than a control group (Hayes et al 1994). This may simply reflect the fact that a significant insult has already occurred which is not remediable to boosting oxygen delivery.

8. In summary, a reasonable form of management is to aim to achieve delivery/consumption goals in cardiovascularly fit subjects undergoing high risk surgery. However, in patients with cardiovascular disease, seek to achieve these goals only using fluid and agents that offload the left ventricle, such as glyceryl trinitrate, thus reducing myocardial work. Prefer to perform this under Swan–Ganz monitoring of cardiac function, transoesophageal echocardiography or the more recent noninvasive oesophageal Doppler cardiac output monitor. For those in whom these goals are unattainable, turn your attention to ensuring an otherwise meticulous perioperative course.

9. Occult hypovolaemia can be detected by measuring gut intramucosal pH (pHi). This has been demonstrated as the area that first suffers during haemorrhagic blood loss (Price et al 1966) and thus is possibly the first to develop acidosis due to anaerobic metabolism. It can be assessed by means of a saline-filled balloon passed into the gut lumen which equilibrates with the carbon dioxide generated in the gut mucosa. From this can be derived the intramucosal pH. This value has been related to outcome following high risk surgery (Mythen et al 1993) and studies are currently being devised to investigate the effects of resuscitating patients to a pHi endpoint. The technology has recently been extended to an automated air-filled balloon in combination with an end-tidal carbon dioxide monitor (Tonocap), thus eliminating user bias due to sampling technique differences. Current trials with this device are in progress.

Quantification of plasma and ECF loss

1. If plasma is lost from the circulation, that remaining still has the same albumin concentration, although the

---

[2]Oxygen delivery = cardiac output × Hb × arterial saturation × 1.34.
[3]Oxygen consumption = cardiac output × Hb × (arterial – mixed venous saturations) × 1.34.

volume is diminished. Since no red cells are lost they become concentrated, resulting in a rise in haematocrit. Plasma is, of course, part of the ECF, so that losses of fluid and electrolytes without protein loss will cause a rise in haematocrit but also a rise in plasma protein concentration (Fig. 9.2). Changes in plasma albumin and haematocrit thus provide a good guide to ECF losses, while only haematocrit is of use in monitoring plasma loss (Robarts et al 1979).

Key point

- **In ECF depletion, the total amount of albumin stays the same, although its concentration goes up.**

Haematocrit and plasma albumin are thus very useful in the assessment of ECF and plasma losses; much more so than the sodium which, though being lost, does not change in concentration.

2. Table 9.5 summarizes the changes in volume and composition of various compartments in:

- isotonic fluid loss
- loss of water in excess of electrolytes
- loss of sodium in excess of water.

The corresponding expansion of compartments is also shown. It is a useful exercise to work through the various boxes predicting what change, if any, will occur. In the case of water loss (from both ECF and ICF) remember that the red cells are part of the ICF, so when water is lost from both compartments the haematocrit may not change. Similarly, when there is hypotonic expansion, red cells increase in volume as part of the ICF, and with the simultaneous expansion of ECF there may again be no change in haematocrit.

Water and electrolyte replacement

Having assessed the amount of deficit, as discussed above, now decide what to give to correct it. The composition of

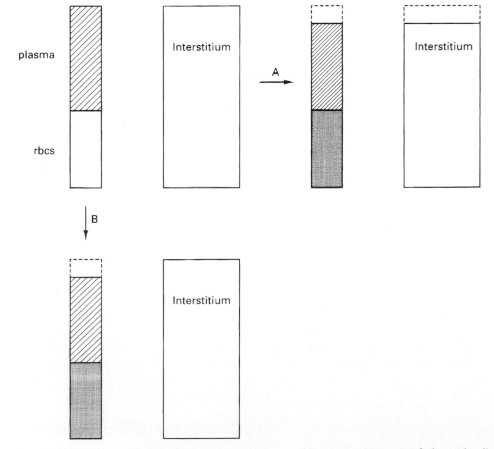

Fig. 9.2 **A** Loss of ECF leading to a rise in albumin concentration and haematocrit. **B** Loss of plasma leading to a rise in haematocrit but no change in albumin concentration.

Table 9.5   Changes resulting from three kinds of expansion and contraction of body fluids

Acute change	Example	Change in ECF vol	Change in ICF vol	Change in [Na]	Change in [Hct]	Change in [protein]
Loss H_2O + NaCl	Cholera	↓	→	→	↑	↑
Loss H_2O > Na	Excess sweating	↓	↓	↑	→	↑
Loss Na > H_2O	Addison's	↓	↑	↓	↑	↑
Isotonic expansion	Saline infusion	↑	→	→	↓	↓
Hypertonic expansion	2 × normal saline	↑	↓	↑	↓	↓
Hypotonic expansion	5% glucose infusion	↑	↑	↓	→	↓

various body fluids (Table 9.6) shows us that ECF losses of water and electrolytes should be replaced either with normal saline or Ringer's lactate with added potassium (see Basal requirements, p. 110). The only hypotonic secretions are saliva and sweat. The sodium content of sweat varies and responds to aldosterone. Gastric secretion, although having a sodium content of only 50 mmol l⁻¹, is isotonic with ECF because of the hydrogen it contains. When the losses are primarily of gastric secretion, such as pyloric stenosis, you might think it necessary to supply hydrogen ions. In fact, the kidney compensates by retaining hydrogen and excreting sodium and bicarbonate so that the net effect is a loss of sodium and chloride. Rehydrate, therefore, with normal saline with potassium.

Plasma replacement and plasma substitutes

1. When you need to replace lost plasma there is a choice between giving plasma prepared from donated blood or one of the synthetic plasma substitutes. Human plasma protein fraction (HPPF) or human albumin solution (HAS) is prepared by separating red cells from donated blood. A bottle contains plasma from several donors and has been pasteurized to prevent the transmission of disease such as hepatitis or human immunodeficiency virus (HIV). It contains 4.5% albumin, has no clotting factors and is stable at room temperature. The main disadvantage is its cost (£46 in the UK, 1999), which reflects its limited availability. The costs of blood and blood derived products are higher. Blood is already leucodepleted to reduce the risk of infection and

transfusion reactions, which significantly adds to the cost of production. A recent meta-analysis suggested that administration of human albumin in the critically ill patient may increase mortality (Schierhout & Roberts 1998). However, this analysis included studies looking at albumin use for both hypoalbuminaemia, which is not common current clinical practice in the perioperative setting, and hypovolaemia. Albumin administration in the management of hypovolaemia is also relatively uncommon because of the high cost, and because the semisynthetic colloids are considered to be at least as effective. This analysis looked at a number of studies, half of which show benefit for this indication, in widely divergent populations and so does not provide a clear message to influence clinical practice. Rather, it suggests the need for a well-designed randomized controlled trial with appropriate outcome goals. A number of solutions containing molecules large enough to stay within the capillaries and generate colloid osmotic pressure are available as plasma substitutes (Table 9.7).

2. *Dextrans* are glucose polymers available in preparations of different molecular weights. There is a large range of molecular weights in the solution. Dextran 70 is so called because the average molecular weight is supposed to be 70 000. In fact, the number-average molecular weight, which is much more relevant to the colloid osmotic pressure, is 38 000 (see footnote to Table 10.7) (Webb et al 1989). Dextran 40 has smaller molecules and can be nephrotoxic. Dextran 110 has larger molecules. Neither of these will be considered further. Dextran 70 is

Table 9.6   Electrolyte content and daily volume of body secretions

	Na	K (mmol l⁻¹)	Cl	Volume (litres daily)
Saliva	15	19	40	1.5
Stomach	50	15	140	2.5
Bile, pancreas, small bowel	130–145	5–12	70–100	4.2
Insensible sweat	12	10	12	0.6
Sensible sweat	50	10	50	Variable

Table 9.7 Characteristics of colloid solutions

Name	Brand name	No. average* mol. wt	Mol. wt range	Na⁺ K⁺ Ca²⁺ (mmol l⁻¹)	$t_{1/2}$ in plasma	Adverse reactions (%)		Effect on coagulation	Cost (UK 1988)
						Mild	Severe		
Human plasma protein fraction	HPPF	69 000	69 000	150 5 2	20 days	0.02	0.004	None	£40
Dextran 70 in saline 0.9% or glucose 5%	Macrodex Lomodex 70 Gentran 70	38 000	<10 000 → 250 000	150	12 h	0.7	0.02	Inhibit platelet aggregation Factor VIII↓ Interfere with crossmatch	£4.78
Polygeline (degraded gelatin)	Haemaccel	24 500	<5 000 → 50 000	145 5 6.25	2.5 h	0.12	0.04	None	£3.71
Succinylated gelatin	Gelofusin	22 600	<10 000 → 140 000	154 0.4 0.4	4 h	0.12	0.04	None	£4.63
Hydroxyethyl starch 6% in saline (hetastarch)	Hespan	70 000	<10 000 → 10⁶	154	25 h	0.09	0.006	>1.5 g kg⁻¹ day⁻¹ can cause coagulopathy	£16.25

*Number-average molecular weight should not be confused with weight-average molecular weight, which is usually quoted by the manufacturers. Number-average molecular weight is more appropriate.

quite a good plasma substitute, but its use has declined in popularity because of its adverse effects on coagulation and crossmatching and the relatively high incidence of allergic reactions.

3. *Gelatin* solutions are prepared by hydrolysis of bovine collagen. They have the advantage over dextrans of not affecting coagulation and of having a low incidence of allergic reactions. Being of smaller average particle size, they stay in the intravascular space for a shorter time. Haemaccel contains potassium and calcium ions, which can cause coagulation if mixed with citrated blood in a giving set. Haemaccel stays for a shorter time in the circulation: 30% of the molecules are dispersed to the interstitial tissues within 30 min. Gelofusin is probably preferable from this point of view.

4. *Hetastarch*, 6% in saline, has become available in the last few years. It has the largest average molecular weight of any of the plasma substitutes and therefore stays in the circulation longer. Limit the dose to 1500 ml 70 kg^{-1}; more can cause coagulation problems. About 30% of a dose is taken up by the reticuloendothelial system without apparent detriment to its function. Smaller molecules (mol. wt <50 000) are filtered by the kidneys. Larger ones are broken down by plasma amylase until small enough for real excretion.

5. *Electrolyte balanced colloid solutions*, such as Hextend, represent a new area of fluid development and it is possible that these solutions offer increased benefit over currently used colloids, due to provision of a more favourable physiological milieu. Indeed, clinical trials to date with balanced colloids (Wilkes et al 2001) suggest those undergoing major surgery benefit from better acid–base profiles and end-organ perfusion than those receiving traditional colloids suspended in 0.9% saline. It is now well recognized that intravenous fluids based on so called 'normal saline' do not represent the physiological composition of plasma and in excess lead to a variety of organ dysfunctions, such as those reported by Wilkes et al, and others including cerebral, renal, gut and metabolic dysfunction. Until recently it has been difficult to explain why, but with new theories of acid–base physiology emerging (see later), the pathophysiology of why 'normal saline' causes acidosis is easy to explain. In essence 0.9% saline (normal saline) is not normal at all. It has approximately 150 mmol of chloride and 150 mmol of sodium per litre. When given in excess, which may be as little as 2–3 litres per 24 h, it can produce high levels of chloride, which in turn lead to the development of a mild acidosis by reducing the strong ion difference (see later).

Choice of solution for plasma expansion

1. The intravascular space can be expanded by using crystalloid solutions such as saline, but because the fluid spreads throughout the ECF, 6 litres of crystalloid are needed to expand the plasma by 1 litre. In an emergency, crystalloid is useful. All the battle casualties in the Falklands War were resuscitated in the field with Hartmann's solution.

2. Do not use 5% glucose from choice as it is distributed throughout both ECF and ICF compartments; thus 13 litres are needed to increase the intravascular space by 1 litre. For most patients with acute hypovolaemia, the best combination of advantages at low cost is offered by succinylated gelatin (Gelofusin). Being relatively short acting, it is particularly useful as a holding measure until blood becomes available. Gelofusin probably stays within the intravascular space for 60–90 min at most.

3. In continuing hypovolaemia, hetastarch gives more prolonged expansion and its larger molecules are better retained in the circulation when the capillaries are leaky, e.g. in septicaemic shock.

4. There is continued debate as to whether it is better to resuscitate with a crystalloid or colloid, the so-called crystalloid versus colloid debate. There have been many meta-analyses that failed to prove any advantage of one over the other for the purpose of resuscitation. Indeed, the most common conclusion is that there are insufficient data available to recommend one rather than the other. A trial of sufficient power to demonstrate a mortality difference using either crystalloid or colloid would need to include over 7000 patients. Trials of that size are currently under way in Australia but are likely to add to the debate rather than resolve it.

Blood loss and blood transfusion

1. So far we have considered plasma loss and plasma expansion. Most of what has been said about the assessment and replacement of plasma volume applies to blood loss. Transfusion of donated blood is possible in most circumstances, but has several disadvantages to be weighed against the fact that only haemoglobin carries oxygen. With a haemoglobin of 14 g dl^{-1}, evolution has equipped us with spare capacity as far as oxygen-carrying capacity is concerned. Indeed, as haematocrit falls, the decrease in oxygen carrying is compensated by better tissue perfusion due to reduced blood viscosity.

2. It has been shown that the best balance between oxygen carrying and viscosity occurs around a haematocrit of 30%. It is also suspected that blood transfusion at the time of surgery for certain cancers leads to immunological suppression and poorer long-term survival. On the other hand, blood transfusion prior to transplant procedures improves graft survival. Because of anxiety over HIV, and with a lack of knowledge of mechanisms of prion transfer relating to bovine spongiform encephalitis

(BSE), there is reluctance by the public to accept blood transfusion. Trials in critical care suggest that restricting transfusion to patients with Hb below 8 g% is associated with a better outcome (Hebert et al 1999).

3. For these reasons, in addition to the hazards of blood transfusion listed in Table 9.8, the expense of blood and rarity of some blood groups, there is reluctance to transfuse blood. In practical terms, operative blood loss up to 500 ml can be replaced with saline, remembering that six times as much will be needed (see above), or plasma substitutes. Only if more than 1 litre of blood has been lost in a healthy adult should you consider giving blood. Point of care testing with Hb analysers or from arterial blood gases will allow you to quantify the need for transfusion; use them when possible. Anaemia alone is a difficult clinical sign on which to base the prescription of blood.

4. Rather than supply whole blood, it is more efficient for the transfusion service to separate it into components (Table 9.9). Blood cross-matched for patients undergoing surgery usually comes as plasma-reduced blood – 'packed cells'. This is more viscous than whole blood so give it with appropriate amounts of crystalloid or colloid solution to restore the volume.

5. Assess the quantity of blood lost by clinical means, as outlined above. At operation, watch the suction bottle and weigh swabs, although this generally underestimates the loss. The only real way of quantifying loss is by arterial blood gases measurement, full blood counts performed in the laboratory, or by bedside testing by, for example, Haemacue when available. In operations such as transurethral resection of the prostate, measurement of haemoglobin in the irrigating fluid gives an accurate measure of blood loss. Haematocrit and haemoglobin concentrations do not change in acute blood loss until the blood remaining in the patient has been diluted by shift

---

Table 9.9   Blood products

- Plasma-reduced blood (packed cells)
- Washed red cells: if transfusion reaction a problem
- Plasma protein fraction (HPPF)
- Fresh frozen plasma (FFP): contains clotting factors more dilute than the concentrates below
- Cryoprecipitate: rich in factor VIII
- Factor VIII concentrate: even richer in VIII
- Factors II, VII, IX and X concentrate
- Factor XI concentrate
- Fibrinogen
- Platelet concentrate

---

of fluid from the interstitial space or intravenous infusion. Plasma-reduced blood and whole blood more than 1 day old, which it almost always is, contain no viable platelets and a few clotting factors. The same applies to plasma protein fraction. In massive transfusion both dilution and consumption of clotting factors make it necessary to send blood for a clotting screen and give platelets and fresh frozen plasma (FFP) according to the results. As a rule, give a unit of FFP for every 4–6 units of stored blood transfused. Contact haematologists for advice (see Ch. 8).

6. As stored blood is generally collected into citrate-containing bags, remember that exogenous calcium may be required after massive blood transfusion, to ensure both adequate haemostasis and a normal vascular response to inotropes.

Intraoperative fluid balance

1. During an operation, many of the problems discussed so far may be continuing. The patient is starved for 6–12 h, there may be blood loss, plasma loss, ECF loss and evaporation of water from exposed bowel. As part of the stress response to surgery the patient retains water and sodium. The importance of careful monitoring in major surgery is obvious, including accurate assessment of blood loss, haemodynamic variables and urine output.

2. As a rule of thumb, in intra-abdominal surgery, give up to 2 litres of Hartmann's solution 5 ml kg^{-1} h^{-1}. This compensates for starvation, ECF loss, evaporation and some blood loss. You may need to give blood or colloids in addition. If the patient is being treated in an attempt to achieve oxygen delivery/consumption goals, in cardiovascularly healthy patients, continually challenge the central venous pressure (CVP) with fluid. In those with cardiac dysfunction, challenge the pulmonary capillary wedge pressure (PCWP) to maintain an optimal haemodynamic state.

Table 9.8   The hazards of blood transfusion

Any transfusion
- Transmission of disease, e.g. AIDS, malaria (donor blood screened for HIV, hepatitis, syphilis)
- Bacterial contamination
- Pyrogenic reactions (antibodies to white cells)
- Incompatibility reactions
- ± Haemolysis (clerical error commonest cause)

Massive transfusion
- Hypothermia
- Hyperkalaemia
- Citrate toxicity
- Acidosis
- Microaggregate embolism, 'shock lung'
- Dilution and consumption of clotting factors

---

3. For the first 36 h postoperatively there is water retention, and there is sodium retention lasting 3–5 days. Obligatory potassium loss of 50–100 mmol per day continues. If you give additional sodium it is simply retained, although the urine may show an increase in sodium output. Provided that intraoperative losses have been replaced by the end of the operation, give the basal requirements: 30–40 ml kg^{-1} day^{-1} H$_2$O + 1 mmol kg^{-1} day^{-1} Na$^+$ and K$^+$, plus additional blood or colloid if there is significant wound drainage.

4. Do not give potassium until urine output is established; the operation of inadvertent bilateral ureteric ligation is not unknown.

ACID–BASE BALANCE

Claude Bernard was the first to recognize that to function effectively the body needs a stable *milieu interieur*. The hydrogen ion concentration is the most important contribution to this. An acid is a hydrogen ion (proton) donor and a base accepts hydrogen ions. Throughout life the body produces hydrogen ions and they must be excreted or buffered to keep the internal environment constant. It is testament to the importance of hydrogen ions that they are regulated on a nanomolar level rather than millimolar as are most of the principle anions and cations in the blood. There are currently two main ways of interpreting acid–base balance. The first or 'traditional view' is the most widespread interpretation and based on work by Severinghaus, Henderson–Hasselbalch and Siggard–Anderson among others. It evolved as technology became more advanced and allowed for the direct measurement of carbon dioxide and hydrogen ion activity and the calculation of those values which were unmeasurable. The 'new' interpretation of acid–base balance takes much of this pioneering work and develops it further on the basis of sound physicochemical principles. For the most part the new theory, proposed by Stewart in the early 1980s, states that there are only three variables that influence pH: carbon dioxide, the strong ion difference (SID) and weak acids. Both methods are described below for completeness.

Traditional view of acid–base balance

Terminology and definitions

Hydrogen ion activity. This is traditionally expressed in pH units, pH being the negative log$_{10}$ of the hydrogen ion concentration:

$$pH = -\log [H^+] = \log \frac{1}{[H^+]}$$

Hydrogen ion concentration can also be expressed directly in nanomoles per litre (Table 9.10). Note that the

pH is a log scale, so that each 0.3 unit fall in pH represents a doubling of hydrogen ion concentration.

Acidosis and alkalosis. The normal ECF pH is 7.36–7.44 (44–36 nmol l^{-1}). Acidaemia is a blood pH below this range and alkalaemia a pH above it. Acidosis is a condition that leads to acidaemia, or would do if no compensation occurred, but the terms 'acidosis' and 'acidaemia' are often used loosely to mean the same thing, which is not strictly correct. Alkalosis and alkalaemia are defined in a similar way.

- *Respiratory acidosis* is a fall in pH resulting from a rise in the Pco$_2$, e.g. opiate overdose leading to hypoventilation causes a rise in Pco$_2$.
- *Respiratory alkalosis* is a rise in pH due to a lowering of the Pco$_2$, such as occurs in hyperventilation.
- *Metabolic acidosis* is a fall in pH due to anything other than carbon dioxide (sometimes referred to as nonrespiratory acidosis). There is a primary gain of acid or loss of bicarbonate from ECF.
- *Metabolic alkalosis* is a rise in pH from non-respiratory causes. There is either a gain in bicarbonate or a loss of acid from the ECF.
- *Compensatory changes.* If the initial problem is respiratory, the result is called a *primary respiratory acidosis* or alkalosis. If the respiratory problem persists for more than a few hours, the kidney excretes or retains bicarbonate to try and compensate for the respiratory disturbance. This is referred to as *secondary* or *compensatory metabolic acidosis* or alkalosis.

Thus a primary respiratory acidosis may be accompanied by a secondary metabolic alkalosis. For example, chronic obstructive airways disease leads to a rise in the Pco$_2$: primary respiratory acidosis. To compensate for this the kidney retains bicarbonate, leading to a rise in ECF bicarbonate: secondary or compensatory metabolic alkalosis.

In the same way, primary respiratory alkalosis (e.g. the hyperventilation that occurs at high altitude) will be compensated by a secondary metabolic acidosis.

Table 9.10 Conversion table for pH units and hydrogen ion concentration

pH unit	H$^+$ (nmol l^{-1})
8.00	10
7.70	20
7.44	36
7.40	40
7.36	44
7.10	80
7.00	100

Where the first disturbance is metabolic, e.g. the buildup of acid in diabetic ketoacidosis, the primary metabolic acidosis will cause hyperventilation (secondary respiratory alkalosis), which will tend to restore the pH to normal. This respiratory compensation for a metabolic change happens much more rapidly than the metabolic compensation for a respiratory problem.

The fourth possible combination of changes is to have a metabolic alkalosis such as loss of H^+ in pyloric stenosis, compensated by a respiratory acidosis. However, hypoventilation (respiratory acidosis) leads to a fall in PO_2, which stimulates ventilation so that, in practice, compensatory respiratory acidosis is not usually seen.

In deciding which is the primary and which is the secondary change, realize that the compensatory changes do not bring the pH back to normal; they bring it back *towards* the normal range. In other words, even after compensation the measured pH is altered in the direction of the primary problem (acidosis or alkalosis). Compensatory mechanisms merely make the disturbance in pH less than it otherwise would have been. It is also important to consider the history. Examiners may give candidates blood gas results to interpret, but in real life blood gases come from patients. Knowing that a patient is an unconscious diabetic breathing spontaneously, rather than an anaesthetized patient on a ventilator, certainly helps one's interpretation.

Buffers. These are substances which, by their presence in solution, minimize the change in pH for a given addition of acid or alkali. Three-quarters of the buffering power of the body is within the cells; the rest is in the ECF. Proteins, haemoglobin, phosphates and the bicarbonate system are all important buffers. The particular importance of the bicarbonate system is that carbon dioxide is excreted in the lungs and can be regulated by changes in ventilation. Bicarbonate excretion in the kidney can also be regulated. The lungs are responsible for the excretion of 16 000 mmol per day of acid and the kidneys for only 40–80 mmol per day. The formation of carbonic acid from carbon dioxide and water is catalysed by carbonic anhydrase (present in red cells). The reaction may go in either direction:

$$H^+ + HCO_3^- \leftrightarrow H_2CO_3 \leftrightarrow H_2O + CO_2$$

The Henderson–Hasselbalch equation is derived from this and expresses the relationship between the bicarbonate concentration, the carbon dioxide and the pH:

$$pH = pK + \log \frac{[HCO_3]}{[H_2CO_3]}$$

The carbonic acid can be expressed in terms of carbon dioxide, so that a more useful form of the equation is:

$$pH = pK + \log \frac{[HCO_3]}{0.03\ PCO_2}$$

As this is a buffer system which minimizes changes in pH, we can see that if the carbon dioxide rises so will the bicarbonate, to keep $[HCO_3^-]/PCO_2$ constant. Similarly, a fall in bicarbonate will be accompanied by a fall in PCO_2 to prevent a change in pH.

Interpretation of acid–base changes

As the patient's acid–base status varies, three things are changing at once: pH, $[HCO_3^-]$ and PCO_2. Blood gas machines measure PO_2, pH and PCO_2 directly. The actual bicarbonate $[HCO_3^-]$ is calculated from the Henderson–Hasselbalch equation. Blood gas machines also derive other variables which help in the interpretation of the acid–base status; however, these all attempt to describe the metabolic derangement. These are as follows:

1. *Standard bicarbonate (SBC)* is the concentration of bicarbonate in the plasma of fully oxygenated blood at 37°C at a PCO_2 of 5.3 kPa (40 mmHg). In other words, it tells you what the bicarbonate would be if there were no respiratory disturbance. Looking at the standard bicarbonate therefore tells you what is going on on the metabolic side. Normal standard bicarbonate is 22–26 mmol l^{-1}. Values above this indicate metabolic alkalosis, and those below, metabolic acidosis.

2. *Base excess (BE)* is the amount of strong base or acid that would need to be added to whole blood to titrate the pH back to 7.4 at a PCO_2 of 5.3 kPa and 37°C. It tells you the same thing as standard bicarbonate, namely the metabolic status of the patient. Normal base excess is obviously zero (±2 mmol l^{-1}). Positive base excess occurs in metabolic alkalosis, and negative base excess (sometimes called base deficit) indicates metabolic acidosis. The base excess is an in vitro determination in whole blood. It is also known as the actual base excess (ABE) or the base excess (blood) (BE b).

3. *Standard base excess (SBE)* is an estimate of the in vivo base excess and takes into account the difference in buffering capacity between the patient's ECF and the blood that was put in the blood gas machine. Interstitial fluid, having less protein and no haemoglobin, has a lower buffering capacity than blood. SBE is therefore 1–2 mmol l^{-1} greater than BE, but this makes very little difference in practice. SBE is sometimes called base excess (e.c.f.).

4. *Total carbon dioxide* (TCO_2) is the total concentration of carbon dioxide in the plasma as bicarbonate and dissolved carbon dioxide.

$$TCO_2 = [HCO_3^-] + (PCO_2 \times solubility)$$

5. *Oxygen saturation* (O_2 sat.). The percentage saturation of haemoglobin by oxygen is derived from the haemoglobin

oxygen dissociation curve and the measured P_{O_2}. The normal value is >95%. Do not rely on this value to be accurate, as other forms of haemoglobin, such as carboxyhaemoglobin, are included as oxyhaemoglobin. If you suspect this, for example in burns patients, then use a co-oximeter to determine the level of oxyhaemoglobin.

6. *P_{O_2} and inspired oxygen (F_{IO_2})*. To interpret the P_{O_2} you need to know the age of the patient and the F_{IO_2}. Normal arterial P_{O_2} declines with age. Roughly speaking P_{O_2} = 100 – age in years/3 mmHg or 13.3 – 0.044 × age kPa.

The expected alveolar P_{O_2} (P_{AO_2}) can be predicted from the inspired oxygen by the simplified alveolar gas equation: $P_{AO_2} = P_{IO_2} – P_{ACO_2}/R$, where R is the respiratory exchange ratio (normally 0.8). In dry gas P_{IO_2} (in kPa) = fractional inspired oxygen (F_{IO_2})%. Alveolar gas is saturated with water vapour (6.3 kPa), for which allowance must be made. If the F_{IO_2} = 40% and the P_{CO_2} = 5.3:

$$P_{AO_2} = \frac{(40 – 40 \times 603)}{100} – \frac{5.3}{0.8} = 30.85 \text{ kPa}$$

As an approximate rule of thumb, deduct 10 from the F_{IO_2}% to give the expected P_{AO_2} in kPa (e.g. if F_{IO_2} = 50% then P_{AO_2} should be approximately 40 kPa). The difference between the estimated P_{AO_2} and the measured arterial P_{O_2} is called the (A – a) P_{O_2} gradient. It is normally 0.5–3 kPa.

Without considering the inspired oxygen it is not possible to comment sensibly on the observed P_{AO_2}. A rough calculation of the (A – a) P_{O_2} gradient should be made when commenting on blood gas results. Some machines even calculate this for you as well!

A blood gas machine usually prints out the variables shown in Table 9.11 There is often a haemoglobin measurement and the temperature of measurement (37°C) is quoted, and in some cases an electrolyte profile may be included.

7. *Temperature correction*. The blood gas machine operates at 37°C. Because gases are more soluble in liquid at lower temperatures (as drinkers of cold lager will know), the blood gases would be different if measured at another temperature. Blood gas machines are programmed to correct the gases if you tell the machine the patient's actual temperature. However, there has been much debate as to whether it is appropriate to correct for temperature. Suffice it to say that the protagonists of not correcting for temperature (the alpha stat theory) hold sway and one should probably act on the blood gases as measured at 37°C and not the temperature-corrected values.

8. *The anion gap*. For electrochemical neutrality of the ECF the number of anions must equal the number of cations. The main cations are sodium and potassium and the main anions are chloride, bicarbonate, proteins, phosphates, sulphates and organic acids.

Normally, only Na^+, K^+, HCO_3^- and Cl^- are measured in the laboratory. Thus, when we add the normal values for these they do not balance:

Cations		Anions	
Na^+	140	Cl^-	105
K^+	5	HCO_3^-	25
Total	145	Total	130

The difference is known as the *anion gap* and represents the other anions not usually measured. Anion gap = $(Na^+ + K^+)$ – $(HCO_3^- + Cl^-)$ = 11–19 mmol l^{-1}. Its significance is that in certain metabolic acidoses (e.g. ketoacidosis or lactic acidosis) the anion gap will be increased by the presence of organic anions. However, in metabolic acidosis in which chloride replaces bicarbonate (e.g. bicarbonate loss due to diarrhoea), the anion gap will be normal. It is simply another way in which to further elucidate the cause of the acidosis.

New insights into acid–base physiology

Conventional methods of interpreting acid–base balance are centred on the Henderson–Hasselbach equation, which describes a ratio of carbon dioxide to bicarbonate to derive the pH. The respiratory component of the equation is easy to comprehend because carbon dioxide is part of the equation, but the metabolic component is less easy to understand. We use surrogate markers of metabolic disturbance, such as base excess, to quantify the degree of metabolic acidosis. There has been an increasing awareness that this model, which works clinically, fails to explain much of the associated pathophysiology, in particular the influence of electrolytes and proteins on acid–base balance. In 1981 Paul Stewart (1981) took a physicochemical approach to acid–base balance and came up with a model, which has subsequently been modified by Fencl, that explained many of these anomalies. He said that for all aqueous systems there must be electrical neutrality and conservation of mass, and that water will dissociate/associate to give/receive hydrogen ions if the

---

Table 9.11   Printout from a blood gas machine with normal values

Temp.	37°C
pH	7.36–7.44 (44–36 nmol l^{-1})
P_{CO_2}	4.6–5.6 kPa (35–42 mmHg)
P_{O_2}	10.0–13.3 kPa (75–100 mmHg)
HCO_3^-	22–26 mmol l^{-1}
T_{CO_2}	24–28 mmol l^{-1}
SBC	22–26 mmol l^{-1}
BE	–2 to +2 mmol l^{-1}
SBE	–3 to +3 mmol l^{-1}
O_2 sat.	>95%
Hb	11.5–16.5 g dl^{-1}

balance of either is altered. He also identified the important factors controlling acid–base balance control.

 Only three independent factors control acid–base balance:

- P_{CO_2}
- **Strong ion difference (SID)**
- **Weak acids (albumin and phosphate).**

All other variables such as hydrogen ions, hydroxide, bicarbonate, etc. change only if one or more of the three independent variables changes.

1. P_{CO_2}. The change in carbon dioxide is self explanatory and influences the pH as predicted by the Henderson–Hasselbach equation.

2. *SID*. Strong ion difference refers to the mathematical difference in charge between the strong ions in solution and is normally between 38 and 42 mmol l^{-1}. Strong ions are those ions which in solution are virtually fully dissociated, e.g Na^+, Cl^-, K^+, Ca^{2+}, Mg^{2+} and, for the purposes of the model, lactate. For example, if NaCl is added to water there is virtually complete dissociation and the only things that exist in that solution are Na^+, Cl^-, H_2O, H^+ and OH^- ions; there are no 'NaCl molecules'. If there is a change in the concentration of one of these ions, that is an increase in the Cl^-, then the SID will be reduced and electrical neutrality has to be restored. This results in the dissociation of water, so producing hydrogen ions and decreasing the pH of a solution. Therefore, increasing the chloride concentration makes the system more acidic. The increase in the hydrogen ion concentration, however, is only in the nanomolar range and does not restore electrical neutrality. The bulk of electrical neutrality is restored by the proteins.

3. *Weak acids*. Albumin and phosphate are the predominant weak acids. If the concentration of albumin decreases, the solution becomes more alkaline. This is a very common occurrence in the critical care patient.

It is therefore possible, if you know the P_{CO_2}, the SID and the weak acid concentration, to work out what the pH will be without having to measure it. It is this degree of quantification that allows physicians working in complicated critical care or postoperative environments to understand the pathophysiology behind the disturbance and work out what and how to treat it effectively.

PLAN FOR INTERPRETING BLOOD GASES

1. Check for internal consistency. Remember that the machine measures only pH, P_{CO_2} and P_{O_2}. If it measures any of these wrongly, which is not infrequent, the derived variables are also wildly abnormal. If the results do not fit with the clinical picture, suspect the machine. Example: a patient on a ventilator in theatre with an end-tidal carbon dioxide of 5% has the following gases:

P_{O_2}	13.0
pH	7.64
P_{CO_2}	5.1
HCO_3^-	37.5
T_{CO_2}	38.5
SBC	39.0
BE	+15
SBE	+16
O_2 sat.	99%

It is much more likely that the pH has been measured wrongly than that the patient has a gross metabolic alkalosis.

2. Look at the pH. Remember the pH change is always in the direction of the primary problem acidosis or alkalosis.

3. Look at the P_{CO_2}. Abnormality of the P_{CO_2} indicates the respiratory component.

4. Look at the base excess or standard bicarbonate. Both give the same information, i.e. the metabolic acid–base status after correcting for the P_{CO_2}.

5. Calculate the anion gap.

6. Look at the P_{O_2} and calculate the A – a gradient.

Examples of abnormal blood gases

pH	7.51	The alkalaemia is due to primary
P_{CO_2}	3.7	respiratory alkalosis (low P_{CO_2}).
P_{O_2}	29	There is no metabolic
HCO_3^-	22.1	compensation (normal base
T_{CO_2}	23.6	excess). The P_{O_2} would be
SBC	25	expected if breathing 40%
BE	+1.1	oxygen $P_{iO_2} - 10 = (40 - 10) = 30$.
SBE	+2	The patient is
O_2 sat.	100%	hyperventilating.
(F_{iO_2} 40%)		

pH	7.28	A respiratory acidosis with high
P_{CO_2}	7.33	P_{CO_2} due to hypoventilation.
P_{O_2}	9.21	Again no metabolic compensation
		(normal SBC and BE). Low P_{O_2}
HCO_3^-	25.2	due to hypoventilation.
T_{CO_2}	28.4	
SBC	22.3	
BE	–1.9	
SBE	–2.5	
O_2 sat.	91%	
(F_{iO_2} air)		

pH	7.35	Again a respiratory acidosis
P_{CO_2}	9.33	(high P_{CO_2}) but this time

P_{O_2}	7.11
HCO_3^-	39.1
T_{CO_2}	41.2
SBC	32.4
BE	+8.2
SBE	+9.1
O_2 sat.	85%
(F_{IO_2} air)	

compensated by metabolic alkalosis (high SBC and positive base excess). This is typical of chronic obstructive airways disease with renal compensation.

pH	7.21
P_{CO_2}	4.0
P_{O_2}	13.3
HCO_3^-	11.5
T_{CO_2}	12.8
SBC	9.3
BE	−15.2
SBE	−16.4
O_2 sat.	99%
(F_{IO_2} air)	

The acidaemia (low pH) is primarily due to a metabolic acidosis (low SBC, base excess −15). Compensatory respiratory alkalosis (low P_{CO_2}), does not return the pH to normal. P_{O_2} normal.

pH	7.36
P_{CO_2}	4.21
P_{O_2}	10.49
HCO_3^-	17.6
T_{CO_2}	18.5
SBC	17.8
BE	−6.2
SBE	−6.9
O_2 sat.	96%
(F_{IO_2} 60%)	

The pH is in the normal range despite low P_{CO_2} (respiratory alkalosis) and low standard bicarbonate (metabolic acidosis). The important thing here is the P_{O_2}. It is apparently in the normal range but not when breathing 60% oxygen. The $(A - a)\ P_{O_2}$ gradient is roughly 40 kPa. These gases are typical of a patient with adult respiratory distress syndrome.

TREATMENT OF ACID–BASE DISTURBANCES

1. As in any other field of medicine, direct treatment at the underlying cause. Correcting the P_{CO_2} is usually possible by taking over the patient's ventilation and adjusting the minute volume to give the desired P_{CO_2}.

2. Treatment of a metabolic acidosis is more controversial. It was traditional to treat a metabolic acidosis by giving sodium bicarbonate according to the formula (base excess × body weight in kg/3) mmol starting by giving half the dose; 8.4% sodium bicarbonate contains 1 mmol ml^{-1}.

3. It is now argued that, particularly in a hypoxic state such as exists following cardiac arrest, bicarbonate administration may do more harm than good (Graf & Arieff 1986). The bicarbonate generates carbon dioxide, which crosses easily into cells, making the intracellular acidosis worse. If ventilation is impaired the carbon dioxide generated is unable to escape via the lungs. The traditional practice of giving 50–100 mmol bicarbonate at

a cardiac arrest is probably unjustified. In metabolic acidosis due to poor perfusion of tissues the best way to manage this is to correct the perfusion defect, which may be achieved, in some instances, by improving oxygen delivery using fluids, vasodilators or inotropes. This may involve the use of invasive monitoring such as Swan–Ganz catheterization in order to guide therapy. Treatment of the metabolic acidosis due to sepsis is controversial and, even though goal-directed therapy may not be universally accepted, most will still try to achieve reasonably high oxygen delivery targets. In sepsis, however, this does not give the anticipated rise in oxygen consumption, after allowing for the rise in oxygen consumption due to increased myocardial work required to achieve the delivery. Sepsis appears to involve a defect in tissue oxygen uptake/utilization.

4. There is still a place for bicarbonate therapy in acidosis due to diarrhoea, renal tubular acidosis and uraemic acidosis, and where an imbalance of the SID exists. As outlined above, use the base excess to calculate the dose; 8.4% sodium bicarbonate is hyperosmolar and must be given into a large central vein. Accidental subcutaneous administration can cause tissue necrosis. Bear in mind that each millimole of HCO_3^- is accompanied by Na^+ and it is easy to overload the patient with sodium.

Key point

- Frequently monitor blood gases and electrolytes during treatment with bicarbonate.

Summary

- Do you have an adequate knowledge of basic fluid physiology?
- Do you recognize that visible fluid deficit is but a small part of the overall problem?
- Are you aware that occult intraoperative hypovolaemia leads to increased postoperative morbidity?
- Will you determine to monitor patients thoroughly to fully understand their fluid status?
- Are you aware that hypovolaemia is the most common cause of intraoperative metabolic acidosis?
- Do you recognize that hypovolaemia is probably the most common *avoidable* cause of multiple organ dysfunction?

References

Boyd O, Grounds RM, Bennett ED 1993 A randomised clinical trial of the effect of deliberate peri-operative increase of oxygen delivery on mortality in high-risk surgical patients. JAMA 270: 2699–2707

Edelman IS, Leibman J 1959 Anatomy of body water and electrolytes. American Journal of Medicine 27: 256, 277

Graf H, Arieff AI 1986 Use of sodium bicarbonate in the therapy of organic acidosis. Intensive Care Medicine 12: 285–288

Grocott MPW, Hamilton MA, Rowan K 2003 Perioperative increase in global blood flow to explicit defined goals and outcomes following surger; issue 1, January, Cochrane Library. Update Software, Oxford

Hamilton-Davies C, Mythen MG, Salmon JB, Jacobson D, Shukla A, Webb AR 1997 Comparison of commonly used clinical indicators of hypovolaemia with gastrointestinal tonometry. Intensive Care Medicine 23: 276–281

Hayes MA, Timmins AC, Yau EH 1994 Elevation of systemic oxygen delivery in the treatment of critically ill patients. New England Journal of Medicine 330: 1717–1722

Hebert PC, Wells G, Blajchman MA et al 1999 A multicenter, randomized, controlled clinical trial of transfusion requirements in critical care. Transfusion Requirements in Critical Care Investigators, Canadian Critical Care Trials Group [see comments] [published erratum appears in N Engl J Med 1999 340(13): 1056]. New England Journal of Medicine 340(6): 409–417

Mattox KL, Maningas PA, Moore EE 1991 Prehospital hypertonic saline/dextran infusion for post-traumatic hypotension. Annals of Surgery 213: 482–491

Mythen MG, Purdy G, Mackie IJ 1993 Post-operative multiple organ dysfunction syndrome associated with gut mucosal hypoperfusion, increased neutrophil degranulation and C-1-esterase inhibitor depletion. British Journal of Anaesthesia 71: 858–863

Price HL, Deutsch S, Marshall BE 1966 Haemodynamic and metabolic effects of haemorrhage in man with particular reference to the splanchnic circulation. Circulation Research 18: 469–474

Robarts WM, Parkin JV, Hobsley M 1979 A simple clinical approach to quantifying losses from the extracellular and plasma compartments. Annals of the Royal College of Surgeons of England 61: 142–145

Shoemaker WC, Appel PL, Kram HB 1988 Prospective trial of supranormal values of survivors as therapeutic goals in high-risk surgical patients. Chest 94: 1176–1186

Starling EH 1896 On the absorption of fluids from the connective spaces. Journal of Physiology 19: 312–326

Staverman A 1952 Apparent osmotic pressure of solutions of heterodisperse polymers. Rec Trav Chim 71: 623–633

Stewart PA 1981 How to understand acid–base. A quantitative acid–base primer for biology and medicine. Edward Arnold, London

Webb AR, Barclay SA, Bennett ED 1989 In vitro colloid pressure of commonly used plasma expanders and substitutes. Intensive Care Medicine 15: 116–120

Wilkes NJ, Woolf R, Mutch M et al 2001 The effects of balanced versus saline-based hetastarch and crystalloid solutions on acid–base and electrolyte status and gastric mucosal perfusion in elderly surgical patients. Anesthesia and Analgesia 93(4): 811–816

10 Nutritional support

J. Payne-James

Objectives

- **Be aware of the incidence, causes, effects and assessment of protein energy malnutrition in surgical patients.**
- **Recognize when and how to administer oral, enteral and parenteral support, and when to stop it.**
- **Be aware of the complications of administering support.**
- **Document your findings and actions.**

INTRODUCTION

The metabolic response to injury, such as major trauma or surgical operation and sepsis, generates increased demand for nitrogen and energy. If the demands are not met, the patient develops protein-energy malnutrition (PEM), which is a significant and often unrecognized problem in hospitals, with up to 40% of patients undernourished, and fewer than half of these having this fact documented in their notes.

Aim to identify actual or potential malnourished patients and correct or improve their nutritional status to minimize the risks of chest, urinary or wound infection, slow healing, wound breakdown or even death. The optimal method of administering additional nutrients is by oral feeding, such as sip feeds and dietary supplements, both in hospital and community practice. A variety of flavours is available in order to make the supplements palatable. When oral feeding is not possible because the patient is incapable, or lacks motivation, seek other routes of administering nutrient substrates to critically ill or postoperative patients.

ASSESSMENT

Key points

- **Assess all patients admitted to hospital, even for elective procedures.**
- **Record the results.**
- **Decide whether or not nutritional support will be required.**

Specific aspects help in classifying nutritional status:

- Record height and weight for comparison with standard charts.
- Estimate from the dietary history and from the assumption that maximum requirements of protein and energy for hospitalized patients are $1.5 \, \text{g kg}^{-1} 24 \, \text{h}^{-1}$, and $40 \, \text{kcal kg}^{-1} 24 \, \text{h}^{-1}$ respectively.
- Assess body composition clinically.
- It may be difficult to identify PEM. Look for and record signs such as loss of muscle power, peripheral oedema, skin rashes, angular stomatitis, gingivitis, nail abnormalities, glossitis, paraesthesia and neuropathy.
- Tests may have poor sensitivity. Compare midarm muscle circumference with tables and measure triceps skinfold thickness, for which you need special calipers. Apply dynamometric tests such as hand-grip strength. Assess serum albumin (normal $36–47 \, \text{g l}^{-1}$), transferrin (normal $2–4 \, \text{g l}^{-1}$) assess the lymphocyte count (normal $1.5–4 \times 10^9 \, \text{l}^{-1}$) and delayed hypersensitivity skin testing.

In the absence of a specific measure, clinically place each patient in one of the following groups:

1. Obvious severe malnutrition, recent or long term (>10% recent weight loss, serum albumin <30 g l⁻¹, gross muscle wasting and peripheral oedema).
2. Moderate malnutrition, with low nutritional parameters, impaired nutrient intake for more than 2–4 weeks, although there may be no obvious physical evidence.
3. Normal or near-normal status but at risk of deteriorating without support in traumatized or ventilated patients.
4. Normal nutritional status which is unlikely to be affected by illness.

If 1, 2, 3 nutritional support maybe needed. If so, determine the best route of administration (Fig. 10.1).

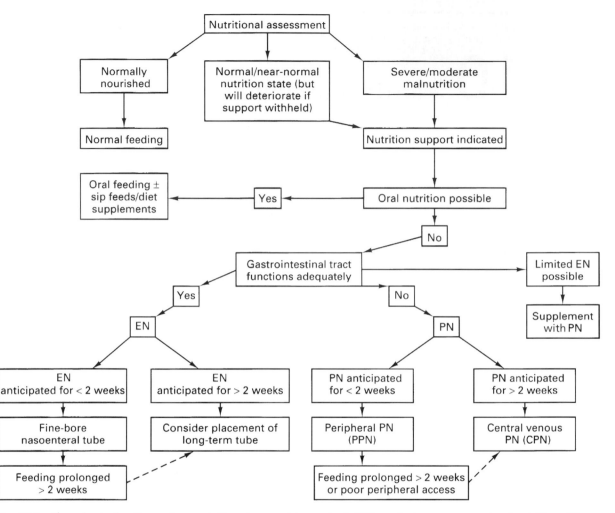

Fig. 10.1 Flow chart of options when nutritional support is required. CPN, central venous parenteral nutrition; EN, enteral nutrition; PN, parenteral nutrition; PPN, peripheral parenteral nutrition.

ENTERAL AND PARENTERAL NUTRITION FOR SURGICAL PATIENTS

 Key point

- **Prefer enteral feeding for all patients with a fully functioning, accessible gastrointestinal tract.**

1. Enteral feeding may improve antibacterial host defences, blunt the hypermetabolic response to trauma, maintain gut mucosal mass, maintain gut barrier function and prevent disruption of gut flora. It may contribute to maintaining splanchnic blood flow and the direct provision of nutrients for enterocytes. The gut was previously considered unimportant during critical illness caused by injury or infection. It is now recognized that the gastrointestinal tract is frequently a reservoir for bacterial translocation across the gut wall. Gut-derived endotoxin may therefore be a link between gastrointestinal failure and multiple organ failure without overt clinical evidence of infection (Fig. 10.2).

2. Research is being carried out to determine whether dietary manipulation, such as provision of glutamine or fibre, can prevent bowel atrophy and maintain intestinal mass, in the hope of reducing morbidity and mortality.

3. For the majority of critically ill patients, including postoperative patients, the gastrointestinal tract is the appropriate route for nutritional support, provided it is functioning normally. Because small intestinal function is better maintained postoperatively than gastric and large bowel function, enteral (small bowel) feeding can start

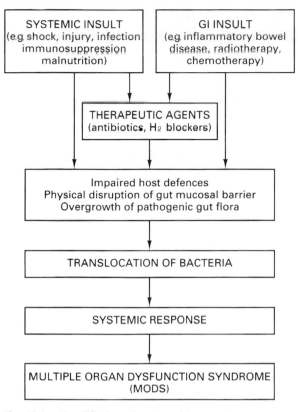

Fig. 10.2   Simplified mechanism of bacterial translocation and multiple organ failure.

early following operation, including major aortic and small bowel surgery, and following head injuries.

4. The benefits of enteral nutrition in patients who would formerly have been given parenteral nutrition have been demonstrated, although patients in whom there is reasonable doubt as to the adequacy of gastrointestinal function should be fed by the parenteral route. There are no differences in major postoperative complications and mortality rates; however, in certain groups (e.g. malnourished gastrointestinal cancer patients) who receive early enteral nutrition, significantly reduced complication rates and shorter duration of postoperative stay may be achieved with enteral nutrition, although parenteral nutrition is better tolerated. In summary total parenteral nutrition is an equally effective alternative to enteral nutrition when a risk of malnutrition is present and enteral nutrition is not tolerated or when gut failure is present.

Preoperative nutritional support

- **Give a severely malnourished (e.g. more than 10% weight loss) patient at least 10 days of** dietary supplementation, enteral or parenteral nutrition.
- **Do not delay operation if the disease is progressing, causing the patient's condition to deteriorate.**
- **Do not delay operation solely on account of borderline or mild malnutrition.**

Postoperative nutrition

1. Consider postoperative nutrition for any patient with an inadequate intake after 5 days.

2. Give parenteral nutrition if oral or enteral nutrition is not anticipated within 7 days post-operation in a previously well-nourished patient and as early as possible in a previously malnourished or critically ill patient.

3. Consider creating access to the gastrointestinal tract via a gastrostomy, a jejunostomy or a central venous feeding line at the time of major oropharyngeal, maxillofacial or upper gastrointestinal operation. This spares the patient a second procedure and the access lines can be disconnected if they are not needed.

4. In extreme circumstances, such as an elderly, malnourished smoker requiring oesophagectomy, provide preoperative nutritional support and arrange to continue it afterwards. By contrast, a patient with perforation of a viscus from inflammatory bowel disease unresponsive to medical management needs operation first, nutritional support afterwards.

ENERGY AND NITROGEN REQUIREMENTS

Many surgical patients in need of nutritional support are metabolically stressed, septic or traumatized by accident or operation. In particular, those with burns or head injuries are likely to be hypermetabolic as a result of neuroendocrine responses. Although precise energy requirements can be determined by indirect calorimetry, this is not a practical approach. Energy requirements to achieve positive energy balance in surgical patients are rarely more than 2200–2400 kcal 24 h^{-1}. Give 35–40 kcal kg^{-1} 24 h^{-1} as a mixture of carbohydrate and fat, which is usually sufficient.

Nitrogen requirements may be considerable; in hypermetabolic, stressed and injured patients it may be impossible to achieve a balance until the underlying cause has been improved. Minimize losses in order not to waste administered nitrogen, maintain lean body mass, allow an adequate supply for repair and allow active repletion of lean body mass in a previously compromised patient. For most adults 14–16 g nitrogen suffices. For those who require even more nitrogen, up to 0.4 g kg^{-1} 24 h^{-1} has been suggested.

When patients are on nutritional support, frequently monitor and chart:

- Diet
- Weight
- Haematology
- Biochemistry.

Keep accurate records of actual as opposed to prescribed intake, in order to identify any nutritional inadequacies promptly. They are particularly important during the changeover to oral feeding. Regularly weigh to ensure that the regimen is satisfactory, especially in those requiring body mass repletion. Weight gain may represent water retention, however, but this is revealed if you regularly monitor haematological and biochemical results. Especially in the first few days and in the malnourished patient, monitor the plasma potassium, phosphate and glucose. Measure vitamin and trace elements in patients on long-term feeding if appropriate. The response to nutritional support may be judged over days and weeks by the levels of plasma proteins, transferrin and thyroid prealbumin.

Although anthropometric and dynamometric measurements are often considered as research tools, they offer sensitive, effective measurements of nutrition, so use them when they are available.

Nitrogen balance

An aim of nutritional support is to try and ensure that the patient is in positive nitrogen balance. This is often difficult or impossible to achieve in patients who are very physiologically stressed or catabolic, the phase of destructive metabolism, in the immediate aftermath of trauma or injury and in the critically ill.

Nitrogen balance depends upon the difference between whole body protein synthesis and breakdown. It is more a measure of the metabolic than the nutritional state. In most patients nitrogen balance can be calculated from urinary and faecal nitrogen losses. Collect 24 h samples of urine, as faecal loss is often negligible. Urinary urea may reasonably be considered to account for 80% of total urinary nitrogen. Adjust for plasma urea levels and for faecal and other routes of loss of 2–3 g.

In a severely ill patient, urinary urea may not represent 80% of urinary nitrogen, because of excessive excretion of ammonia and other non-urea nitrogenous products. If chemiluminescence measurement of total urinary nitrogen is available, there is no need to estimate output from urea values.

ENTERAL NUTRITION

Types of diet

Polymeric (Greek *polys* = much, many + *meros* = part) *diets* contain whole protein as a nitrogen source, triglycerides and glucose polymers for energy, together with standardized amounts of electrolytes, trace elements and vitamins. Standard polymeric diets contain approximately 6 g nitrogen l^{-1} with an energy density of 1 kcal ml^{-1}. Energy (nitrogen dense) diets contain 8–10 g nitrogen/l and an energy density of 1–1.5 kcal ml^{-1}. These diets are suitable for more than 90% of patients with normal or near normal gastrointestinal function. In those with impaired intraluminal hydrolysis from severe pancreatic exocrine insufficiency or intestinal failure from short bowel syndrome, give a predigested or elemental diet.

Predigested or elemental diets have nitrogen sources derived from amino acids or oligopeptides. Their benefit over standard diets in acute pancreatitis has been established. Glucose polymer mixtures with polymers predominantly of chain length more than 10 glucose molecules provide energy. A combination of long- and medium-chain triglycerides provides the fat component.

Some *disease-specific diets* have been developed. High carbohydrate loads increase carbon dioxide production in patients with respiratory failure who are on ventilators; diets containing a higher fat energy component may allow the patient to be weaned from the ventilator as a result of decreased carbon dioxide production and reduced respiratory quotient.

Research is underway to design diets that modify or modulate stress and the immune response. No general recommendations are yet available but specific groups such as the critically ill may benefit.

Route of administration

Most patients require nutritional support for less than 1 month. For these, a fine-bore nasogastric tube suffices. Ensure that the tube is correctly positioned, especially if the patient has altered swallowing, diminished gag reflex, or has had surgery of the pharynx or upper airway. Confirm that the tube is correctly placed by aspirating gastric contents. If the patient is unable to cooperate, confirm the position of the tube tip radiologically. It should preferably be sited beyond the pylorus if gastric atony and regurgitation are likely. Advance the tube using a combination of manipulation and administration of a motility stimulant such as metoclopramide. Longer term feeding may be provided by percutaneous endoscopically placed gastrostomy or needle catheter jejunostomy. These techniques are valuable for undernourished patients at presentation, those undergoing major upper gastrointestinal operation, adjuvant radiotherapy or chemotherapy, and those undergoing laparotomy following major abdominal trauma. Anticipate the problem at operation by placing the tube at the time; sometimes pharyngostomy or oesophagostomy may be used.

Anticipate and prepare for gastric atony or paresis in:

- Critically ill and recumbent patients and following head injury
- Patients being ventilated or needing intensive care
- Following abdominal surgery
- Diabetes with neuropathy
- Hypothyroidism
- Neuromotor deglutition disorder

Preferably administer enteral diet from a large reservoir holding up to 2 litres, from a sterile closed system, especially if the patient is immunosuppressed or critically ill. Change the reservoir and giving set every 24 h. Prefer continuous to intermittent bolus feeding, so avoiding bloating and diarrhoea. Use gravity feed or a peristaltic pump. A starter regimen of undiluted full-volume diet does not, as is commonly thought, provoke gastrointestinal side-effects in patients with normal bowel, or those with inflammatory bowel disease. Starting with reduced volume or diluting the feed limits the intake, thereby prolonging the duration of negative nitrogen balance. In most adult patients with no other metabolic or fluid balance problems, prescribe 2–2.5 litres of diet each day from the beginning.

Complications

1. Feeding tube blockage most usually occurs when the giving set is disconnected and the residual diet solidifies. Prevent it by flushing out the tube with water after disconnecting it. Unblock it by instilling pancreatic enzyme or cola. The tube may be malpositioned or be inadvertently removed.

2. Diarrhoea, occurring in about 10% of patients, is multifactorial, often associated with concomitant antibiotic treatment or hypoalbuminaemia. Only rarely do you need to discontinue feeding, as codeine phosphate or loperamide is usually effective. Review the drug chart frequently and stop antibiotics if they are no longer required.

3. Nausea and vomiting are rarely caused by the feeds but may develop because of slow gastric emptying; try giving antiemetics. Too rapid administration, or bolus feeding, may produce bloating, abdominal pain or cramps. Regurgitation and pulmonary aspiration occasionally occur.

4. Anticipate and prevent vitamin, mineral and trace element deficiencies.

5. Enteral diets react with enterally administered drugs such as theophylline, warfarin, methyldopa and digoxin, especially if the patient is fed orally. If drug therapy that was effective fails during enteral feeding, assume it results from the enteral feeding unless proved otherwise.

Key point

- Exclude complications of infection originating in the diet, reservoir or giving set.

PARENTERAL NUTRITION

The successful use of intravenous parenteral (Greek *para* = besides + *enteron* = gut, intestine) nutrition was first demonstrated three decades ago. Parenteral nutrition (PN) (often termed TPN – total parenteral nutrition – although this is only true if all macronutrients and micronutrients such as electrolytes, vitamins and trace elements are included) is required for any patient with intestinal failure (short term or long term). It is essential for some acutely ill patients, although the increasing preference for the enteral route is reducing this. About 25% of hospitalized patients requiring nutritional support need it to be administered parenterally. Consider it for actual or potential malnourished patients with a non-functioning, partially functioning and/or inaccessible gastrointestinal tract. When in doubt about gastrointestinal function, use parenteral nutrition until you are reassured about gastrointestinal function.

Access

Parenteral nutrition solutions generally have high osmolalities (Greek *otheein* = to push; the tendency of water to pass through a semipermeable membrane from the side of lower concentration to the side of higher concentration, to equalize the concentrations). Hypertonic solutions infused into peripheral veins damage the endothelium, causing thrombosis. This is overcome by introducing them through a catheter passed into a large central vein, such as the vena cava, where the concentrated fluid mixes rapidly with the large volume of blood and is diluted.

The risk of introducing sepsis demands the highest level of technical care. The catheter is usually passed through a subcutaneous tunnel before entering the vein, to distance the vein entry from the surface. If a patient with a central venous catheter develops pyrexia and raised leucocyte count, and has no detectable cause after a rigorous search, assume it is catheter related.

The development of lower energy regimens in which lipid provides a substantial part of the required calories allows the administration of parenteral nutrition via peripheral veins. Peripheral parenteral nutrition (PPN) without provoking thrombophlebitis is facilitated by using fine-bore cannulas, the use of heparin, in-line filtration, cortisol, buffering and the local application of glyceryl trinitrate patches. In addition, most courses last no more than 10–14 days.

Nutrients

Macronutrients, larger molecules, contain glucose and lipid emulsions, usually 50:50 with nitrogen sources in the form of L-amino acids. New lipids with better stability in solution are now available; they can modulate immune functions, inflammatory processes and metabolism, and promise to become more widely used.

Micronutrients include electrolytes, trace elements and vitamins. Commercial all-in-one bags contain mixed macro- and micronutrients which can safely be infused over 12–24 h. They can be safely stored for several weeks. They suit almost 80% of patients and are widely used. Ready-to-use standardized formulations, either made up in pharmacies or presented as commercial multichamber bags, simplify administration, and the most appropriate formula best approximating the patient's needs can be chosen.

Key points

- **Monitor blood glucose 6-hourly for the first week to detect insulin resistance; you may need to give exogenous insulin by injection or infusion.**
- **Monitor electrolytes daily so you can detect and correct imbalances.**
- **Monitor liver function to check serum albumin and hepatobiliary dysfunction, which inevitably results from parenteral nutrition in some patients.**

Complications

Metabolic complications of parenteral nutrition, in descending order of frequency are: hyperglycaemia, hypoglycaemia, hypophosphataemia, hypercalcaemia, hyperkalaemia, hypokalaemia, hypernatraemia, hypo-

natraemia. In the longer term, anticipate deficiencies of folate, zinc, magnesium, other trace elements, vitamins and essential fatty acids.

Home parenteral nutrition

Some patients require long-term nutritional support by virtue of loss of bowel by disease or resection. Such parenteral or enteral support demands commitment by you as part of the surgical team, by skilled carers and by the patients. Although patients can often be monitored locally, overall management must be undertaken at a special centre. The principles are the same as for inpatient management but long-term monitoring and specific complications are more complex. Those in need of home nutritional support ahould be referred at an early stage.

NUTRITION SUPPORT TEAM

In hospital, the best way of optimizing nutritional care is with a multidisciplinary support team, each member providing specialty expert care. They receive input from clinicians, dieticians, pharmacists, nurses, chemical pathologists and microbiologists. A central support team can establish specialized teams to attend to specific needs in, for example, intensive care and paediatrics.

Summary

- How does malnutrition affect surgical outcome?
- How do you assess the nutritional state of your patients?
- How do you identify and treat malnourished patients?
- What methods are available and how do you select them?
- What is the make-up of a nutritional support team?

Further reading

Payne-James JJ, Wicks CW 2002 Key facts in clinical nutrition, 2nd edn. Greenwich Medical Media, London

Payne-James JJ, Grimble GK, Silk DBA (eds) 2001 Artificial nutrition support in clinical practice, 2nd edn. Greenwich Medical Media, London

11 Clinical pharmacology

J. Robin

> **Objectives**
>
> - **Understand how drugs are developed and licensed.**
> - **Know how to select drugs rationally, according to efficacy, safety, convenience and cost.**
> - **Learn to prescribe safely and effectively.**
> - **Be aware of the use of drugs in special situations.**
> - **Beware of drug interactions whenever you prescribe.**

INTRODUCTION

Almost all doctors prescribe drugs. As a budding surgeon, you are no exception. You use drugs extensively perioperatively. You also use drugs as first line therapy for some conditions referred to you. Many of your patients have an extensive list of medications prescribed for coexisting diseases, some of them unfamiliar to you. You often continue to prescribe these drugs while the patient remains under your care.

This chapter aims to teach you the principles of selecting drugs rationally, and using them safely and effectively. The *British National Formulary* (BNF) is a source of much useful information for prescribers. Keep it to hand as you study this chapter so you can refer to it. You need to understand the various factors that influence your decision to prescribe a particular drug to your patient, and the consequences that flow from that decision. A drug (the word is of uncertain origin) is any substance used in the composition of a medicine.

DRUG DEVELOPMENT AND LICENSING

As a prescriber, you need to have a basic understanding of the process of drug development and marketing.

1. New drugs are continually developed and marketed by the major pharmaceutical companies. Development begins with the pharmaceutical company identifying an 'unmet medical need', such as diseases for which no effective therapy is available, or conditions for which the existing therapy is considered suboptimal in terms of efficacy, tolerability or both.

2. Once the need is identified, the drug company synthesizes novel compounds that might have some useful pharmacological activity, called 'new chemical entities' (NCEs). Any NCEs showing promise are immediately protected by a patent, giving the company 20 years exclusive rights to develop and market the drug. The attrition rate for NCEs is high, the majority being discarded because they do not work or are too toxic. Drug development is expensive and time consuming: it can take up to 10 years to bring one to the market.

3. Once a drug is successfully developed the manufacturers apply for a product licence, the marketing permit, with specific indications, specific patient groups and for specific doses. Indications may be a symptom, disease or a physiological derangement.

4. If a specialist chooses to prescribe a drug outside the terms of its product licence (an unlicensed indication), the prescriber, not the drug company, is responsible for any harmful consequences.

> **Key point**
>
> - **Do not prescribe a drug outside its product licence. Consult your senior colleagues.**

SELECTING DRUGS

The BNF contains thousands of established drugs for a multitude of indications. Each year many existing drugs gain new indications and hundreds of new drugs or new formulations of existing drugs are added to the BNF. For some indications the choice of drugs may be bewildering and the marketing claims made for them

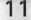
may be very impressive at first glance. Sensibly evaluate the real worth of drugs.

Key point

- **Select drugs for their proven efficacy (effectiveness), safety, convenience and cost, not on the basis of claims made for them.**

Efficacy

1. In order to gain a product licence, the pharmaceutical company must provide evidence from clinical trials that a drug is at least more effective than placebo (Latin 'I shall please'; treatment that pleases the patient rather than exerts a curative effect). It need not demonstrate that the drug is better than existing therapy.

2. The benefits of a drug over existing therapy may be relatively small. To demonstrate a small clinical advantage over existing therapy, a large, lengthy and very expensive clinical trial is often required.

3. The size, length and cost of a clinical trial can be reduced by employing surrogate (Latin *sub* = in place of + *rogare* = to ask; substitute) as opposed to real endpoints. A surrogate endpoint is some measurement or test that plausibly suggests, but does not prove, genuine benefit to patients, such as reduction in prostate size in benign prostatic hypertrophy. Real endpoints (something the patient will notice and is likely to bring benefit, such as a reduction in prostatic symptoms) provide a much more secure basis for determining the clinical efficacy of a drug. Read claims critically (see Chs 12, 45, 46).

Key points

- **Ensure the trial patient group represents the likely clinical patients, not younger or healthier.**
- **Has the new drug been tested against and shown to be more effective than existing therapy, using real endpoints?**

4. Efficacy data are often presented in the most favourable light. Reductions in relative risk are more impressive than reductions in absolute risk, but reduction in absolute risk is most important. To get a feel for the benefit of a drug, consider the number needed to treat (NNT):

- Consider two drugs compared using relative risk. Drug **A** reduces the relative risk of disease **X** by 50%. Drug **B** reduces the relative risk of disease **Y** by 10%. Which is the more effective drug? Drug **A** perhaps?
- It is impossible to say without knowing the absolute risks of diseases **X** and **Y**. If the absolute risk of disease

X is 1%, drug **A** will reduce absolute risk by 0.5%. The number of patients that need to be treated for one to benefit (NNT) will be 100/0.5 = 200. However, if the absolute risk of disease **X** is 50%, drug **A** will reduce absolute risk by 5%. The number of patients that need to be treated for one to benefit (NNT) will be 100/5 = 20.

- Now which is the most effective drug?

Assessing safety

1. So you have decided that a new drug offers a genuine and clinically significant advantage over, or in addition to, existing therapy. You must now investigate the drug's safety profile. When you assess comparative safety over placebo or existing therapy, again make sure that the selected patient group is representative of the patients that you actually treat. Relatively young and otherwise healthy individuals are less likely to experience significant side-effects compared with the elderly patients with comorbidity that you might treat. Just as the concept of absolute and relative risk may paint different pictures in terms of benefit, they may also do so in terms of harm.

- Consider a new drug that is stated to increase only the absolute risk of an adverse effect by 5% only. How safe is the drug?
- It is impossible to say without knowing the absolute risk of the adverse effect in patients not taking the drug. If this risk is 20%, the drug will increase the relative risk by 25%, but if it is 1%, the drug will increase the relative risk by 500%!

2. Also, make sure that, when compared to existing therapy, equivalent doses in terms of efficacy were used. Have low doses of existing therapy been used when making comparisons of efficacy and high doses when comparing safety and tolerability?

Surely the adverse effects are already known?

1. Most new drugs are purposely designed to enhance target selectivity. This is often an important part of the marketing message. Indeed, such an approach can potentially minimize adverse effects and enhance tolerability.

2. New drugs, no matter how well designed, also have a distinct disadvantage. Prior to gaining a licence, it is unusual for a drug to have been tested in more than a couple of thousand patients. It is often many fewer. While dose-dependent, or predictable, adverse effects may have been designed out during development, idiosyncratic (Greek *idios* = one's own + *syn* = together + *krasis* = a mixing; individual mental or physical constitution) adverse effects may not yet have occurred with sufficient frequency to be noticed. Idiosyncratic adverse effects are often serious and sometimes fatal.

3. Postmarketing surveillance is used to detect these adverse effects as quickly as possible. In the United Kingdom, the basis of postmarketing surveillance is the Yellow Card Scheme. It is quite common for a new 'wonder drug' to be withdrawn a few months later as an unacceptable side-effect profile becomes apparent through the postmarketing surveillance.

Key points

- **New drugs are not necessarily safer than existing therapy.**
- **Moderately rare adverse effects are only detected after the drug is marketed through the process of postmarketing surveillance.**

The Yellow Card Scheme

1. This is a scheme that encourages doctors and pharmacists to report all suspected adverse effects of new drugs (marked with an ▼ in the BNF) and serious and life-threatening adverse effects of existing drugs.

2. Because the scheme is not compulsory, it is underused and only 10% of adverse effects are reported.

Key points

- **Be alert to the possibility of unexpected adverse effects, especially when prescribing drugs marked ▼ in the *British National Formulary*.**
- **Report all suspected adverse effects of new drugs.**
- **Report all serious and life-threatening adverse effects of established drugs.**

Convenience and cost

1. Sometimes a drug company freely admits that its new drug is no safer or effective than existing therapy but claims that it is more convenient. For instance, a drug may need to be taken only once rather than twice daily. It is suggested that it will improve patient compliance. In fact, there is little evidence that once-daily preparations achieve significantly better compliance than twice-daily preparations, although both are better than three or more times-daily drugs.

2. As a result of technological advances, a plethora of expensive long-acting or slow-release formulations are now marketed. As well as reducing dosing frequency, it is often also claimed that they achieve smoother plasma drug concentrations, which improves either efficacy,

tolerability, or both. Is there genuine clinical evidence to support these claims?

3. The cost of a new drug should not be a primary consideration in your decision whether or not to prescribe it to an individual patient, but remember that a newer, and inevitably more expensive, drug is not necessarily better. You should be persuaded to prescribe an expensive new drug only if you are convinced that it offers a genuine and worthwhile advantage over existing therapy.

4. A number of very similar drugs may be developed simultaneously for the same indication by different companies. In such cases, it is sensible for you to select the cheapest.

Key points

- **Once- or twice-daily dosing improves compliance compared with more frequent regimens.**
- **Long-acting or slow-release formulations are more expensive and may not necessarily confer any clinical advantage.**
- **Prescribe a more expensive new drug only if it offers worthwhile benefit over cheaper existing therapy.**
- **When a range of very similar drugs exist, select the cheapest in the class.**

Gaining reliable information about drugs

1. Many sources are available. They are not all helpful, some may be misleading. Review articles or journal editorials are usually balanced, but sometimes the authors have links with the manufacturers. Carefully read the small print at the end of the article stating the author's potential conflicts of interest.

2. Recommendations from expert bodies are usually but not always reliable.

3. Colleagues may be a useful source of information or guidance.

4. Consult independent assessments, which are available nationally through the *Drug and Therapeutics Bulletin* (DTB) and National Prescribing Centre (NPC). Locally, hospital committees select new drugs from those available to list in the hospital formulary. Except in very exceptional circumstances, use drugs on that list.

5. Consult guidance produced by the National Institute for Clinical Excellence (NICE) on relevant drugs. Such guidance recommends what drug technology should be made available, but rarely how particular drugs should be integrated with other treatment you wish to offer. You remain responsible for deciding where and when to use the drug.

Key point

- Obtain and critically evaluate the best and most reliable information available about drugs.

USING DRUGS

Favour prescribing from a personal selection of formulary drugs with which you are familiar. From time to time, as new evidence becomes available, you might rationally add or substitute new drugs according to the principles outlined above. You will also know that your patients vary in their individual clinical response to drugs. Therefore, in order to use drugs both safely and effectively, you should carefully tailor your prescribing to the characteristics of the individual patient. Individual variability is manifested in both *pharmacodynamic* ('what the drug does to body' including both desired and adverse effects) and *pharmacokinetic* ('what the body does to the drug') responses, according to such factors as age, disease, genetic background and other drugs the patient is taking.

Elderly

1. Patients of advanced age consume most of the drugs that are prescribed. Although no drugs are specifically contraindicated in the elderly, exercise particular caution when prescribing drugs to this group. In particular, be aware that the elderly are often more sensitive to both the effects and adverse effects of a drug. There are many reasons for this. Drug elimination becomes progressively impaired with age, causing drug accumulation. In addition, the adverse effects of many drugs are blunted by physiological compensatory responses. These compensatory responses are less efficient in the elderly.

2. Elderly patients are more likely to have coexisting disease that may alter their response to drugs. Other diseases mean that other doctors are involved and frequently this results in them taking a long list of drugs, often with little rational justification – 'polypharmacy' – (Greek *polys* = much, many). This significantly increases the potential for drug interactions.

3. Before prescribing, ask yourself whether your elderly patient really requires an additional drug? If so, perhaps this is a good time to ask a medical colleague specializing in the care of the elderly to rationalize the patient's therapy. If you do decide to prescribe, start with the lowest possible dose and titrate the dose gradually upwards until the desired effect is achieved. Some drugs

may even have a lower starting dose for elderly patients, so check the BNF.

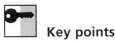

Key points

- The elderly are more sensitive to the effects and adverse effects of drugs.
- Polypharmacy in the elderly increases the potential for drug interactions.
- Avoid prescribing additional drugs to elderly patients unless absolutely necessary.

Children

1. As paediatricians continually point out, children are not just small adults. This is especially true for the way children respond to drugs, both in the nature and the extent of the response. Not surprisingly, neonates are the most different and, as children develop, they gradually respond more like adult patients. Some drugs are specifically contraindicated below a certain age and, of those medicines that are considered suitable, few have been formally tested in children. This means that they are unlicensed for paediatric use.

2. Paediatricians are well aware of these difficulties. Over the years, they have learnt from experience what are suitable drugs and suitable doses for children. Most hospitals have a **paediatric formulary** incorporating this experience; this will often give more age-specific dosing information than standard references like the BNF. Therefore, always refer to the paediatric formulary and always ask a paediatrician for help if you are at all unsure, or if you wish to prescribe a drug not contained in the paediatric formulary.

Key points

- Children may respond very differently to drugs compared with adults.
- Most drugs are unlicensed for paediatric use.
- Be guided by the local paediatric formulary.
- Always be willing to seek specialist advice.

Pregnancy

1. The problems with thalidomide in the 1960s have understandably made doctors very wary about prescribing drugs when a patient is, or might become, pregnant. The drug was prescribed to pregnant women to relieve morning sickness, and resulted in the birth of babies with aplastic or hypoplastic limb deformities – phocomelia (Greek *phoke* = seal + *melos* = limb; from the resemblance

to a seal's flipper). Many commonly used drugs are known or suspected to be harmful to the fetus, or have never been prescribed in pregnancy. There is, however, a small group of older drugs that accumulated clinical experience suggests are relatively safe.

2. Often the extent and nature of the harm depends on the trimester of pregnancy during which the drug is prescribed. Drugs harmful in the first trimester are potential teratogens (Greek *teras* = monster + *gennaein* = to generate), whereas those prescribed in the second or third trimesters may adversely effect fetal development or metabolism. Drugs prescribed late in pregnancy may also affect labour and harm the child in the peri- and postnatal periods.

3. As far as possible, avoid prescribing any drugs in pregnancy, but where prescription is inevitable, restrict yourself to those drugs that are regarded as relatively safe. On every occasion check in the BNF (Appendix 4) that the drug is appropriate for the stage in pregnancy of your patient.

4. What happens if the mother is seriously ill and you have to prescribe a drug that may harm the fetus? This can be justified because the well-being of the fetus is secondary to the well-being of the mother. If you are faced with such a situation, always try to seek advice from a fetal medicine specialist in order to minimize risk to the unborn child.

Key points

- **If possible, avoid all drugs in pregnancy or in women who might become pregnant.**
- **If you must prescribe, specifically check in the BNF that the drug is considered safe.**
- **If in doubt, or when a potentially harmful drug is indicated, seek specialist advice.**

Disease

Many drugs are known to have the potential to harm organs or to exacerbate certain diseases. Potential organ damage will be listed as a specific adverse effect of a particular drug. A disease exacerbated by the drug will be listed in the BNF as a specific **contraindication** to prescribing the drug.

Liver and kidney disease

1. The kidneys and the liver are the organs principally involved in drug elimination. This means that both the liver and kidney are particularly susceptible to the harmful effects of drugs (hepatotoxicity and nephrotoxicity). It also means that pre-existing liver and renal disease may adversely affect the body's handling of some drugs, leading to drug accumulation and increased adverse effects.

2. When prescribing hepatotoxic or nephrotoxic drugs, carefully consider whether the potential benefits to the patient outweigh the potential risks. If you do prescribe, monitor for organ toxicity. In those patients with either pre-existing liver or renal disease, the risks are usually so great that you should avoid prescribing drugs that are potentially toxic to the affected organ. However, in some cases, such prescribing is inevitable. If this is the case, make every attempt to minimize exposure to the drug by reducing dose and duration of therapy. Rigorously monitor any biochemical changes signalling worsening organ impairment.

3. With pre-existing liver or renal disease, even if you prescribe drugs that are not directly toxic to the affected organ, you may still face difficulties due to impaired drug elimination. In general, reduce the dose and/or frequency of the prescribed drug. Appendices 2 (liver) and 3 (kidney) of the BNF suggest appropriate dosage reductions according to the degree of organ impairment.

Key points

- **The liver and the kidneys are especially likely to be harmed by drug therapy.**
- **Where the potential for harm exists, carefully monitor for toxicity.**
- **Pre-existing liver and renal disease often causes drug accumulation and increase adverse effects.**
- **Adjust the dose according to the BNF.**
- **If possible, avoid prescribing potentially hepatotoxic or nephrotoxic drugs to patients with impairment of those organs.**
- **If such prescribing is inevitable, take every step to minimize additional harm.**

Genetic background

It is increasingly recognized that multiple genetic factors are responsible for much of the individual variability observed in patients' pharmacodynamic and pharmacokinetic responses to drugs. New drugs are increasingly designed to minimize such genetically determined variability but, for the vast majority of patients, we have not reached a point where a patient's precise genetic make-up is a factor to consider when prescribing. The only area where is does matter is when prescribing for patients with rare single-gene disorders which affect their response to a wide range of drugs. The best known of these disorders are porphyria and glucose-6-phosphate dehydrogenase deficiency (G6PD deficiency). Many drugs are recognized to aggravate these conditions. If you have a patient with either of these disorders you should make sure (by checking the BNF) that the drug and dose that you prescribe is not regarded as potentially harmful.

Interactions

In practice, it is often drug interactions due to the co-prescription of other drugs that cause the most problems. The possibilities for interactions increase exponentially with each new drug that is added. Drug interactions can be either pharmacodynamic or pharmacokinetic.

Pharmacodynamic interactions

1. *Additive* – where two drugs combine to produce a greater effect. You may on occasion exploit this interaction clinically to enhance a desired effect, but it also can unwittingly produce enhanced toxicity.
2. *Antagonistic* – where one drug cancels or diminishes the effects of another. Again, you may sometimes wish to exploit this interaction clinically, particularly in the case of overdose.

Pharmacokinetic interactions

Any stage of the pharmacokinetic process (absorption, distribution, metabolism and excretion) has potential for drug interactions. The most common and important interactions involve drug metabolism and, in particular, induction and inhibition of the hepatic cytochrome P450 (CYP450) enzyme system. This is a family of the hepatic enzymes responsible for the metabolism of a wide variety of commonly used drugs, referred to as CYP450 substrates. These enzymes can be either inhibited or induced by other drugs.

1. In the presence of a *CYP450 inhibitor*, the substrate drug is metabolized more slowly, causing the plasma levels to rise. Examples of CYP450 inducers are cimetidine, ciprofloxacin and erythromycin. To compensate, reduce the dose of the substrate drug.

2. In the presence of a *CYP450 inducer*, the substrate drug is metabolized more rapidly, causing the plasma levels to fall. Examples of CYP450 inhibitors are phenytoin, carbamazepine, rifampicin and alcohol. Increase the dose of the substrate drug to compensate.

3. In practice, interactions due to CYP450 inhibition or induction are most likely to cause you problems when the CYP450 substrate drug has a *narrow therapeutic index*. This means that there is only a narrow range of plasma concentration in which the drug is neither subtherapeutic nor toxic. Common CYP450 substrates with a narrow therapeutic index include theophylline, ciclosporin and warfarin. Your safe and practical solution with such drugs is to monitor the plasma level (or International Normalized Ratio (INR) in the case of warfarin). This monitoring should be more extensive (i.e. daily) when starting or stopping CYP450 inhibitors and inducers.

Key points

- Drug interactions can be either pharmacodynamic or pharmacokinetic.
- Potential drug interactions are listed in Appendix 1 of the BNF.
- Identify and carefully monitor drugs with a narrow therapeutic index.

Summary

- Are you aware that, even as a surgeon, prescribing drugs is likely to be a common and important part of your practice? In order to prescribe effectively for your patients, you must be able to select drugs rationally and use them safely. Despite the marketing claims, new drugs may not necessarily be more effective than existing therapy and will often be much more expensive. Before prescribing, you should look for objective and clinically relevant evidence of benefit from well-designed clinical trials. New drugs are not always safer than existing therapy. In fact, precisely because they are new, there is significantly less clinical experience than with older drugs. For this reason, new drugs are subjected to intensive postmarketing surveillance for adverse effects that are too rare to have been detected in prelicensing clinical trials.
- Do you recognize the need to rely on the hospital formulary when you prescribe, not on your memory? Consult the BNF unless you are absolutely sure about a drug. Always use the BNF when prescribing for difficult patients, especially those who are at the extremes of age, pregnant, have coexisting disease (especially hepatic and renal) or are receiving other drugs. Always seek to minimize the number of drugs a patient is receiving and weigh up carefully the risks and benefits of using a particular drug. You should be alert to the problems of drug toxicity and interactions. If these occur, act quickly to prevent further harm. In difficult situations, never be afraid to seek advice from specialists who have more experience. Remember, they will be very keen to seek your help with surgical problems.

Further reading

British National Formulary. *Published 6-monthly by the British Medical Association and the Royal Pharmaceutical Society of Great Britain, London*
Drug and Therapeutics Bulletin. *Published monthly, and free to all NHS doctors, by Which Ltd, London, DTB reviews new and existing therapies. The articles are concise, independent and well respected and should be considered essential reading*
Ritter JM, Lewis LD, Mant TGK 1999 A textbook of clinical pharmacology, 4th edn. Edward Arnold, London

Useful links
www.bnf.org   *British National Formulary*
www.nice.org.uk   National Institute of Clinical Excellence
www.npc.co.uk   National Prescribing Centre

12 Evidence-based practice

J. W. McClenahan

Objectives

- **Understand the purpose and nature of valid, important and applicable evidence to augment personal experience.**
- **Recognize the factors that help and hinder more widespread application of 'evidence-based practice' to surgery.**
- **Identify some suggestions for action that you or your colleagues could take.**

INTRODUCTION

You already use evidence (Latin *e* = from + *videre* = to see; hence, that can be seen) of many kinds in your surgical practice. The more systematically you can do that, the better a surgeon you can become. The encouragement given to evidence-based practice (EBP) seeks to enhance the role that systematic, critical review of valid, reliable and applicable evidence can play in enabling you to:

- Perform more appropriate surgery
- Inform patients better about the probable benefits and risks of surgery for their condition – both in general, and in relation to their own personal circumstances
- Enlarge the range of surgical interventions that have been *reliably* shown to be worthwhile, by participation in higher quality research.

WHAT IS 'EVIDENCE-BASED PRACTICE'?

1. Different authors will give varying definitions of what the phrase means, or even limit it to evidence-based medicine (excluding other clinical professions such as nursing or therapies). The following definition from McKibbon et al (1995) is the one I prefer.

Evidence-based practice is:

An approach to health care that promotes:

- **the collection, interpretation and integration (into clinical practice) of**
- **valid, important and applicable**
  - **patient-reported**
  - **clinician-observed, and**
  - **research-derived evidence.**

2. There are several points of note about this definition. It is an *inclusive* approach to health care as a whole, not a narrow limitation to research-derived evidence, let alone just to evidence from randomized controlled trials (RCTs).

3. It acknowledges the potential validity of patient perceptions, your clinical observations, and the use of judgement to integrate the different sorts of evidence.

4. However, randomized controlled trials remain the 'gold standard' of evidence. They are applicable if the types of patients included in them adequately match the real world of your clinical practice.

5. The definition also emphasizes the importance of building the use of evidence into your routine clinical practice. Do not see it just as an 'off-line' educational or research activity done by others. Furthermore, it implies the development of skills and judgement to decide what is valid, important and applicable, both to the individual patient you are considering now, and the whole range of patients you are or should be treating.

6. Evidence-based practice constitutes an intellectual revolution in the practice of medicine (in the broadest sense, i.e. what doctors of all kinds, including surgeons, do). It has been fuelled in the last decade or so particularly by five interrelated factors:

a. The *knowledge explosion* – the exponential growth in published research and knowledge.

b. The particular technique of *meta-analysis* – pooling the results of multiple clinical trials to derive more robust conclusions than any one alone can support.

c. The rapid evolution of *systematic review* – now a fomalized, thorough and reproducible (but resource-intensive) method of finding virtually all evidence on a topic, grading it by quality and relevance, and summarizing the results in a form able to be peer reviewed, and used by busy clinicians.

d. The organization of the *International Cochrane Collaboration*. This links researchers, information analysts, and practising clinicians worldwide. In the UK, two centres of particular importance are the Cochrane Centre in Oxford, and the Centre for Reviews and Dissemination in York. The collaboration helps to resource systematic reviews and engages with others in doing so worldwide.

e. Technological developments in *knowledge distribution* – particularly CD-Rom and the Internet – which make knowledge widely accessible easily and relatively cheaply. Increasingly, this means in the ward, operating theatre, diagnostic department, outpatient clinic, clinical staff's own offices and GP surgeries, as well as in libraries, postgraduate centre and people's own homes.

7. Evidence-based practice aims to improve clinical effectiveness – doing the right things for the right people at the right time in the best known way in routine practice. This means translating the findings of research which demonstrated *efficacy* – that there was a difference in a controlled trial in favour of one intervention over another – into *effective use* for a real population of patients.

 ### Achieving clinical effectiveness requires:

- **Professional staff who have up-to-date knowledge and skills, together with appropriate attitudes**
- **Working together in a cohesive and coordinated fashion within clinical teams**
- **The support of managers to meet both patient needs and strategic needs of the organization (Batstone & Edwards 1997).**

For surgeons, this can mean some significant personal changes or even challenges. Only those with strong individual egos seem to become surgeons, and surgery has a competitive culture. Acknowledging the importance of teamwork is perhaps easier now than allowing that managers have a valid role to play, but both run counter to many stereotypes if not the reality of modern surgery. Some of your behaviours may have to be unlearned!

Weren't we doing it anyway?

1. No conscientious medical practitioner I know wants to perform badly, and most make strenuous efforts to keep up to date. So it hurts to be told that your practice could be improved if you were to change the way you approach the use of evidence. You think that you already do the best you can with your limited time and, with help from your colleagues, you already use evidence – you were taught to do so by your professors or consultants or you have been challenged by your up-and-coming juniors. Well, yes … up to a point.

2. The reality, as opposed to the aspiration, is that there are often long delays between the production of convincing research evidence and its widespread adoption. The proponents of EBP believe, often with justification, that these delays could and should be shortened.

3. Things are getting better, however. A historical perspective illustrates the point. Prevention of scurvy took roughly two centuries between the first evidence of efficacy in 1601 (James Lancaster) and its routine adoption by the British Navy from 1775–1814. In this century, thrombolytic therapy after myocardial infarction took about two decades (from the 1970s to the 1990s) to be acknowledged as appropriate. Only then did it gain general acceptance as what ought to be done, even though the application is still uneven (see, for example, Antman et al 1992). Surfactants to relieve respiratory distress syndrome from hyaline membrane disease for neonates were adopted even more quickly – in part because their effects were obvious and dramatic, and in part because they went 'with the grain' of clinical culture and experience.

What EBP is not, but is feared to be

1. *Just cost cutting, or being banned from doing certain procedures?* Many doctors fear that EBP is just an attempt to reduce costs. They therefore react negatively. However, careful interpretation of the evidence may suggest that *different* things be done, some of which may cost more, some less, and some about the same. Part of your task when you are a senior surgeon will be to balance the many competing demands on resources. Evidence of effectiveness must play a bigger part in future decisions (see Ch. 42).

2. *Another reduction in clinical freedom, or 'cook-book' medicine?* Appropriate integration of research evidence into clinical practice poses no threat to clinical freedom (using the McKibbon et al definition), except to help you avoid unnecessary or indefensible mistakes. Is that the freedom you want to retain?

3. *Central diktats will determine local guidelines and protocols and 'the way we do things here'?* These should rather be determined locally, but using centrally collated and validated evidence. By establishing more clearly your own and your colleagues' understanding of what is known with reasonable certainty, based on research evidence, experience and patient feedback, you can make

Table 12.1 Examples and issues

Nature of evidence	Examples	Issues
Evidence convincing, widely accepted, but not universally applied	Early thrombolytic therapy for AMI	(Often mistaken) belief that 'we already do it here' – local and national audits often show otherwise Achieving organizational change to allow it
Evidence readily available but not sought	Which surgical patients benefit from DVT prophylaxis? Whom should we treat for atrial fibrillation?	Shifting professional attitudes to seeking evidence CPD (continuous professional development) Interpretive skills (critical appraisal training)
Evidence sought, but not locally accessible at the relevant time or place	As above, and ... Adjuvant therapy following surgical removal of cancers	Organizational and technical infrastructure Information and library facilities and staffing Technical skills training
Evidence actively sought, not found, equivocal or disputed	When should we remove catheters after paediatric cardiac surgery?	Establishing effective local guidelines, and local audit or research projects Feedback to national R&D priority setting or local academic centre

commonplace practice more consistent, and higher quality easier to deliver, audit and sustain. This leaves more, not less, freedom and time to use your judgement in areas where the circumstances are not routine, the research-based evidence is absent or equivocal, or the patient's individual preferences are uniquely out of the ordinary.

4. *Just for doctors, or just for clinical staff?* Evidence-based practice is as relevant for patients and their families or carers, and for managers, as it is for you. Media attention and the internet now make much more of the evidence widely available. Sessions with non-clinical staff, including managers and non-executive directors from NHS organizations, demonstrate that they can quickly and intelligently appraise even technical papers against systematic appraisal criteria. They can reach clear conclusions about the strength and interpretation of the evidence for themselves (from my personal experience with such groups at the King's Fund).

 Who needs information on evidence-based practice?

- **Patients to discuss options and risks with you.**
- **Professionals to improve their practice.**

- **Providers to improve effectiveness for their organizations.**
- **Purchasers, now primary care trusts (PCTs) in the NHS; more generally, commissioners of health care, to obtain the best quality service they can afford.**
- **Public for assurance that all of the above is happening properly in their interests.**

HOW CAN EVIDENCE MAKE A DIFFERENCE?

1. Evidence can impact practice in several different ways, and what needs to be done to improve things depends on the nature of the evidence, and what sort of barriers prevent its use. Examples (not exhaustive) are shown in Table 12.1.

2. What helps or hinders change? The 'change equation' (adapted from Beckhard & Harris 1987) is shown in Figure 12.1. You need to pay attention to all four boxes to maximize the likelihood of successful use of evidence to change practice. Acknowledge that you may be able to work on the *perception* that others have of the proposed

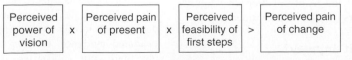

Fig 12.1 Beckhard's change equation. In order to change practice you need to take account of all four boxes. Present a clear, persuasive view of how things might be, show the present drawbacks, devise feasible initial changes and minimize 'discomfort' of change perceived by those affected

changes as well as the 'real' content of the change, as, for them, their perception *is* the reality.

3. To succeed:

a. Present a clear and persuasive view of how things might be (the vision) in terms relevant to the intended audience.

b. Show the drawbacks of the present circumstances (perhaps unsatisfactory or even dangerous), and ensure that other people become as uncomfortable with it as you are yourself.

c. Devise some initial changes that people see as feasible to get started (so make them as easy to adopt as possible).

d. Minimize the discomfort of the change as it will be *perceived* by individuals or groups affected.

4. Changing clinical practice is a multistage process. It does not happen all at once, and different influences work at different stages of people's readiness for change.

Key point

- **Do not presume that a rational argument, clearly and forcefully presented, will of itself predispose people to change, especially if they are not yet emotionally ready even to believe it is necessary at all.**

5. Figure 12.2 shows one model of individual change (based on Prochaska & DiClemente 1984) that may be helpful in understanding where you and your colleagues stand. It is crucial to acknowledge the importance of the early stages – initial awareness of the possibility of change

and recognition of a need to change. This can often take time (months, or occasionally years) to work through.

Where the major personal block is an emotional one, restating the rational case ever more forcefully is positively unhelpful. Ask rather than tell, and try to find out what emotion is being triggered by your proposal (or your own reaction to others' proposals) and seek to deal with *that* first.

6. Organizational change is a slower process than you expect – be patient. You may be used in your surgical team to making decisions and seeing them implemented very quickly or even instantly, if the power to change lies wholly within the surgical team. However, much of the improvement in clinical practice suggested by research evidence requires change on a broader organizational front. Many people with different professions, personal backgrounds, beliefs and values may have to be persuaded. Evaluation of change 'in the field' in response to evidence suggests four major hindrances to change at a scale larger than a single clinical team:

a. *Getting momentum going.* Raising awareness and recognition of the need to change takes time, patience, and repeated application as the 'cast of characters' is constantly changing in the hectic pace of NHS reorganization.

b. *Staff turnover.* Original sponsors of change may leave the organization.

c. *Action.* Getting guidelines agreed and accepted is more difficult than most people initially believe is possible.

d. *Implementation and maintenance.* If you think getting guidelines agreed is the hard part, think again. After that is when the most difficult (but ultimately rewarding) part really starts. To engage others more widely beyond the enthusiasts, you or a small group around you, need yet more patience, careful planning, wide consultation and

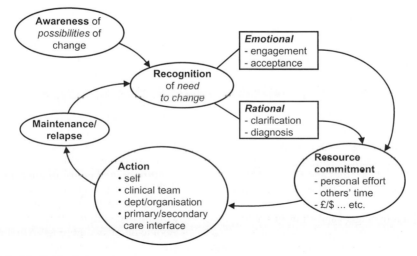

Fig 12.2 A model of individual change

listening, and adequate resource to see your proposals into widespread and sustained use. Grol (1997) has a useful review of the different types of approach that could be adopted, and the evidence for their effectiveness.

7. You need other sorts of information, some relatively obvious, others perhaps unexpected:

a. Local demographics (population size, density and distribution), and prevalence of the disease or condition of interest. How many people does it affect? How seriously?

b. Actual local practice. Audit of current practice, and open discussion with colleagues may reveal unexpected differences between what you believe *should* happen or *think* is already happening, and what actually *does* happen.

c. Patients' and service users' views. Have you asked them, or looked for previous evidence of their views, rather than what you think their views are, or ought to be?

d. Understand the organizational context. How does the diagnostic, treatment and care process actually work at present, and who would be affected by proposed changes? How are referral decisions influenced? How could you change that?

e. Local 'political insight'. Who has a stake in this process? What do they think about the issues? What else is on their agenda that may help, or hinder, progress in the direction you want?

f. Where might resources be obtainable? Change is unlikely to be completely neutral in resource terms, such as time, energy, money and facilities. How may they be freed up to pump prime change, or where can additional resources be sought with some chance of success?

Key points

- **We can all identify what is wrong.**
- **Merely stating problems is ineffective. Devise solutions.**
- **The goal is not just devising solutions but implementing them.**

WHAT HELPS?

1. In our own research into the process of implementing evidence-led change in North Thames region (Smith & McClenahan 1997, 1998; Haines and Evans 2000; Wye and McClenahan 2000), six factors seem to make progress more likely:

a. Support from both managers and clinicians at a senior level

b. Adequate resourcing in relation to the scale of ambition

c. A project management approach, with clarity about lead roles, and clarity of objectives for the change process on a realistic scale (neither overambitious nor too modest)

d. Having, or putting in place, the right organizational infrastructure to support clinical service improvements

e. An understanding of change management as a process

f. Closing the loop properly – auditing whether clinical *processes* have changed to match those associated with efficacy in a research environment. It is usually not possible or necessary to audit *outcomes* themselves – that was what the research was about.

2. Depending on your present level of seniority and influence, consider some of the following ways of making a difference:

a. What is your own attitude to the possibility of improvement to your own practice? Talk it over with colleagues. Analyse your emotional reactions as well as the practical and rational ones.

b. Access information sources (particularly the Cochrane database (CD-Rom), Medline, CINAHL and the internet) and learn how to make use of them. Encourage *all* your staff to use them. Get help from others with the relevant skills.

c. Seek local training (if you have not already had some) in *critical appraisal* – the process of reviewing published research evidence to assess its quality and relevance to your own patients' circumstances. Practise it in your routine work.

d. Try to make or reinforce connections between the clinical governance or clinical effectiveness committee (or its local equivalent) and its subgroups; clinical audit; library and information services; multidisciplinary team working; education and training; Continuous Professional Development/Continuing Medical Education; guideline development; and patient information provision (see Chs 42, 43).

e. Seek management support for implementing desired change processes: in your own team; across departments; for common clinical conditions; and across organizational boundaries with primary and tertiary care and where relevant, social care and support organizations.

f. For the real enthusiast: take part in a systematic review of an area of practice that interests you.

Summary

- Recognize that evidence based practice encompasses not just the application of randomized controlled trials but all aspects of health care.
- Question your practice and consider how much is justifiable on reliable evidence.
- Can you offer your patients firm evidence on which you base your advice?
- Do you accept that you can enlarge your range of surgical interventions by seeking trustworthy evidence and by participating in high quality research?

References

Antman EM, Lau J, Kupelnick B, Mosteller F, Chalmers TC 1992 A comparison of results of meta-analyses of randomized control trials and recommendations of clinical experts. Treatments for myocardial infarction. JAMA 268: 240–248

Batstone G, Edwards M 1997 Challenges in promoting clinical effectiveness and the use of evidence. In: Harrison A (ed.) Health care UK, 1996/7. King's Fund Policy Institute, King's Fund, London

Beckhard R, Harris RT 1987 Organizational transitions: managing complex change, 2nd edn. Addison Wesley, Reading, MA

Grol R 1997 Beliefs and evidence in changing clinical practice. BMJ 315: 418–421

Haines A, Evans D (eds) 2000. Evidence based change in healthcare. Churchill Livingstone, Oxford

McKibbon et al 1995: see Useful links

Prochaska J, DiClemente C 1984 The transtheoretical approach: crossing traditional boundaries of therapy. Dow Jones–Irwin, Homewood, IL

Smith L, McClenahan JW 1997 Putting practitioners through the paces: initial findings in our evaluation of putting evidence into practice. King's Fund and North Thames R & D Directorate, London

Smith L, McClenahan JW 1998 Snakes and ladders: levers, obstacles and solutions to putting evidence into practice. King's Fund and North Thames R & D Directorate, London

Wye (née Smith) L, McClenahan JW 2000 Getting better with evidence. King's Fund and North Thames R & D Directorate, London

Useful links

hiru.mcmaster.ca/hiru/medline/mdl-ebc.htm McKibbon K, Wilczynski N, Hayward RS, Walker-Dilks C, Haynes RB 1995 The medical literature as a resource for evidence based care

www.kingsfund.org.uk/eLeadership/html/publications.html King's Fund Publications, London

www.doh.gov.uk/ntrd/pdf/getbtr.pdf Department of Health, London

13 Decision making

R. M. Kirk, K. Cox

> **Objectives**
>
> - Recognize the complex, multiple, interacting factors that need to be taken into account when making a decision. Even though you may not be able to evaluate all of them, do not ignore them.
> - Good decisions demand the best available evidence. Critically search out and use discriminant information in preference to equivocal and dubious evidence.
> - Decisions are valid only at the time they are made. Be prepared to revise them if the circumstances change.
> - Remember that your patient must be fully informed, *and understand the information*, in order to participate in the decision making and give informed consent. Furthermore, your patient's evaluation of a successful outcome may not be the same as yours.

Good surgery is 25% manipulative skill and 75% decision making.

Adapted from the distinguished
American surgeon F. C. Spencer

INTRODUCTION

This chapter forms the fulcrum of the book. What has gone before is the knowledge and evidence that you should have available. What follows are the actions and consequences of the decision or decisions that you take.

As a surgeon you cannot merely follow a set of rigid instructions. You are a professional who searches for information, appraises it, makes decisions, acts on them, monitors the outcomes and accepts responsibility for them to your patients, your peers and your own conscience. However, decision making depends on a multi-plicity of factors, many of which may be unknown or even unknowable. Some are not susceptible to scientific or statistical evaluation, and because they are disparate, they cannot be listed in a ranked sequence of graded importance. In the past there was little appreciation of risk analysis, cost effectiveness and the patient's assessment of quality of life following treatment.

Our challenge is to identify the important, discriminant elements from the inconsequential ones, but oversimplification is dangerous. You must not concentrate on the components in isolation but consider the patient as a whole, not merely as an aggregation of individual parts. The whole has qualities beyond those of the parts. The term *Gestalt* (German = form, build, fashion), was coined in 1890 by a group of German psychologists to denote experiences that require more than basic sensory capacities to comprehend.

Within a simple linear system the whole behaves precisely and predictably as the sum of the parts. A change of one factor produces a consistent, predictable effect. We are composed of multiple biochemical, cellular, physiological and psychological systems which interact by means that include biochemical and neuroendocrine feedback loops. Within such a complex system a change in one unit may produce unforeseeable, seemingly capricious, collective behaviour. The emerging 'complexity theory' takes account of the fact that complicated, self-organizing systems continuously adapt to and change their environment, but in ways that are impossible to predict. The theory is not yet a fully developed science, but seeks to identify, with the intention to predict, the emergence of characteristics that are not present in the individual components. For these reasons, reliable clinical decisions cannot be made by adhering to rigid rules. There is often an element of uncertainty (Plsek & Greenhalgh 2001, Wilson & Holt 2001).

Data derived from linear systems is often 'Yes or No,' and 'Black or White.' In complex biological systems it is more frequently, 'Perhaps, depending on a number of factors,' and 'A shade of grey.' We do not judge the evidence before us with open minds because we are already conditioned by our previous knowledge and experience.

Our subjective assessment may differ from that of others with a different knowledge background and experience. Our own judgement may vary, resulting from a recent success, or series of disasters. This is not a defect in us; we learn to recognize patterns and make tentative prejudgements – 'prejudices'. Prejudices are reprehensible only if they are inflexible.

Some surgeons are more successful than others at making correct decisions. Their results are superior to those of others, not only following operation when their superior skills can be invoked, but also in the one-third of surgical cases that are treated conservatively. They usually cannot give a rational explanation for their judgement and often attribute it to a 'gut feeling'. Such surgeons appear to anticipate and evaluate the possible risks instinctively. Perhaps they take time to consider all the possibilities, rather than settling on the first course that presents itself. We surgeons like to think of ourselves as men and women of action, that is, 'decisive'. Not all decisions need to be taken instantly. The increasing requirement to display the arguments for or against the possible courses of action to colleagues and to patients should have a beneficial effect on decisions.

It is remarkable that most of our major decisions are not made rationally. Consider your own life decisions. Can you logically defend your choice of profession, your life partner, or always justify the clinical judgement to ask advice, enlist assistance, conclude that you must proceed, or relinquish responsibility to someone better able to care for your patient?

Previous generations of autonomous surgeons made decisions and presented them to their team and patients without discussion. Attitudes have gradually undergone a transformation. As a result, we first make our assessment on the basis of our training, experience and access to scientific and professional information. We consult other members of our team and specialist colleagues. When dealing with certain conditions, such as complex tumours, we form specialized groups in order to bring together all relevant experts. We can now offer an appraisal for discussion with the patient, in terms that are comprehensible, in order to reach a mutually agreed course of action and receive informed consent (see Ch. 14). This entirely appropriate change has, of course, added yet greater complexity to the factors that must be taken into consideration. The change has been from what was a virtual statement of intent, into a complicated group negotiation.

Surgeons formerly dealt with a wide range of conditions and a single surgeon might see relatively few cases of any particular condition, making it difficult to make judgements for the future. Individual decisions may be impossible to assess in retrospect. The outcome could be poor in spite of good judgement and expert care, owing to factors that are unknown, unmeasurable or over which there is no control. Conversely, a robust patient may survive incorrect or inadequate management.

As a result of specialization, the formation of teams, specialist groups, and national and international exchange of information, large numbers of similar cases can be accumulated and the outcome following different methods of treatment can be compared.

The initial assessment and decision resemble the strategy (Greek *stratos* = an army + *agein* = to lead) of an army general. He is not, though, able to predict the response of the opposing general to his planned moves, so must closely observe and react by rearranging his plans; this is tactics (Greek *tactikos* from *tassein* = to arrange, hence rearrange). Very few decisions in life are once and for all.

ESSENTIALS OF SURGICAL DECISION MAKING

Information

1. Since you cannot incorporate all the information into a balanced judgement, you must discriminate by choosing what is relevant and reliable, what must be borne in mind, what can be left out of consideration for the time being, and what can be rejected as invalid or irrelevant.

2. Can the published literature be applied to your patient? No two patients are exactly the same and some factors may exclude your patient from being comparable with the tightly selected patients assessed in statistical trials. However, some of the aids to decision making may be less constrictive (see later).

3. Following carefully considered initial judgement, determine to anticipate and react to subsequent changes so you do not endanger recovery.

4. Determine to monitor, analyse and record the circumstances and outcome of your strategic planning and subsequent management, so you can in future adjust your decisions.

Joint decision making with the patient

1. First decide what is the professional opinion you will offer the patient. You should review the possible methods of management, with the benefits and risks. Patients expect you to have your facts marshalled, otherwise you cannot give them a clear picture. Informed consent (see Ch. 14) implies that patients are well informed.

2. Match your explanation to patients' comprehension. At all costs avoid scientific terms or jargon that are likely to confuse rather than instruct them. From time to time check that they understand you by asking them to tell you how they view the situation (see Ch. 47).

3. Although patients wish to participate, you are the professional adviser. How you pass the information inevitably influences their judgement.

4. Many patients faced with the presence of disease and the necessity for treatment, including perhaps an operation, are not in the best state of mind to make important choices. For this reason, whenever there is time, state the various possibilities and likely outcomes as simply as possible, then suggest that the patient returns after an interval to ask any supplementary questions and then reach a decision.

5. As you point out the consequences of the proposed management, your measures of success are not necessarily in line with those of your patients. Powerful fears for many patients, beyond length of survival, are constant pain, loss of the ability to care for themselves, and loss of dignity. However, it is often difficult for them to anticipate what will be their reaction to the effects of the proposed management.

6. Recognize your patient's right to ask for treatment that differs from that advised by you but do not agree to treatment that is harmful, ineffective or offends against your own moral code.

Cost effectiveness

This was often ignored in the past when making decisions, the only consideration being for what treatment best met the patient's needs. It is now openly accepted that in no society can treatments be offered without taking into account the economic implications, and the likely cost-benefits of other treatments (see Ch. 44).

Key points

- **Prepare yourself; learn from experience, experts, surgical literature and other sources of evidence-based information.**
- **Do not overburden yourself with unreliable, irrelevant data – favour proven, discriminant facts.**
- **Do not obsessively limit your study to one possible choice. Assess the benefits and risks of other management options.**
- **Follow your patients: study the outcomes in the hope of improving your results.**

OBSTACLES TO GOOD DECISION MAKING

1. Clinicians are rarely able to concentrate on a single problem. You always have many tasks to fulfil. Make sure that you allocate each one a ranked place in order of priority, and that you reconsider the order from time to time. Try not to attempt too many tasks at once – but in an emergency be willing to abandon a less important one and undertake one that is urgent.

2. We hope to select available information with open minds but there is a temptation to seek and select evidence that confirms our prejudice. Make a deliberate effort to stand away from the problem so you may become aware of incongruities that make you revise your first assumption.

3. Very few questions can be answered positively – 'Yes or No,' or 'Black or White'; the particular shade of grey is a subjective opinion.

4. All clinical decisions demand some simplification of the multiplicity of factors, but do not lightly leave anything out of consideration. Albert Einstein stated, 'Everything should be as simple as possible, but not simpler'. The difficulty is in allotting importance to disparate influences on diagnosis, extent of disease and management options.

5. Measuring individual aspects separately does not provide a complete picture. You must also look at the patient as a whole.

6. It is usually accepted that experience leads to better decision making. We learn to recognize familiar patterns. However, there is a temptation to identify resemblances early and overconfidently, thus not fully checking the remainder of the available evidence. Two similar clinical situations are rarely identical, and so may call for different action.

EMERGENCIES

A sudden, urgent, unexpected incident puts great strain on your judgement. You are often put under pressure to 'do something', and 'doing something' may be inappropriate. Although this is an emergency (Latin *e* = out of + *mergere* = to plunge, to thrust suddenly), it does not inevitably demand instant action. Except for standardized situations like cardiopulmonary arrest, be willing to take sufficient time to assess the situation and make a decision. Is the required action within your capability, and is the required assistance and equipment available? If the action is beyond your normal capability, but if there is no one more capable, are there any effective measures you can perform? In such circumstances, when there is no alternative, people have achieved near miracles.

AIDS TO DECISION MAKING

Clinical skills

1. In case of difficulty, when there is no urgency, be willing to defer making a decision and give yourself time

to think about the possibilities, discuss it with a trusted colleague, and refer to the literature to check the recent reports.

2. In an emergency be willing, if time permits, to review the features after a short interval – they sometimes change dramatically.

3. In case of doubt, ask a colleague who has no commitment to the patient's outcome, whose opinion you respect, to carry out a fresh and independent examination.

Educational value

1. Use every opportunity to learn by studying how each decision is reached and how it can be justified.

On many surgical firms it is common practice for the senior surgeon to make an on-the-spot decision, which is not questioned. Complex, controversial problems should be used as valuable educational aids. Each member of the team studies the literature, considers the possibilities, and reaches and justifies a conclusion at a meeting chaired by the senior surgeon. When each participant has presented a well-argued viewpoint, try to reach a consensus judgement. Subsequently, review the outcome to decide if the decision was correct, or whether a different conclusion should be reached when a similar case is encountered. At intervals, review all the patients who have been treated for the condition under consideration (see Ch. 42).

2. Can useful guidelines be drawn up for future consultation – and regular review?

3. How do the results compare with those from other units?

RISK MANAGEMENT

Organizational risk management

1. Do not make your decision solely on clinical grounds. Surgical treatment demands a wide range of complex facilities. Your own competence, and confidence that the patient can withstand the proposed procedure, are not the only considerations when judging how to proceed.

2. Before investing in an unknown business, some commercial firms ask for a report on its perceived strengths, weaknesses, opportunities and threats (SWOT). This stimulates the informant to stand away from individual problems and consider the overall picture. The threats in surgical decision making do not merely refer to patient survival versus recovery. There are many possible sequelae, such as unexpected findings, absence of vital staff, and failure of some important

equipment. In making your decisions, ensure that you consider all the possibilities and take precautions against possible difficulties.

3. There are many aspects to risk management. Many of the procedures carried out have health and safety implications. Make sure that you know the correct precautions with electrical, radiation and other equipment (see Ch. 17). Ensure, when making your decision, that your requirements will be adequately met.

4. Do you have the required support of expert staff, with necessary equipment such as intensive care beds fully staffed?

Key points

- **Surgeons previously accepted serious support deficiencies, adding to the risk, because there was no alternative.**
- **Do not undertake procedures when the circumstances are not ideal, except in dire emergency.**

Clinical risk management

1. Prognostic risk scores. A number of scoring methods have been proposed so that the chances of recovery can be estimated. In this way the success of various methods of treatment can be compared. These methods were developed for comparing groups rather than individuals but their use has often been extended to assess individual risks.

a. The American Society of Anesthesiologists (ASA) produced a five-grade risk assessment, on to which can be added the effects of age, operative severity, respiratory, cardiac and nutritional state.

b. The Acute Physiology and Chronic Health Evaluation (APACHE) score is helpful in assessing the outcome for a group of patients but less so for individual cases. In the United Kingdom the modification, labelled APACHE II, is most commonly used.

2. The Physiological and Operative Severity Score for the enUmeration of the Mortality and morbidity (POSSUM) and Portsmouth modification (P-POSSUM) are particularly valuable for assessing the operative risks in the two-thirds of patients who require surgical treatment (Jones & de Cossart 1999). They incorporate an operative severity score as a predictor of outcome. Proposed use of POSSUM and P-POSSUM for comparative audit is deprecated (Bann & Sarin 2001). Trauma and sepsis scores can also be calculated. Biological age offers a better assessment of risk than does calendar age (Farquharson et al 2001).

TYPES OF DECISION

Codified decisions

If facts and experience can be measured and then compared with the findings in other similar situations, it becomes possible to make decisions for future guidance when faced with similar problems (Wyatt 2001). As a result of reviewing series of cases, various standardized methods of management have been devised. If the problem complies with previously assessed cases, a plan can be developed so that succeeding problems can be dealt with according to predetermined directions:

- *Algorithm* (Arabic *al-Kwarazmi*, modern Khiva in Uzbekistan). In this city lived the 9th century mathematician Abu Ja'far Mohammed ben Musa, who developed a rule for solving a problem in a finite number of steps. The sequential steps are followed automatically and algorithms are embodied in computer software.
- *Protocol* (Greek *protos* = first + *kolla* = glue; a glued-on first leaf of a manuscript). Among other things it is a set of rules, or uniform method, of approaching a problem, sometimes displayed as a flow chart, with alternative pathways to treat differing circumstances and outcomes.
- *Guidelines* offer a viewpoint agreed by an authoritative person or body. They are not as reliable as evidence based on prospective, double-blind, trials that have produced statistically significant results; however, they are less rigid. The issuing of guidelines is contentious because those who, for good reason, do not follow the guidelines, may feel vulnerable to criticism if the outcome in a particular case is poor. Because guidelines vary in their power, they may be graded (Harbour & Miller 2001).
- Decision trees are valuable in displaying and evaluating possibilities and outcomes. Risks of treatment mortality and long-term survival are available for many conditions in the medical literature or from reviews such as the Cochrane collaboration or on the internet. In the future the National Institute for Clinical Excellence (NICE) will issue reports on a wide range of treatments.

All the probable outcomes should add up to 1 (Fig. 13.1). In addition to the objective outcome measure, there is a subjective value, called a 'utility;' your evaluation and the patient's may differ – but it is the patient's valuation that must prevail. However, it may be difficult or impossible for the patient to anticipate the effect of the outcome on the quality of his or her life, often calculated as quality adjusted life years (QALYs). The quality of each year of life is subjectively judged by the patient. A year during which the patient enjoys full fitness is 1 QALY. A 2 year survival, each judged to have provided 50% of full fitness and enjoyment, is also judged to be 1 QALY. You may be able to advise, or put the patient in contact with others who have been treated for the same condition. The sum of the probability and utility produces a figure for the 'expected utility', and the course of management earning the highest mark is the preferred one (Fig. 13.2) (Birkmeyer & Welch 1997).

Although the objective evidence for all the possible courses of action may not be available, forming a decision tree is a valuable exercise for displaying the range of possibilities.

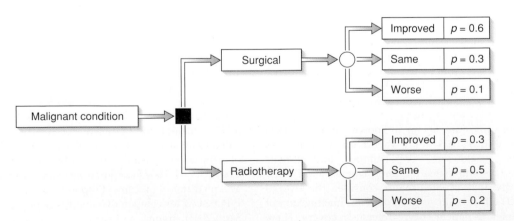

Fig. 13.1 A simple decision tree comparing the probability (*p*) of outcomes for two methods of treating a malignant condition. ■ Denotes a decision node; ○ denotes possible outcomes.

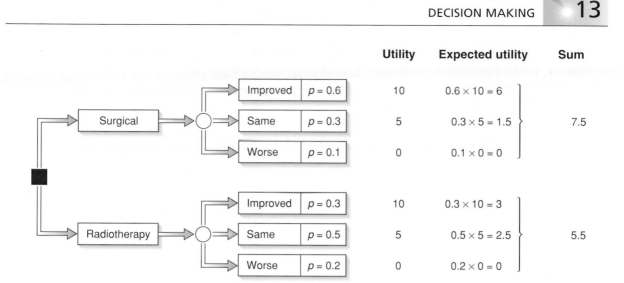

			Utility	Expected utility	Sum

Fig. 13.2 The utility (subjective benefit or disability) resulting from the outcome is graded from 10 (good) to 0 (bad). The product of probability (*p*) and utility is the 'expected utility'. Finally, the sum of the expected utilities for each decision can be compared. The course scoring the highest mark is the preferred one, in this case surgery. ■ Denotes a decision node; ○ denotes possible outcomes.

Key point

- Review guidelines, algorithms, protocols and decision trees from time to time (Fig. 13.3). They may require modification in the light of audited results of previous outcomes, comparison with published data from other units, and advances in diagnosis and management.

Personalized decisions

1. Many decisions are complex and cannot be made in a standardized, codified manner. The condition may be complicated by cofactors, or may have unusual features. The decision is unique and may be challenging or even controversial. Some of the factors may be indefinable and difficult to weigh in the balance. It is in such circumstances that opinions differ between specialists because of individual selection of evidence and the importance given to it.

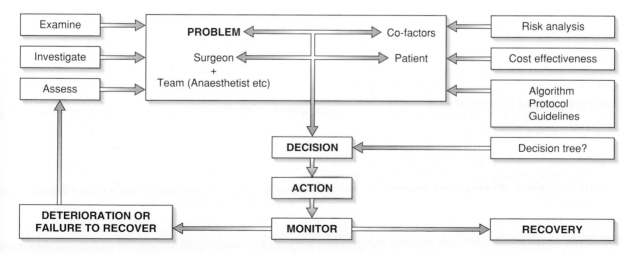

Fig. 13.3 Some of the complex, and disparate, considerations to be taken into account when making a decision, acting on it and monitoring the result.

2. Knowledge that cannot be transferred verbally can be labelled 'tacit' (Wyatt 2001) (Latin *tacere* = to be silent). The decision-maker cannot justify the decision in scientifically acceptable terms. Some surgeons produce better results than average; they may be technically superior, but an alternative or additional reason is that they make a higher proportion than average of correct decisions.

3. The likelihood is that good decisions are made by an intuitive selection of the most important factors, while discounting less important factors. Combined with this is the selection of treatment that is appropriate for that particular patient. Some surgeons say, 'I know what I can get away with'; others are overoptimistic of their ability to achieve success with poor risk patients subjected to overaggressive treatment. Other surgeons are dissuaded from embarking on potentially highly successful treatment for fear of failure, or of 'spoiling' their results. Such reluctance may increase if the outcomes for individual surgeons or units become accessible to the general public.

4. Personal experience, especially of rare problems, is a powerful influence on decisions, so that senior surgeons are usually trusted to deal with them. A particular example is the recognition of postoperative complications, or of failure to recover as expected; if you are inexperienced, you do not know how to recognize what is normal and what is important. In some cases the experienced colleague may be unable to explain a suspicion, but may just acknowledge a 'gut feeling' that all is not well.

Key point

- It is wasteful of resources for every decision to be made on a one-to-one basis if the problem conforms to a standardized pattern for which guidelines, algorithms, protocols or decision trees have already been published. The guides must be regularly reviewed and authenticated. Unless there is additional evidence, or circumstances that differ from the standardized description, hesitate to make a heterodox decision. Will you be able to justify it to your patient, your colleagues, and to your own conscience, if there is an adverse outcome?

Summary

- How many influences and factors can you list that must be brought into the process of clinical decision making? How many of them can be scientifically assessed? Can you rank them in terms of their importance of effect on outcome?
- What are discriminant features? Can you list such features for some of the common clinical conditions with which you deal?
- Do you know the published outcomes for three common conditions? Where would you look for the information in order to create a decision tree?
- Can you name examples of decisions for which there are well-authenticated pathways to follow, and also those that are exceptional and demand your best judgement – or the advice of an experienced expert?
- Can you recall the important considerations necessary when informing patients and making joint decisions with them?
- As a surgeon committed to taking decisions and acting upon them, how would you justify demanding the facilities, throughout your career, to acquire and critically evaluate new information, both verbally and by association with leading colleagues?

References

Bann SD, Sarin S 2001. Comparative audit: the trouble with POSSUM. Journal of the Royal Society of Medicine 94: 632–634

Birkmeyer JD, Welch HG 1997. A reader's guide to surgical decision analysis. Journal of the American College of Surgeons 184: 589–595

Farquharson SM, Gupt A, Heald RJ, Moran BJ 2001. Surgical decisions in the elderly: the importance of biological age. Journal of the Royal Society of Medicine 94: 232–235

Harbour R, Miller J 2001. A new system for grading recommendations in evidence based guidelines. BMJ 323: 334–336.

Jones HJS, deCossart L 1999. Risk scoring in surgical patients. British Journal of Surgery 86: 149–157

Plsek PE, Greenhalgh T 2001. The challenge of complexity in health care. BMJ 323: 625–628

Wilson T, Holt T 2001 Complexity and clinical care. BMJ 323: 685–688.

Wyatt JC 2001. Management of explicit and tacit knowledge. Journal of the Royal Society of Medicine 94: 6–9

Further reading

Cox K 1999 Doctor and patient: exploring clinical thinking. Phase 3: Deciding what to do. University of New South Wales Press, Sydney, pp 185–270. *This thoughtful readable book is an account of the way in which we think and make our decisions*

O'Connor AM, Rostom A, Fiset V *et al* 1999 Decision aids for patients facing health treatment or screening decisions: system review. BMJ 319: 731–734. *Patients may need help when they are deciding between treatment options*

Polanyi M 1958 Personal knowledge. Routledge and Keegan Paul, London. *References and explanations throughout of tacit knowledge and acquisition of skills. A masterpiece from a Hungarian-born polymath, investigating the special wisdom of the expert. It explores those skills that cannot as yet be verbalized but need to be passed on during the master–apprenticeship relationship*

PREPARATIONS FOR SURGERY

14 Consent for surgical treatment

L. Doyal

Objectives

- **Recognize the need to establish trust and confidence in patients under your care.**
- **Understand that a signature on a consent form is not legal proof that informed consent has been given.**
- **Realize that you must warn patients of the hazards as well as the benefits of surgical treatment.**
- **Identify and deal appropriately with difficulties in gaining consent. Respect the confidentiality of your dealings with patients.**

INTRODUCTION

For surgery to be successful, there must be a relationship of trust and confidence between you and your patients, otherwise they are likely to be reticent in presenting for treatment or in divulging the detailed personal information required for recording accurate case histories and making successful diagnoses. Aside from the belief that their care will conform to a high clinical standard, the trust of patients also depends on their belief that their autonomy will be respected – that they will have the right to decide their own medical destiny, whatever anyone else may think.

Moral rights are like that. They indicate claims that individuals can legitimately make against others who have corresponding duties to respect those claims. To the degree that we believe that the right to make such a claim exists, then those on whom it is properly made must respect it and act accordingly, irrespective of their preferences. Examples of often-cited moral rights emphasize the entitlement of individuals to self-determination – to be able to pursue life goals and perceived interests in ways in which the individual has chosen – provided that others are not harmed in the process. Moral rights might or might not be backed up by the force of law. For example,

the legal right of women to choose to have an abortion under certain circumstances is regarded as immoral by those who believe that a fetus has the rights of a born child. In short, our beliefs about who has a right to what inform our decisions about how we should act toward others if our actions are to be deemed morally, and perhaps legally, acceptable.

The general right of surgical patients to self-determination can be subdivided into three further rights: to informed consent, to the truth and to confidentiality. The latter two clearly follow from the first. Choices cannot be properly informed on the basis of deception and cannot be respected if what patients deem private is made public. Therefore, it is the principle of informed consent itself which is fundamental and on which both the mortality and the legality of good surgical practice partly depend.

THE MORAL IMPORTANCE OF INFORMED CONSENT

Key point

- **The moral unacceptability of anyone exercising unlimited power over others is at the heart of many of our liberal values.**

It is our capacity for rational choice that differentiates humans from other creatures. Respect for this capacity – especially our right to be the informed gatekeepers of our own bodies – is an indication of the seriousness with which we respect the humanity and dignity of others.

What is informed consent?

For patients to give their informed consent to surgery – to be able to make a considered choice about what is in their personal interests – they must receive sufficient accurate information about their illness, the proposed treatment and its prognosis. For this to be more than a moral abstraction, you must complete four general tasks:

1. Describe the procedure itself, including information about its practical implications and probable prognosis.
2. Reveal the probability of specific associated risks or complications.
3. Do not assume that the patient already knows the risks of other aspects of the proposed surgical procedure, such as the complications that might result from a general anaesthetic, bed rest, intravenous fluids or a catheter.
4. Outline other surgical or medical alternatives to the proposed treatment, including non-treatment, along with their general advantages and disadvantages.

Ideally, the amount of such information should be that which a mentally competent patient requires to make informed choice a realistic possibility. Think of competence here as the ability to understand, retain and deliberate about such information and to accept its personal applicability. You must remember that the amount of information the patient is obligated to divulge may well change, depending on what you should know about your patient as an individual. For example, it may not be necessary for a manual labourer to be told of an extremely small operative risk of minor stiffness in one finger. This would obviously not be true of a concert pianist, underlining the importance of recording the patient's employment in case notes and referring to it in the presentation of case histories.

Good consenting practice

1. As much as possible, ensure that the physical surroundings during the discussion between you and your patient are conducive to easy, quiet conversation. Ideally, choose somewhere private and free of disturbances and interruptions by junior staff or medical students following in retinue on a busy Nightingale ward. Do not stand threateningly over the patient in bed, and avoid giving the appearance of being rushed by other duties. Empathy with the patient is crucial.

2. Use the simplest possible language, avoiding needless technicalities. If the patient permits it, have a relative or friend of the patient present when serious matters are being discussed. This is both for support and to help ensure that the patient really does understand – both at the time the information is given and later when the patient returns home. In the hospital ward, nurses familiar to the patient can often fulfil this role effectively. Appropriate leaflets or booklets can be helpful, as is innovative work using audiorecording of interviews; patients can be encouraged to take the recording home to discuss with others.

3. Having attempted to provide clear information, now determine whether or not the patient has actually understood it. No doubt there are time constraints on doing

both. However, it is clear that you are morally responsible for attempting both to an acceptable standard. To achieve this, ask the patient to repeat in personal terms what has been said, and at various times invite questions. The more confident you are in exercising these skills, the less time is needed to obtain effective consent.

4. We often limit the amount of information we give to patients on the grounds that it is potentially distressing. If your long-term aim is to keep the patient in ignorance, this is not acceptable. All competent individuals have a right to decide what is and is not in their best interests, even if what they decide is not endorsed by their professional advisors. It would not be morally acceptable for a solicitor or accountant to delude their clients on the grounds that they did not want to distress them about the possibility of losing a court action or of going bankrupt. Why should your moral obligations be any different?

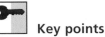 **Key points**

- **It is your responsibility to provide clear information, and to determine whether it has been understood.**
- **It is the patient's right to decide what is in his or her best interest, not yours.**

The consent form

1. In principle, the consent form signed by the patient before operation is a public and permanent affirmation of agreement. All competent patients who are 16 years or older should sign the form for all surgical procedures involving a general anaesthetic. You should obtain signed consent for procedures under local anaesthetic if there is a risk of significant sequelae; for example, an excision of skin lesions. You should also sign the form after obtaining consent to indicate that, to the best of your knowledge, the patient has both received and understands the information necessary to make a considered judgement.

2. However, it is unnecessary for a competent patient to sign for all surgical interventions. A simple investigative procedure such as venepuncture, involving minimal risk, can be undertaken after oral explanation of, and consent to, what it physically entails. Consent can be assumed to be implied if the patient then accepts the procedure.

3. The consent form is not legal proof that consent has been given. Always bear this in mind if you are tempted to cut corners as regards good practice in obtaining consent. It is merely one piece of evidence that some attempt was made to obtain informed consent, not that it was a morally or legally satisfactory attempt.

THE LEGAL IMPORTANCE OF INFORMED CONSENT

 Key point

- In addition to the general and clinical importance, your legal obligation is to respect the patient's right to consent to treatment.

Battery

1. Battery is a violation of the civil law forbidding intentionally touching other persons without their consent. For example, a woman won damages in the UK for this reason because she was given a hysterectomy to which she did not agree in the aftermath of a gynaecological operation for another problem. In Canada, a woman who made it clear that she wanted to be injected in one arm successfully sued when she received the injection in the other! The harm resulting from battery is not necessarily physical. In law, a battery can be deemed to have occurred without such harm having taken place. Here, harm should be construed as the violation of the right of persons to exercise autonomous control over their own bodies.

2. In many situations involving minor surgical procedures or tests, it is not possible or advisable specifically to ask for consent every time you touch a patient. If this were the case, surgery would become impossible. But it does not follow that the patient's consent is legally irrelevant. Rather, as we have just seen, a patient can be said to have given implied consent by virtue of presenting for treatment and accepting what is offered. A man once argued in the USA, for example, that a ship's surgeon had committed a battery because he was vaccinated without having given specific verbal permission for the injection to be administered. He lost on the grounds that his consent was implied because he was in a queue of people who were clearly waiting to be injected and he held out his arm when his turn came!

3. Clearly, there will be many less clear-cut situations. Is there a risk of battery if a patient claims that surgery would have been refused if more information had been given beforehand? If you informed the patient in broad terms of the general nature of the condition and the proposed operation to try to correct it, if you did not deliberately deceive and the patient gave no indication of desiring not to proceed by asking for more information, and signed the appropriate consent form, then the answer is probably no. This presupposes that you have not deprived the patient of information that was specifically requested, and, returning to our example of an unwanted hysterectomy, you have not usurped a clinical choice legally regarded as remaining with the patient.

Negligence

1. Battery is not the only legal action you risk for inadequately respecting your patient's right to informed consent. In an important case, Mrs Sidaway suffered paralysis resulting from spinal surgery to relieve pressure on a nerve root without being told that the operation carried a small risk of paralysis. Here, it was judged that she had not been a victim of battery because, again, she had given her general consent to the surgery in question. However, her solicitors then claimed negligence, the legal action now recommended in such cases. Negligence a potential breach of duty, concerns your professional duty properly to advise patients not just about the proposed surgery but also about its potential hazards. In such cases, patients argue that, had they known the risks in question, they would not have proceeded with the surgery.

2. Do not assume that in these circumstances you are protected from such accusations by a signed consent form for treatment. The patient might still successfully argue that, even having signed the form, he or she was not given enough relevant information to make an informed decision before signing and/or was unaware of the significance of the form. There is no escaping your general duty to disclose information about potentially harmful side-effects and to do so in a way that the patient can understand in principle. For example, in all cases other than those of acute emergencies, you must take care to provide translations for non-English-speaking patients.

3. How can we establish whether or not compliance with this duty has been sufficient – whether or not enough information has been disclosed about risks so that the rights of patients are respected? Legal judgements concerning negligent standards of adequate disclosure in the UK are still primarily determined by the profession itself. Suppose that expert witnesses for the defence are regarded by the court as constituting a recognized body of professional opinion. If they agree that they would have communicated the same amount of information in similar circumstances as the defendant, this should be sufficient to ensure that the claimant will lose the legal action. In other words, in such actions the judge does not decide which expert witnesses are right – those for the claimant or defendant. All that is required to exonerate the latter is for a responsible body of professional opinion to endorse the action in dispute, even if the endorsement does not represent the views of the majority of members of the profession.

4. Recent legal developments have underlined this 'professional standard' in the determination of what constitutes negligent informed consent. In the Sidaway case, for example, a majority of the judges in an appeal to the House of Lords agreed with this approach to determining negligence, as have other judges since. However, many have also warned of the dangers of completely equating the right of patients to information with standards set by the profession. Indeed, in the Sidaway case, one judge stated in a minority opinion that there will be some information about surgery, for example serious hazards, which any 'prudent' patient would wish to know before giving consent to proceed. A similar legal standard of negligence as regards informed consent is found in North America and has largely become accepted good practice by the medical profession in the UK.

5. Therefore, do not look to the law for advice on how much information about risks and side-effects is morally required by the right of your patients to informed consent. Ask instead what a reasonable person would want to know under similar circumstances, especially in the context of any other personal information you have about the patient and his/her public and private interests. Disclose the same amount of information about risks to your patients as you would wish to be communicated to your close friends and relatives. The fact that an adequate amount of information for informed consent may be legally acceptable does not entail that this should be regarded as professionally or morally acceptable.

The unconscious adult patient

1. Suppose that you are a surgeon in the accident and emergency (A & E) department, confronted with the victim of an automobile accident who requires an immediate operation to save life or to prevent permanent and serious disability. Here, there is a clear duty to treat, despite the fact that it is impossible to obtain the patient's consent, and there would be no risk of battery if operation proceeded. This is not because you become the proxy of the patient and so make a substituted judgement on his or her behalf, one which attempts to anticipate the choice the patient would make. It is because it is your moral and legal responsibility to act in the patient's best interests – to do what is 'necessary', as there is no way of knowing for certain what the patient might choose.

2. Indeed, no adult in the UK can legally consent to surgery on behalf of another, including close relatives. Do not ask relatives to sign consent forms on behalf of unconscious or otherwise incompetent adults. It would be both

a misrepresentation of the law and a liability risk, if the surgical outcome is poor. The relatives may inappropriately and harmfully blame themselves.

3. The only circumstance that justifies surgery without consent is the dramatic need of patients, coupled with their inability to give consent. Inconvenience will not suffice. For example, the arrest of a life-threatening haemorrhage in an otherwise healthy patient would clearly be in order, while the same could not be said of the repair of a hernia. Of course, if the patient is conscious and evidently capable of rational judgement, then even in an emergency offer advice on the condition and the proposed treatment. If it is physically possible, have the patient also sign a consent form, as would be the case in normal circumstances. Verbal consent is adequate if the patient's condition precludes giving written consent. However, in these circumstances, if possible, ask another health worker to act as a witness and to record the verbal consent in the notes.

Children

1. Ordinarily, obtain consent for elective surgery on young children from someone – usually the parent – deemed competent to make informed choices about the child's best interests. However, this does not suggest that you must always be guided solely by parental wishes. If you believe such a decision is necessary to save the child's life, the parents' wishes can be overridden. If there is time, apply to the court for the appropriate order. If not, you can still proceed. If the parents propose long-term treatment or non-treatment options which you regard as similarly inconsistent with the best interests of the child, again you can apply for them to be overriden by an appropriate court order.

2. The legal age for medical consent is normally 16. However, it is legally acceptable for you to treat adolescents under the age of 16 years without parental consent, just as it is for general practitioners to prescribe contraceptives. If you intend to do this you must ensure that the young person is competent – mature enough to understand, retain and deliberate about information concerning the nature of the illness, the prognosis, proposed treatment and any important associated risks. The patient must also be able to believe that this information applies personally to her or him. Before proceeding without parental consent, encourage the young person to discuss the proposed treatment with the parents and so be assured that the treatment is in the best interests of the child.

3. Nevertheless, regard treatment without parental consent as exceptional. Unless the adolescent has specifically refused permission, attempt if possible to find and

consult the parents if they are not already approachable. In the case of life-threatening illness, even young people below the age of 18 years do not have the right to reject treatment on their own which might save their lives. Only those with parental responsibility can exercise such judgement, in agreement with you. Paradoxically, the law appears to be that the right of a competent adolescent to consent to life-saving treatment does not entail the right to refuse it. As regards elective surgery which is not life saving or will not prevent serious and permanent injury, the law is the same. Morally, however, the wishes of the competent young person not to proceed should be and are commonly respected, even where the parent disagrees. If surgical treatment is forced upon such patients without consent, it might undermine the relationship of trust and the willingness to comply with future treatment, both of which will be important for sustained clinical success. Such force can be argued not to be in the best clinical interests of the child.

4. Quite young children often have a good grasp of their prospects and treatment, especially when they have already experienced distressing surgical therapy for an illness which they have had for some time. In such circumstances, before further surgery is undertaken, attempt to consult such a child about his or her wishes. Where there is disagreement between parent and child about the best course of action, especially in instances of potentially terminal disease, arrange counselling for both about what appears clinically to be in the child's best interests. Such counselling is particularly important when there is disagreement between you and the parent about the most appropriate way to proceed. Again, in the unusual event that you believe parental choice dramatically conflicts with the medical interests of the child, approach the court for a judgement.

Mental handicap and psychiatric illness

1. In the case of adults who are judged incompetent to choose for themselves, we have seen that no one may legally act as a proxy for this purpose. However, decisions about incompetence are complex. For example, incompetence to consent to surgery does not follow from severe psychiatric illness. Just because individuals may be incompetent in one respect due to illness does not mean that they are incompetent in all respects. People may be detained under the 1983 Mental Health Act on the grounds that, because of the seriousness of their psychiatric illness, they are a potential danger to themselves or others. As a result they may be given psychiatric treatment without their consent. However, this does not hold for ordinary surgical treatment. In such circumstances, attempt to obtain the patient's consent, even when communication is difficult and certainty of understanding not

assured. For example, in a recent legal case in Britain, a judge accepted that a detained patient suffering from schizophrenia was competent to refuse to have a foot amputated if it became terminally gangrenous.

2. With the exception of specific and extreme interventions such as psychosurgery, there are circumstances when surgical treatment can be given to a detained psychiatric patient who cannot consent due to extreme illness. There are two conditions:

a. the treatment must be deemed necessary to protect life or to avoid permanent and serious disability

b. the patient must be diagnosed as unable to give informed consent as a direct result of the psychiatric illness.

As a consequence of psychotic delusion, for example, patients may believe that you are going to kill them and that the diagnosis of a life-threatening condition is a sinister plot. Here, necessary treatment can proceed, provided that you and the relevant psychiatric team agree that it is in the best interests of the patient. Note that this exception to the consent requirement would not ordinarily apply to elective surgical care, as the assumption should be that there will be time for patients to make up their own minds when their competence to do so is no longer being impaired by their illness.

3. Some patients in need of surgery suffer not from psychiatric illness but from permanent mental disability. This may severely impair competence to give informed consent for either life-saving or elective surgery. The fact remains, however, that in such circumstances no adult can act as a legal proxy for another as regards the provision of such consent. The only person who can make the decision that surgery is in the best interests of severely mentally handicapped patients is yourself in consultation with the principal carers, including close relatives. Take great care. As regards elective surgery, responsibility for promoting the interests of mentally handicapped patients can be a heavy burden, especially if there is dispute among carers about what these actually are. The sensitivity of these issues is witnessed by the fact that the courts sometimes refuse to permit the sterilization of mentally handicapped women under the age of 16 years, even if the surgeon has agreed to perform the procedure.

TWO PRACTICAL PROBLEMS

The general obligation to disclose information about both proposed surgery and its hazards is not open to debate. However, putting this moral and legal imperative into practice does involve discretion and is not always easy, for two reasons.

Limitations on the understanding of patients

1. It is sometimes unclear whether or not consent has really been obtained, even if you have taken care to explain the proposed procedure and its potential hazards. The comprehension of competent patients can be compromised by their illness, their educational and social background and by other aspects of their personalities which may make them overly anxious or unwilling to listen. Difficult as such instances of impaired autonomy can be, especially for patients facing acute and complex surgery, you must still be able to show that they have disclosed adequate information for proper consent to be possible.

2. Practically speaking, therefore, how should you demonstrate to yourself, and if necessary to a judge, that you have done your best in this regard? Most important of all, you need to work constantly to improve your ability to communicate. Both the General Medical Council (GMC) and the British Medical Association (BMA) stress this point, and its importance is underlined by the increasing emphasis placed on communication skills within medical education (see Ch. 47). You can do no more than your best.

3. Keep a written record in the case notes of the main points about treatment which have been communicated prior to the signing of the consent form. Follow the model of the reasonable patient outlined above. Give information on what will be done and why, along with significant risks of mortality and other hazards to bodily functions relevant to normal social participation, such as swallowing, speaking, continence, mobility, pain and sexual performance. Record that each of these variables has been mentioned and will provide evidence that may be useful if the fact is denied by the patient in a context of a medicolegal dispute.

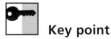

Key point

- Consider reinforcing information about proposed treatment and possible side-effects with written information.

4. Even after you have followed good practice in obtaining consent, you may conclude that your patient still cannot be said to have given proper consent to treatment. Apart from life-saving emergencies, your most appropriate choice is to postpone treatment until you have achieved better communication. This may be inconvenient, but it is necessary to protect the patient's rights and to demonstrate that you have taken your moral and legal duties seriously.

Limitations on the right of patients to consent

Key points

- **The right of a patient to consent to surgery does not entail (imply as an inevitable consequence) a right to demand and receive it.**
- **You do not have a professional duty to provide requested surgery for a patient who has no need for it.**
- **You may also refuse to carry out an operation that will be futile, no matter how much the patient may want it.**

1. What happens if the patient clearly needs operation but does not want it? Here, respect for the autonomy of patients may well conflict with your other moral obligation to protect life and health. This conflict is most acute when, in considered and unambiguous terms, a patient refuses life-saving surgery. The moral and legal emphasis on respect for autonomy within surgery is so strong that, even in such circumstances, you must not undertake treatment without consent, again assuming that the patient is conscious and competent. This fact is sometimes obscured because patients who are terminally ill and do not wish further treatment are reticent about refusing it. It becomes very clear, however, in the case of a Jehovah's Witness, who will only proceed with surgery on the understanding that no transfusion will be given in the event of haemorrhage. Legally, a competent patient has every right to make such a demand. If you ignore this you risk an action for battery.

2. It is not suggested that you have to operate on patients who place stipulations on the types of life-saving treatment they will accept. In principle, and assuming that there is time, you may refer them to others who are more sympathetic and willing to undergo the stress that such restrictions inevitably carry. Equally, we have already seen that, if a patient is unconscious or incompetent for some other reason you must do what is necessary to try to save life. However, even this is changing in the face of so-called 'advance directives' or 'living wills', which are now regarded by expert opinion in the UK as having legal force. Thus any competent adult can draft a document specifying in advance which life-saving treatments are and are not acceptable if the patient becomes incompetent and contracts specific types of illnesses. Ideally, an advance directive should be witnessed and you should act upon it. Such documents are common in North America and will eventually be so in the UK.

3. After consultation with you, a competent patient may, therefore, decide that further treatment is pointless,

given the irreversible and terminal character of the particular disease. If you comply with such a request to omit or to stop treatment, it can be argued to be neither actively killing nor aiding and abetting suicide. It is reasoned that, unlike the potential suicide, competent patients may well want desperately to live, but not at any cost to their quality of life. Furthermore, as we have seen, to treat them against their will constitutes a battery. Whatever the correctness of these arguments, what patients cannot expect is for active steps to be taken to end their lives, although they do at times request this as well.

4. Yet to go along with a patient's refusal of surgery when it is clear that the consequence will be death is a very serious moral and legal matter. Take great care to ensure that the patient fully understands the implications of refusing life-saving treatment and is competent to make an informed judgement, especially if the refusal is followed by a lapse into unconsciousness. A mistake, either about the patient's understanding or wishes, cannot be corrected. Therefore, respect prior refusal only if you judge it to be an autonomous decision intended to apply in the circumstances that have arisen. For example, a young adult woman in the UK refused a blood transfusion on the grounds of her acceptance of the doctrine of the Jehovah's Witnesses, despite the fact that she was not a Witness herself. She lost consciousness and the court overruled her refusal on the grounds that she had been unduly influenced by her mother and that her decision was based upon inadequate information about her prognosis.

INFORMED CONSENT AND SURGICAL RESEARCH

1. The availability of surgical options is dependent on the experimental research which makes them possible. Yet researchers must be careful. Without enthusiasm and conviction about the importance of their work, they will not have the commitment that successful research requires. However, such commitment can lead to an underestimation of the risks or discomfort of experiments. Research can be either therapeutic and to the potential benefit of participants, or non-therapeutic with no such promise. Participants in the former will be patients, and in the latter either patients or healthy volunteers.

2. Patients involved in research have a right to informed consent for the same reasons described above. By allowing them to make an informed evaluation for themselves, they exert a regulating influence on experimental zeal; this has unquestionably led to moral abuses in the past. A clear example is the notorious and needless experiments inflicted by some Nazi doctors and surgeons on Jewish prisoners. However, there have been more recent illustrations involving patients, some of

whom have died as a result of their participation in research.

3. The Nuremburg Code was adopted internationally as a result. It declared that 'the voluntary consent of a patient is essential' in any medical research. The later Declaration of Helsinki is also explicit. It states: 'In any research, each potential subject must be adequately informed of the aims, methods and anticipated benefits and potential hazards of the study and the discomfort it may entail.' After this, participants' consent must be obtained.

4. The enforcement of the Helsinki Declaration in the UK is entrusted to research ethics committees. These are administered by health authorities and are responsible for evaluating all surgical research involving humans, wherever it might be undertaken. Under no circumstances should research proceed without the approval of the appropriate ethics committee, and academic journals usually publish the results only when such approval has been given. In principle, research ethics committees are supposed to ensure that the proposed protocol makes good scientific sense and poses no further risks than those of the best available treatment. Only then should patients be asked to consent to participate, on the basis of being given appropriate information about the research that the committee has also approved.

5. There is, however, one remaining, significant problem concerning surgical research and informed consent. As a result of differing ability and willingness to understand and to question medical authority, we have seen that patients vary in their ability to assimilate the details of clinical information. Consequently, enthusiastic researchers are in a position, wittingly or not, to manipulate patients to subject themselves to procedures that might not be proposed in ordinary treatment. Patients may be encouraged to agree to participate in the development of surgical procedures, for example, without realizing how experimental they are. Here, the general guidelines concerning informed consent must be followed with extra vigilance. For example, take care to identify surgical procedures that might not be regarded as standard professional practice and proceed only when the patient gives informed and written consent with the knowledge that this is the case. When in doubt about whether or not a procedure is standard, consult the research ethics committee. You must not pretend that a surgical innovation that goes beyond a minor incremental variation on already standard procedures is not research that requires further ethical evaluation before proceeding.

6. In non-therapeutic research with patients or healthy volunteers, you must be equally stringent to avoid confusing agreement to participate with informed consent to do so. Try to ensure that the moral legitimacy of the

consent of the volunteer is not obtained under financial, social or professional duress. In the UK, for example, the difficulty of doing so has led to surgical research not ordinarily taking place among the prison population.

INFORMED CONSENT AND CONFIDENTIALITY

1. As a corollary of their right to informed consent, patients have the right to control access to information which they give to you for the purposes of treatment. The General Medical Council (GMC) supports this right through the importance it attaches to the principle of confidentiality – obtaining the permission of patients before revealing clinical information about them to others. Few acts can more quickly lead to you being professionally disciplined than a proven breach of confidence in unwarranted circumstances.

2. There are two types of justification for this emphasis. First, the right to be the moral gatekeeper of one's own body extends to information divulged in clinical consultations. Second, if patients are frightened that their confidence might be breached, they may not be willing to provide the honest information on which successful diagnosis depends, or even to turn up for treatment at all. This can pose a severe danger to them and possibly to the general public.

3. It is in the area of potential conflict between the freedom of the individual and the interest of the public that circumstances may arise in which you either must or might divulge information otherwise regarded as private. The same professional codes which stress the importance of confidentiality (the 'Duties of a Doctor' of the GMC, for example) also outline the exceptions to the rule. These fall into two general categories.

The public interest

1. Suppose that in a clinical consultation in the accident and emergency department you discover that a highly agitated patient is armed, has committed a robbery and has killed a bank clerk and a customer as a result. Here, it seems straightforward that the confidence should be broken and the police informed. The patient may strike again. Indeed, it is legally mandatory to breach confidentiality where patients are suspected of involvement in terrorism within the UK or where they are found to be suffering from a highly infectious and notifiable disease.

2. How serious must a risk to the public actually be to breach confidentiality legitimately? For example, are you just as willing to report someone who confesses in confidence to stealing a badly needed winter coat? It is not always easy to balance the interests of the patient against those of the public. This can create difficult dilemmas for you when the two seem in direct conflict and when, as is often the case, there is considerable professional discretion as to how morally to proceed. Debates about HIV and AIDS have recently underlined these issues.

3. Two things are clear.

a. First, it does not follow from a claim that the public interest demands a breach of confidence that it actually does. For example, the police have no right to disclosure or to access clinical records that may provide evidence of a crime. A judge may issue a warrant legally authorizing such access or a subpoena demanding disclosure in court. However, even this does not make it morally mandatory. Some clinicians have felt so strongly about the immorality of breaking a patient's confidence that they have risked being charged with contempt of court for refusing to do so. Do not fuse the law and morality, even though they often do overlap.

b. Second, patients have no right to harm others through the exercise of their right to confidentiality. There is an obvious link between this right and the right of individuals to control the use of their private property. Yet just as the legitimate exercise of this property right stops at the point at which the safety of others is threatened, the same can be said about clinical information. Therefore, if you discover that maintaining confidentiality will lead to the threat of serious harm to another known individual – the suspicion of a general threat is not sufficient – then a breach of confidence may be warranted. For example, although the legal precedent does not apply in the UK, a psychiatrist in the USA was successfully sued for negligence for not informing a young woman that he had clearly been told by a patient that he was going to kill her. He did. If you do consider a breach of confidence to a third party in these circumstances, it is always important to warn the patient that this is what you intend.

The interest of the individual patient

1. Breaches of confidence may not just be in the public interest. They may also be necessary in order to obtain information vital for successful treatment. Because of the physical or psychological effects of their illness, some patients are unable to communicate clearly about their medical history. Under such circumstances, you may need to consult relatives or friends, especially in emergencies.

2. This said, still make strong attempts to obtain the patient's consent and to verify the identity of any others from whom information is sought. Reveal no more information about the patient's condition than is necessary for the clinical purposes at hand. Keep knowledge confidential concerning prognosis and treatment, for example. Remember how its unwarranted spread might drastically

affect the patient's private and public life. Never communicate clinical information over the phone to those not involved in treatment, unless it is with the patient's prior consent and there is a reliable way of identifying the person to whom you give the information.

3. The interests of patients are also served if you share clinical information they have given you, with colleagues whose assistance you require. Patients are presumed to consent to such revelations by virtue of their general agreement to treatment. Given the complexity of its division of labour, surgery is an essentially cooperative exercise and its success depends on the free flow of relevant information. This said, allow access to information only to those professionals involved – something which requires caution, especially on open wards.

MORAL INDETERMINACY, INFORMED CONSENT AND OPEN COMMUNICATION

1. Thus far, we have examined the general principles governing informed consent that are endorsed by the surgical profession and which are reinforced by statute and case law. Yet, clear as these are, their correct interpretation may be much more obscure in practice. Such rules do not interpret themselves: you must interpret them as an individual when faced with the complexities of specific cases.

2. In the majority of cases there is a consensus among the surgical team about the most appropriate interpretation. It will be reasonably clear, for example, how much information should be communicated to knowledgeable patients about the hazards of a particular treatment and whether or not they have understood enough of it to warrant proceeding. Yet in some situations, such agreement does not exist and interpretations are conflicting. Reference to the facts of the case themselves cannot solve the problem. Their openness to conflicting interpretation is what poses it.

3. Suppose, for example, that despite careful attempts to communicate the considerable risks of an urgently needed operative procedure there is still disagreement within the surgical team about whether or not the patient has fully understood. Against the background of the necessity to come to a quick decision, there may be no 'right' interpretation as to how to proceed ethically.

4. Another illustration might be conflicting beliefs about whether or not to operate urgently on a Jehovah's Witness who refuses a blood transfusion but seems to be doing so partially under pressure from family or congregation.

5. What is crucial in such circumstances is that, despite their disagreements, individual members of the surgical team accept that the final decision about how to proceed is reached after an open and reasoned discussion. Everyone then has the chance to present their arguments. As a result, clinicians are more willing to cooperate in the search for a common view, even though it involves a degree of what may be perceived as moral compromise. Open communication does not have to conflict with the recognition that it is the senior clinician who takes responsibility for the final choice. If you are a surgeon in authority, always try to create space for such discussions, a practice that is increasingly common in the face of taxing moral dilemmas that have to be resolved in short periods of time – for example, those concerning the withdrawal of life sustaining treatment.

Summary

- Do you respect the right of patients to give or withhold consent to surgical treatment?
- Will you provide patients with sufficient information to make informed choice possible?
- Even in surgical emergencies, will you avoid overriding the right of conscious and capable patients to decide on treatment?
- Will you continue to respect the rights of all patients, including children, and those who are unconscious, mentally handicapped or psychiatrically ill?

ACKNOWLEDGEMENTS

Many thanks to John Cochrane, Robert Cohen, Lesley Doyal, John Dickenson, Arlene Klotzko, Alastair McDonald, Rosanne Lord, Paul Lear, Norman Williams, Daniel Wilsher, Christopher Wood and Richard Wood. Special thanks to Ian Kennedy.

 Further reading

Alderson P 1993 Children's consent to surgery. Open University Press, Buckingham

Beauchamp T, Childress J 1994 Principles of biomedical ethics. Oxford University Press, New York

Brazier M 1992 Medicine, patients and the law. Penguin, Harmondsworth

British Medical Association 2001 Withholding and withdrawing life-prolonging medical treatment. BMJ Books, London

British Medical Association 2001 Consent, rights and choices in health care for children and young people. BMJ Books, London

Buchanan A, Brock D 1989 Deciding for others: the ethics of surrogate decision making. Cambridge University Press, Cambridge

Doyal L, Tobias J (eds) 2000 Informed consent in medical research. BMJ Books, London

Harris J 1985 The value of life. Routledge, London

Kennedy I, Grubb A 2000 Medical law. Butterworths, London

Lipkin M, Putnam S, Lazare A (eds) 1995 The medical interview: clinical care, education and research. Springer, New York

McHale J, Fox M 1997 Health care law – text and materials. Sweet and Maxwell, London

McLean S 1989 A patient's right to know: information disclosure, the doctor and the law. Dartmouth, Aldershot

Mason J, McCall Smith R 1999 Law and medical ethics. Butterworths, London

Montgomery J 2002 Healthcare law. Oxford University Press, Oxford

Rothman DJ 1991 Strangers at the bedside: a history of how law and bioethics transformed medical decision making. Basic Books, New York

Royal College of Surgeons 1997 The surgeon's duty of care. Royal College of Surgeons, London

Wear S 1993 Informed consent. Kluwer, Dordrecht

15 Preoperative preparation for surgery

S. Bhattacharya, G. M. H. Wray

Objectives

- **Understand the general principles of preoperative preparation.**
- **Appreciate how, in high risk patients, preoperative preparation may lower the risk.**
- **Understand the principles of preparation for specific types of operation.**
- **Appreciate the value of protocols and routines, and the importance of adhering to them, even in emergency situations.**

To obtain satisfactory results in surgery, a careful preoperative preparation of the patient is vital. Attention to detail is the key to success. The importance of this preparation becomes more evident as the surgical procedure performed becomes more complex.

ROUTINE PREOPERATIVE PREPARATION

Evaluation

1. Take a full history and exclude any significant medical problems (see Ch. 6).

2. Check clinical signs against the planned surgical procedure, in particular noting the side involved. Confirm that the planned operative procedure is appropriate.

Key point

- **During the interval between the decision to operate and the actual operation, the disease may have progressed, making the intended operation inappropriate; seek advice from a senior colleague.**

3. Take a full drug history with specific enquiry regarding allergic responses to drugs, latex and skin allergies. Continue medication over the perioperative period, especially drugs for hypertension, ischaemic heart disease and bronchodilators. Give patients on oral steroid therapy intravenous hydrocortisone. Stop oral warfarin anticoagulation 3–4 days preoperatively and check the prothrombin time prior to surgery. If the prothrombin time remains unacceptably high, the patient may require an infusion of fresh frozen plasma. Those on warfarin who have had a life-threatening thrombotic episode (e.g. pulmonary embolus) within the previous 3 months should be switched to heparin intravenously until 6 h before surgery; the heparin can usually be recommenced 4 h after surgery. Patients taking aspirin or other antiplatelet medication (e.g. clopidogrel) may have an increased risk of bleeding; stop these drugs for at least 48 h preoperatively for major surgery. Stop drugs, over the perioperative period, that may interfere with anaesthetic agents, including monoamine oxidase inhibitors, lithium, tricyclic antidepressants and phenothiazines. If possible, stop the oral contraceptive pill 4 weeks prior to any major surgery. Postmenopausal patients on hormone replacement therapy do not need to have their medication stopped before an operation.

4. There is a clear correlation between malnutrition in the preoperative period and an increased morbidity and mortality from surgery (see Ch. 10). Nutritional assessment can be based on total body weight loss, anthropomorphic measurements such as skinfold thickness to assess the amount of subcutaneous fat, or biochemical tests that reflect protein deficiency, such as the measurement of serum albumin, prealbumin or transferrin. Such preoperative nutritional assessment may detect patients in whom malnutrition is a major concern for their operative procedure, but the correction of this malnourished state, which in part reflects their underlying disease process, may be impossible in the preoperative period. Highlight the problem to allow you to commence nutritional support at an early stage and consider inserting a feeding enterostomy or a designated central venous feeding line at the time of operation. Do not consider

correcting a low preoperative serum albumin level with human albumin solution except as an adjuvant to full parenteral or enteral nutrition. It is an ineffective and expensive method of providing nutritional support.

5. Young and fit patients undergoing minor procedures do not require any preoperative investigations (see Ch. 4). In older patients or those with significant medical problems, standard investigation would include a full blood count, urea and electrolytes, chest X-ray and electrocardiogram. For a critical evaluation of routine preoperative investigations see Velanovich (1994).

Routine preoperative measures

1. Each clinical firm evolves a standard protocol for preoperative preparation appropriate for its patients. Adhere to the protocol followed by your firm. Use a checklist – these are very useful to ensure that you do not leave out an important step.

2. Prohibit solid diet to adult patients for 6 h, and clear fluids for 4 h, prior to an elective general anaesthetic. Fasting times for children vary in different hospitals and they are also age dependent. A suggested regimen is summarized in Table 15.1.

3. The operation site must be prepared by the removal of hair, if this is necessary for access, using a depilatory cream. Shaving or clipping hair from the operation site increases the risk of infection, unless the skin preparation is carried out immediately prior to surgery.

Table 15.1 Preoperative fasting times for children

Babies under 1 year
No breast milk for 2–3 h before anaesthesia
No formula feed for 6 h before anaesthesia
Clear fluids may be given up to 3 h before anaesthesia

Children over 1 year
No food/milk for 6 h before anaesthesia
Clear fluids up to 3 h before anaesthesia

Key point

- **Mark a unilateral operation site on the skin with an indelible marker pen.**

4. Explain to the patient (or guardian) the procedure and any likely complications, answer questions the patient may have, and only then have them sign the consent form. If you are unable to answer the patient's questions, seek help from a senior colleague. It is good practice for the operating surgeon to obtain the patient's consent; failing that, it may be done by another member of the team who is familiar with the operation and its aftercare. Consent should ideally be obtained from patients not immediately before an operation but some time ahead, so that they may have a period of reflection, and an opportunity to ask further questions that may arise.

5. Antibiotic administration is guided by the surgical procedure involved and is discussed below, as is prophylaxis against deep vein thrombosis.

6. If specific services, such as frozen section histopathology or intraoperative radiography are likely to be required during the operation, organize these in advance.

THE USE OF ANTIBIOTICS

1. As a general rule, treat patients with clinical infection using systemic antibiotics before they undergo operation.

2. Antibiotic prophylaxis for an elective operation depends on the procedure being performed (Table 15.2).

3. Clean procedures, as for varicose veins, do not require antibiotic prophylaxis. Abdominal operations not associated with significant contamination, such as cholecystectomy, demand only a single dose of prophylactic antibiotic given on induction of anaesthesia.

Table 15.2 The risk of infection

Type of wound	Description	Incidence of wound infection (%)
Clean	No violation of mucosa No inflammation No drains	2
Clean–contaminated	Incision of mucosa but no spillage, *or* Clean procedure in immunocompromised	10
Contaminated	Pre-existing infection Spillage of viscus contents	20–40

---

4. Procedures in a contaminated field, such as appendicitis, require a preoperative dose and two postoperative doses. This regimen is also satisfactory for most other gastrointestinal tract procedures, including gastric surgery, and colonic operations on prepared bowel.

5. The choice of antibiotic prophylaxis is determined by the surgical procedure itself. Operations potentially contaminated by skin flora require prophylaxis against staphylococcal infection with flucloxacillin 500 mg intravenously. Procedures involving the bowel require broad-spectrum cover for Gram-positive and Gram-negative organisms and anaerobes. Commonly used regimens include co-amoxiclav or a cephalosporin with metronidazole. Biliary tract procedures rarely involve anaerobic contamination: a cephalosporin alone is satisfactory.

Key point

- If a patient has a penicillin allergy, avoid not just penicillin but also drugs such as ampicillin and amoxicillin. Cephalosporins have a 10% chance of crossreactivity in patients with penicillin allergy; prescribe them with caution.

PROPHYLAXIS AGAINST DEEP VEIN THROMBOSIS AND PULMONARY EMBOLI

Pulmonary emboli are a major cause of mortality for surgical patients, accounting for 10% of inpatient deaths in the United Kingdom. Recent operation, immobilization and trauma were responsible for 50% of deep vein thrombosis (DVT) in a review by Cogo et al (1994), but there are other important predisposing factors, such as the high oestrogen content oral contraceptive pill, and significant obesity (Table 15.3). Many risk factors cannot be avoided, but take measures to avoid propagation of any thrombosis:

1. Subcutaneous heparin may reduce the incidence of DVT by 50%; it is generally well tolerated but very occasionally causes thrombocytopenia. Systemic anticoagulation effects of low dose subcutaneous heparin are minimal and haemostasis is not impaired. Newer low molecular weight heparins (LMWHs), as effective as standard heparin, need only once a day dosage.

Key point

- Epidural anaesthesia? Take precautions against epidural haematoma.

Table 15.3   Risk factors for deep vein thrombosis
Recent surgery
Immobilization
Trauma
Oral contraceptive pill
Obesity
Heart failure
Arteriopathy
Cancer
Age > 60 years
Adapted from Cogo et al (1994).

Epidural (or spinal) anaesthesia significantly reduces postoperative morbidity and mortality (Rodgers et al 2000) and is used for perioperative analgesia (see also Chs 16, 35). Insertion and removal of epidural catheters have been associated with the development of epidural haematomas in anticoagulated patients with potentially serious neurological consequences. Current recommendations are to delay insertion or removal of an epidural catheter for 12 h after a dose of LMWH. Delay subsequent doses of LMWH for 2 h following catheter insertion or removal (Wheatley & Veitch 1997).

2. Graduated compression stockings and intraoperative intermittent pneumatic calf compression are also effective in reducing deep venous thrombosis.

PREPARATION OF HIGH RISK PATIENTS

For the management of specific preexisting comorbidity, such as heart disease or diabetes, see Chapter 6. Risk assessment is an important part of the preoperative anaesthetic assessment. You may use the ASA (American Society for Anesthesiologists) scoring system to assess the overall risk (Table 15.4). The functional status of patients with cardiac disease may be stratified using the NYHA (New York Heart Association) classification (Table 15.5). Risk stratification in patients in intensive care may be done using more complex systems such as the APACHE (Acute Physiology and Chronic Health Evaluation) score (Knaus et al 1985).

Emergency surgery

1. The results of emergency surgery are less satisfactory than those of elective procedures. The emergency nature of the surgery may not allow sufficient time for investigation and treatment of associated medical problems. Do not cut corners, and adhere to your elective preoperative protocols as far as possible. These patients are commonly dehydrated and hypovolaemic; if that is the

Table 15.4	American Society for Anesthesiologists (ASA) status	
Category	Description	Perioperative mortality (%)
I	Healthy patient	0.1
II	Mild systemic disease – no functional limitations	0.2
III	Severe systemic disease – definite functional limitation	1.8
IV	Severe systemic disease that is a constant threat to life	7.8
V	Moribund patient not expected to survive 24 h with or without surgery	9.4

Table 15.5	New York Heart Association classification
Class	Description
I	No functional limitation
II	Slight functional limitation. Fatigue, palpitations, dyspnoea or angina on ordinary physical activity but asymptomatic at rest
III	Marked functional limitation. Symptoms on less than ordinary activity, but asymptomatic at rest
IV	Inability to perform any physical activity, with or without symptoms at rest

case, their initial management must include insertion of wide-bore venous access lines and prompt rehydration. Consider inserting a central venous line, and also a urinary catheter to assess the adequacy of rehydration. Such patients may have sepsis, requiring systemic antibiotic treatment. Insert a nasogastric tube if there is insufficient time to allow for the usual period of fasting, or if you suspect bowel obstruction.

Key point

- **As far as possible adhere to your elective preoperative routines.**

2. Carefully judge the timing of the operation, and involve senior colleagues in the decision making. The morbidity and mortality audit (National Confidential Enquiry into Perioperative Deaths, NCEPOD) performed by the Royal College of Surgeons of England (Campling et al 1993) suggests that the majority of patients with acute surgical problems are better managed by active resuscitation prior to operation performed on a scheduled operating list by an experienced surgeon.

Very high risk patients

1. Some patients are at particularly high risk because they have significant comorbidity and may require a major or emergency operation. If possible, admit them to a high dependency unit (HDU) or intensive care unit

(ICU) preoperatively to undergo 'preoptimization'. The value of this high standard of care has been recognized for many years.

2. Survival following operation requires adequate cardiac reserve. It is possible that the perioperative course can be improved by setting targets for improving circulating blood volume and cardiac function measured by cardiac output, oxygen delivery and oxygen consumption. The targets were originally defined by Shoemaker et al in 1988, and are known as 'Shoemaker's goals':

- Cardiac index (CI) > 4.2 ml min^{-1} m^{-2}
- Oxygen delivery (D_{O_2}) > 600 ml min^{-1} m^{-2}
- Oxygen consumption (V_{O_2}) > 170 ml min^{-1} m^{-2}

They were chosen as representing 'survivor values' when high risk surgical patients were studied retrospectively and are claimed to improve survival if achieved preoperatively (Wilson et al 1999, Takala et al 2000). This involves the insertion of a central line or pulmonary artery catheter sufficiently early before operation to allow manipulation of haemodynamics using fluid resuscitation, with or without the addition of an inotrope such as dopexamine. Beware of the risks of using high levels of inotropic drugs to achieve Shoemaker's goals in those who fail to respond to treatment or are in the late stages of septic shock.

PREPARATION FOR SURGERY OF SPECIFIC PATIENT GROUPS

Preparation must be tailored to the procedures to be performed and the stage of the underlying pathology.

Large bowel operations

1. Most surgeons consider bowel preparation essential to reduce the risk of sepsis, although some recent controlled studies failed to prove any benefit from it. For elective operations, institute a liquid diet for several days and administer oral purgatives on the preoperative day. Sodium picosulphate (Picolax) 10 mg morning and night, or polyethylene glycol/sodium salts (Klean-Prep) four sachets in 4 litres of water taken 250 ml every 15 min, are suitable. If they fail to cleanse the bowel, combine them with mechanical washouts via a rectal tube. Elderly patients may require intravenous hydration while undergoing bowel purgation to compensate for associated fluid loss. Bowel preparation is usually contraindicated in obstructed patients, although some surgeons advocate on-table colonic lavage with the infusion of fluid through a caecostomy or appendicostomy; the effluent drains through a wide-bore tube inserted proximal to the obstruction.

 Key point

• **Warn all patients undergoing bowel surgery of the possible need to create a colostomy or ileostomy.**

2. Before operation ask the stoma care nurse to select and mark the most practical site for a colostomy on the abdominal wall.
3. Counsel patients undergoing rectal surgery about the risks of pelvic nerve injury with consequent impotence and loss of bladder control.
4. Inform patients with Crohn's disease of the possibility of recurrence and anastomotic breakdown. Similarly, discuss with patients undergoing pouch surgery the likelihood of bowel frequency and incontinence. Those undergoing anal surgery, especially for high fistula, need to know about the risks of incontinence.

Upper gastrointestinal surgery

1. Patients may be anorexic, in a poor nutritional state, requiring correction by enteral or parenteral feeding before and after operation. If the patient is vomiting, detect and correct dehydration, electrolyte depletion and possible acid–base imbalance. If there is evidence of gastric delay or obstruction, insert a nasogastric tube to empty the stomach and prevent aspiration at the time of induction of anaesthesia. Vomiting may be associated with episodes of aspiration so assess and if necesssary correct respiratory function.

2. The oesophageal lumen becomes rapidly contaminated in the presence of disease or partial obstruction. For 24 h before operation give 10 ml of 0.2% chlorhexidine mouthwash and swallow, 6-hourly.

Liver, biliary and pancreatic operations

1. Jaundiced patients may be deficient in the vitamin K-dependent clotting factors II, V, VII, IX and X, resulting in a bleeding tendency. Give vitamin K (10 mg intramuscularly or intravenously) to patients with obstructive jaundice prior to surgery, if their prothrombin time is abnormal. Be ready to give fresh frozen plasma to those in whom there is a significant coagulopathy and who require urgent operation.
2. Preoperative insertion of a biliary endoprosthesis to correct obstructive jaundice in the hope of reducing operative risk is controversial. There is also little evidence that routine preoperative biliary stenting or drainage by endoscopic retrograde cholangiopancreatoscopy (ERCP), or percutaneous transhepatic cholangiography (PTC), is helpful in these patients. However, consider preoperative drainage in patients who are elderly, deeply jaundiced or with biliary tract sepsis.
3. Avoid or reduce renal failure secondary to obstructive jaundice (hepatorenal syndrome) by ensuring adequate preoperative hydration; do not stop oral fluids pre-operatively without intravenous fluid replacement. The value of the osmotic diuretic mannitol and the inotrope dopamine (in a low dose resulting in renal vasodilatation) to prevent hepatorenal failure is unproven.
4. Infective complications are common after operations for obstructive jaundice, so always give antibiotics as prophylaxis.
5. Acute cholangitis demands systemic administration of fluids, antibiotics and urgent biliary tract drainage, either endoscopically or percutaneously. Patients with biliary obstruction who undergo an unsuccessful ERCP (where the duct is entered but not stented) are at a high risk of developing cholangitis. They require antibiotic cover and urgent consideration of a PTC.
6. If you intend that the procedure will be carried out laparoscopically on a patient with severe pulmonary disease, take advice from the anaesthetist. Inducing pneumoperitoneum increases intra-abdominal pressure and may render ventilation difficult.

 Key point

• **Before laparoscopic biliary operations, inform the patient about the possibility of conversion to an open procedure.**

7. Hepatic cirrhosis is a particularly high risk disorder, requiring treatment by an experienced team. Clotting is often deranged, and may need elective correction with vitamin K or emergency infusion of fresh frozen plasma and clotting factors.

8. The presence of portal hypertension raises operative risks. The operation may be technically difficult, with excessive venous bleeding. Patients tolerate major fluid shifts badly and become encephalopathic as a consequence, or may develop renal failure. Avoid operating on those with decompensated cirrhosis (Child–Pugh C) unless it is absolutely essential.

9. In patients requiring pancreatic resection, consider giving octreotide (a somatostatin analogue that suppresses pancreatic secretion) in the perioperative phase to reduce the risk of leakage from the pancreatojejunal anastomosis. Several trials have shown probable but not certain benefit. In operations on the pancreatic tail, with the possibility of splenectomy, be prepared to inject the patient preoperatively with vaccines against pneumococcal, meningococcal and *Haemophilus influenzae* type B infections.

Endocrine surgery

1. Thyrotoxic patients require preoperative treatment to reduce thyroid activity, such as carbimazole 10–15 mg three times daily, and a beta blocker such as propranolol 20–40 mg, 8-hourly for 10 days preoperatively, to prevent thyrotoxic crisis.

2. Have the movement of the vocal cords checked by indirect laryngoscopy prior to operation, to exclude an unsuspected idiopathic unilateral palsy.

3. Demonstrate the extent of a retrosternal goitre with computed tomography.

4. Patients with phaeochromocytoma require preoperative medication to block the α- and β-adrenergic effects of catecholamines, and may require admission a week before operation. As a rule, start with α-blockade using phenoxybenzamine, followed 48 h later by β-blockade with atenolol or metoprolol.

Paediatric patients

1. The common surgical procedures in childhood are often performed by general surgeons with special training and interest in paediatric surgery. Complex congenital defects and surgery in neonates require specialist surgical expertise and specific preoperative preparation.

Key point

• **Manage all paediatric patients together with a paediatrician.**

2. Although comorbidity is unusual in children, exclude upper respiratory tract infection or cold, which can cause potentially life-threatening laryngeal spasm due to the sensitivity of the inflamed airway. Discuss this with the anaesthetist and be willing to postpone any but an emergency operation.

3. Arrange elective procedures for children at the beginning of the operating list to minimize the period of fasting. If operation is delayed, give fluids intravenously; insert venous cannulae after applying topical anaesthetic cream to reduce discomfort. Administer fluids according to body weight (40–60 ml kg^{-1} 24 h^{-1}). Heparin and antibiotics are not required for routine clean surgical procedures.

Thoracic surgery

1. Arrange preoperative lung function tests in patients with severe functional limitation due to chronic airway disease, including arterial blood gases on room air and measurements of forced expiratory volume in 1 min (FEV$_1$) and forced vital capacity (FVC). Patients with FEV$_1$/FVC below 50% of the predicted value are at a high risk of respiratory failure.

2. In patients requiring lung resection, assess the likely impact of this on postoperative lung function using radioactive isotope perfusion scans of the individual lungs.

3. Arrange active preoperative physiotherapy, treatment of any respiratory infection with antibiotics and good postoperative analgesia in order to minimize the risk of postoperative respiratory failure. In this patient group, seek evidence of associated atherosclerotic coronary and cerebral vascular disease and obtain the advice of a cardiologist if necessary (Goldman et al 1977).

4. Anticipate the possibility of pulmonary emboli and give routine subcutaneous heparin.

Vascular surgery

1. Atherosclerosis is a generalized disease so search carefully the complete vascular system for evidence of widespread insufficiency, such as cerebral, coronary, renal and peripheral arterial disease. Arrange for expert advice and management before undertaking any operation for peripheral vascular disease. In elective circumstances be willing to await improvement of severe ischaemic heart disease with drugs, angioplasty or coronary artery grafting. An operation within 3 months of a myocardial infarction carries a 20–30% risk of a perioperative infarct. This risk decreases to 10–20% between 3 and 6 months, and 4–5% after 6 months. This compares with a risk of 0.1–0.2% risk of infarction in patients with no evidence of a previous myocardial infarct. Remember that the risk of

death from perioperative myocardial infarction is extremely high, at around 70%.

2. Diabetic patients with limb ischaemia require diabetes control and treatment of infected skin lesions before operation.

3. Since smoking is a common predisposing factor to atherosclerosis and it reduces small vessel blood flow, ask the patient to stop it preoperatively. Smoking also predisposes to chronic obstructive airways disease and bronchial carcinoma, so carefully assess respiratory function. If there is a productive cough, send sputum for culture, antibiotic sensitivity and cytology. In addition, check the serum lipid profile to exclude correctable hyperlipidaemia.

Orthopaedic surgery

1. The most common orthopaedic operations are for the treatment of joint abnormalities secondary to osteoarthritis. Many patients are elderly, with comorbidity such as ischaemic heart disease and chronic obstructive airways disease. Diagnose, assess and treat them appropriately (see Ch. 6).

2. Crossmatch blood for joint replacement, as there may be significant blood loss.

3. The increased use of prostheses (Greek *pros* = to + *thesis* = putting) in orthopaedic surgery allows early mobilization, but infection is a serious risk around the foreign material. Administer antibiotic prophylaxis against contamination from skin commensals such as staphylococci and streptococci.

4. Since thromboembolism is a major cause of mortality in orthopaedic patients, especially following pelvic surgery, routinely give prophylaxis with standard heparin or LMWH.

Patients with latex allergy

Latex allergy is becoming more prevalent and is thought to result from true anaphylaxis to latex proteins. It can pose a serious risk to life from both anaesthetic and surgical equipment. There is an increased incidence in those exposed repeatedly to latex, such as healthcare workers, patients with spina bifida who have had repeated catheterization, atopic (Greek *atopia* = strangeness; hypersensitivity) individuals and people with banana or avocado allergy (crossreactivity with similar proteins). Plan operations on these patients so that all concerned in the operating theatre and hospital ward use appropriate equipment. The operating theatre should have a checklist of equipment that is safe to use in such patients, and

ideally there should be a 'latex allergy box' containing most of these items.

Summary

- Do you realize the importance of preoperative preparation with close attention to detail?
- Are you aware of the specific needs of different patients undergoing different procedures?
- Can you recognize the need to identify high risk patients early so you can institute appropriate measures at once?
- Do you accept the need for a multidisciplinary approach, requiring good communication within the team?

References

Campling EA, Devlin HB, Hoile RW, Lunn JN 1993 Report of the national confidential enquiry into perioperative deaths 1991/1992. King's Fund Publishing, London

Cogo A, Bernardi E, Prandoni P et al 1994 Acquired risk factors for deep vein thrombosis in symptomatic outpatients. Archives of Internal Medicine 154: 164–168

Goldman L, Caldera DL, Nussbaum SR 1977 Multifactorial index of cardiac risk in noncardiac procedures. New England Journal of Medicine 297: 845–850

Knaus WA, Draper EA, Wagner DP et al 1985 APACHE II: a severity of disease classification system. Critical Care Medicine 13: 818–824

Rodgers A, Walker N, Schug S et al 2000 Reduction of postoperative mortality and morbidity with epidural or spinal anaesthesia: results from overview of randomized trials. BMJ 321: 1493–1497

Shoemaker WC, Appel PL, Kram HB et al 1988 Prospective trial of supranormal values for survivors as therapeutic goals in high-risk surgical patients. Chest 94:1176–1186

Takala J, Meier-Hellman A, Eddlston J et al 2000 Effect of dopexamine on outcome after major abdominal surgery: a prospective, randomized, controlled multicentre study. Critical Care Medicine 28: 3417–3423

Velanovich V 1994 Preoperative laboratory screening based on age, gender and concomitant medical diseases. Surgery 115: 56–61

Wheatley T, Veitch PS 1997 Recent advances in prophylaxis against deep vein thrombosis. British Journal of Anaesthesia 78: 118–120

Wilson J, Woods I, Fawcett J et al 1999 Reducing the risk of major elective surgery: randomized controlled trial of preoperative optimization of oxygen delivery. BMJ 318: 1099–1103

16 Preoperative assessment and anaesthesia

M. W. Platt

> **Objectives**
>
> - Understand the role of the preoperative assessment in the work-up for surgery.
> - Gain a general understanding of the function of the anaesthetist, the effects of anaesthesia and the perioperative medical management of the patient.
> - Realize the importance of analgesia in minimizing the stress response and its significance in reducing postoperative complications.
> - Understand the basic pharmacology and toxicology of local anaesthetic agents and their use.

PREOPERATIVE ASSESSMENT AND PREMEDICATION

Ideally, an anaesthetist should assess all patients preoperatively. Often, daycare (or ambulatory care) patients attend the hospital only on the morning of operation. The anaesthetist carries out the assessment in the ward just before the list begins, or even in the anaesthetic room. Patients with significant intercurrent disease have normally been assessed at a booking clinic and admitted before the day of surgery to optimize their physical state. An anaesthetist is usually asked to assess risk factors involved.

The anaesthetic assessment evaluates the patient's physiological status, vital organ functional reserve and any concurrent disease states, including diabetes, thyroid and cardiac diseases (see Chs 6, 15). This is in order to judge the patient's ability to withstand the stress of surgery and anaesthesia, and to check that the patient has not eaten or drunk for 4 h, although this is slightly modified for young children by allowing clear, glucose-containing fluids up to 2 h preoperatively. Physical examination focuses on the cardiovascular, respiratory, hepatic, renal, and central nervous systems.

> **Key point**
>
> - Are there any drug allergies, intercurrent medications, history of personal or family anaesthetic problems?

The anaesthetist then prescribes premedication, the drugs administered preoperatively, including any essential intercurrent medication. They are usually prescribed by the anaesthetist at the preoperative visit to allay anxiety, relieve pain and, occasionally, to dry saliva and oral secretions.

Intercurrent medication

Many patients requiring operation have other medical problems that are treated by a variety of different drugs (see Ch. 6). Especially consider those on antihypertensive therapy, antiarrhythmic therapy, anticoagulation regimens, oral or insulin therapy for diabetes, endocrine replacement therapy (particularly thyroxin), adrenocortical replacement or augmentation therapy, asthma or chronic obstructive airways disease treated with bronchodilators and allied drugs, cardiac failure therapy, and those requiring diuretics. Because of fasting, or the operation itself, it may not be possible to continue the medication. Many drugs must be continued up to the time of operation and some agents can be administered parenterally. Antihypertensives, anticonvulsants, antiarrhythmics and other essential medications can often be given 2 h preoperatively with a small sip of water.

Anaesthetic premedication

Anxiolysis (Table 16.1)

Patients attending for surgery are normally anxious about the outcome. They may have a fear of the unknown, of pain, of dying, of cancer, or non-specific fears. Although the preoperative visit by the anaesthetist does much to allay anxiety by reducing the unknown element, waiting for an operation may be unpleasant. Anxiolytics calm the

Table 16.1	Anxiolytic agents in common use	
Agent	Dose	Approx. duration (h)
Benzodiazepines		
Diazepam	0.05–0.3 mg kg^{-1}	36–200
Temazepam	0.15–0.5 mg kg^{-1}	5–20
Lorazepam	0.015–0.06 μg kg^{-1}	10–20
Midazolam	0.07–0.08 mg kg^{-1}	0.5–2
Phenothiazines		
Promethazine	0.2–0.5 mg kg^{-1}	8–12
Prochlorperazine	0.1–0.2 mg kg^{-1}	8–12

Table 16.2	Analgesic agents in common use	
Agent	Dose (mg kg–1)	Approx. duration, i.m. (h)
Morphine	0.1–0.2	4
Diamorphine	0.05–0.1	4
Papaveretum	0.2–0.4	3

Notes
1. Papaveretum is a mixture of alkaloids which contains morphine (45–55% dry weight), codeine, papaverine, thebaine and noscopine. It should not be used in women of child-bearing age, because noscopine has been shown to be a gene toxin.

Papaveretum is most commonly used as a premedication in combination with hyoscine, and comes in a premixed ampoule containing papaveretum 20 mg ml^{-1} and hyoscine 0.4 mg ml^{-1}.
2. Morphine, often used alone for both its sedative and analgesic properties, is usually combined with a drying agent such as atropine (also useful to prevent bradycardia), or in combination with an antiemetic drug.

patient and help to reduce time spent 'dwelling' on fears. Agents specifically used for anxiolysis are the benzodiazepines, particularly the shorter-acting agents such as temazepam, usually given orally 2 h preoperatively. Midazolam can be given intranasally, intramuscularly or intravenously. It is a potent benzodiazepine and often produces unconsciousness! Opioid analgesics calm and sedate the patient and are used especially if analgesia is required (see below).

Phenothiazines are usually given in combination with an opioid. Promethazine is frequently combined with pethidine. These agents are useful, especially in the elderly, as they calm but do not oversedate. Phenothiazines are also appropriate in atopic individuals, such as asthmatics; their antihistaminic action may be useful. Prochlorperazine has combined sedative and antiemetic properties.

Analgesia (Table 16.2)

There are two main reasons for using opioid analgesia as part of the anaesthetic premedication, apart from the excellent sedative properties. These analgesics ease patients with painful conditions such as fractured hips and other types of trauma for comfortable transfer to theatre. They also provide a continuous background of analgesia to aid the anaesthetic and extend analgesia into the postoperative period. Recent evidence suggests that preoperative medication with analgesics such as opioids or non-steroidal anti-inflammatory drugs reduces postoperative analgesic requirements. Recent evidence also suggests that preoperative administration of cyclooxygenase (COX) 2 inhibitors, such as rofecoxib, can significantly reduce postoperative pain, probably by reducing neurosensitization by prostaglandin release. Take care when using these drugs, as they can aggravate renal failure and may cause gastric bleeding, although this is much less than with COX 1 drugs.

Opioid premedication is usually combined with anticholinergic agents, such as glycopyrrolate, to dry secretions and, in the case of hyoscine, to potentiate sedation.

The choice of premedication depends very much on the individual patient. A moribund patient does not benefit, and may indeed suffer, from such side-effects as respiratory or cardiovascular depression. In contrast, a young, fit, anxious patient could benefit from anxiolysis or sedation, besides possible analgesic requirements, especially in trauma.

Drying secretions (Table 16.3)

When ether anaesthesia was used, it was important to dry oral secretions, because ether stimulates salivary secretions on induction, with the risk of laryngospasm. With modern anaesthesia it is less of a requirement, although it may be useful to dry secretions before dental surgery,

Table 16.3	Drying agents in common use	Approx. duration	
Agent	Dose (mg kg^{-1})	i.v.	i.m.
Atropine	0.02	15 30 min	2–4 h
Hyoscine	0.008	30–60 min	4–6 h
Glycopyrrolate	0.01	2–4 h	6–8 h

bronchoscopy, operations on the lung, and for paediatric patients in whom salivation can be troublesome. In addition to drying secretions, muscarinic receptor antagonists also prevent bradycardia, a common side-effect of general anaesthesia, especially in very young children.

Hyoscine, in contrast to atropine, contributes to the sedative properties of premedication. Glycopyrrolate does not cross the blood–brain barrier, and is an inhibitor of salivary secretions, with little effect on the vagus nerve and hence on the heart rate. Atropine has also been shown to have a small antiemetic effect, presumably by inhibiting vagal activity, as well as a slight bronchodilator effect.

GENERAL ANAESTHESIA

1. The anaesthetist is responsible for managing the patient peroperatively. This includes managing acute blood loss, maintaining normal cardiorespiratory physiology and protecting organ function. It may include minimizing the stress response to surgery and the effects of the stress hormones on organ function, such as the heart and kidneys. General anaesthesia is a reversible, drug-induced state of unresponsiveness to outside stimuli, characterized by lack of awareness, by analgesia and relaxation of striated muscle. Older agents such as ether need to be given in high dosage, and take a long time for induction and recovery.

2. The mechanisms of general anaesthesia are complex and ill understood. Current knowledge suggests that general anaesthesia is produced when certain molecules interact with multiple hydrophobic pockets, often within complex protein molecules, such as those forming part of the potassium channel of a cell membrane, as well as certain neuron receptors, such as those for the inhibitory transmitter gamma-aminobutyric acid (GABA). It is clear that short-term memory mechanisms are disrupted, in addition to 'normal' brain function. These changes are completely reversible, as normal function resumes on removal of the anaesthetic agents. General anaesthesia is an 'all-or-none' phenomenon, as the patient is either anaesthetized or not, with no in between state.

3. Deep anaesthesia obtunds (blunts) the neurohumoral stress response to surgery. Modern anaesthesia is usually at a much lighter plane, and some responses may be seen. Ultrashort-acting opioids help inhibit the stress response; this is believed to be better for the patient. Alternatively, regional anaesthetic techniques prevent the stress response by blocking afferent nerve fibres.

4. Sedation is not general anaesthesia. Agents used include benzodiazepines (for example midazolam), or propofol in subanaesthetic doses. The patient continues to respond to spoken command, but may not remember the procedure later.

5. The advent of newer, more specifically acting agents, such as the muscle relaxants, has enabled modern general anaesthesia to be considered as a balance between the triad of 'relaxation', 'analgesia' and 'hypnosis' (lack of awareness).

Phases

A general anaesthetic may be considered in three phases, analogous to an aircraft flight. I shall consider each part of the triad separately, under the heading of each phase of the anaesthetic.

'Take off': *induction of anaesthesia*

1. Hypnosis (Greek *hypnos* = sleep) at induction of anaesthesia. In the anaesthetic room patients are induced using one of several intravenous anaesthetics. In approximate order of frequency, those shown in Table 16.4 are the most commonly used agents. When drugs are taken up in the bloodstream, initial distribution is to 'vessel-rich' tissues and those taking a large fraction of the cardiac output. Thus the brain, which is vessel-rich and also taking a large fraction of the cardiac output, receives a considerable portion of intravenous anaesthetic given as a bolus. Subsequently, drugs diffuse out of the brain, down a concentration gradient formed by the falling blood concentration, and are redistributed to other vessel-poor tissues. This results in an initial short redistribution half-life. The longer elimination half-life of a drug represents its metabolism and elimination from the body. In some instances, this can appear to take a long time, due to the slow leaching out of drug from vessel-poor fat tissues.

2. *Thiopental*, a very short-acting barbiturate, was the first widely used intravenous induction agent. It was first used to great effect on casualties from the bombing of Pearl Harbor in 1942. However, its ability to depress the myocardium was tragically evident in the deaths of young sailors already shocked from hypovolaemia. It was soon

Table 16.4	Anaesthetic agents		
Drug	Dose (mg kg^{-1})	Distribution half-life (min)	Elimination half-life (h)
Thiopental	3–5	3–14	5–17
Propofol	1–3	2–4	4–5
Etomidate	0.3	2–6	1–5
Ketamine			
i.v.	1–2	10	2–3
i.m.	5–10	15	2–3
Midazolam	0.03–0.3	6–20	1–4

appreciated that the dose should be reduced, giving only enough to cause sleep (a 'sleep dose'), titrated carefully for each patient, especially those with a low cardiac reserve.

3. *Propofol* has a very short half-life, and is used particularly in daycase surgery, where rapid recovery is necessary. It is also used to abate the effects of procedures which occasionally cause laryngospasm, such as laryngeal mask placement and anal stretching. It is sometimes infused intravenously to maintain anaesthesia, because of its short half-life. The initial bolus of propofol sometimes causes a profound fall in blood pressure and inhibits compensatory increases in heart rate; this can be attenuated by administering glycopyrrolate or atropine before the induction. Small doses of propofol are sometimes used to produce sedation for procedures carried out under local anaesthetic.

4. *Etomidate* is indicated only for induction of anaesthesia. As a side-effect, it causes a reversible suppression of an enzyme in the adrenal cortex, leading to inhibition of cortisol secretion – this is especially important if it is used as an infusion. It is indicated in patients with poor cardiac reserve, or those in whom a fall in cardiac output could prove catastrophic, because it tends to maintain cardiac output. It is relatively long acting, and may cause postoperative nausea and vomiting.

5. *Ketamine*, structurally related to LSD, is used in shocked patients because it stimulates the sympathetic nervous system and prevents a fall in cardiac output. However, patients who are already on full sympathetic drive still suffer a reduction in cardiac output and blood pressure. It produces a state known as 'dissociative anaesthesia' with profound analgesia.

6. *Benzodiazepines*, and particularly midazolam, which is the most efficacious in this respect when given intravenously, are occasionally used to induce or assist induction of anaesthesia and are commonly used for sedation.

7. *Opioids* in very high doses are used to induce anaesthesia in some situations. The most commonly used agents for this are the highly potent synthetic derivatives fentanyl, alfentanil and sufentanil. Fentanyl is used in a dosage of up to 1.0 mg kg^{-1}, particularly in cardiac anaesthesia, as it avoids hypotension and maintains cardiac output. Unless other agents are added, awareness may occur. Chest rigidity, preventing adequate ventilation, occasionally occurs but is easily reversed using muscle relaxants.

Key point

- **Apart from the exceptions mentioned, all intravenous anaesthetic agents depress the myocardium.**

Relaxation at induction

Muscle relaxation is necessary at induction to facilitate tracheal intubation. Relaxation during maintenance of anaesthesia is discussed below.

Suxamethonium is a depolarizing relaxant used primarily for difficult intubation and crash induction. It lasts only approximately 5 min following a dose of 1.5 mg kg^{-1}. It is essentially two acetylcholine molecules joined together. This similarity to acetylcholine results in activation of the receptor and depolarization of the muscle membrane, lasting some 5–10 min, and muscles become unresponsive to acetylcholine. Because of its short action it is useful, apart from intubation, for very short surgical procedures. Side-effects include the following.

- Histamine release. 'Scoline rash' is very common following intravenous administration of suxamethonium. An erythematous rash is seen spreading over the upper trunk and lower neck anteriorly. Very occasionally, suxamethonium will cause bronchospasm and other more severe sequelae.
- Bradycardia (Greek *bradys* = slow) occurs particularly if a second or subsequent dose is given, especially in children. Give atropine to prevent or reverse this effect.
- Generalized somatic pain of unknown cause may result from widespread fleeting muscle contractions, termed 'fasciculations', caused by the depolarization of muscle fascicles.
- Hyperkalaemia (Greek *kalium* = potassium) results because suxamethonium causes the release of potassium from muscle cells and can lead to cardiac arrest.
- Persistent neuromuscular blockade may occur from the genetically related deficiency or abnormality of plasma pseudocholinesterase. The result is prolonged action of suxamethonium, sometimes called 'scoline apnoea'. The completely silent gene is rare, occurring in approximately 1:7000 of the population.
- Malignant hyperthermia occurs in some 1:100 000 of the population. It is a reaction to certain anaesthetic drugs, of which suxamethonium and halothane are the commonest. Muscle metabolism becomes uncontrolled because of an abnormality of intracellular calcium flux. Body temperature rises at the rate of at least 2°C every 15 min, and Pa_{CO_2}, reflecting the massively raised metabolic rate, also increases with alacrity. Treat with ventilation, surface cooling and intravenous dantrolene sodium (Dantrium), given promptly before death ensues.

'Crash induction'

1. This is necessary when you assume that the patient has a full stomach (see below). The technique consists of a rapid-sequence intravenous induction, cricoid pressure

and tracheal intubation, with the aim of preventing regurgitation and aspiration of stomach contents.

2. Immediately following a preplanned dose of thiopental ($3-5$ mg kg^{-1}), give suxamethonium (1.5 mg kg^{-1}), currently the fastest muscle relaxant, acting within one circulation time. Rocuronium, a newer non-depolarizing relaxant, is also used, but has a longer duration of action. Have a trained assistant apply pressure to the cricoid cartilage, simultaneously compressing the oesophagus between the cricoid ring and the vertebral column. Intubate the trachea with a cuffed tube, and inflate the cuff. When the anaesthetic circuit is attached and cuff seal confirmed, only then have the cricoid pressure relaxed.

3. The following patients are at risk of aspiration of stomach contents on induction of anaesthesia:

a. All non-fasted patients

b. Patients with a history suggestive of hiatus hernia

c. In an emergency, any traumatized patient, as trauma slows stomach emptying

d. Those with intestinal or gastric obstruction or stasis

e. Pregnant women in whom stomach emptying is slowed and the cardiac sphincter relaxed

f. Those with intra-abdominal tumours that may slow gastric emptying.

'Cruising': *maintenance of anaesthesia*

1. Hypnosis during anaesthesia is usually maintained with volatile agents, which are hydrocarbons, liquid at room temperature, with high saturated vapour pressures and lipid solubility. Diethyl ether, inflammable and explosive, was the earliest agent used, and is still popular in some parts of the world. The addition of fluoride and other halogens makes the hydrocarbon molecule much more stable. Modern agents are non-flammable, non-explosive, and much more potent than ether. Being less soluble in blood, as indicated by the blood/gas partition coefficient, they also have a much faster uptake and elimination time than diethyl ether. Table 16.5 shows the most commonly used anaesthetic volatile agents, with ether as a comparison.

2. *Halothane* is a hydrocarbon with fluorine, chlorine and bromine atoms. It was the first modern volatile non-flammable and non-explosive anaesthetic agent. Synthesized in 1951 and first used clinically in 1956, it was the most commonly used anaesthetic agent for 30 years. It is a potent anaesthetic, allowing a smooth induction, especially important for gaseous induction of children, and with relatively rapid onset of anaesthesia. In the body, up to 20% is metabolized by the liver, the majority being eliminated unchanged via the lungs. The recovery time from halothane anaesthesia is also relatively brisk and smooth. The most common side-effects of halothane result from its effects on the heart. Halothane

Table 16.5   Anaesthetic volatile agents

Agent	Structure	MAC	Blood/gas partition coefficient
Diethyl ether	$CH_3CH_2-O-CH_2CH_3$	1.92	12
Halothane	$CF_3CHClBr$	0.75	2.3
Enflurane	CHF_2O-CF_2CHFCl	1.68	1.9
Isoflurane	$CHF_2O-CHClCF_3$	1.05	1.4
Sevoflurane	$(CF_3)_2CHO-CF_2F$	2.0	0.6
Desflurane	$CF_3CFHO-CF_2H$	$6-9$	0.42
Xenon	Xe	71	0.14

Notes

1. MAC: the minimum alveolar concentration of a gas or vapour in oxygen required to keep 50% of the population unresponsive to a standard surgical stimulus (opening of the abdomen). MAC is expressed as a percentage concentration.

2. Blood/gas partition coefficient: indicates how rapidly a gas or vapour is taken up from the lungs. The higher the blood solubility, the longer it takes for the brain to gain adequate anaesthetic concentrations.

3. Summary of effects of modern vapours on organ systems:

a. *Heart*: generally cause depressed contractility: halothane > enflurane > isoflurane (halothane causes more arrhythmias)

b. *Blood vessels*: generally cause vasodilation: isoflurane > enflurane > halothane

c. *Respiration*: depressed by all agents: enflurane > isoflurane > halothane

d. *Brain*: all may cause vasodilation and raised intracranial pressure: halothane > enflurane > isoflurane (isoflurane safe up to 1 MAC).

slows the sinoatrial node, slowing heart rate and causing variations in the PQ interval. It reduces myocardial workload. Like verapamil, halothane produces these effects by blocking calcium channels in the heart. However, it also sensitizes the heart to catecholamines and may precipitate arrhythmias – especially important in the presence of adrenaline (epinephrine)-supplemented local anaesthesia and if the arterial carbon dioxide tension, $Pa\text{CO}_2$, is elevated. By reducing cardiac output, halothane attenuates splanchnic blood flow, diminishing hepatic blood flow and possibly aggravating its effects on the liver. With the aid of very fine indicators of hepatic performance, it has been shown that even the briefest exposure to halothane causes some degree of liver dysfunction, probably related to the large amount, up to 20%, of halothane that is metabolized. An idiosyncratic (Greek *idios* = one's own + *syn* = together + *krasis* = a mixing;

hence a personal peculiarity), reaction, which occurs after halothane exposure in some patients, is known as 'halothane hepatitis'; it is a fulminant centrilobular hepatic necrosis which appears 2–5 days postoperatively. The incidence is 1:35 000 of the population (National Halothane Study, USA, 1966), with a mortality of over 50%. Halothane is now used in only 10% of anaesthetics given in the UK, mainly for paediatric anaesthesia.

3. *Enflurane* is an ether synthesized in 1963 and first used in 1966. It is halogenated with fluorine and chlorine atoms to render it non-explosive and non-flammable. Enflurane is more efficacious in reducing peripheral vascular resistance and is less likely to cause cardiac arrhythmias, nor does it sensitize the heart to catecholamines; however, its pungent odour makes it unsuitable for gaseous induction in children. Enflurane causes greater respiratory depression than halothane or isoflurane, and so it is less suitable for maintaining anaesthesia in the spontaneously breathing patient. Enflurane is only slightly metabolized by the liver (up to 2.5%) and appears not to cause hepatitis.

4. *Isoflurane* was synthesized in 1965 and first used in 1971. It is a structural isomer of enflurane, but with different properties. Isoflurane tends to act on the peripheral vasculature as a calcium antagonist, reducing peripheral vascular resistance. Although it has minimal effects on the heart, isoflurane may cause 'coronary steal', whereby blood is diverted from stenosed coronary arteries to dilated unblocked coronary arteries, possibly compromising ischaemic areas of myocardium. This is still a controversial area and isoflurane generally causes minimal depression of contractility. In the brain, isoflurane has the least effect on cerebral blood flow, causing no significant increase up to 1 MAC (minimum alveolar concentration). Isoflurane causes least respiratory depression and is suited to the spontaneously breathing patient. Up to 0.2% only of isoflurane is metabolized by the liver and no cases of hepatitis have been reported.

5. *Desflurane* is popular for anaesthetizing daycare patients because of the rapid recovery; however, it is very pungent, often causing patients to cough, so it is unsuitable for gaseous induction. It is useful for patients with large amounts of adipose tissue, as it has the lowest fat solubility of all the agents used, resulting in a more rapid recovery, with little accumulation.

6. *Sevoflurane* is very popular as a gaseous induction agent, especially in children, because of its rapid onset and non-pungent characteristics. It has a low volatility, so is cheaper to use at low gas flow rates, as less liquid is used. It is now probably the most commonly used anaesthetic agent. Both desflurane and sevoflurane are characterized by remarkable molecular stability, with very little hepatic metabolism. They also have a very low blood gas solubility coefficient, resulting in very rapid onset and recovery.

7. *Xenon* (Greek *xenos* = stranger, guest), a rare, heavy gas, is currently under trial as an anaesthetic agent. It is an extremely stable molecule and gives excellent cardiovascular stability with a rapid onset and offset, and no metabolism. However, it is very expensive and has required the development of special anaesthetic machines which allow the gas to be recycled for further use.

8. *Nitrous oxide* (N_2O), unlike the volatile agents, is a gas at atmospheric pressure and room temperature. It has a MAC of 103% at sea level. The requirements of keeping the patient well oxygenated mean that it can never be relied upon to provide anaesthesia in its own right. It is, however, a very potent analgesic agent. Fifty per cent N_2O is equivalent in efficacy to approximately 10 mg morphine sulphate. It continues to enjoy popularity as the main background anaesthetic gas, usually given as 70% in oxygen. In concentrations greater than 50% it causes amnesia and contributes significantly to the overall anaesthetic.

9. General anaesthesia can also be maintained intravenously using a continuous infusion of anaesthetic agents such as propofol, which are non-cumulative and are rapidly cleared. This is usually supplemented with an infusion of a short-acting opioid such as remifentanil or alfentanil. This is termed 'total intravenous anaesthesia (TIVA)'.

Relaxation during anaesthesia

1. To allow the surgeon access to intra-abdominal contents, or to allow artificial ventilation of the patient in chest surgery, for example, muscle relaxation (paralysis) is required.

2. Agents used specifically to relax muscles are called relaxants; they are agents which block acetylcholine receptors on muscle endplates. There are two types of relaxant:

a. Depolarizing muscle relaxants. The only one still in common use is suxamethonium, which is described above in relation to induction.

b. Non-depolarizing muscle relaxants. There are many different relaxants available today. Because of the side-effects of suxamethonium, researchers continue to seek a non-depolarizing relaxant with a very rapid onset and very short half-life. They have a usual onset time of 2–3 min, and last from 20 to 60 min. They are competitive inhibitors of the acetylcholine receptors on muscle endplates, preventing access of acetylcholine to receptor, blocking transmission of nerve impulse to muscle. Curare was the first relaxant of this class, developed from an arrow poison used by the indigenous people of the Amazonian rainforests to kill animals for food. The dextrorotatory isomer alone is active; the term 'tubo-' refers to the bamboo tubes in which it is carried – D-tubocurarine. Modern relaxants tend to be shorter acting, with fewer side-effects (Table 16.6).

Table 16.6	Non-depolarizing muscle relaxants		
Agents	Dose (mg kg^{-1})	Duration of effect (min)	Side-effects
Pancuronium	0.01	45–120	Vagolytic: tachycardia, increases blood pressure
Vecuronium	0.01	30–45	Bradycardia
Rocuronium	0.05	30–45	Rapid onset
Atracurium	0.06	15–40	Histamine release
Cisatracurium	0.15	30–45	No histamine release

Notes

1. With the exception of atracurium and cisatracurium, all these agents require renal and hepatic function for their clearance.

2. Atracurium and cisatracurium are excreted by two mechanisms: Hoffman elimination (up to 40% with atracurium, up to 70% with cisatracurium) and hepatic metabolism. Hoffman elimination results in breakdown of the molecule as a result of pH and temperature. It is used in those patients with renal failure.

3. The duration of effect with each agent varies slightly according to anaesthetic technique. The use of volatile agents, particularly enflurane and isoflurane, potentiates the effect of non-depolarizing muscle relaxants. Hypothermia also potentiates non-depolarizing relaxants.

4. The shorter-acting agents atracurium and vecuronium are often used as infusions for long cases and in intensive care.

5. Muscle relaxants have no intrinsic anaesthetic effect.

Analgesia during anaesthesia

The final part of the triad of general anaesthesia during its maintenance consists of analgesia. The anaesthetized patient derives analgesia from three potential sources: from the premedication, from anaesthesia supplementation with opioids, and from the analgesic properties of volatile and gaseous agents.

1. *Premedication.* Opioids used in premedication, as discussed earlier, tend to last intraoperatively and into the postoperative period. In this way, premedication affects both the anaesthetic and postoperative analgesia.

2. *Anaesthetic opioid supplementation* is often administered intraoperatively to deepen the effect of the anaesthetic, or to reduce the amount of volatile agent used (often because of their side-effects such as hypotension). To limit the effects of opioids to the perioperative period, anaesthetists often use highly potent short-acting agents such as fentanyl, alfentanil or sufentanil. Recently, the ultrashort-acting remifentanil has become available, and is given only by infusion. These agents are all much more potent than morphine, and much shorter acting, of the order 20–30 min. They may need to be reversed at the end of the operation, to facilitate spontaneous respiration. However, this is at the expense of analgesia. Longer acting opioids such as morphine, papaveretum or pethidine may also be used, especially if postoperative analgesia may be a problem.

Modern non-steroidal anti-inflammatory agents, such as diclofenac, are used for postoperative analgesia, either on their own for minor surgery or in combination with opioid techniques to give a much better quality of analgesia. Side-effects include renal failure (prostaglandin inhibition may lead to renal shutdown), gastric ulceration and bleeding (inhibition of platelet function). Different agents have different degrees of complications, but their careful use has revolutionized the aftercare of patients, particularly after daycare surgery. The development of COX 2 antagonists, such as rofecoxib, will reduce the problems of gastric bleeding but will still be a problem for renal function.

3. *Analgesic properties of volatile agents.* Modern volatile anaesthetic agents have poor analgesic properties and contribute little to this part of the anaesthetic. However, nitrous oxide is a very good analgesic (see above) and is also used for analgesia during labour as a 50% mixture with oxygen, known as Entonox.

'Landing': recovery from anaesthesia

At the end of the operation, anaesthesia is terminated. Volatile agents and nitrous oxide are turned off on the anaesthetic machine and oxygen alone administered. Anaesthetic gases and vapours diffuse down concentration gradients from the tissues to the alveoli of the lungs and out via the airway.

1. Reversal of muscle relaxation: competitive muscle relaxants usually need to be reversed to ensure full return of muscle power. The degree of neuromuscular blockade can be monitored with a peripheral nerve stimulator.

2. Neostigmine (0.05 mg kg^{-1}) or edrophonium (0.5 mg kg^{-1}) is given intravenously. They block acetylcholinesterase in the neuromuscular junction, resulting in accumulation of acetylcholine. This overcomes the competitive blockade of the relaxant molecules in favour of acetylcholine. However, both neostigmine and edrophonium cause acetylcholine accumulation at both muscarinic and nicotinic sites. Muscarinic receptors are those cholinergic receptors in the heart, gut, sweat glands, etc. Therefore, to prevent bradycardia, profuse sweating and gut overactivity, atropine (0.02 mg kg^{-1}) or glycopyrrolate (0.01 mg kg^{-1}) must be given with the anticholinesterase.

3. Full reversal of muscle relaxation is only apparent from appropriate neuromuscular monitoring, or when the patient is able to maintain head lifting. This aspect of recovery from anaesthesia is crucial, as full muscular control is necessary for coughing and for good control of the airway. Indeed it highlights the importance of adequate recovery facilities in the theatre suite.

POSTOPERATIVE ANALGESIA

It is important to continue good analgesia into the postoperative period and to continue to have a stress-free patient. The anaesthetist will usually ensure that sufficient longer-acting opioid such as morphine or diamorphine has been administered towards the end of the procedure for adequate postoperative analgesia. This can be topped up as necessary in recovery. If an epidural or other regional block such as a brachial plexus block is sited, the analgesia can be continued with a continuous infusion of local anaesthetic combined with a short-acting opioid. The surgeon may be asked to inject local anaesthetic locally at the site of wounds to minimize postoperative discomfort.

There are several methods of managing postoperative pain, which can be considered as follows:

- Systemic analgesia: intravenous, intramuscular, subcutaneous, oral, nasal or sublingual application of analgesics
- Regional analgesia: usually placed before surgery, as part of the anaesthetic technique – continued into postoperative period
- Other techniques (TENS, acupuncture): not very effective for acute pain – used more for chronic pain.

Pre-emptive analgesia may reduce postoperative analgesic requirements. This involves the preoperative administration of: nerve blocks/regional analgesia; premedication with opioids; use of supplementary agents with specific spinal actions such as α_2-agonists.

The World Health Organization produced a simple pain ladder for the administration of analgesia. Originally designed for cancer pain, it is also appropriate for acute postsurgical pain:

- Minor pain: paracetamol, aspirin, other non-steroidal analgesics
- Moderate pain: above combined with minor opioids – co-proxamol (propoxyphine), co-dydramol (codeine); minor or intermediate opioids alone, e.g. tramadol, buprenorphine
- Severe pain: opioids – morphine, diamorphine, oxycodone, etc.

The 'minor opioids' consist of propoxyphene, codeine and tramadol. Propoxyphene and codeine are often combined with paracetamol. Tramadol has the least effect on respiratory depression and is not a class A drug. It is roughly equivalent to codeine in its action.

The 'intermediate opioids' mainly consist of buprenorphine, which is well absorbed sublingually.

The 'major opioids' include morphine, diamorphine (heroin), oxycodone, fentanyl, sufentanil, alfentanil and remifentanil.

The dose of the major opioids, of which morphine and diamorphine are the most commonly used, is whatever is required! The dosage should be carefully titrated intravenously. Long-term chronic and cancer pain in those who can swallow can be titrated orally and converted to long-acting drugs such as morphine continus tablets or capsules. Initially, the required loading dose, titrated, should be given. Care may need to be taken with subsequent dosage, especially in the elderly, as the half-life may be extended. Opioids can be given by a number of different routes: intravenous, intramuscular, infusion, regional (including spinal). They may be used in combination therapy with non-steroidal anti-inflammatory drugs, or with local anaesthetics. Opioids act on μ & δ receptors in the brain and spinal cord. Mu receptors also cause nausea, vomiting and respiratory depression. Delta receptors are found mainly in the spinal cord.

Non-steroidal anti-inflammatory drugs block the cyclo-oxygenase (COX) pathway. There are two forms of the enzyme: COX 1 and COX 2. COX 1 is always present, but COX 2 is only induced by inflammation, such as occurs with surgery or in chronic inflammatory conditions. They both also have a central role, where both COX 1 and COX 2 are found as neurotransmitters. COX 2 antagonists are preferable where there is a high risk of peptic ulceration/bleeding, however, there is still not a 100% guarantee! Currently the second generation of COX 2 antagonists are being released, some of which will be available for parenteral administration, enabling easier peroperative administration.

REGIONAL ANAESTHESIA

1. Regional (local) anaesthesia is the reversible block-ade of nerve conduction by regionally applied agents, for the purpose of sensory ablation either of traumatized tissue or to enable minor surgery. These agents are referred to as 'local anaesthetics'. Both motor and sensory nerves may be blocked, depending on the agent used and the anatomical region where the agent is applied.

2. Nerves may be blocked anywhere between the central nervous system and the site of required sensory loss. Local anaesthetics are used to block pain fibres as they enter the spinal cord: epidural, spinal and paravertebral techniques. They may also be blocked along their anatomical route in the neurovascular bundles: field blocks, or specific nerve blocks. Finally, local infiltration around the required site may be performed (for example, skin and subcutaneous infiltration) to block conduction at the nerve endings.

3. Types of nerve fibre: the speed with which local anaesthetic agents are taken up by nerve fibres depends on their size and whether they are myelinated. Nerve fibres are classified according to their size and speed of conduction (Table 16.7).

4. Sensitivity to local anaesthetics: the smaller fibres are more sensitive to local anaesthetic agents than the larger fibres. Hence, 'C' fibres conducting pain are more sensitive than motor fibres in the 'A' group. This is why patients may still be able to move limbs, even during regional anaesthesia. The reason for the difference is most likely to be due to more rapid absorption and uptake of local anaesthetic into the smaller fibres within neurovascular bundles.

Local anaesthetic agents

Drugs used as local anaesthetics all tend to have 'membrane-stabilizing' properties. They act by inducing a blockade of nerve transmission in peripheral nerve impulses. This occurs as a result of obstruction to sodium channels in the axon membrane, preventing ingress of sodium ions necessary for propagation of an action potential.

Local anaesthetic agents belong to one of two chemical classes according to their structure, which consists of an amide or ester linkage separating an aromatic group and an amine:

Aromatic group ⇌ Amine group
Amide or ester

Ester class

The only ester still in frequent use is cocaine, which is an ester of benzoic acid. It is generally used only for topical anaesthesia of mucous membranes in the nose and sinuses. Amethocaine is still used as a topical agent, as is benzocaine.

Amide class (Table 16.8)

- *Lidocaine (lignocaine)* was the first amide to be synthesized. It was shown to be safer than cocaine and has remained a mainstay for local anaesthetic practice. The maximum dosage is 4 mg kg^{-1} alone or 7 mg kg^{-1} with adrenaline (epinephrine).
- *Prilocaine* has the highest therapeutic index, and is considered the safest agent for intravenous blockade. The maximum dose is 6 mg kg^{-1}. Other amides in common use include bupivacaine, levo-bupivacaine and ropivacaine.
- *Bupivacaine* is longer acting than lignocaine and is commonly used in epidural analgesia.
- *Levobupivacaine*, the isomer, is safer than the racemic bupivacaine in terms of cardiotoxicity and has a similar dosage profile.
- *Ropivacaine* has less motor blockade than bupivacaine when used epidurally.

Lidocaine (lignocaine), bupivacaine and levobupivacaine: maximum dose 2 mg kg^{-1}.

Table 16.7	Types of nerve fibre			
Fibre	Type	Function	Conduction velocity (ms)	Diameter (μm)
A	α	Motor, proprioception	70–120	12–20
	β	Touch, pressure	30–70	5–12
	γ	Motor (spindles)	15–30	3–6
	δ	Pain, temperature, touch	12–30	2–5
B		Preganglionic autonomic	3–15	<3
C		Dorsal root: pain, reflexes	0.5–2	0.4–1.2
		Sympathetic: postganglionic	0.7–2.3	0.3–1.3

Table 16.8 Amide class		
Drug	Maximum dose (mg)	Side-effects
Lidocaine (lignocaine)	300 (500 + adr.)	No unusual features. CNS excitation with toxicity
Prilocaine	600	Least toxic. Methaemoglobinaemia > 600 mg
Bupivacaine	175 (225 + adr.)	Sudden cardiovascular collapse. Not indicated for intravenous blockade
Levobupivacaine	175 (225 + adr.)	Less cardiotoxicity
Ropivacaine	2.5 per kg is recommended (e.g. 30 ml of 5% ropivacaine in a 60 kg patient)	Less motor blockade in epidural administration
Cocaine	150	Cardiac arrhythmias. CNS excitation. Topical use only

Notes

1. The table includes only those agents currently in common use and maximal doses relate to adult size (70 kg body weight). The dosages in parentheses refer to maximal doses in the presence of adrenaline (epinephrine).

2. All local anaesthetic agents have membrane-stabilizing properties. Their toxic effects therefore relate to this property and involve mainly the cardiovascular and central nervous systems.

   Toxic effects on the central nervous system include fitting and coma, leading to death from hypoxia without adequate resuscitation. Cardiovascular effects from toxicity include hypotension, cardiac arrhythmias and acute cardiovascular collapse.

   Bupivacaine has a high affinity for cardiac muscle cells – a property which is thought to be responsible for the high incidence of cardiovascular collapse associated with its use for intravenous blockade (Bier's block), for which it is no longer recommended.

3. Toxic effects may also occur with the accidental intravascular injection of drug.

4. Concentration of local anaesthetic agents varies. Bupivacaine and levobupivacaine comes as 0.5% or 0.25%, with or without adrenaline (epinephrine). Lidocaine (lignocaine) generally comes as 0.5, 1.0, 2.0% concentrations, again plus or minus adrenaline (epinephrine). The higher concentrations obviously have lower maximum safe volumes (1% = 10 mg ml^{-1}, 2% = 20 mg ml^{-1}).

5. Local anaesthesia techniques should always be performed where adequate resuscitation facilities are present.

6. Adrenaline (epinephrine) and other vasoconstricting agents, such as felypressin, allow higher doses of local anaesthetic to be used, the vasconstriction resulting in reduced absorption.

Clinical application

1. Local infiltration is used for surgery alone or in combination with general anaesthesia. Used with adrenaline (epinephrine), it reduces bleeding at the operative site. It also produces good postoperative analgesia. EMLA (eutectic mixture of local anaesthetics), a mixture of lignocaine and prilocaine, produces good analgesia when applied topically to skin. It is useful for insertion of intravenous lines, arterial lines and removal of minor skin lesions. It needs to be applied some 2 h before the procedure. Tetracaine (amethocaine) 4% gel (Ametop) can also be used in the same way.

2. 'Field' blocks and nerve blocks are useful for producing wider areas of anaesthesia and analgesia, for example in inguinal hernia repair, brachial plexus blockade for the upper limb, and femoral and sciatic blocks of the lower limb.

3. Spinal, epidural and paravertebral blockade produce widespread anaesthesia and analgesia. The pain of labour and childbirth involves nerve roots of lower thoracic, lumbar and sacral regions of the spinal cord. Epidural techniques, involving the epidural placement of a catheter, allow continuous analgesia or anaesthesia, alleviating pain from all these groups of fibres. Regional anaesthesia such as this is frequently employed for urological and other surgery in the lower half of the body. It should be noted, however, that spinal and epidural techniques also block sympathetic ganglia at the appropriate levels. Hypotension will occur unless adequate precautions are taken.

RECENT ADVANCES

1. Pre-emptive analgesia has gained popularity with the recent publication of data suggesting that the

administration of analgesia preoperatively, either systemically as with an opioid, or regionally as in use of local anaesthetic techniques, reduces the patient's need for analgesia postoperatively. This has been reinforced by the finding that using epidural analgesia for 3 days prior to leg amputation produces a marked reduction in the incidence of phantom limb pain. Thus the use of regional techniques combined with general anaesthesia is becoming more popular.

2. The widespread development of acute pain services is enabling the continuation of regional local analgesic techniques from the operating theatre into the general wards, improving the standards of postoperative pain control and perhaps reducing the incidence of postoperative nausea and vomiting secondary to opioids.

Further reading

Atkinson RS, Rushman GB, Lee A 1987 A synopsis of anaesthesia, 10th edn. Wright, London

Barash PG, Cuplen BF, Stoelting RK 1989 Clinical anaesthesia. Lippincott, Philadelphia

Gilman AG, Goodman LS, Rall TW, Murad F 1985 Goodman and Gilman's pharmacological basis of therapeutics, 7th edn. Macmillan, London

Miller RD 1990 Anesthesia, 3rd edn. Churchill Livingstone, Edinburgh, vols I–II

Nimmo WS, Smith G 1989 Anaesthesia. Blackwell Scientific, Oxford, vols I–II

Stoelting RK 1987 Pharmacology and physiology in anesthetic practice. Lippincott, Philadelphia

Vickers MD, Morgan M, Spencer PSJ 1991 Drugs in anaesthetic practice, 7th edn. Butterworths, Oxford

---

Summary

- What are the risks of failure to carry out preoperative assessment before an anaesthetic is administered?
- Can you describe the functions of premedication?
- What are the phases of general anaesthesia? With what other activity has it been compared?
- What is a 'crash' induction?
- What are the common types of local anaesthetic? Do you know their maximal dosage?

17 Operating theatres and special equipment

M. K. H. Crumplin

> **Objectives**
>
> - **Learn the safe positioning, movement and care of patients while they are unconscious.**
> - **Respect and understand the principles of diathermy, laser, cryosurgery and X-ray usage in a theatre environment.**
> - **Comprehend principles of the use of all equipment you use, including laparoscopic insufflation principles and instrumentation, fibreoptics and microscopes.**
> - **Understand the prevention of sepsis in the theatre.**

OPERATING THEATRE DESIGN AND ENVIRONMENT

Introduction

1. A large proportion of your life is spent within the environment of an operating theatre. There are physical, chemical and infective hazards to yourself and your colleagues, nurses and patients, thus making the operating department the most hazardous part of the hospital. You must gain an understanding of this environment and the risks to both staff and patients. In the operating theatre the patient is totally helpless, and under full control of the theatre staff.

2. The operating theatre environment must provide a safe, efficient, user-friendly environment that is as free from bacterial contamination as possible. Operating suites should be sited near to each other for efficient flexibility of staff movement, preferably on the first floor, away from the main hospital traffic. They should be on the same level as, and close to, intensive care units and surgical wards. The suite should incorporate the theatre sterile supply unit.

3. There should be minimum distance between operating rooms and the accident and emergency (A & E) unit and X-ray facilities, which will both be sited on the ground floor. Your hospital has a multidisciplinary user committee to optimize efficiency and safety, comprising surgeons, anaesthetists, operating theatre and anaesthetic nurses, microbiologists, a manager and a finance officer, in line with updated Department of Health recommendations.

4. Operating theatres now have an incident reporting system in place to audit adverse incidents in theatre. This is not designed to be punitive (Latin *punire* = to punish), but educational. Joint audit sessions between anaesthetists and surgeons allow adverse incidents to be discussed in an open and constructive way.

5. An attempt was made by the Department of Health and Social Security in 1978 to introduce the nucleus concept, providing hospitals with theatre suites appropriate to the average district general hospital requirements. Orthopaedic, cardiac, neurosurgical, laser and other specialist requirements make it necessary to adjust the standard design. Examples are the Charnley tent, controlled areas for laser therapy, and the provision of a pump preparation room beside a cardiac bypass theatre.

The antiseptic environment

Zones

- An outer, or general access zone for patient reception area and general office.
- A clean, or limited access zone between the reception bay and theatre suite, and dispersal areas, corridors and staff rest room.
- Restricted access zone, for those properly clothed personnel engaged in operating theatre activities, including the anaesthetic room, utility and 'scrub up' rooms.
- An aseptic or operating zone – the operating theatre. Keep the number of people to a minimum, as the bacteriological count is related to the number of persons and their movement.

Air flow

Directional air flow (laminar air flow) may be vertical or horizontal. In addition to normal turbulent air flow through theatre, which is necessary to maintain humidity, temperature and air circulation, an increased rate of air change is necessary to reduce the number of contaminated particles over the patient, that is aerobic counts of less than 35 microorganism-carrying particles per mm^{-3}. Air is pumped into the room through filters and passed out of vents in the walls of the operating room; it does not return into the operating suite. Most theatres have 20–40 or more air changes per hour.

Operating suit and tent environment

In this system there is a high vertical laminar flow within a tent or designated area marked on the floor, and clean air from above the table is expelled down to floor level in a funnel shape, thereby reducing contamination. The number of air changes may be increased to 400–600 per hour or more in the vertical laminar flow system of a Charnley tent. Orthopaedic surgeons may wear airtight suits and helmets, and work in a high velocity vertical air flow environment, which has limited access to other personnel. By using suitable exhaust suits and such tents, infection in hip replacement may be kept as low as 0.5%.

Wearing of disposable, non-woven fabrics

Reusable, comfortable cotton operating gowns, sterilized by heat, have the disadvantage that when they are wet, bacteria can pass through onto the operative field. Disposable gowns of less permeable fabrics reduce dispersal of bacteria-laden particles that may emanate (Latin *emanare* = to flow) from the operating or nursing staff (see Ch. 18). Optimally, everybody should wear these gowns, but they are costly. Although masks are not essential for the surgeon or nurses, wear them when the patient is particularly susceptible to infection, when a prosthesis is being inserted, or when you or the nurse has an upper respiratory tract infection.

Skin preparation

Prefer a non-spirit-based skin preparation such as Betadine, to minimize the risk of explosion. If you shave the patient, carry it out as late as possible. Skin drapes have limited benefit in preventing wound infection but help keep the skin towels in place. To prevent the ingress of skin bacteria apply an iodine-impregnated adhesive skin sheet.

Temperature and humidity control

These should be controlled as part of an integral air conditioning system to maintain a comfortable atmosphere, with a higher temperature for neonates, children, elderly patients and if the operation is prolonged. The temperature range is 20–22°C (68–71.6°F), with approximately 20–40 air changes per hour. Patients become hypothermic if the temperature falls below 21°C (69.8°F) during prolonged procedures. Reduce heat loss by laying warming blankets on the sorbo-rubber table surface, wrap the patient in aluminium foil and infuse warmed intravenous fluids. Pass the blood, crystalloid or colloids through a coiled plastic infusion pipe within a heated waterbath. Minimize postoperative heat loss by wrapping the patient in metal foil. Increasing the humidity to 50% reduces cooling by evaporation.

OPERATING TABLES

Operating tables need to be heavy and stable, easily manoeuvrable, comfortable for the patient and highly adjustable in terms of positioning the patient correctly for a particular operative procedure. There are two basic types of operating table. Most commonly they are completely mobile, thus allowing replacement if necessary. A second type has a fixed, permanently installed column in the centre of the operating room on which a variety of table tops can be mounted; they are usually expensive and can be remotely controlled. The problem is that if a fault develops the table and theatre will be out of service; the advantage is that interchangeable table tops allow efficient patient handling and flexible operating-room scheduling.

Ensure that the surface is sympathetic to the contours of the patient who is placed on it. This is achieved by using soft, moveable, easily cleaned sorbo-rubber padding that moulds to the patient. It raises the patient clear of the metal table.

Key point

- **It is imperative that no part of the patient comes into contact with the metallic structure of the table or any metal object attached to it.**

There should be a radiolucent section on tables used for general surgery and urology to allow for static X-ray films or the use of an image intensifier. Built-in, adjustable lumbar supports may be useful; alternatively, use partially filled intravenous fluid bags. Make sure that motorized or hand-operated controls are easily accessible. The table should be capable of two-way tilt, and breaking at its centre to allow operations such as lateral nephrectomy, or jack-knife positioning. The bottom half of the table must be easily removed to allow various types of leg support and stirrups to be employed for gynaecological, urological, orthopaedic and pelvic operations. A variety of armrests, screen support bars and shoulder and pelvic supports should be available.

Safety

When using limb supports, avoid overstressing or producing localized pressure upon joints, ligaments, nerves, blood vessels, skin or any point of the patient's limbs. Various nerves are at risk from injury or pressure due to inappropriate positioning on the table. The brachial plexus may be stretched during arm movements, the ulnar nerve damaged at the elbow during pole insertion into the canvas sheet before transferring the patient, and the common fibular and saphenous nerves may be damaged by pressure against a leg support bar. Osteoarthrosis may be aggravated by rough handling during transfer, excessive joint movement, or distortion during the operative procedure, such as cervical extension during thyroid surgery.

 Key point

- **Before induction of anaesthesia, rehearse a stressful position on the table with patients suffering from spinal or joint disorders.**

Be particularly careful when moving patients on and off the operating table. Check that attached tubing will not be dislodged. Transfer is best carried out using the Patslide, a tough plastic board, which acts as a bridge, on which the patient is slid from trolley to table, or vice versa. At least three people should be involved in moving an unconscious patient.

Remember your own comfort in theatre. Always have the table adjusted so that you are not stooping or uncomfortable. You should have the table at such a height that your elbows are flexed at about a right angle to your field of work.

Operating table fixtures for specialist procedures

Orthopaedic surgery

There is a great variety of limb attachments to an operating table, enabling circumferential access to a limb and manoeuvrability, and also allowing the surgical team to use the image intensifier following fixation or reconstructive procedures.

Neurosurgery

Access to the cranial cavity may be optimized by having the patient sit up, while keeping the head comfortably fixed using an appropriate padded head support placed opposite the surgical field.

 Key points

- **Make sure the table is secure and the patient is safely positioned before you start operating.**
- **Have the table at a comfortable height for surgery.**

SPECIAL EQUIPMENT

Tourniquets

Abuse of tourniquets may lead to vascular damage or thrombosis. Soft tissue and nerve injury may also occur. Avoid these problems by:

1. Exsanguinating the limb using an Esmarch bandage
2. Applying the tourniquet cuff over soft padding at the appropriate site
3. Inflating the tourniquet above the systolic blood pressure
4. Recording the time when the tourniquet is inflated and not allowing it to remain inflated for more than 2 h.

Diathermy

Principles and effects

A high frequency alternating current (AC) is passed through body tissue; where the current is locally concentrated (a high current density), heat is produced, resulting in temperatures up to 1000°C. Low frequency alternating current such as mains electricity (50 Hz), causes stimulation of neuromuscular tissue. The severity of the 'electrocution' depends on the current (amperes) and its pathway through the body. Five to ten milliamps (mA) can cause painful muscle contractions, while 80–100 mA passing through the heart causes ventricular fibrillation. Increasing the current frequency reduces the neuromuscular response; at current frequencies above 50 000 Hz (50 kHz) the response disappears. Surgical diathermy involves current frequencies in the range 400 kHz to 10 MHz. Currents up to 500 mA may then be safely passed through the patient. Heat is produced wherever the current is locally concentrated.

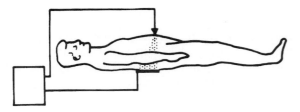

Fig. 17.1 Monopolar diathermy.

Monopolar and bipolar diathermy

Monopolar diathermy is the most common configuration (Fig. 17.1). High frequency current from the diathermy generator (or 'machine') is delivered to an active electrode held by you. Current density is high where this electrode touches body tissue, producing a pronounced local heating effect. The current then spreads out through the body, returning to the diathermy generator through the patient plate electrode (incorrectly called the 'earth plate'). Having shaved an area of skin, make sure that the plate is in good contact over at least 70 cm^2, and preferably more than twice this area, to ensure that the current density at the plate is so low that there is minimal heating.

Key point

- **Misapplication of the patient plate is by far the most common cause of inadvertent diathermy burns.**

Bipolar diathermy (Fig. 17.2) avoids the need for a plate and uses considerably less power. You hold forceps connected to the diathermy generator. The current passes from one limb of the forceps through the contained piece of tissue to be coagulated, and then back to the generator through the other limb of the forceps. This inherently safer system has not gained wide use for two main reasons:

1. It cannot be used for 'cutting' (see below), as this involves a continuous arc (spark) between the active electrode and the tissue involved. In bipolar

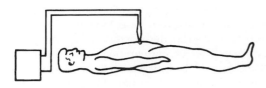

Fig. 17.2 Bipolar diathermy.

diathermy an arc can be struck only between the limbs of the forceps. Increasingly, surgical dissection is now carried out with diathermy and harmonic scalpels.
2. It will not work when a haemostat has grasped a vessel and is then touched with the active diathermy electrode. Bipolar current passes directly from one diathermy forceps limb to the other and no current passes through the tissue held by the haemostats.

Cutting, coagulating and blend

For cutting, the generator produces a continuous output, causing an arc to be struck between the active electrode and tissue and creating temperatures up to 1000°C. Cell water is instantly vaporized, causing tissue disruption with some coagulation of bleeding vessels. Coagulating diathermy current is a pulsed output resulting in desiccation (Latin *sicca* = dry) and the sealing of blood vessels with the minimal tissue disruption. Most diathermy generators have a 'blend' facility, functioning only when in cutting mode, allowing a combination of cutting and coagulation waveforms, increasing the degree of haemostasis.

Earth-referenced and isolated diathermy generators

Earth-referenced generators. Older diathermy generators, some of which are still in everyday use, have valves and spark gaps to generate high frequency current. These unsophisticated circuits produce a wide frequency range, which includes frequencies above 1 MHz, and large earth leakage currents are unavoidable. The patient plate on these generators is earthed via a capacitor. The capacitor allows easy passage of high frequency current, such as in diathermy, but presents a large resistance to low frequency currents, such as mains electricity. (The patient is therefore not earthed for mains (50 Hz) current to reduce the risk of electrocution.)

As long as the patient plate is correctly applied, the patient is kept at earth (zero) potential for alternate sites such as electrocardiogram (ECG) electrodes or a drip stand accidentally touching the patient's skin. Unfortunately, if the patient plate is omitted, or has become displaced, diathermy current will still flow (though a higher setting may be required) using the ECG electrodes or drip stand for the return pathway. An ECG electrode or drip stand presents skin contact of 1–5 cm^2, so a severe burn is inevitable.

Isolated generators. The more modern, often smaller, generators use transistors and 'solid-state' circuitry to produce the high-frequency current. Sophisticated electronics result in a much tighter frequency range

(400–600 kHz) and a considerable reduction in earth leakage currents. Some of these solid-state generators (but by no means all) are designated 'isolated': the diathermy circuit is not earthed. This type of generator is inherently safer than an earth-referenced machine. Diathermy current can only pass back to the generator via the patient plate; there is no pathway back via earth. If the plate is omitted, no current will flow.

Safety

General safety. Ensure that whenever electrical equipment is to be used on patients it meets the required safety standards and is properly maintained. Everyone using the equipment should be properly trained in its use. At the very least, you should read the user's manual: all diathermy machines are supplied with one.

Responsibility. The decision about who has overall responsibility for surgical diathermy is often ignored until a diathermy disaster occurs. The diathermy is set up by nurses or operating department orderlies and the anaesthetist is usually the only doctor present when the patient plate is applied. Few surgeons check the diathermy before use.

Key points

- **You are responsible for using this equipment correctly. Check the alarm wiring, the patient plate and its positioning before use.**
- **Only the surgeon wielding the active electrode should activate the machine.**
- **Always replace the electrode in an insulated quiver after use.**
- **If diathermy performance is poor, carefully check the patient plate and lead rather than increasing the dial settings.**

Alarms. Monopolar diathermy depends on the patient plate for its safety. If the plate is not connected to the machine (plate continuity alarm), all diathermy machines in use will alarm when switched on; only a few possess an alarm system that ensures the plate is attached to the patient. Rigidly adhere to the safe, correct procedures: first connect the patient plate to the patient, connect the return lead to the plate, switch on the diathermy machine so the plate continuity alarm sounds. Only now is the return lead connected to the diathermy machine, thus silencing the continuity alarm. Never do this in the reverse order. At the end of every operation undo all these connections and switch off the diathermy machine.

If the continuity alarm fails to silence, change the patient plate and lead first, not the machine. Some modern diathermy generators, such as the Eschmann and Valleylab, possess systems that monitor the patient–plate interface. These systems are explained in the user's manual. Never disregard these alarms – check the patient plate contact carefully.

The patient plate. The most common cause of accidental diathermy burns is incorrect application of the patient plate. It may not be applied at all, but more often there is a failure to follow guidelines. Site the plate as close as possible to the operation site, while ensuring that diathermy current is moving away from ECG and other monitoring electrodes. Make sure that the area under the plate has a good blood supply to remove any heat generated. Avoid bony prominences and scar tissue. The whole area of the plate must make good skin contact, so, shave hairy skin and ensure the plate is not kinked or crinkled. Do not allow skin preparation fluids to seep under the plate.

The patient. The second most common cause of diathermy burns occurs when the patient touches earthed metal objects such as drip stands, uninsulated 'screens' and parts of the operating table. These small skin contacts offer alternative return pathways for the diathermy current, and the local current densities may be sufficient to cause a burn.

If you have used an alcohol-based skin preparation, it may pool, be ignited by the diathermy current and cause a fire. As a rule avoid such skin preparations.

Key points

- **Beware of using diathermy on or inside the intestine – its gas contains hydrogen and methane, both are inflammable and explosive.**
- **Beware of using diathermy on appendages such as salpinx or penis, or isolated tissue such as testis; high current density can persist beyond the operative site.**
- **Remember that diathermy can damage other structures, such as sutures and endotracheal tubes and their balloons**

If a burn occurs. Diathermy burns are often poorly investigated and remain unexplained. Other skin lesions, such as chemical burns from preparation solutions or pressure sores, may masquerade as diathermy burns. Definite electrothermal burns usually occur because of lapses in procedure, rarely from faults in the diathermy machine. The operating theatre record for all patients subjected to diathermy should include the site of the patient plate; and when the plate and monitoring electrodes are removed the underlying skin should be inspected. If a possible burn is discovered, the patient and all attached equipment should remain in the operating theatre while you summon the electromedical safety officer. If the alleged burn is discovered after the patient has left the theatre, contact all those involved in the procedure and determine the precise arrangement of equipment and patient plate. All electrical equipment used should be tested, including the patient plate lead.

Diathermy burns are usually full thickness and will require excision. Inform the patient of the misadventure.

Diathermy and pacemakers. There are two possible dangers:

1. The high frequency diathermy current may interact with pacemaker logic circuits to alter pacemaker function, resulting in serious arrhythmias, or even cardiac arrest.
2. Diathermy close to the pacemaker box may result in current travelling down the pacemaker wire, causing a myocardial burn. The result will range from a rise in pacemaker threshold to cardiac arrest.

For safe use of diathermy with pacemakers, contact a cardiologist and ask about the type of pacemaker, why and when it was inserted, whether it is functioning properly, and what the patient's underlying rhythm is, so you will know what will happen if the pacemaker stops functioning.

Key points

- **Avoid diathermy completely if possible. If not, consider bipolar diathermy.**
- **If monopolar diathermy must be used, place the patient plate so that diathermy current flows away from the pacemaker system.**
- **Use only short bursts, and stop all diathermy if any arrhythmias occur.**

Laparoscopic procedures. Sometimes the working space can be 'crowded', and inadvertent contact may be made between an instrument and the bowel, especially if there is contact between the electrode and another metal instrument, which is touching bowel. In a similar way, current can pass along an organ, which is resting against the gut, and pass out via the indifferent electrode. An adequate view, carbon dioxide pneumoperitoneum, and use of well-insulated instruments should be the aim. Apply careful technique by avoiding excessive use of the diathermy, and 'tent' structures into space before applying current. Use lower voltage currents or

bipolar diathermy to minimize spread of current and sparking.

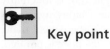

Key point

- **Ensure that the insulation of instruments is complete and undamaged, and avoid sparking between bowel wall and electrode.**

Lasers

The laser is a device for producing a highly directional beam of coherent (monochromatic and in phase) electromagnetic radiation, which may or may not be visible, over a wide range of power outputs.

Laser is an acronym for Light Amplification by the Stimulated Emission of Radiation. This describes the principle of operation of a laser. Energy is pumped into the lasing medium to excite the atoms into a higher energy state to achieve a population inversion in which most of the atoms are in the excited state. A photon emitted as a result of an electron spontaneously falling from the excited to the ground state stimulates more photons to be emitted and lasing action starts. After reflection back and forth many times from a pair of mirrors at opposite ends of the resonant optical cavity containing the lasing medium, the number of photons is amplified, that is, the light intensity or power is increased. One of the mirrors is only partially reflecting and allows a small part of the laser light to emerge as the laser beam. The lasing medium is commonly gaseous, such as argon or carbon dioxide, but may be crystalline, such as neodymium, yttrium, aluminium garnet (NdYAG). It is the lasing medium which determines the wavelength emitted. It is mainly the wavelength of the laser which determines the degree of absorption in tissue. However, surgical applications also depend on the power density: the duration of exposure should be just sufficient to produce the required effect. Delivery systems are designed to allow the laser beam to be transported, aimed and focused onto the treatment site. Argon and NdYAG lasers, for example, are transmitted down fibre-optic cables to a slit lamp or into an endoscope. Carbon dioxide laser light is usually routed via a series of mirrors through an 'articulated arm', and thereafter through a micromanipulator attached to a microscope or colposcope.

Types

1. Carbon dioxide infrared laser light has a wavelength of 10.6 μm. It is invisible and is rapidly absorbed by water in tissue and has very little penetration. It is therefore useful for vaporizing the surface of tissue, and water or

wet drapes can be used as a safety barrier. There is a very small margin of damaged tissue and healing is rapid, with minimal scarring. Treatment is relatively pain free.

2. The NdYAG laser penetrates more deeply, to 3–5 mm. The wavelength is 1.06 μm and is in the invisible infrared light range. It is useful for coagulating larger tissue volumes and leaves behind an eschar of damaged tissue.

Both the above types require a visible guiding beam which is usually a red helium/neon beam.

3. Argon laser light is blue/green and hence absorbed by red pigment. The principal wavelengths are 0.49 and 0.51 μm. It is used principally in ophthalmology and dermatology.

Clinical applications

Gastrointestinal tract. The NdYAG laser is frequently used in the treatment of gastrointestinal pathology. It can be employed for vaporizing and debulking recurrent or untreated advanced oesophageal carcinoma. Its use is predominantly in fairly short malignant strictures and may be superior to intubation. However, expanding covered metal stents may well prove to be a better palliative alternative. Laser ablation is labour intensive and requires treatments every 6–8 weeks. This laser can be used for controlling gastrointestinal haemorrhage from the stomach, oesophagus and duodenum, destruction of small ampullary tumours in the duodenum and palliative resection of advanced rectal carcinomas. In the future, photosensitization may prove to be of value. The use of lasers in laparoscopic surgery is, perhaps, less frequent at present. There is a risk of carbon dioxide gas embolism.

Urology. The NdYAG laser can be used to treat low grade, low stage transitional cell lesions in the bladder and is suitable for treating outpatients under local anaesthetic. Here again, photosensitizing agents such as haematoporphyrin (Hpd) may be used in conjunction with a laser light wavelength of 630 nm. The beam is directed at sensitized tissues which are then more easily destroyed.

Ophthalmology. The NdYAG laser can be used to destroy an opaque posterior capsule during or following extracapsular cataract extraction. The argon laser may be employed for trabeculoplasty, to decrease intraocular pressure in patients with open-angle glaucoma. Laser photocoagulation is becoming standard treatment for patients with various retinal diseases such as diabetic retinopathy, and as a prophylactic measure in patients at risk from retinal detachment. Most ophthalmic photocoagulators are argon lasers.

Otolaryngology. A carbon dioxide laser may be used for haemostasis, removal of benign tumours and premalignant conditions. The argon laser has been used in middle ear surgery.

Vascular surgery. Laser angioplasty (carbon dioxide, NdYAG and argon) has been used to vaporize atheromatous plaques. Only approximately 50% of patients benefit, and significant complications are reported, such as perforation of vessel wall.

Plastic surgery. Pulsed ruby lasers may be used to remove tattoos, and port wine stains selectively absorb the argon laser beam. The carbon dioxide laser may be employed to resect atretic bony plates in congenital bony choanal atresia.

Gynaecology. There are several uses in gynaecology. Perhaps the most frequent is the treatment with a carbon dioxide laser of cervical and vulval precancerous lesions that have been identified by colposcopy.

Classification

Lasers are classified according to the degree of hazard:

Class 1 (low risk). These are of low power and are safe. The maximum permissible exposure (MPE) cannot be exceeded.

Class 2 (low risk). These are of low power, emitting visible radiation. They have a maximum power level of 1 mW. Safety is normally afforded by natural aversion responses, such as the blink reflex.

Class 3a (low risk). These emit visible radiation, with an output of up to 5 mW. Eye protection is afforded by natural aversion. There may be a hazard if the beam is focused to a point, as through an optical system.

Class 3b (medium risk). These emit in any part of the spectrum and have a maximum output of 0.5 W. Direct viewing may be dangerous.

Class 4 (high risk). These are high power devices with output in any part of the spectrum. A diffusely reflected beam may be dangerous and there is also a potential fire hazard.

 Key point

- **Use high risk lasers with caution. Most medical lasers are in this class.**

Hazards

The manufacturers are required to classify and label the product according to hazard level.

1. *Patient hazard:* inevitably, burning of normal tissue or perforation of a hollow viscus may occur with increasing depth of treatment (e.g. perforation of

oesophagus) or damage to trachea or lungs during ear, nose and throat (ENT) procedures.

2. *Operator hazard*: usually the operator is not exposed to laser beams, but if you are accidentally exposed, it is frequently your eyes or skin that are damaged. Always wear eye protection since some laser beams will penetrate, and be focused on, the retina. Corneal burns or cataract formation have also occurred with less penetrating beams.

Safety measures

1. There should be a laser protection advisor (LPA) to consult on the use of the instruments throughout the hospital and to draft local rules.

2. A laser safety officer (LSO) should be appointed from the staff of the appropriate department using each laser. This person may well be, for example, a senior nurse and will have custody of the laser key.

3. Everybody using the laser should be adequately trained in its use and be fully cognizant of all safety precautions.

4. There should be a list of nominated users.

5. A laser controlled area (LCA) should be established around the laser while it is in use, with control of personnel allowed to enter that area. The entrance should be marked with an appropriate warning sign, usually incorporating a light that illuminates while the laser is functioning.

6. While in the laser controlled area adequate eye protection, appropriate to the type of laser in use, must be worn. The laser should not be fired until it is aimed at a target, and usually there is an audible signal during laser firing.

7. The laser should be labelled according to its classification. Lasers in classes 3a, 3b and 4 should be fitted with a key switch and the key should be kept by a specified person. The panels which constitute the side of the laser unit should have an interlocking device so that the laser cannot be used if the panels are damaged.

There are various safety features that are required by way of shutter devices and emergency shut-off switches. Foot-operated pedals should be shrouded to prevent accidental activation. Medical lasers require a visible low power aiming beam, which may be an attenuated beam of the main laser, if this is visible, or a separate class 1 or 2 laser, such as helium/neon. The laser must be regularly maintained and calibrated.

8. Environment: reflective surfaces should be avoided in the laser controlled area. However, matt-black surfaces are not necessary. Adequate ventilation must be provided and should include an extraction system to vent the fumes produced. These fumes are known as the 'laser plume'.

Key point

- **Pay particular attention to avoiding fire. Class 4 lasers ignite dry drapes or swabs. Damp drapes effectively stop carbon dioxide laser beams.**

Fibre optics

Flexible instruments

Fibre optics have undoubtedly made an immense impact on patient management. There is little evidence, however, that the instruments that incorporate fibre optics necessarily reduce mortality. Their value is in allowing accurate diagnosis and assessment of, for example, upper gastrointestinal bleeding or oesophageal obstruction. Most hollow viscera or tubes, even very narrow ones, may now be inspected. Diagnostic and therapeutic procedures can be performed under clear vision, such as exploration of a ureter for tumour or stone, or subfascial ligation of incompetent perforating veins. Thin fibreoptic instruments are integral to the development of minimal access surgery, such as 5 mm telescopes used for retrieving bile duct stones.

In the 1950s, Professor Harold Hopkins of Reading University, UK, developed the earlier work of John Logie Baird, the inventor of television, to further the design of fibreoptic bundles, which could not only transmit a powerful light beam but also, when suitably arranged, deliver an accurate image to the viewer. In the 1960s, urological instruments were developed incorporating multiple flexible glass-fibre rods. Each fine fibre rod is constructed of high quality optical glass and transmits the image, or light beam, by the process of total internal reflection. This principle allows light to travel around bends within the fibre. Each fibre is only 8–10 μm in diameter, and to achieve the principle of total internal reflection it must be coated with glass of low refractive index, to prevent light dispersion. Many such coated fibres are bound together in bundles which can bend. For light transmission, fibres may be arranged in a haphazard manner (non-coherent). For clear-image transmission, the fibres must be arranged in a coaxial manner (coherent) (Fig. 17.3). The following are examples of currently available flexible endoscopes utilizing fibreoptic light bundles:

- Oblique (for endoscopic retrograde cholangiopancreatography (ERCP) and end-viewing gastroscopes
- Laryngoscope
- Bronchoscope
- Fibreoptic sigmoidoscope and colonoscope
- Cystoscope (pyeloscope)
- Choledochoscope
- Arterioscope.

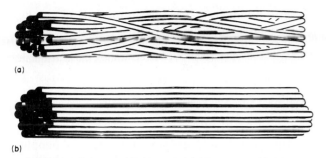

Fig. 17.3 (a) Non-coherent fibre bundles for light transmission. (b) Coherent fibre bundles for viewing. Reproduced from Ravenscroft & Swan (1984) by permission of Chapman & Hall.

Each instrument has similar design principles incorporating the following:

- Coherent fibre bundles for high quality visual image transmission
- Non-coherent fibreoptic bundles for light transmission
- A lens system at the tip and near the eyepiece of the instrument
- A proximal control system to manoeuvre the tip of the instrument and also to control suction and air/water flow
- Channels for blowing air or carbon dioxide and water down the instrument, and for suction – the latter doubles as a biopsy channel
- A wire guide incorporated to control tip movement, which takes place in four directions, each usually allowing a deformity of greater than 180° movement
- A cladding, consisting of a flexible, jointed construction, covered by a tough outer vinyl sheath.

Figures 17.4 and 17.5 show the basic structure of a typical endoscope, and Figure 17.6 shows the tip of an instrument, illustrating the lenses for light transmission and viewing, a suction channel, which should be large so it can be used in the presence of gastrointestinal haemorrhage, and a small nipple directed over the lens, to enable the wash solution to clear the lens of debris.

Light sources should emit a powerful beam and the intensity is usually 150 W. Many light sources employ a halogen bulb, which needs to be fan cooled.

Rigid endoscopes

Optical systems in rigid endoscopes also employ the principle of total internal reflection, but there are several lens systems in addition. The objective lens systems are nearest the image, and the relay lens systems are nearer the eyepiece of the rigid instrument, through which the observer

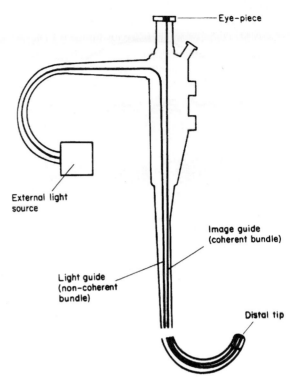

Fig. 17.4 Basic design of a fibreoptic endoscope. Reproduced from Ravenscroft & Swan (1984) by permission of Chapman & Hall.

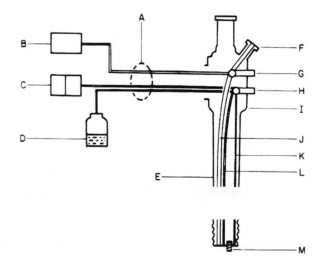

Fig. 17.5 Further details of the basic design of a fibreoptic endoscope. A, endoscopic 'umbilicus'; B, suction pump; C, air pump; D, water reservoir; E, endoscopic insertion tube; F, biopsy port; G, suction button; H, air/wash button; I, endoscope control head; J, combined suction biopsy channel; K, water channel; L, air channel; M, combined air/water port. Reproduced from Ravenscroft & Swan (1984) by permission of Chapman & Hall.

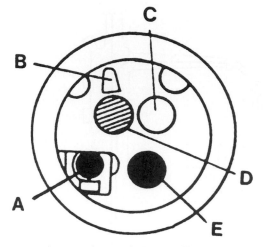

Fig. 17.6 The top of an end-viewing fibreoptic instrument. A, forceps raiser; B, wash jet; C, image guide; D, light guide; E, biopsy/suction channel. Reproduced from Ravenscroft & Swan (1984) by permission of Chapman & Hall.

views a rectified and magnified image. Light is transmitted through a cable of non-coherent fibres or liquid electrolyte solution. Vision is through coaxial fibres which direct the light coaxially through a lens system in the rigid tube. Some of the longer lenses are made of high quality optical glass and act as a single large optical fibre for image transmission. Examples of rigid instruments are:

- Cystoscope, urethroscope, pyeloscope, ureteroscope
- Choledochoscope
- Laparoscopes.

The lenses at the far end of the instruments vary to allow different fields of view and minimize peripheral field distortion.

Care of fibreoptic instruments

1. They must be properly cleaned and disinfected before use. Debris may block channels and make suction and insufflation of air and liquid difficult. After use, the instruments should be cleaned internally by utilizing one of several automatic cleansing machines, and externally with a suitable detergent solution. 'Q-tips' may be employed to clean lenses. Instruments should be soaked for at least 5–10 min between patients, often in a 2% gluteraldehyde solution, although 70% alcohol and low molecular weight povidone–iodine are alternatives.

2. In order to avoid instrument damage, endoscopies are usually performed in dedicated units under expert care. Damage is more likely to occur when a variety of people handle and clean instruments. Guard against

forcible distortion, dropping and, particularly, of crushing from biting by patients' teeth; always insert the peroral endoscope through a suitable mouth gag. Broken fibres appear as black dots when viewed through the instrument.

 Key point

- **Ensure that only competent and careful people use and care for these expensive and valuable instruments.**

Autologous cell salvage

With recent anxieties over transmitted disease, expense, religious views and the occasional scarcity of blood, autologous (blood derived from the same individual) blood transfusion may be used. The advantages are considerable: it avoids blood-related disease transmission, transfusion reactions, immnunosuppression and the need for grouping. A rapidly obtainable supply is available. The blood is collected via a sucker from the wound site, anticoagulated, filtered and then passed through a washing phase, using saline. Washing removes all but the red cells, which are concentrated to an acceptable haematocrit and then reinfused. This technique is of particular use in cardiothoracic, vascular and orthopaedic surgery, especially when the loss of blood is expected to exceed 1 litre. It is a safe procedure provided you follow the rules. As a rule, do not use blood contaminated with septic fluids and malignant cells. Never use blood contaminated with bile, gut contents, meconium, urine or amniotic fluid. Cell salvage cannot be used if the blood is likely to mix with fluids which would lyse red cells, such as water, hydrogen peroxide, alcohol, povidone-iodine antiseptic, fibrin glue or antibiotics that are unsuitable for parenteral use.

The alternative is predonation.

Cryosurgery (syn. cryotherapy or cryocautery)

Any application of an instrument that touches tissue at an extreme of temperature produces cell death. Cryosurgery (Greek *kryos* = frost) is the freezing of tissue to destruction. Although cells are destroyed at –20°C, they may recover at higher temperatures than this. After freezing, the destroyed tissue sloughs off and reveals a clean, granulating base. The treatment is relatively pain free and minimizes blood loss. The object is to destroy abnormal tissue and preserve adjacent, healthy areas. You achieve this by producing an ice ball at the tip of a cryoprobe (Fig. 17.7). You must watch the size of the resulting ice ball, to control the volume of tissue destroyed. The size of

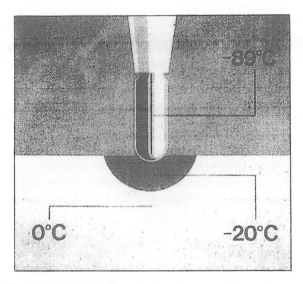

Fig. 17.7 An ice ball at the tip of a cryoprobe. Reproduced by permission of Eugene A. Felmar, Santa Monica Hospital Medical Center, USA.

the lesion produced by cryosurgery is related to the temperature at the tip of the ice probe, the size of the tip and the number of freeze–thaw sequences. The size of the iceball increases until the heat loss at the edge of the iceball is too small to permit further freezing of adjacent tissues. The size of an iceball and the extent of destruction can then be increased by a further freezing sequence. As a rule, allow the iceball to spread 2–3 mm into healthy tissue to ensure adequate destruction of the diseased area. Inevitably, freezing a wart on the sole of the foot is less

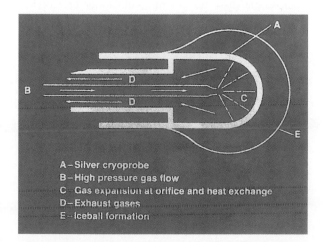

A – Silver cryoprobe
B – High pressure gas flow
C – Gas expansion at orifice and heat exchange
D – Exhaust gases
E – Iceball formation

Fig. 17.8 Cross-section of a cryoprobe tip, illustrating the Joule–Thompson principle. Reproduced by permission of Eugene A. Felmar, Santa Monica Hospital Medical Center, USA.

critical than reattaching a retina. Various probe tips are available for the different tasks demanded of cryosurgery.

Principles of therapy

According to the Joule–Thompson principle, when gas expands, heat is absorbed from the surrounding matter. The simplest example of this is spraying ethyl chloride vapour on skin, which, as it releases gas, subsequently freezes. With a cryoprobe, however, the liquid gas, usually nitrogen or carbon dioxide, is sprayed against the inside of a hollow metal probe. The gas then expands in the tip and freezes the tissue on contact (Fig. 17.8).

Cell injury with cryotherapy

1. *Immediate phase*: ice crystals form in the cell, rupturing the cell membrane. This is most effective with rapid freezing at greater than $5°C\ s^{-1}$.
2. *Intracellular dehydration*: results in increased and toxic levels of intracellular electrolytes.
3. *Protein denaturation*: occurs in the lipoprotein structure of the cell membrane, nucleus and mitochondria.
4. *Cellular hypometabolism*: results in enzyme inhibition.

Later in the course of injury there is also a loss of blood supply, causing tissue necrosis, and the resultant slough, before separation, protects the tissues deep to the injury. When the slough separates it leaves a clean ulcer.

As nerve endings are susceptible to cold injury, painful lesions can be rendered insensitive. Also, the treatment is not particularly painful for the patient, and local analgesia is usually unnecessary. Adjacent neurovascular structures are relatively safe, as collagen and elastic tissue resist freezing. Thus, the advantages of cryotherapy are that it is a relatively pain-free and simple method of destroying tissue, usually leaving clean wounds, often with a reasonable scar.

The disadvantages of the technique are that frozen tissue cannot be analysed histologically, and thus this method of treatment is unsuitable for any lesion for which you will require microscopic examination. It may sometimes be difficult to gauge the exact penetration in the depth of the tissues treated. Thus, its use may be limited in curative treatment of malignancy, and is of value in palliation. Occasionally there is some bleeding, and later discharge after the slough separates following, for example, cryosurgical treatment of haemorrhoids.

Clinical applications

Since there are various shapes of probe tips, a reasonable variety of therapeutic applications is available. To ensure that freezing occurs, there must be a wet contact to allow thermal conductivity. Two or three freeze–thaw cycles may be applied, with overlap of the treated areas if necessary.

Examples of the clinical application of cryosurgery include the following:

- Proctology: haemorrhoids and warts
- Gynaecology: cervical erosions and warts
- Dermatology: warts, low grade skin cancers, herpetic lesions
- ENT: pharyngeal tonsillar remnants, carcinoma of the trachea, hypophysectomy
- Ophthalmology: cataract extraction, glaucoma, detached retina
- Neurosurgery: Parkinson's disease and cerebral tumours.

Microwave ablative techniques

You can use this technique on prostatic tissue, for benign prostatic hypertrophy, and the endometrium – usually for menorrhagia. The principle of treatment depends on the transfer of energy by the use of microwaves, which are a form of electromagnetic energy. Penetration depths depend on the electrical properties of the tissues, and the frequency of the electromagnetic wave. Conventional microwave kitchen ovens use energy at a frequency of around 2.45 GHz, which, in tissue with a high water content, would penetrate to a depth of approximately 18 mm. The microwave applicator has a strength of 9.2 GHz, uses 30 W of power and the treatment takes about 2–4 min. For endometrial ablation performed under general or regional anaesthesia, the cervix is dilated, the length of the uterine cavity is measured, and the calibrated and non-adherent probe is inserted to the fundus and withdrawn with side-to-side movements. Temperature measurement is monitored and probe temperatures of 80–95°C are reached to ablate the endometrium to a depth of 4–6 mm. Interestingly, with this range of endoluminal temperature, there is little serosal heating.

This treatment may be safer than endometrial resection and hysterectomy, as there are fewer complications. The few serious complications of the procedure have been endometritis, cervical splitting during dilatation, and in one instance perforation of a retroverted uterus. There are other methods of endometrial ablation. This is merely used as an example of microwave energy, and you should not confuse it with radiofrequency endometrial ablation (RAFEA).

Ultrasound

Diagnostic

Ultrasound probes provide a valuable aid during abdominal surgery to identify tumour deposits and anatomical landmarks such as blood vessels. Clear guidance may be obtained as to the resectability of tumours or the presence of clinically undetected metastatic deposits. Hand-held ultrasound probes can be employed at open operations; for example, small islet cell tumours of the pancreas may be located accurately.

Small laparoscopically inserted instruments are also used for staging and anatomical purposes when performing operations with minimal access (see Ch. 23). They compensate to some extent for the inability to palpate structures. During laparoscopic cholecystectomy, a probe may be used not only to identify structures but also to locate common bile duct stones.

Surgical aspirator

There are various ways in which the liver parenchyma may be dissected with minimal blood loss. One of these is the CUSA (Cavitron UltraSonic Aspirator). The operating titanium tip of the instrument vibrates longitudinally at 23 000 oscillations per second (23 kHz). The instrument works by converting electromagnetic energy to mechanical movements. An electrical coil wrapped around metal laminations sets up a magnetic field, thus causing the metal to vibrate. The fine hollow tip of the instrument disrupts solid parenchyma by its fine vibrations and the heat this generates. When debris is shed, it is mixed with fluid jetting from the instrument and the mixture is sucked away. More solid and fibrous structures, such as ducts and blood vessels, are not disrupted, and may then be clipped with haemostats or ligated. Not only may this instrument be useful for open, solid parenchymal dissection, but it may also be used during laparoscopic dissection of the gallbladder or mobilization of the colon.

Ultrasonic harmonic scalpel

Increasing use of this instrument attests to its ability to aid safe, careful dissection with less bleeding than accompanies diathermy dissection. The instrument works by transforming electrical energy from a generator into mechanical energy through a set of piezoelectric ceramics, which are contained in a hand piece. The mechanical energy is passed through a disposable element, often a hook or clip, which vibrates at approximately 55.5 kHz. The energy spreads a small distance around the instrument tip. The extreme vibrations fracture internal cellular bonds. Proteins are denatured and reorganize to form a sticky coagulum. Vessels up to 2 mm in diameter can be safely divided. Soft tissue coagulation occurs at temperatures below 100°C, producing minimal charring and smoke or vapour.

A real advantage of this equipment is that it reduces the number of instrument changes during an operation, such as haemostats, staples, scissors and ligatures. It is a multifunctional instrument facilitating precise cutting with minimal lateral thermal damage. It does not use electricity, with all its potential risks. It was introduced in the mid-1990s and is used in, for example, the specialities of gastrointestinal surgery, gynaecology, urology and otolaryngology. Do not use it for incising bone or for contraceptive tubal ligation.

The harmonic scalpel system is valuable for soft tissue incisions where you require good haemostasis and minimal thermal injury. The instrument can be used for open or laparoscopic surgery as an adjunct to, or substitute for, diathermy, lasers or steel scalpels.

Argon beam (plasma) coagulator (Valleylab)

This instrument offers a thermal technique for sealing blood vessels from large, raw areas such as the cut surface of the liver and kidney. It works by passing an electrical current through what is called a 'plasma arc', created in argon, not air. When electrons are fired into the gas, ionization occurs, which in turn produces further electrons. These then ionize more gas and a 'domino' effect takes place. The plasma thus consists of free electrons, positive ions and neutral atoms (Fig. 17.9).

The coagulator can be valuable in controlling bleeding resulting from coagulation disorders. It applies a direct, high frequency electric current to the target tissue without direct contact. The effect is well defined and has a self-limiting depth of penetration. There is minimal charring of the treated tissues, producing a thin and flexible eschar. As a result there is a minimal tendency for rebleeding. Because there is no contact between the instrument and the coagulated area, the coagulum is not pulled off and so is unlikely to rebleed. The tissue which has been treated by this technique develops a spongy appearance and enlarges the tissue surface.

X-rays

Preoperative findings

 Key point

- **It is negligent and dangerous to start an operation without having available all the radiological results and films (see Ch. 4).**

Place essential films, with the names, date and hospital number checked, correctly orientated, on the screen so you can refer to them as necessary.

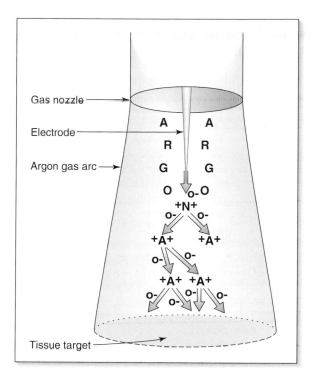

Fig. 17.9 Argon-enhanced coagulation. This is in effect a bipolar diathermy with the pathway from the active electrode to the tissue completed through argon gas. An arc or beam is produced with argon gas from the nozzle, which makes contact with the target tissue. Electrons are fired into it from the electrode, producing ionization, which, in turn, produces further electrons; these produce more ionization and so generate a domino or self-generating effect. The plasma arc is thus partly converted into positive ions and free electrons – in effect passing a current without instrument contact. The conventional active diathermy electrode adheres to the coagulum and may pull it off as it is withdrawn. The argon beam carrier overcomes this disadvantage, as there is no physical contact with the tissue coagulum. Capital letters indicate argon gas; capital letters such as +A+ indicate ionized argon, o- indicates electrons. It overcomes the disadvantage of adherence of the active diathermy electrode to the tissue coagulum.

Intraoperative procedures

Diagnostic help. An example is on-table cholangiography. Use sufficiently dilute contrast medium to allow one to 'see through' the common bile duct on the film. Fill the biliary tree adequately to show the main intrahepatic ducts as well as the common bile duct. Contrast medium is heavier than bile and tends to gravitate to dependent ducts. If the ampulla is patent, contrast medium flows into the duodenum, which is clearly recognizable by its mucosal pattern. Remember to put a 20°

lateral tilt on the table to eliminate the overlap of contrast on the vertebral column.

Intraoperative angiography can be performed following a steady intra-arterial injection, and provides adequate films. Adverse reactions to modern contrast media when the patient is generally anaesthetized are very rare.

Therapeutic use. Imaging using fluoroscopy may facilitate therapeutic procedures. It is valuable for simple procedures, including fracture reduction. Complex techniques include interventional uroradiology. Many of these techniques can be performed either in the operating room or in the X-ray department; facilities for fluoroscopy are usually better in the X-ray department, but asepsis is better in the operating theatre. X-ray machines are difficult to clean and are potential sources of crossinfection. In specialist centres, dedicated complex X-ray rooms may be organized in a fashion similar to operating theatres, or the facilities for radiology may match those in the X-ray department.

Key points

- **Discuss problems beforehand with a radiologist and subsequently report the outcome and anatomical findings.**
- **Give adequate warning to the radiographer of the need for X-rays in the operating theatre.**

Equipment

This is more likely to be mobile than static. The use of image intensification avoids the need for you to allow your eyes to become dark-adapted. Mobile image intensifiers for use in the operating theatre are mounted on a small C-arm. The table top must be radiolucent, with space beneath as well as over the table for the X-ray tube and the image intensifier. If films alone are required, the table top must have a 'tunnel' that admits the X-ray cassette beneath the patient. Alternatively, the cassette may be draped in sterile towels. This may be necessary, for example, if you need to carry out intraoperative mesenteric angiography on bowel lifted out of the abdomen at laparotomy. For a small field, the X-ray cassette can be placed on the image intensifier itself to obtain a film. Some modern machines can produce dry silver images directly from the television monitor.

Biplane screening is not usually available in the operating theatre. The mobile C-arm is, nevertheless, quite versatile and the effect of 'parallax' can be used to aid the judgement of depth.

Mobile X-ray sets operate from designated 13 A sockets that are on a separate ring main from other essential equipment. Modern mobile sets use 'sparkless' switching to avoid the danger of igniting inflammable gases. It is

desirable to keep the mobile X-ray machine in the operating suite.

X-rays and the law

X-rays, as well as scalpels, become weapons of assault if not used with care. Medical staff clinically directing examinations employing ionizing radiation are required to have obtained a certificate demonstrating that they have received some training in radiation protection. This should eventually be included in the undergraduate curriculum. Equipment must be regularly serviced and calibrated, and 'local rules' applied. In case of doubt, contact the hospital radiation protection supervisor.

Key points

- **Only radiologists, radiographers or others holding an approved qualification may direct exposures.**
- **Look after yourself, other staff in the theatre and the patient. Use the lead aprons.**

Safety

- Remember that the patient 'scatters' the X-ray beam. The inverse square law applies, so staff should not be unnecessarily close. Be aware of the screening time and record it.
- Do not X-ray the abdomen of pregnant patients unless absolutely necessary. Establish the date of the last menstrual period before the patient is anaesthetized.

Key point

- **Take an interest in imaging, as 'a picture is worth a thousand words'.**

Microscopes

Spectacles have been available for nearly 700 years and the compound microscope for about 300 years, but it was only 70 years ago that a microscope was used in theatre, and only 30 years ago that its use became more widespread. Although they were introduced very gradually to the operating theatre, they have now become indispensable in a wide variety of surgical fields. They offer improved views of the surgical field, more precision, greater flexibility, and less trauma to delicate tissues. They provide good stereoscopic appreciation of depth, through a narrow surgical approach, much smaller than your own unaided interpupillary distance allows.

A Swedish otolaryngologist, Nylen, introduced his monocular microscope in the surgical treatment of otosclerosis in 1921. A year later his chief, Professor Holmgren, used a binocular microscope for the same condition. In 1925, Hinselman used a microscope for colposcopy, but aside from this for three decades otolaryngologists alone continued to use microscopes. In Chicago, Perritt used a microscope for ophthalmic surgery in 1950, and Zeiss started to mass produce their MiI surgical microscope in 1953. Clinical applications then expanded: Jacobson in vascular surgery in 1960; Kurle in neurosurgery and Burke in plastic surgery in 1962. With the increased employment of free transfer flaps and microvascular anastomosis, the use of the operating microscope reaches several surgical disciplines.

Features of an operating microscope

- *Eyepieces* provide an adjustment for interpupillary distance and each eyepiece has a range of 5 dioptres.
- *Binocular tube* may be straight or inclined.
- *Beam splitter* allows for the connection of extra viewing tubes for observation and assistance. It also makes the use of still and video cameras possible as teaching aids.
- *Magnification system.* Magnification is available as a galilean system, variable in steps (e.g. ×6, ×10, ×25, ×40), or as a zoom system.
- *Objective lens* allows the working distance to be altered by changing lenses with variable focal lengths. For example:

$f = 150, 175, 200$ for ophthalmology and plastic surgery
$f = 250$ for otology and vascular surgery
$f = 250$ or 300 for gynaecological tubal surgery
$f = 300$ or 400 for neurosurgery
$f = 400$ for laryngoscopy.

- *Depth of field.* The stereoscopic depth of field is less at higher magnification. Focus at higher magnification first, then reduce to the working magnification so as to have the best focus at the centre of the depth of field.
- *Light.* A powerful coaxial halogen light is incorporated in the body of the microscope. Oblique light is available for eye surgery.

Instruments used with microscopes

Each speciality has developed microsurgical instruments for its own needs; however, the following basic instruments are common to many specialities:

- *Spring-handled needle holder* such as Borraquer or Castrovieso, ophthalmic.
- *Spring-handled microscissors*, straight or curved. The straight are for cutting vessels and the curved for cutting tissue and thread.

- *Jewellers' or watchmakers' forceps* in a wide variety.
- *Microsurgical clips* such as Scoville Lewis, or fine Heifetzs neurosurgical clips, can be used for vessel anastomosis.
- *Microelectrode*: monopolar or bipolar cautery is necessary.
- *Suture material*: (1) blood vessel anastomosis: 9/0 or 10/0 nylon on a 3–6 mm needle with a tapered end; (2) nerve anastamosis: as above, but the needle has a cutting point; (3) fallopian tube work: 7/0 or 8/0 absorbable non-reactive suture with a 4 mm or 6 mm reverse cutting needle.
- *Sterilization*: sterile rubber cups or drapes are available to cover the controls.
- *Adjustment*: versatility in position demands several interlocking arms and counterbalanced vertical movement, as well as a geared angled coupling between the microscope carriage arm and body. This enables you to swing the microscope from side to side while mounted in an oblique axis.
- *Mounting*: can be on a solid, well-balanced mobile floor stand, or a fixed ceiling mounting. Wall-mounted microscopes are also available.

Control of tremor

Counteracting surgical tremor is of vital importance. The instrument or the limb on which it is held must be firmly supported as close to the point of work as possible.

The future

The combination of the laser with a micromanipulator to the objective lens of the microscope will enhance the use of both instruments in the future.

Summary

- Are you familiar with the requirements of behaviour and technique to obviate operating room infection?
- Have you learned the methods of positioning and moving unconscious patients to avoid injuring them?
- Do you accept that you are in charge of the tourniquet, diathermy, laser, cryoprobe and X-rays in theatre?
- Will you lead by example in the operating room, by adopting careful and responsible attitudes to delicate and potentially dangerous equipment?

ACKNOWLEDGEMENTS

I am deeply grateful for help with writing this chapter to: Mr John Bancroft for the diathermy section; Dr David Parker for the section on X-rays in theatre; Mr Derry Coakley for the section on microscopes; and to my wife for her help in the section on lasers. I should also like to thank Miss Sharon Langford for typing the manuscript. I am grateful to Ethicon Endosurgery (a Johnson & Johnson Company) for information on the Harmonic Scalpel System; to the Microsulis Group for data on their Microwave Endometrial Ablation System; to Frigenis for help with the Autologous Transfusion Cell Salvage System; and to Valleylab for guidance on the use of the argon beam coagulator.

 Further reading

Brigden RJ 1988 Operating theatre technique, 5th edn. Churchill Livingstone, Edinburgh

Douglas DM (ed.) 1972 Surgical departments in hospitals: the surgeon's view. Butterworth, London

Johnston IDA, Hunter AR (eds) 1984 The design and utilization of operating theatres. Edward Arnold, London

Cell salvage

Duguid JKM 1999 Review. Autologous blood transfusion. Clinical and Laboratory Haematology 21: 371–376

Diathermy

Dobbie AK 1974 Accidental lesions in the operating theatre. NAT News December

Earnshaw JJ, Keene TK 1989 Gastric explosion: a cautionary tale. BMJ 293: 93–94

Editorial 1979 Surgical diathermy is still not foolproof. BMJ 12: 755–758

Pearce JA 1986 Electrosurgery. Chapman & Hall, London

Fibre optics

Ravenscroft MM, Swan CMJ 1984 Gastrointestinal endoscopy and related procedures – a handbook for nurses and assistants. Chapman & Hall, London

Lasers

1982 General guidance on lasers in hospitals. Medical physics and bioengineering working group. Welsh Scientific Advisory Committee (WSAC)

1983 Guidance on the safe use of lasers in medical practice. HMSO, London

Murray A, Mitchell DC, Wood RFM 1992 Lasers in surgery – a review. British Journal of Surgery 79: 21–26

Microscopes

Taylor S 1977 Microscopy. Recent advances in surgery. Churchill Livingstone, Edinburgh, ch. 8

X-rays

Ionizing radiation regulations 1985, 1988

Mound RF 1985/1988 Radiation protection in hospitals (Medical Sciences Series). Adam Hilger, Bristol

18 Adjuncts to surgery

A. L. G. Peel

> **Objectives**
> - Recognize the importance of good theatre management.
> - Ensure basic understanding of usage and care of theatre instruments, accessories and special equipment.
> - Appreciate the place of implants and tissue glues in modern surgical practice.

INTRODUCTION

In health service economics an operating suite requires large capital and revenue budgets and this is favourably influenced by careful management of utilities. Good care of quality instruments ensures their long use; appropriate ordering and stocking means the shelf-life of equipment is not exceeded; wastage due to change in practice is reduced to a minimum; and storage space is efficiently used. The avoidance of an unnecessarily wide range of equipment and materials allows better use of capital.

From the medicolegal aspect, the establishment of simple protocols aids efficient management within the theatre complex and helps to reduce errors, such as breakdowns in sterility or retention of swabs or instruments in patients.

A practical example of the rapidly changing scene in surgical practice is illustrated by orthopaedic surgery, where considerable expansion has occurred, particularly in prosthetic joint replacement, and in this field infection can result in very costly failure in terms of patient morbidity and financial implications to the health service.

In the attempt to 'abolish' infection to elective orthopaedic surgery the following factors are considered important.

Patient screening for occult infection

Give particular attention to:

- Possible urinary tract infection in females
- Carrier status – postpone elective surgery until pathogens are eliminated, for example nasal *Staphylococcus aureus*.

THEATRE MANAGEMENT

1. *Orthopaedic theatre* should be dedicated to 'clean' orthopaedics, where no dirty or contaminated orthopaedic operations and no general surgery is carried out.
2. *Clean air enclosures.* The routine use of clean air enclosures has reduced the infection rate in prosthetic joint surgery of hip and knee by more than half compared with conventionally ventilated theatres. Unidirectional air systems, especially with a downflow direction, reduces bacteria-carrying particles from 400–500 m^{-3} to 30–40 m^{-3}. Power tools produce additional problems because they create an aerosol spray, which effectively disseminates bacteria and viral particles.
3. *Theatre gowns.* Airborne bacterial dispersion can be further reduced by the use of appropriate fabric clothing. It is not widely appreciated that, in either conventional or unidirectional airflow theatres, the use of disposable fabric gowns alone in lieu of cotton gowns has not achieved a significant reduction in bacteria-carrying particles.

Drawbacks to conventional clothing

- Bacteria from you, the surgeon, tend to be pumped by air through or out of cotton pyjamas and gowns into theatre air.
- Bacteria from you are drawn through wet clothing by capillary action, contaminating the sterile operative area.
- Contamination of you with patient's fluids.

Alternative clothing

It has been stated that pharmaceutical manufacturing areas would be closed down if they used clothing currently worn in the majority of operating rooms. The choice includes:

- The total exhaust gown, developed by the outstanding orthopaedic surgeon Sir John Charnley, which is well established for clean orthopaedic surgery.
- Disposable non-woven clothing such as Sonta (manufactured by DuPont Ltd), which has been shown to be effective.
- Breathable plastic membrane clothing which requires seals at the neck and trouser openings, with the result that the wearer soon becomes hot and uncomfortable.
- Close woven polyester or polycotton fabrics which are expensive but represent a significant improvement over conventional garments. The cost must be equated with the significant costs of morbidity from infection.

Theatre technique

1. Make sure you 'scrub up' in the prescribed manner. Protect your skin 'envelope'; gently scrub your nails but wash the remainder of skin with a suitable agent such as 20% chlorhexidine gluconate solution (e.g. Hibiscrub) or 10% aqueous povidone-iodine solution (e.g. Betadine) starting from fingertips, washing proximally, avoiding subsequent contamination.
2. Use closed gloving technique.
3. Double glove when carrying out orthopaedic implant procedures or when using power tools.

 Key points

- **If your gloves become contaminated or pierced, change them.**
- **At the conclusion of the operation check your gloves carefully before removing them. You may have sustained an unnoticed needlestick injury.**

DRESSINGS

Make sure you appreciate why you are applying dressings, what you expect from them and how often they should be changed.

1. If you have closed the wound and it is sealed and dry, a dressing may be unnecessary, or be merely collodion, modern plastic spray or adherent plastic strip.
2. For acute open wounds that are not contaminated the best dressing is closure by suture, flaps, grafts or temporary synthetic non-adherent non-allergenic dressings.
3. Open wounds that are producing exudate require absorbent dressings. If these become soaked through to the surface, bacteria may penetrate through from the surface. Consequently, ensure that the absorbent dressings are changed regularly. Tulle (net – named after the French town near Limoges) of paraffin gauze or plastic, sometimes containing a bacteriocidal, such as chlorhexidine or povidone-iodine, may be applied to allow exudate to pass through it. The exudate can be absorbed into dressings placed on the tulle. Some starch-containing hydrogel dressings also absorb exudate. Hydrocolloid seals the wound, provides a moist environment and can be left for up to 1 week. Bead dressings also absorb exudate. Plastic foam can be cut from a sheet or poured in to set, creating a shaped filling for a defect.
4. Infected wounds need bacteriological assessment, careful debridement of all dead tissue, and in some cases the application of appropriate substances or dressings. Eusol (Edinburgh University solution of lime) was formerly popular but is now discouraged as damaging to tissues. Normal saline dressings, sodium hypochlorite solutions and hydrogen peroxide solutions may be applied.
5. For the treatment of slow-healing wounds, topical negative pressure has been tried over an open cell foam dressing or saline-moistened dressing. A negative pressure of 125 mmHg can be exerted continuously for 48 h and then intermittently.
6. A wide range of materials and substances is now available for managing chronic wounds. Of course, you must first exclude an underlying cause and ensure that the blood supply and oxygenation are satisfactory. Apart from skin grafts or flaps, biological techniques in use include:
   a. Growth factors
   b. Hyperbaric oxygen
   c. Allograft skin – prepared from porcine skin
   d. Amniotic membrane, which is thought to entrap inflammatory cells
   e. Chitosan – prepared from the chitin of organisms with an exoskeleton, used as an occlusive dressing
   f. TransCyte – human newborn fibroblasts cultured on nylon mesh
   g. Procuren – prepared from the patient's own blood platelets to stimulate wound healing.

INSTRUMENTS

Surgeons and instrument makers have combined to produce a wide range of instruments. Some, such as certain scissors, forceps and retractors, may be used in several different fields of surgery. Others have more specific functions, for example, those used in anal surgery, such as Park's anal retractor and Lockhart–Mummery fistula probes. Consider what your requirements are for instruments and appreciate the range and potential of different instruments. One advantage of a training rotation scheme is that it allows you to experience a number of surgical disciplines and permits you to observe instruments being used in a variety of procedures. You can then reapply this knowledge to particular problems in whatever field you subsequently work.

Instruments are a sound investment; whenever possible use those of the highest quality. Of equal importance is the investment in maintenance care, mechanical and chemical cleansing, particularly of hinge joints, adjustment of misalignment and regular sharpening of cutting instruments. Although you cannot control the maintenance, you do have a responsibility to avoid damage to the instruments by not dropping them or using them inappropriately.

Sterilization

The majority of instruments are autoclaved (moist heat under pressure for a prescribed time) and this process needs constant monitoring, with care in the packing of the autoclave and verification that the temperature, pressure and time are correct.

Where steam autoclaving is impracticable and may cause damage, alternatives include (see Ch. 19):

- Formaldehyde autoclave.
- Ethylene oxide.
- Gluteraldehyde 2% solution with prolonged immersion. It is rendered ineffective by organic debris. The substance is toxic and causes skin irritation so the procedure must be carried out in a well-ventilated room. Alternatives are being developed.
- γ-Irradiation, widely used for the commercial sterilization of plastic instruments.

Instrument sets

It is advantageous to have the instruments required for a particular surgical procedure packed and sterilized in a single set. As far as possible, each type of instrument should be included in multiples of five. Each design or size of artery forceps is grouped in separate fives or tens, scissors of differing size and design are grouped in fives.

A standardized typed, numbered, contents list is included in the sterilized set for each operation. This reduces the number of single-packed instruments that need to be opened and, more importantly, simplifies the instrument count at the beginning and end of each procedure.

Develop a close liaison with the central sterile supply department (CSSD) and theatre management to ensure adequate supplies of trays to meet the demands of a full schedule of operating lists. The organization is put particularly under strain when carrying out many minor procedures with a quick turnover.

LIGATURES, SUTURES, STAPLES AND CLIPS

When selecting a ligature or suture, consider several factors with regard to the material itself.

1. Is the material to be absorbed? Catgut has been withdrawn because of fears that it may contain prions (coined from 'protein'), which are inheritable or mutant, transmittable 'rogue' proteins associated with, in particular, bovine spongiform encephalopathy (BSE) and scrapie in sheep. New synthetic materials are absorbed more reliably than formerly, so the strength remains long enough for healing to be well advanced before a suture is absorbed. In some situations, absorbable sutures have replaced non-absorbable threads; for example, abdominal wounds are often closed using reliable, slowly absorbed, synthetic sutures. The synthetic threads may be monofilamentous, such as polydioxanane (PDS), polyglyconate (Maxon) and glycomer 631 (Biosin), or multifilamentous, such as polyglactin (Vicryl), polyglycolic acid (Dexon) and lactomer 9-1 (Polysorb).

2. Non-absorbable natural threads, such as silk and linen, are still used. Polyesters, polypropylene and polyamides are synthetics that retain their strength indefinitely. Polytetrafluoroethylene (PTFE, Gortex) is also popular. Stainless steel was formerly popular but the synthetic polymers have largely replaced it.

3. Modern suture materials have good strength-to-thickness properties, so ligatures and sutures tend to be less bulky than formerly.

Handling properties vary. Synthetic threads are extruded (Latin *ex* = out + *trudere* = to thrust); a liquid is forced through a hole and solidifies as a thread. If the surface of the resulting thread is damaged, it seriously weakens it. Monofilamentous extruded synthetics may be rather stiff and often have a 'memory' so they spontaneously tend to return to the straight form in which they were created; because the surface is so smooth it binds less firmly to itself. These factors make the knots less secure than those tied using flexible and rougher materials.

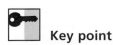

Key point

- **Do not injure the smooth surface of extruded synthetic threads – it fatally weakens it.**

4. Needles are now almost universally curved and inserted using a 'no-touch' technique on a needle holder. This protects your hands from the danger of needle stick injury. The needles are simple round-bodied or sharp-edged cutting needles for penetrating tough tissues. The majority of sutures are now 'atraumatic', being swaged into eyeless needles. This facilitates passage through the tissues.

5. Catgut was absorbed by creating an inflammatory reaction. Modern absorbable materials are often absorbed by hydrolysis and so provoke very little inflammatory reaction.

6. Metal clips are valuable alternatives to ligatures where access is difficult. They were originally made of stainless steel and were frequently used to demarcate an area for subsequent radiotherapy, or to assess radiologically the response of a neoplasm to treatment by radiotherapy or chemotherapy. Stainless steel clips may produce a stellate shadow, obscuring detail in computed tomography (CT) scans, so they are now made from titanium.

7. Sutures or clips may be unnecessary for skin closure, provided the tissues are perfectly apposed. Dry the edges and apply plastic adhesive strips across the wound.

8. A variety of staples are used in visceral tissues, offering changes in practice. Be aware of the range, the indications and contraindications for each type of instrument, including staple size, and the differences in design between manufacturers. Remember that surgical technique may need to be adapted as compared with the standard suture procedure. However, staple techniques are not as versatile as suturing. Reserve staple techniques for circumstances when:

a. The procedure can be carried out with greater safety, for example, reducing anastomotic leakage

b. Operative time is significantly reduced and this is an important factor

c. The incidence of late complications (stenosis) is low; for example, low anterior resection of the rectum or oesophagogastric anastomosis high in the chest.

SWABS AND PACKS

1. All cotton or fabric swabs and packs used during operations have radio-opaque thread marking. Choose the size appropriate to the procedure and defined purpose. You may need small 'patty' swabs for neurosurgical procedures and narrow swabs for tonsillar surgery. Use large packs or gauze rolls for retaining abdominal

viscera out of the operative field, for limiting gross contamination and for haemostatic control of raw surfaces.

2. Although haemostasis is usually achieved by electrocoagulation, ligation, undersewing or the use of clips, in some situations it is invaluable to use manufactured haemostatic agents in the presence of a slow ooze. There is a choice between Surgicel, Oxycel or Sterispon; gain experience of the particular properties of each of them. Surgicel applied to the gallbladder bed, with overlying pressure from a warm, moist swab, controls a slow persistent ooze following cholecystectomy. When you carefully remove the overlying swab, the haemostatic agent remains undisturbed. In neurosurgery you may prefer the more delicate Sterispon.

DISPOSABLE ACCESSORIES

Included in this category are accessories that remain on the surface of the body, skin or epithelial lining, and those that attain access to the interior of the body, usually for a limited period. Remember that they cause tissue irritation and create a break in the body's defence system.

Categories

1. Vascular cannulae, catheters and specialized equipment (e.g. Fogarty embolectomy catheters, Swan–Ganz catheters).
2. Urological catheters and stents.
3. Alimentary tract stents and catheters, for example:
   a. Straight, curved, cuffed or expansile stents for oesophageal and biliary malignant stricture
   b. Balloon dilating catheters for strictures
   c. Enteral feeding tubes.
4. Stoma appliances.

Key point

- **Avail yourself of the skill of a stomatherapist so your patient benefits from the correct appliance in the right place.**

5. Neurological valved shunts.
6. Drains.

Key point

- **Define the purpose and, therefore, duration of use. Use closed systems.**

ENDOSCOPES

1. Endoscopes are continuously being developed, together with new applications for diagnosis and therapy. Instruments can be passed in the upper and lower respiratory tracts, the upper and lower alimentary tracts (including the biliary tree and pancreas), the upper and lower urinary tracts, the female genital tract, and into joints, the peritoneal cavity and along blood vessels. Design modifications have resulted in a wide range of instruments with considerable therapeutic capabilities, often with the use of specialized accessories.

2. Ensure that they are carefully stored, maintained, cleaned, decontaminated and expertly disinfected, otherwise there is a risk of transmitting infection, particularly viruses such as hepatitis B and C and human immunodeficiency virus (HIV). Flexible instruments are usually disinfected by immersing them in a buffered 2% solution of gluteraldehyde for 20 min. Modern cystoscopes, for instance, may now be autoclaved.

3. Do not neglect to master the use of the simple proctoscope, anal retractor, such as Park's or Eisenheimer's retractors, and sigmoidoscope.

IMPLANT MATERIALS

1. Prosthetic (Greek *pros* = to + *thesis* = putting; the fitting of artificial parts into the body) surgery continuously expands. Perhaps the greatest impact is in orthopaedic surgery, where successful joint replacement is well established in the hip, knee, interphalangeal joints and, to a more limited extent, the shoulder and elbow joints.

2. Prosthetic implants are widely used in general, vascular, cardiac, urological, plastic and other branches of surgery, and there is wide variation in the materials used. Basic considerations and principles apply. They must be easily and reliably manufactured at reasonable cost. The strength and durability must be reliable, especially for cardiac valves, pacemakers and joint replacements.

3. There must be no adverse reaction between prosthetic materials themselves and the body tissues; for example, between the metal and plastic components of certain artificial hip replacements or between the joint prosthesis, cement and the bone. Another example is platelet aggregation and plasma protein precipitation around intravascular prostheses.

4. The degree of incorporation into the body may be important; for example, metallic and silicone implants are isolated within a collagen capsule but polytetrafluoroethylene (PTFE, Goretex) allows the ingrowth of fibroblasts.

Implant materials in orthopaedic surgery

1. Surgical-grade stainless steel is used for joint replacement-bearing surfaces, plates, screws and wires.

2. Alloys, including Vitallium, are also used in joint replacement surfaces, wires and, less frequently now owing to the preference for compression steel plating for internal fixation, in plates.

3. High density polyethylene (ultrahigh molecular weight) is used for joint replacement-bearing surfaces to articulate with steel or Vitallium.

4. Silicone is used for hinge-type joint replacement, but not in bearing surfaces where debris produces a synovitis. It has been used very successfully in metacarpophalangeal and proximal interphalangeal joints.

5. Dacron and PTFE are materials that can be used under tension (e.g. synthetic ligament repair). Carbon fibre has been abandoned as a result of fragmentation and foreign body reaction.

The risk of infection

This is one of the most serious complications of prosthetic surgery. Risk factors include:

- Immune compromised host
- Active infection present elsewhere in the host or in contacts
- Positive carrier state in patient or staff
- Crossinfection in hospital
- Failure of sterilization and/or packaging
- Inadequate air ventilation in the operating theatre and ineffective operating theatre clothing
- Poor operative technique with contamination, poor haemostasis or ischaemic tissue
- Inadequate antimicrobial prophylaxis.

The time scale of presentation is of significance. Late infection may develop, up to a year or more after surgery, particularly with a deeply inserted prosthesis. A smooth-surfaced implant is bacteriostatic and non-wettable, whereas a textured surface allows the entrapment of blood, serum, particles and bacteria in the crevices.

Deep infection around implants, such as of a hip replacement with *Staphylococcus aureus*, produces a capsular thickening; *S. epidermidis* produces a polysaccharide slime. The prosthesis becomes loose, causes pain and may need to be removed.

Do not use an implant unless there is no natural alternative. Thus, in vascular surgery prefer vein grafts for lower limb arterial bypass surgery such as infrainguinal bypass and especially for below-knee femoropopliteal bypass. Synthetic materials, Dacron (collagen-coated knitted Dacron) or Goretex (PTFE) may be used, particularly where large vessels need to be bypassed or replaced.

Tissue response to foreign material

1. Tissue reaction varies according to the material and the roughness of the surface. Marked inflammatory response, with microabscess formation, occurs around a buried silk or linen knot. By comparison, minimal response occurs around polypropylene, with not only a reduced likelihood of bacterial infection but also increased tensile strength, depending on the material used, and a lack of surrounding tissue inflammatory infiltrate.

2. Silicone generates the formation of a capsule. Fibroblasts orientate themselves to the surface of the foreign material and the collagen is laid down in mirror image to the specific surface; as it matures, it contracts. Fibroblasts cease to secrete collagen when they are in contact with other fibroblasts, but not when in contact with other cells. Thus, over a smooth surface sheets of collagen are produced with increased contractile force of the capsule. Gradually, fibroblastic activity on the free surface subsides, collagen deposition is completed and moulding takes place, producing a mature capsule at approximately 3 months after surgery. Collagen production against the smooth inner capsular surface continues because the fibroblasts are not in contact with each other and, as a result, the cavity diameter decreases and the contractile force increases.

3. By comparison, roughened surfaces allow fibroblasts to conform to the crevices; the fibres of collagen are then orientated at random with counteracting contractile forces and the fibroblasts lie in different planes and directions, allowing a greater chance of contact with each other, thus reducing the collagen deposition and resulting in a thinner capsule. Silicone particles are found in phagocytes in the capsule wall adjacent to lymphatic vessels, in the outer layer of capsules, and may reach the lumen of lymphatic vessels, as they are found in regional lymph nodes.

4. Metal-on-metal joint replacement produces small particulate debris which is incorporated into the synovium, producing foreign-body giant cells.

5. Acrylic cement (polymethylmethacrylate), used in the fixation of prostheses, becomes encapsulated by fibrous tissue, the inner layer of which is sometimes hyaline and acellular and sometimes contains histiocytes and multinucleate giant cells. There is no evidence for malignant transformation or chronic inflammatory reaction with sinus formation (Charnley 1970). Revisional surgery of the cemented prosthesis is difficult. Alternatives under trial are based on isoelastic or mesh coating of the prosthesis to allow fibrous tissue to grow in.

The controversy over the safety of silicone mammary prostheses

In 1992 in the USA a moratorium (Latin *mora* = delay) was placed on the use of silicone gel breast implants because of the possible association with connective tissue disorders. In the UK, an independent expert advisory group reported to the Department of Health in 1993 that there was no evidence of an increased risk in implanted patients (Park et al 1993). In 1994, the Medical Devices Directory supported the Chief Medical Officer in stating that there was no evidence for a change in policy. As always, absence of evidence is not evidence of absence. Since the incidence of connective tissue disorders in the population is low and the latent period is long, large numbers and prolonged follow-up are needed. Silicone, like any foreign body, may initiate an antibody and cell-mediated inflammatory response, but this is not in itself suggestive of an adverse effect on the immune system. There is currently no evidence that breast-implanted patients have an enhanced risk of developing either autoimmune connective tissue disease or mammary carcinoma. Silicone implants do, however, reduce the value of mammography. Alternative filler substances, developed to allow mammograph and avoid silicone reaction locally, include triglyceride and saccharides. They were withdrawn because of adverse reactions in some patients (Medical Devices Agency 2001) and patients are advised to have them removed, to be replaced by silicone gel or saline filled prosthetics if desired. All of them have textured silicone shells.

TISSUE GLUES

Glues have been used for many years. Collodion, a cellulose nitrate, has been used for many years as a wound seal. Karaya gum is routinely used to attach stoma bags to the skin; it has also been used as a slow release vehicle for caffeine and diclofenac. Cyanoacrylate 'instant glue' is used as a tissue glue. Gelatine-resocinol-formaldehyde has been used, for example, as an adhesive to fix a patch sealing an intraventricular septal defect.

Research into new methods of surgical tissue repair has yielded the prospect of wide use of tissue glues. One such method is fibrin adhesion, based on the conversion of fibrinogen into fibrin on a tissue surface by the action of thrombin. The fibrin is then crosslinked by factor XIIIa to create a firm stable fibrin network with good adhesive properties. Fibrin foam may be valuable in controlling tumour bleeding. The addition of aprotinin prevents premature dissolution of the fibrin clot by plasmin. In the presence of heavy bleeding the fibrin glue tends to be washed away before sufficient polymerization of the fibrin has occurred. The use of collagen mesh sheet with fibrin glue dispersed over the surface has been of considerable practical value. Note that the sheet should be kept in contact with the surface by gentle pressure for 3–5 min. The indications are for tissue adhesion, haemostasis and suture support (Table 18.1).

Concern has been expressed that the use of human fibrinogen and factor XIII might allow the transmission of viral agents such as hepatitis B, hepatitis C or HIV. Commercial inactivation of a virus is achieved by pasteurization with purification of the proteins and then heating the solution for 10 h at 60°C. Laboratory studies demonstrated that this process not only inactivates the hepatitis B and HIV viruses, but also herpes simplex virus and cytomegalovirus. Particular care is taken to use human fibrinogen from hepatitis B antigen-negative,

anti-HIV-negative and anti-hepatitis C-negative plasma of healthy donors.

Marked arterial or venous bleeding renders the system ineffective. Hypersensitivity reactions have been described. The process is under evaluation in the UK.

Table 18.1 Examples of the use of tissue glues

- *General surgery*
  Trauma to or surgery of liver, spleen, pancreas
  Haemostasis in gallbladder bed (cheaper agents
     currently available)
  Support anastomosis e.g. pancreaticojejunal
     anastomosis
- *Neurosurgery*
  Repair of dural tear, sealing cerebrospinal fluid
     leak
  Peripheral nerve anastomosis
- *Orthopaedic surgery*
  Acetabuloplasty (cement-free prosthesis)
  Tendon repair
  Re-attaching osteochondral fragments
- *Cardiovascular and thoracic surgery*
  Prosthetic implant in combination with collagen
     sheet to seal lung air leaks
- *Ophthalmic surgery*
  Cataract operations
- *ENT surgery*
  Tympanic membrane surgery
  Sealing CSF leaks
- *Urology*
  Haemostasis, especially after TURP
- *Plastic surgery*
  Attaching skin grafts

Summary

- Do you recognize the safety factors and cost effectiveness of good theatre management for you and your patient?
- Do you know the basic principles of sterilization?
- Will you contribute to cost savings by using only the smallest range of effective instruments, equipment and consumable materials?
- Implants can transform a patient's quality of life but the surgery is costly and complications can be serious and prolonged.

Further reading

Detweiler MB, Detweiler JG, Fenton J 1999 Sutureless and reduced suture anastomosis of hollow vessels with fibrin glue: a review. Journal of Investigative Surgery 12: 245–262

Gosden PE, MacGowan AP, Bannister GC 1998 Importance of air quality and related factors in the prevention of infection in orthopaedic surgery. Journal of Hospital Infection 39: 173–180

Harding KG, Jones V, Price P 2000 Topical treatment: which dressing to choose. Diabetes/Metabolism Research Reviews 16 (suppl. 1): S47–S50

References

Charnley J 1970 Acrylic cement in orthopaedic surgery. E and S Livingstone, Edinburgh

Park AJ, Black RJ, Watson ACH 1993 Silicone gel breast implants, breast cancer and connective tissue disorder. British Journal of Surgery 80: 1097–1100

19 Prevention of infection in surgical practice

K. E. Orr, F. K. Gould

Objectives

- **Appreciate the importance of surgical sepsis as a significant cause of morbidity.**
- **Understand the principles of infection control and its role in preventing infections.**
- **Be aware of methods by which asepsis and antisepsis are achieved, and when they are necessary.**
- **Know when antibiotic prophylaxis is desirable and when it is not.**
- **Recognize the benefit of infection audit with feedback to surgeons as a means of reducing the infection rate.**

INTRODUCTION

The Hungarian obstetrician Ignaz Semmelweiss was the first to demonstrate the importance of antisepsis, working in Vienna in the early 1850s. He found that on his obstetric ward attended by medical students almost one-fifth of all his patients died, usually of puerperal (Latin *puer* = child + *parere* = to bear) sepsis. On another ward, without medical students, the mortality was about 3 in 100. He realized that the medical students came straight from the autopsy room and proceeded to examine his patients without so much as washing their hands. Having insisted that each student should do so with soap and water and then in chlorinated lime solution before entering the ward, he saw the mortality rate drop to less than 2 in 100. Despite this dramatic result, Semmelweiss was largely ignored and even ridiculed. It was not until Joseph Lister built on Pasteur's germ theory of disease in Glasgow in the late 1860s that antisepsis was looked at seriously.

Since then, the improved prevention and management of infections in surgical practice has been one of the most important factors allowing the development of surgery as

we now know it. Even so, surgical wound infections remain an important cause of morbidity. Over 70% of hospital-acquired infections occur in patients who have undergone a surgical procedure. Of these, wound infections are those that increase hospital costs and length of hospital stay the most. On average, wound infections prolong the hospital stay of the patient by 7 days.

Surgical wounds are traditionally classified as follows:

Clean (Class I)

These are wounds created during surgical procedures in which the respiratory, genitourinary or gastrointestinal tracts have not been entered. The usual causes of infections in these wounds are airborne or exogenous bacteria that have entered the wound during surgery, or, in the case of prosthetic implants, the patient's own skin flora. The infection rate should not exceed 2%.

Clean-contaminated (Class II)

This term (Latin *con* = together + *tangere* = to touch; hence, soiled) describes wounds in elective surgery where the respiratory, gastrointestinal or genitourinary tracts have been entered. The primary cause of infection is the endogenous flora of the organ that has been breached surgically. The infection rate has been found to be approximately 5%.

Contaminated (Class III)

These are wounds where acute inflammation (but not pus) was found at surgery, or where there was spillage of gastrointestinal contents. They become infected with bowel/endogenous flora at a rate of about 20%.

Dirty (Class IV)

These are wounds where pus was found at operation, usually following organ perforation, although this category also includes contaminated traumatic wounds. The infection rate is up to 40%.

Not only are surgical infections extremely important to the outcome for individual patients and costly for hospitals, but they have also assumed medicolegal significance. All departments and surgeons should ensure that their infection rates are compatible with those in other units, using methods that will be discussed later in this chapter.

You cannot reduce infection by concentrating attention in a single area

- Control resistant organisms in all areas within the hospital.
- Unfailingly adhere to aseptic and antiseptic principles.
- Practise the highest standards of surgical technique.
- Use prophylactic antibiotics logically.
- Audit your results to maintain and improve standards.

CONTROL OF RESISTANT ORGANISMS

1. Antibiotics have been in use for more than 50 years and many organisms are now resistant to the older agents. For example, in many hospitals more than 50% of isolates of *Escherichia coli* are resistant to ampicillin. The development of newer agents with increased activity and wider spectrum has allowed the benefits of antimicrobial therapy to be maintained and even improved. However, increasing use of these has led to the emergence of resistance in some important pathogen groups.

2. The most obvious example is methicillin-resistant *Staphylococcus aureus* (MRSA). This is resistant to the commonly used antistaphylococcal agent flucloxacillin and has to be treated with drugs such as the glycopeptides, vancomycin and teicoplanin. As well as being more toxic, these agents penetrate less well into soft tissues and wounds, can only be given parenterally and are expensive. MRSA is of particular concern in fields such as burns, plastic surgery and orthopaedics where tissue penetration of the antibiotic is of paramount importance and where an infection may result in removal of a prosthesis or failure of a graft. Even more worrying is the reported emergence in Japan and the USA of vancomycin intermediate *S. aureus* (VISA) with reduced susceptibility to vancomycin. So far this does not appear to be a common cause of clinical infections, however there is a danger that in the future we shall again be unable to treat *S. aureus* infection.

3. Enterococci are also posing major problems with resistance; glycopeptide-resistant enterococci (GRE) are now found in many UK hospitals and, although they are less virulent than MRSA, they may cause life-threatening infections in immunocompromised patients.

4. Gram-negative organisms such as *Pseudomonas aeruginosa* may also be multiresistant. The increasing use of third-generation cephalosporins appears to be encouraging the emergence of Gram-negative bacilli such as *Klebsiella pneumoniae* and *Enterobacter cloacae* resistant to these and other beta-lactams.

Key point

- Make every effort to keep the prevalence of resistant organisms within the unit to a minimum, and prevent their spread between patients.

5. Handwashing and basic infection control practices cannot be overemphasized. Handwashing has been highlighted in recent national evidence-based guidelines for preventing healthcare-associated infections (Pratt et al 2001). Most hospital acquired (nosocomial from Greek *nosos* = sickness + *komeein* = to tend; hospital) infections are transmitted on the hands of staff and many studies have shown that handwashing is the single most important and successful method of controlling the spread of infection in hospital. Wash your hands before and after physical contact with any patient, and after any activity where they are likely to become contaminated. Wash them with soap, detergent, or with alcohol rubs or gels if your hands are not visibly soiled. Before carrying out aseptic procedures, wash with an antiseptic solution such as povidone-iodine or chlorhexidine.

Key points

- Wash your hands, and see that all members of your team do so, before and after contact with every patient.
- Rigorously apply universal precautions when appropriate, to minimize risk of infection for colleagues and patients (see Ch. 20).

6. Screen at-risk patients to identify those who are colonized. Reserve this, as a rule, for detecting MRSA so you can implement precautions to prevent spread of the organism to other patients, and also to reduce the risk of infection in those planned for high risk surgery such as

vascular graft procedures and prosthetic orthopaedic surgery. Take swabs of nose, throat and perineum. Colonized patients are asymptomatic and do not require systemic antibiotic treatment unless they show clinical evidence of infection. Consider using topical agents in an attempt to eradicate MRSA carriage in colonized patients; however, this is unlikely to succeed in the presence of foreign bodies such as percutaneous feeding tubes, and persisting wounds. If there is evidence of an outbreak on your unit, the infection control team may advise you to screen the unit staff, in case there are carriers. In most UK hospitals the management of patients and staff in units affected by MRSA is based upon national guidelines (Duckworth et al 1998).

7. Isolate patients found to be colonized with a significant multiresistant organism, usually in a side room – 'wound and enteric' or 'source' isolation. All staff wear disposable gloves and aprons when in contact with the patient. You and your medical colleagues remove your white coats before entering the side room. Ideally the same nurses should care for the patient throughout the shift. All other staff, such as porters, physiotherapists, phlebotomists and domestics, must be aware of, and take relevant precautions for, 'wound and enteric/source isolation.'

8. Control the movement of colonized patients between departments. Whenever possible, arrange for those carrying multiresistant organisms to be operated upon at the end of the surgical list, so that the theatre can be cleaned thoroughly afterwards with minimum disruption. Warn the theatre staff of the patient's status in advance. The same applies to visits to other departments, such as radiology, physiotherapy and the gymnasium. Keep patient movement within the hospital to a minimum and transfer patients between wards only when absolutely necessary.

9. Use antibiotics judiciously, only when there is evidence of clinical infection or as part of a policy regarding perioperative prophylaxis. Choose the antibiotic rationally; if in doubt, consult the microbiologist earlier rather than later. Overuse of antibiotics encourages development of resistance in exposed organisms. It also destroys patients' normal flora so they are more susceptible to colonization with hospital organisms. Furthermore, it predisposes to infection with *Clostridium difficile*, which can lead to pseudomembranous colitis: third-generation cephalosporins are notorious for this.

Key point

- **Adopt locally agreed guidelines for antibiotic prescribing, and audit your infection rates.**

ASEPSIS AND ANTISEPSIS

The term 'asepsis' (Greek *a* = deprive + *sepsis* = sepsis = putrefaction) describes methods preventing contamination of wounds and other sites by ensuring that only sterile objects and fluids come into contact with them; the risks of airborne contamination are minimized. Antisepsis (Greek *anti* = against) is the use of solutions, such as chlorhexidine, iodine or alcohol, for disinfection.

Theatre clothing

1. *Gowns*. Woven cotton clothing is relatively ineffective at preventing the passage of bacteria. Choose disposable non-woven fabric, Goretex or tightly woven polycottons. The Charnley exhaust gown is of some benefit in prosthetic implant surgery. It is an important part of theatre discipline to change into fresh theatre clothing when entering the theatre suite because clothing worn in ward areas has been shown to be more heavily contaminated with microorganisms than freshly laundered 'scrub suits'.

Normal cotton clothing does little to prevent the passage of bacteria, especially those on skin scales, as the diameter of holes at the interstices of the cloth is usually greater than 80 μm. In addition, once cotton material is wet its barrier properties are much reduced, allowing bacteria to penetrate through from the wearer's skin; therefore, if clothes become wet, change them. 'Soak through' of blood has been shown to occur in over one-third of orthopaedic and general surgical operations and may present a risk to the wearer. Reduce the risk by using impermeable gowns or by wearing plastic aprons under linen gowns in situations where 'soak through' is likely.

Materials that reduce the dispersal of skin scales and bacteria are restrictive to wear so a compromise has to be reached. Clothing made from disposable non-woven fabric is suitable but expensive, as the whole team must wear it to obtain a benefit. Breathable membrane fabrics such as Goretex, or other materials such as tightly-woven washable polycottons are also suitable. Pay special attention to the design of the clothing so that bacteria are not 'pumped out' at the neck or the ankles. Most effective of all is the Charnley exhaust gown, which for maximum benefit must be used in conjunction with a unidirectional high efficiency particulate air (HEPA) filter system. It is also very restrictive and so rarely used by general surgeons. However it can be valuable in orthopaedic prosthetic surgery.

2. *Mask* use is controversial. Few bacteria are discharged from the mouth and nose during normal breathing and quiet conversation, and it is argued that for general abdominal operations masks are not required for

the protection of the patient, particularly by staff members in theatre who are not directly assisting. If you wear a mask, change it for each operation; reuse and manipulation simply contaminates the outside of the mask with skin commensals. Masks have been shown to reduce airborne contamination in ultraclean air theatres and should therefore be worn in prosthetic implant surgery.

An efficient mask must be capable of arresting low velocity droplets. Paper masks become wet within a few minutes and lose their barrier qualities, so do not use them. Disposable masks made of synthetic fibres are better and contain filters made of polyester or polypropylene. Surgical antifog masks with flexible nosebands are available; they follow facial contours and retain a high efficiency of filtration.

Masks continue to be worn to provide protection for the wearer against blood-borne viruses as part of a policy of universal (or standard) precautions. Full-face visors also afford similar protection.

3. *Eye protection/visors* also protect mucous membranes. Wear them during any procedure that is likely to generate droplets of blood or other body fluids, in order to protect your mucous membranes from blood-borne viruses. A variety of lightweight anti-fog goggles, glasses and visors are available that do not obstruct vision.

4. *Tie up long hair* and cover hair completely with a close-fitting cap made of synthetic material. Cover beards fully with a securely tied mask and hood of the balaclava type. This is especially important for prosthetic implant surgery.

5. *Footwear* has a minor role in spreading infection. There is little evidence that the floor plays a significant role in the spread of infections in hospital. Wear clean, comfortable, antislip and antistatic shoes. If there is a risk of fluid spillage, as in genitourinary surgery, wear ankle-length boots that can be cleaned with warm soapy water. Make sure your footwear fits well and does not produce a 'bellows' effect. Make sure they are sufficiently robust to protect your feet from sharps injury. Overshoes are not required for visitors who do not enter the operating or preparation rooms.

6. *Gloves* protect both you and your patient from blood-borne viruses (see Ch. 20) and prevent the wound from becoming contaminated with your skin flora. Wear single-use surgical gloves from a reputable source, sterilized by irradiation.

Surgical gloves made of natural rubber (latex) are increasingly reported to cause hypersensitivity reactions. Non-latex gloves without powder are available. Worryingly, many gloves are found to have pre-existing holes prior to use, as a result of inadequate quality control and poor manufacture. Furthermore, during the operation, around 20–30% develop holes of which the wearer is often unaware. Therefore inspect them at the end of each operation. Avoid needlestick injury; if you sustain one, let it bleed, and wash well with soap and water. As soon as possible fill in the accident form and report to the occupational health department.

Double-gloving affords extra protection but at the expense of reduced sensitivity and dexterity, and possible discomfort. In appropriate circumstances protect your fingers with armoured gloves or thimbles, in addition to protective clothing.

Theatre air

1. Air-borne bacteria are generally believed to be a source of postoperative sepsis, although this has been unequivocally proved only in the case of prosthetic orthopaedic implant infections. The number of circulating bacteria is directly related to the number of people in theatre, and their movements, which should both therefore be minimized. It is also affected by the type of theatre clothing worn.

Carefully balanced ventilation systems will not operate optimally if theatre doors are left ajar.

2. General operating theatres are equipped with *positive pressure* or *plenum* (Latin = *full*) ventilation systems, with the pressure decreasing from theatre to anaesthetic room to entrance lobby. Thus air-borne microorganisms tend to be carried out rather than in. In a conventional plenum system there should be a minimum of 20 air changes per hour. Routine checks of bioload are not required. Guidelines regarding theatre air ventilation and theatre design can be found in the Department of Health documents Health Technical Memorandum 2025, *Ventilation in Health Care Premises*, and Health Building Note number 26, *Operating Department*.

3. Ultraclean air systems are advocated for prosthetic implant surgery. In these systems, instead of the turbulent airflow associated with plenum pressure systems, there is unidirectional or *laminar* airflow at about 300 air changes per hour. The air is recirculated through high efficiency particulate air (HEPA) filters. This produces a reduction in circulating microorganisms compared with a conventional system. In these theatres regular bacteriological assessment should be undertaken.

A large multicentre study in prosthetic orthopaedic surgery demonstrated that the incidence of deep periarticular infections was reduced from 3.4% to 1.6% by the use of ultraclean air conditions. With the addition of prophylactic antibiotics, the infection rate was reduced further to 0.19%. Bear in mind that, if the level of asepsis is otherwise only moderate, the impact of ultraclean air systems may be lost. Their role in clean surgery other than prosthetic implant surgery is uncertain.

Surgeon preparation

1. Most theatre-acquired infections are of endogenous origin, but the scrub team must ensure that they do not put their patients at risk. In order to minimize the risk of transmitting infection to patients, you must all satisfy local occupational health requirements before entering the operating theatre. For example, you must not operate with bacterial pharyngitis, during the prodromal (Greek *pro* = before + *dromos* = run, course; hence, incipient) period of a viral illness or with chronic or infected skin conditions. Try to avoid operating if you have cuts, cracks, sores or rashes on your hands or forearms. If in doubt take advice from the occupational health department. The Department of Health has issued comprehensive guidance regarding healthcare workers infected with blood-borne viruses (see Ch. 20).

2. The term 'scrubbing up' is unlikely to disappear from surgical practice but repeated scrubbing is counterproductive because it results in skin abrasions and more bacteria being brought to the surface. At the start of a list have an initial scrub of 3–5 minutes; thereafter, use effective handwashing with an antiseptic between cases. Skin antiseptics act rapidly and some have a cumulative effect. Use sterile, single-use brushes of polypropylene, not with wood or bristles. Do not shower prior to operating, it increases the number of bacteria shed from the skin.

3. Antiseptics commonly used are:

a. Chlorhexidine gluconate 4% (Hibiscrub), which is rapidly active, broad spectrum and persists with a cumulative effect, even under surgical gloves. It is easy to use but the detergent-like effect must be washed off with running water. Some surgeons are allergic to it and can use hexachlorophane or povidone-iodine.

b. Hexachlorophane (pHisoHex), which is effective only against Gram-positive bacteria and has a slow action but a cumulative effect.

c. Povidone–iodine (Betadine), which acts more rapidly than hexachlorophane and has a broader spectrum but does not have a prolonged effect.

4. Dry your hands thoroughly using single-use sterile towels. Hot-air drying machines are not recommended.

Preparation of the patient

1. The longer a patient stays in hospital before operation, the greater the likelihood of a subsequent wound infection. Keep hospital stay as short as possible and carry out as many tests as possible beforehand, as an outpatient. Cultures from postoperative wound infections often suggest that organisms are transferred from other areas of the patient to the operative site (endogenous transfer) despite the use of antiseptics. Ensure that the patient is socially clean prior to operation. The value of routine preoperative showering with antiseptic solutions remains unproven. Infections at other sites increase the risk of surgical wound infection; therefore, diagnose and treat pre-existing infections before elective operation. Similarly, consider eradicating MRSA carriage in colonized patients prior to elective surgery.

2. The patient can be transported to theatre in bed directly, after being changed into a clean operating gown. Remove ward blankets before entering theatre. There is no need for a special transfer area, changing trolleys, porters putting on plastic overshoes, or passing the trolley wheels over a sticky mat. Trolleys must be cleaned daily.

3. Shaving of the operation site increases wound infection rates because of injury to the skin. If hair removal is necessary, use clippers or depilatory cream. If it is essential to shave the area, it should be performed as near as possible to the time of operation, preferably by you, prior to scrubbing up.

4. Prepare the skin area around and including the operation site. First scrub it with a sponge or swab impregnated with detergent. After the skin has been cleaned and degreased in this way, use antiseptic solutions. For intact skin consider alcoholic solutions of chlorhexidine or povidone-iodine rather than aqueous solutions. However, take care when applying alcohol solutions if you use diathermy; if it pools in the umbilicus or under the perineum, you may cause fire hazard. For vaginal or perineal disinfection consider a solution of chlorhexidine and cetrimide (Savlon).

5. Traditionally the periphery of the proposed incision site was protected with sterile cotton drapes; however, these soon become wet, diminishing their protective properties. Incisional plastic drapes have been advocated but Cruse & Foord (1980) showed that applying adhesive plastic drapes to the operation area does not decrease the wound infection rate; this has since been confirmed in a study of caesarean section.

Cleaning and disinfection

1. Decontamination, or the process of removing microbial contaminants, can be carried out by cleaning, disinfection or sterilization. The appropriate method of decontamination is determined by the risk of infection associated with the object or procedure.

a. Cleaning is a process that removes visible contamination but does not necessarily destroy microorganisms. It is a necessary prerequisite to effective disinfection or sterilization.

b. Disinfection is a process that reduces the number of viable microorganisms to an acceptable level but may not inactivate some viruses, hardy organisms such as mycobacteria and bacterial spores. A topical disinfectant that may safely be applied to epithelial tissues is known as an antiseptic.

Where an interventional procedure is planned for a patient known, suspected or at risk of suffering from a transmissible spongiform encephalopathy (TSE) such as Creutzfeldt–Jakob disease (CJD) or variant CJD, seek advice from the infection control team and sterile service department.

2. Disinfection of heat-tolerant items can be achieved reliably by exposure to moist heat; for items such as surgical equipment and bedpans it can be carried out using a washer-disinfector. Recommended time–temperature combinations are 71°C for 3 min, 80°C for 1 min or 90°C for 12 s. Boiling water kills bacteria, some viruses (including human immunodeficiency virus (HIV) and hepatitis B virus (HBV)) and some spores. It does not sterilize. Soft water at 100°C at normal pressure for 10 min is satisfactory. Suitable instruments include specula, proctoscopes and sigmoidoscopes. This method is now rarely used in secondary care.

3. Chemical disinfection can be used where heat cannot. A good example is the use of glutaraldehyde 2% (Cidex) to decontaminate flexible endoscopes. It is rapidly active against most vegetative bacteria and viruses (including HIV and HBV), and slowly effective against tuberculosis and spores. It is toxic, irritant and allergenic.

Other chemical disinfectants include hypochlorite solutions, chlorine dioxide, superoxidized water and peracetic acid.

Those involved in the purchase and development of new instrumentation for surgery or investigation need to consider how it may be decontaminated at the end of the procedure. Recent years have seen the introduction of increasing numbers of instruments that cannot be sterilized and can be disinfected only with difficulty. As sterilization by heat is the most reliable and easily monitored method, choose reusable instruments that will withstand autoclaving, if possible. Reprocessing of disposable equipment is hazardous and must not be carried out.

Antiseptics include chlorhexidine, iodophors such as povidone-iodine, triclosan and 70% alcohol.

Sterilization

This is defined as the complete destruction of all viable microorganisms, including spores, viruses and mycobacteria. It is, in practice, defined in terms of the probability of a single viable microorganism surviving on 1 million items. The term sterilization (Latin *sterilis* = barren) can be applied only to equipment and not to the skin, where antisepsis alone can be achieved.

1. Steam under pressure attains a higher temperature than boiling water and the final temperature is directly related to the pressure. Instruments can be cleaned, then reliably sterilized by steam under pressure using autoclaves. The process can kill bacteria, including *Mycobacterium tuberculosis*, viruses and heat-resistant spores. The preferred cycle is 134°C at 2 atmospheres for a holding time of 3 min, which entails a total cycle time of at least 30 min to reach the required temperature. Autoclaves should be centralized in specialized units, e.g. the sterile service department (SSD) or theatre sterile service unit (TSSU) and maintained by highly trained personnel. Maintenance and performance tests are very strictly controlled. In the future there will be a requirement for systems tracing the decontamination processes of surgical instruments.

Small portable autoclaves are used in some theatres for convenience. There is a potential danger in that they are used by staff untrained in scrutinizing and maintaining them. Many portable autoclaves are unsuitable for processing wrapped instruments or those with a narrow lumen.

In patients at risk of TSE, for procedures not involving high risk tissues, use the autoclave, after thorough cleaning of the instruments, with a cycle of 18 min at 134°C or six cycles of 3 min.

2. Destroy instruments used for invasive procedures on patients known to have TSE, using incineration (ACDP 1998). The same applies to instruments used on patients suspected of having TSE, unless an alternative diagnosis is established, and for instruments coming into contact with high risk tissues, such as brain, spinal cord or the eye, in patients at risk of developing TSE. Therefore, when possible use single-use instruments.

3. Sterilization can be achieved by dry heat at 160°C for a holding time of 1 h. The process is inefficient compared with steam sterilization, but has the advantage of being able to treat non-aqueous liquids, ointments and airtight containers. It is also useful for avoiding corrosion of non-stainless metals and instruments with fine cutting edges, such as ophthalmic instruments. Do not use it for aqueous fluids or for materials that are likely to be damaged by the process, such as rubber and plastics. This equipment is subject to rigorous checks and maintenance.

4. Sterilants are chemical compounds that, under defined conditions, are able to kill bacterial spores:

a. Ethylene oxide (EO) is a highly penetrative, non-corrosive agent with a broad cidal (Latin *caedere* = to kill) action against bacteria, spores and viruses; however, it is also flammable, toxic, irritant, mutagenic and potentially carcinogenic, and should not be used when heat sterilization is possible. Its main uses are for wrapped and unwrapped heat-sensitive equipment: it is ideal for electrical equipment, flexible-fibre endoscopes and photographic equipment. Do not use it for ventilatory equipment. It is inappropriate for items with organic soiling. EO sterilization is a mainly industrial process for single-use medical devices. There are a limited number of NHS regional units. It is expensive, has a slow turnaround time, is potentially dangerous and must be carefully controlled and monitored.

b. Glutaraldehyde: shorter immersion times provide disinfection, but 3–10 h of exposure to 2% alkaline glutaraldehyde is required for sporicidal activity.

c. Other sterilants include peracetic acid, superoxidized water, gas plasma and chlorine dioxide; however, validation processes have not yet been established by the Department of Health for some of these newer technologies.

5. Irradiation employs gamma rays or accelerated electrons. It is an industrial process suitable for sterilizing large batches of similar products, such as catheters and syringes.

Spillages

Have body fluid spillage removed as soon as possible. Gloves and a plastic apron should be worn. First, cover spills with an appropriate disinfectant such as hypochlorite granules (Presept), then absorbent paper towels. Discard as clinical waste. Do not use chlorine-releasing agents on urine spills or chlorine gas will be released.

Waste disposal

Sort hospital waste to ensure it is correctly disposed of. Place 'sharps' in approved containers, and clinical waste in yellow plastic bags. These are disposed of, usually by incineration, separately from domestic waste, which may be sent for landfill. Other categories of waste requiring segregation include pharmaceuticals and radioactive or cytotoxic waste.

SURGICAL TECHNIQUE

Postoperative infection rate is influenced by the following factors.

- The longer the operation, the more likely is the wound to become infected. Perform operations as expediently as safety allows.
- Keep operative trauma to a minimum and handle tissues gently.

- Make incisions with sharp instruments – they are less likely to become infected than those produced, for example, by cautery; however, cautery may reduce the need for sutures, which can act as a nidus for infection. Use the finest suitable ligature.
- Haematomas are at risk of becoming infected.
- Necrotic or ischaemic areas are at risk.
- Avoid leaving a dead space.
- Avoid unwarranted prophylactic drains, which increase the risk of infection. Insert a necessary drain through a separate stab, not through the wound. Use an entirely closed system to decrease the chance of ascending infection, and remove it as soon as possible.

Key point

- **Why do some surgeons performing standard operations have minimal infection? Their technique is impeccable!**

PROPHYLACTIC ANTIBIOTICS

It has been shown that, for many contaminated and clean-contaminated procedures, postoperative infection can be avoided by using appropriate prophylactic antibiotics given prior to surgery. The general principles of antibiotic prophylaxis (Greek *pro* = before + *phylax* = a guard) are as follows:

1. Use antibiotic prophylaxis only when wound contamination is expected or when operations on a contaminated site may lead to bacteraemia. It is not required for clean-wound procedures except:

a. When you insert an implant or vascular graft

b. In valvular heart disease to prevent infective endocarditis

c. During emergency surgery in a patient with pre-existing or recently active infection

d. If an infection would be very severe or have life-threatening consequences.

2. There is no evidence that prolonged prophylaxis has any advantage over short courses – 24 h. Prolonged administration may lead to superinfection. Normally in a clean operation one dose is sufficient. In contaminated operations three doses are often given.

3. Administer the antibiotic parenterally, immediately prior to operation to achieve effective tissue levels. If you give them soon afterwards they do not prevent infection. If the procedure continues for more than 3–4 h, or if there

is excessive blood loss, give a further dose in theatre or tissue levels may no longer be effective. Acrylic cement containing gentamicin has been used successfully in joint replacement surgery.

4. Select antibiotics to cover relevant organisms after discussion with the microbiologist regarding likely contaminants and local resistance patterns. For example, in orthopaedic surgery the main pathogens are staphylococci, but in bowel surgery cover is required for anaerobic and Gram-negative aerobic bowel flora. Work together with the microbiologist to develop standard policies for the unit, and follow them strictly when they are in place.

FEEDBACK TO YOU AND THE UNIT

Using these four strategies, aim to keep your postoperative infection rate to a minimum. Both you and the unit must keep aware of your infection rates and determine to keep them comparable with rates in other similar units. Achieve this by surveillance and infection audit.

Surveillance

This is the systematic collection, collation, analysis and distribution of data and it has been shown to be valuable in the prevention of infection. The Study on the Efficacy of Nosocomial Infection Control (SENIC) was carried out in the USA over 10 years in the 1970s. A random sample of 1000 patients from each of 338 hospitals was studied and details about each patient were recorded and analysed. It was found that infections of the urinary tract were the most common nosocomial infections but, as already mentioned, wound infections were the most costly, both financially and in terms of delayed discharge from hospital.

SENIC data measured intensity of surveillance, control efforts, policy development and teaching and whether or not infection rates were fed back confidentially to individual surgeons. In hospitals with optimal performance in all these categories the wound infection rate was 38% lower. The key factor in this reduction appears to be confidential feedback to individual surgeons. This is known as the Hawthorne effect.

There are a number of different types of surveillance of nosocomial infection and no clear consensus regarding the optimal method. Continuous hospital-wide surveillance may be expensive and time consuming, while targeted surveillance may be more practical and cost effective. Whichever method is employed, it is essential that the definitions of infection are clearly understood and reliably applied. Despite the drawbacks, surveillance is useful not only for feedback but also for identifying changes in epidemiology or a rise in infection rates, or for assessing the effect of implementing new preventive strategies.

Due to the increase in day surgery and shorter hospital stays, there is evidence suggesting that the majority of surgical wound infections will present after hospital discharge. The addition of postdischarge surveillance will therefore provide a more accurate reflection of the true healthcare-associated infection rate.

Infection audit

Although a record of overall infection rates by surveillance is the ideal, this may not always be practical, as discussed above. Clinical audit is a way of reviewing clinical practice and outcomes and it has also been shown to be useful in surgical practice. All UK NHS units are required to carry out audit of their practices. It is important to audit infection rates. An acceptable standard exists and steps can be taken to improve rates in the process of closing the audit loop.

Summary

- Do you recognize that postoperative wound infections cause serious morbidity to patients and expense to hospitals?
- Can you classify surgical wounds? What are the infection rates you would expect for each type of surgical wound?
- Can you outline the main strategies for minimizing the risk of surgical wound infection?
- What is the single most important measure for preventing the spread of infection between patients?
- What do the terms asepsis, antisepsis, sterilization and disinfection mean? Name two antiseptics.
- Can you list the main aseptic precautions taken in theatre?
- Can you list the major methods of sterilization and disinfection, and give examples of when to use them?
- Can you describe the principles of antimicrobial prophylaxis and give examples?
- What is the value of surveillance of hospital-acquired infection to surgical practice?

References

ACDP, Advisory Committee on Dangerous Pathogens Spongiform Encephalopathy Advisory Committee 1998 Transmissible spongiform encephalopathy agents: safe working and the prevention of infection. HMSO, London

Cruse PJE, Foord R 1980 The epidemiology of wound infection: a 10-year prospective study of 62 939 wounds. Surgical Clinics of North America 60: 1

Duckworth G et al 1998 Revised guidelines for the control of methicillin-resistant *Staphylococcus aureus* infection in hospitals. Report of a combined working party of the British Society for Antimicrobial Chemotherapy, the Hospital Infection Society and the Infection Control Nurses Association. Journal of Hospital Infection 39: 253–290

Pratt RJ, Pellowe C, Loveday HP et al 2001 Standard principles for preventing hospital acquired infections. Journal of Hospital Infection 47S: S21–S37

Further reading

Ayliffe GAJ, Fraise AP, Geddes AM, Mitchell K (eds) 2000 Control of hospital infection, 4th edn. Arnold, London

Morgan D (ed.) 1995 A code of practice for sterilization of instruments and control of cross infection (amended). British Medical Association, London

Philpot-Howard J, Casewell M 1995 Hospital infection control. Saunders, London

20 The risks to surgeons of nosocomial virus transmission

D. J. Jeffries, I. Ushiro-Lumb

Objectives

- **Understand the main surgically important viruses.**
- **Appreciate the sources and methods of viral transmission.**
- **Recognize how to reduce the risks of transmission during surgical treatment.**
- **Know what action to take if exposure to infection has occurred.**

INTRODUCTION

Many different viruses have been associated with nosocomial (Greek *nosos* = disease + *komeein* = to tend; relating to hospital) spread and healthcare workers frequently become infected as part of a hospital outbreak. It may be difficult to define the extent of an outbreak of a nosocomial virus infection due to a virus such as influenza or respiratory syncytial virus, as there is usually evidence of a parallel outbreak in the community and new infections are likely to be introduced repeatedly by patients, visitors and staff. Some viruses (e.g. herpes simplex, varicella-zoster and viral haemorrhagic fever viruses) may be spread to healthcare workers by close patient contact, while others may be widely disseminated in a ward or outpatient unit, e.g. winter vomiting due to small round structured viruses (SRSVs). The risk of acquiring a nosocomial virus infection is reduced by the following measures:

1. Education and awareness of the risks
2. Isolation or cohorting of patients when appropriate
3. Good hygiene and adherence to infection control procedures
4. Immunization, if vaccines are available
5. Postexposure measures if available.

Close collaboration between microbiologists, virologists and other healthcare workers ensures that staff are aware of the risks from individual infected patients and of the appropriate procedures necessary to control these risks. All healthcare workers in contact with patients or their samples are exposed to nosocomial virus infections and, provided that adequate protective clothing and other facilities are available, the risk of occupationally acquired infection is accepted as part of the job. Surgeons are at no greater risk of acquiring most of the recognized nosocomial virus infections than any other healthcare worker (for detailed reviews of specific infections and their control see Breuer & Jeffries (1990) and Jeffries (1995a)). The nature of your work exposes you to the risk of infection from blood-borne viruses, particularly human immunodeficiency virus (HIV), hepatitis B virus (HBV) and hepatitis C virus (HCV). All of these viruses may lead to a prolonged infectious carrier state, and demonstration of persistent infection in a surgeon may lead to the need to change his or her practice to avoid exposure-prone invasive procedures or, if this is not possible, it may be necessary to change to another speciality. There are potentially serious outcomes from blood-borne virus infections that may be occupationally acquired; this chapter is therefore focused on these agents.

THE BLOOD-BORNE VIRUSES

Blood-borne viruses posing the highest risk of nosocomial crossinfection are those associated with a chronic carrier state, where continuous viral replication leads to persistent viraemia. Currently, the three most important agents to consider in this setting are HIV, HBV and HCV. Seek expert advice if other, less common, blood-borne viruses are being considered.

The main features of HIV and the hepatitis viruses are presented in the 1995 publication from the Advisory Committee on Dangerous Pathogens (ACDP), entitled *Protection Against Bloodborne Infections in the Workplace*, and in a review by Jeffries (1997).

Human immunodeficiency viruses (HIV-1, HIV-2)

The first cases of the acquired immune deficiency syndrome (AIDS) were recognized in 1981 and in 1983 a retrovirus (HIV-1) was identified and was subsequently shown to be the causative agent. In 1985, a second human immunodeficiency virus (HIV-2) was isolated from individuals from West Africa and this has now spread to other parts of Africa, India and Europe. The two viruses are very similar and their modes of spread and clinical effects are identical, although there is some evidence that disease progression is slower in HIV-2 infection. In this chapter the two viruses are referred to collectively as HIV. HIV contains RNA and during the course of its replication the genetic material of the viral particle is reverse-transcribed by an enzyme, reverse transcriptase, into a DNA copy, which is inserted into the chromosomes of an infected cell. This integrated package of viral genetic material (or provirus) produces new viral particles, which are available to infect other cells. Thus, following primary infection with HIV, the virus persists within cells for the life of the cells and, because of continual transfer to other cells in the immune system and central nervous system, the infection persists for the life of the individual. Recent work indicates that an HIV-infected individual produces very high levels of virus, 10^9–10^{10} virus particles per day, and is consequently potentially infectious to others for life. In health care, the nature of the viral particle, which is surrounded by a lipid-containing envelope, means that it is easily destroyed by heat, disinfectants and detergents. At ambient temperatures, however, the virus is protected from desiccation and may persist in dried blood or secretions for several days.

The major cellular receptor for HIV is the CD4 antigen which is present on helper T lymphocytes and cells of the antigen-presenting series. These are the main target cells for the virus and gradual depletion of these cells over a period of years leads to the opportunistic infections and tumours that are characteristic of AIDS. Potent and complex combinations of antiretroviral drugs have been in use for many years now, with an ensuing decline in morbidity and mortality among individuals who achieve long-term viral suppression.

Hepatitis B virus (HBV)

Hepatitis B virus is a DNA virus which causes acute hepatitis; because of its long incubation period (45–180 days, mean 75 days) it was previously known as long-incubation hepatitis (or serum hepatitis). During the acute infection, and in carriers of HBV, viral particles released from the liver are present in the circulation. The surface coating of the particles is present in excess and this material, hepatitis B surface antigen (HBsAg), is identified by serological tests as the main indicator of active infection. A second antigen, HBeAg, which is derived from core particles of the virus present in the liver, indicates continuing activity of the virus in the liver, and the presence of HBeAg in the

blood correlates with high levels of infectivity. Note, however, that precore mutants of HBV exist, which are unable to express HBeAg but continue to produce infectious viral particles. Individuals carrying such HBV variants may have high levels of viraemia despite undetectable serum HBeAg, which ultimately translate into higher levels of infectivity than previously thought. The implications of this HBV variant in the healthcare setting will be further addressed when discussing the infected healthcare worker.

As with all types of viral hepatitis, the degree of illness produced is variable and ranges in different individuals from asymptomatic infection to acute hepatic failure. The immune response is a major factor in determining the severity of disease. In the immunologically immature or immunocompromised, asymptomatic infections are common, but the risks of proceeding to long-term carriage of the virus are high. The long-term carrier rate following neonatal infection is >90%, in children aged 1–10 years it is 23%, and in adults 5% or less become carriers. This high rate of persistence following infection in early life largely explains the estimated 250–300 million carriers in the world, the majority of whom are in resource-deprived countries, where 15–20% of the population may be infected.

The carrier of HBV presents a potential risk of horizontal transmission to others, predominantly via sexual intercourse and blood transfer. The HBV-positive mother is also likely to infect her baby during delivery, with the highest risk amongst HBeAg-positive carriers (up to 90%). Vertical transmission is in fact a very important route of HBV spread in parts of the world where the virus is highly endemic.

Persistent replication of HBV in the liver of HbeAg-positive carriers carries a risk of progressive liver damage, leading to chronic active hepatitis, cirrhosis and an increased risk of hepatocellular carcinoma.

Hepatitis C virus (HCV)

Following the identification of HBV, the continued occurrence of post-transfusion hepatitis led to the realization that there were other blood-borne hepatitis viruses (termed non-A, non-B hepatitis). The RNA virus, HCV, is now recognized as the major cause of non-A, non-B hepatitis, with an estimated 170 million people infected worldwide. Hepatitis C is predominantly blood borne and infection is common in injecting drug users and recipients of unscreened blood and/or blood products. The acute phase of HCV infection is usually asymptomatic and only approximately 10% of individuals have overt hepatitis. Following primary infection, however, the majority (about 80%) proceed to become persistent carriers of the virus and, as with HBV infection, there is a long-term risk of chronic liver disease with cirrhosis (10–30%) and hepatocellular carcinoma. In the industrialized world, chronic HCV infection is the leading cause of chronic liver disease and the most common indication for liver transplant.

SOURCES OF INFECTION

As the term implies, the major blood-borne viruses, HIV, HBV and HCV, are found predominantly in the circulation and most occupational infections occur as a result of exposure to blood. Other body fluids may contain infectious virus, however, and these are listed in Table 20.1. Percutaneous inoculation is the major route of infection in health care; there is no evidence of transmission of any of the common blood-borne viruses by the airborne route or from occupational or social contact that does not involve body fluid exposure.

RISKS OF INFECTION

Transmission of blood-borne viruses from patient to healthcare worker most commonly occurs following percutaneous exposure to infected blood through a 'sharps' injury. Although transmission may also result from contamination of broken skin, or of mucous membranes of the eyes or mouth, the risks are much lower.

HIV

The overall risk of acquiring HIV following a single percutaneous inoculation with HIV-infected blood is approximately 0.36% (1 in 275). The results of a case–control study of 31 healthcare workers infected occupationally, compared with 679 control subjects, identified several factors that affected the risks of percutaneous transmis-

sion of HIV (Centers for Disease Control 1988). These are listed in Table 20.2. Note from the table that, in this case–control study, the use of the antiviral drug AZT reduced the transmission rate by 80%. This will be returned to later. The risk of acquiring HIV from mucous membrane or conjunctival exposure to blood from infected individuals is lower than from percutaneous inoculation. One seroconversion was reported on follow up of 1107 exposures (Jeffries 1995b).

HBV

Hepatitis B immunization has dramatically altered the level of risk to surgeons and other healthcare workers. Before the introduction of safe and potent HBV vaccines and subsequent checks of immune status, the risk of infection could be as high as 30% after percutaneous injury involving the blood of an HbeAg-positive patient. Transmission of HBV has also been associated with mucous membrane exposure to blood and with bites from HBV-infected patients but the risk of infection from these routes has not been quantified.

HCV

The risk of percutaneous transmission of HCV has not been clearly defined and rates of 0–10% have been reported. In a small study of 68 healthcare workers in Japan, who sustained percutaneous exposure to the blood of HCV RNA-positive patients with chronic renal failure or HCV-related liver disease, seven (10%) developed markers of infection. In a survey of 3267 orthopaedic surgeons in the USA, HCV antibodies were present in 0.8%. The antibody prevalence increased from 0% in the 20–29 year age group to 1.4% in those over 60 years. For comparison, 12% had evidence of past or current HBV infection (ranging from 2.9% in the 20–29 year age group to 26% in those 60+) and two surgeons were HIV positive (both had other risk factors apart from surgery).

Table 20.1 Body fluids, etc. that should be handled with the same precautions as blood

1. CSF
   Semen
   Vaginal secretions
   Breast milk
   Amniotic fluid
   Peritoneal fluid
   Pleural fluid
   Pericardial fluid
   Synovial fluid
2. Any other body fluid containing visible blood
3. Unfixed tissues and organs

Table 20.2 Factors affecting percutaneous transmission of HIV during occupational exposure		
Factor	Odds ratio*	95% CI
Deep injury (intramuscular)	16.1	6.1–44.6
Visible blood on device	5.2	1.8–17.7
Needle used in a blood vessel	5.1	1.9–14.8
Source patient with AIDS	6.4	2.2–18.9
AZT prophylaxis used	0.2	0.1–0.6

*Significant at $p < 0.01$.

Adapted from Centers for Disease Control (1988).

REDUCING THE RISKS OF INFECTION

General measures – universal precautions

It is neither cost effective nor reliable to embark on routine screening of patients for blood-borne viruses. The marker tests for infectivity, HIV and HCV antibodies and HBsAg become positive up to 12 weeks, 26 weeks and 26 weeks, respectively, after infection and a patient may be highly infectious before positivity is demonstrated. Similarly, it is unreliable to attempt to identify carriers of the viruses by designation of 'risk groups'. Although the blood-borne viruses HIV and HCV were originally associated with homosexuality and drug use, the spread of infection outside of perceived risk groups, and control of infection in those previously perceived to be in risk groups by education, needle exchange schemes, etc., means that 'risky activity' by anyone should raise the suspicion of possible infection. Faced with the ever present risk of occupational infection, you should adopt a policy of 'universal precautions' with regard to carrying out procedures with a risk of contact with high risk body fluids and tissues (see Table 20.1). The basis and procedure of using universal precautions was presented by the Centers for Disease Control (1987, 1988, 1991) and by the UK Health Departments (1990, 1998). As percutaneous inoculation is the major route of infection, take care when handling sharp instruments. In some studies, approximately 40% of inoculation injuries of staff have occurred during attempts to resheathe needles.

Key points

- **Always pass sharp instruments to others through the vehicle of a rigid container, never directly.**
- **Do not attempt to resheath needles unless there is a resheathing device available. Discard them into a 'sharps' container.**

Do not leave suture needles and scalpels on trays for others to clear away. Cover cuts and abrasions with waterproof dressings and wear disposable gloves if there is a risk of contamination of your hands with blood. Wear protective eyewear and a mask if there is likely to be any splashing with blood or other body fluids.

It is possible to produce guidelines for the use of protective clothing on the basis of an assessment of likely exposure to blood (Table 20.3).

Attend to blood spillage on to a surface promptly, by first covering it with disposable towels, and apply a suitable disinfectant, such as sodium hypochlorite (10 000 parts per million available chlorine), in accordance to local infection control guidelines.

Immune prophylaxis

While neither passive nor active prophylaxis is available for HIV and HCV, HBV infection is preventable by immunization with the current, safe, genetically-engineered

Table 20.3	Categorization of procedures according to risk of exposure to blood	
Category	Examples of procedures	Protective measures
A(i) Contact likely: risk of uncontrolled bleeding	Major surgery Gynaecology Obstetrics	Full range of protective clothing (gloves, water–repellent gown and apron, protective headwear, mask, protective eyewear, protective footwear)
A(ii) Contact probable; splattering unlikely	Intra-arterial puncture Insertion/removal of intravenous/ intra-arterial lines Dentistry	Gloves to be worn Masks/protective eyewear to be available
A(iii) Low likelihood of blood contact	i.m., i.d., s.c. injections	Gloves available
B No risk of blood contact	Most ward/clinic work	None necessary
Adapted from UK Health Departments (1990).		

vaccines. All staff likely to be exposed to blood, tissues or other body fluids in the course of their work should be immunized and their antibody levels should then be checked to ensure that they have developed protective immunity. If response to the vaccine is inadequate, the healthcare worker's hepatitis B status should be investigated to exclude current or past HBV infection. Those who are susceptible to HBV and fail to mount an antibody response to the vaccine must be made aware that they are non-responders and, in the event of exposure to known or suspected HBV-positive blood, they should be offered passive protection with HBV immunoglobulin (HBIG).

Reducing blood exposure of you and your patient during operation

In an observational study by Tokars et al (1992), the rate of inoculation injury was recorded during the course of different types of surgical operation. Percutaneous injury rates to the main operator per 100 procedures were 4 for orthopaedics, 8 for general surgery, 9 for coronary artery bypass grafting, 17 for gastrectomy and 21 for vaginal hysterectomy. Inspection of gloves after operation has revealed a perforation rate for single glove use of 11–54% (Church & Sanderson 1980, Brough et al 1988, Maffulli et al 1989, Smith & Grant 1990, Palmer & Rickett 1992). The wearing of two pairs of surgical gloves has been reported to result in perforation of the inner glove in 2% of operations (Matta et al 1988). Penetration of the glove material by a sharp instrument or needle has a significant wiping effect and this reduces the volume of blood and amount of virus transferred. Studies using a paper prefilter model in vitro and an ex vivo porcine tissue model demonstrated a reduction of blood transfer of 46–86%, depending on whether a solid or hollow needle was used and on the gauge of the latter (Mast et al 1993). Thus, although standard disposable latex gloves offer no protection against needle penetration, this evidence of reduction of exposure to blood provides strong support for the use of gloves, even in simple procedures such as venepuncture, if there is a risk of injury to the operator, for example in the case of an uncooperative patient.

A number of aspects of surgical technique are worthy of appraisal in the interests of reducing the risk of percutaneous injury.

Key points

- **Whenever possible have one person only working in an open wound or body cavity at any one time.**

- **Favour the 'hands-free' technique, in which the same sharp instrument is not touched by more than one person at the same time.**

The need for care in passing instruments to others has already been stressed. Needles, scalpels and other sharp instruments should not be left in the operating field. Have them removed promptly by the scrub nurse after they have been deposited in a neutral zone, such as a tray or kidney dish. Use instruments rather than fingers for retraction and holding tissues during suturing. Remove scalpel blades from handles with instruments and direct all needles and sharp instruments away from your own non-dominant, or your assistant's hand. Remove suture needles before tying sutures, or use instruments rather than fingers for tying.

In addition to the discipline of carrying out surgical techniques, in appropriate circumstances consider using alternative equipment. Electrocautery, blunt-tipped needles and stapling devices may reduce the need for sharp instruments and needles. Avoid using sharp clips for surgical drapes. Prefer blunt clips or disposable drapes incorporating self-adhesive film. Employ scalpels which are disposable, have a blade release device or retractable blades, to remove the risk of injuries associated with assembly or disassembly of these instruments.

The risk of contact with infected blood varies depending on the local prevalence of infections and the nature of the patient population. With the current distribution of blood-borne viruses, however, all operating theatre staff are exposed from time to time. The decision to introduce double-gloving for all surgical procedures may depend on a local risk assessment, but other measures to reduce exposure to blood and other body fluids can be applied to all operative procedures.

Postexposure measures

Key point

- **As soon as possible after percutaneous inoculation or, in the case of operative surgery, as soon as the patient is stable and can be left to the care of others, wash the site of injury liberally with soap and water.**

Avoid scrubbing, encourage bleeding. Do not use antiseptic preparations, as the effect of these on local defences is unknown. Wash out splashes into the eye or mouth by irrigating with copious volumes of water.

Complete an incident form and contact the occupational health department or another doctor designated with the responsibility of caring for staff, as specified in the local guidelines.

Key point

- **Seek advice at once; if postexposure prophylactic drugs for HIV are to be considered, they should be started without delay, and ideally within 1 h of exposure.**

It is normal practice to take a blood sample from the staff member at this time as the stored serum can then be used as a baseline for further testing. Laboratory testing of the source patient, after pretest discussion and obtaining fully informed consent, will aid further management by clarifying the risks, if any, of exposure to blood-borne viruses.

Key point

- **Decisions on postexposure prophylaxis should not await results of testing the source patient. Immediate assessment of risk of transmission must include the source patient's history and the type and severity of the exposure.**

HIV

Guidelines for the use of postexposure chemoprophylaxis to prevent HIV infection of healthcare workers were issued in the UK in June 1997 (UK Health Departments 1997). Postexposure prophylaxis is recommended when there has been significant exposure to material known, or strongly suspected, to be infected with HIV. Significant routes of exposure are percutaneous inoculation, exposure of broken skin or contact with mucous membranes, including the eye, and high risk material (listed in Table 20.1). As in equivalent guidelines issued in the USA, the first-line drugs for postexposure prophylaxis are currently combined zidovudine (AZT) 300 mg and lamivudine (3TC) 150 mg b.d., and nelfinavir 1250 mg b.d. Treatment should start as soon as possible, ideally within 1 h of exposure, and should be continued for 1 month. A negative test for HIV antibody 6 months after the exposure confirms the absence of occupationally acquired infection.

HBV

If the source patient is known or suspected to be an HBV carrier, the prophylactic regimen will depend on the immune status of the healthcare worker. Those who have never had vaccine should receive hepatitis B immunoglobulin (HBIG) within 48 h of exposure and a course of hepatitis B vaccination should be started as soon as possible. In those who have been vaccinated, the recommendation of the occupational health adviser is likely to depend on the record of the person's antibody response. If there is a recorded antibody response of more than 100 min ml^{-1} within the previous year, no further action is necessary. If the person's blood has not been tested within the year, or if a lower titre was recorded, a booster dose of vaccine followed by retesting of antibody status may be necessary. Healthcare workers who have failed in the past to respond to the vaccine should be offered protection with HBIG.

HCV

There is currently no prophylaxis for HCV and follow up consists of monitoring liver function and testing for anti-HCV antibodies and HCV RNA. There is, however, growing evidence to suggest that commencement of antiviral therapy with interferon-α during the acute phase of HCV infection can prevent chronic carriage (Jaeckel et al 2001), and occupational exposure to HCV is potentially the ideal indication for interventions of this nature.

INFECTED HEALTHCARE WORKERS

Guidelines issued by the General Medical Council, General Dental Council and the United Kingdom Central Coordinating Committee for Nurses, Midwives and Health Visitors (UKCCC) stress the importance of healthcare workers who consider that they have been at risk of infection with HBV or HIV seeking appropriate pretest discussion and testing. If found to be infected, they have a responsibility to be under regular medical supervision. Guidelines issued in the UK recommend that those who are infected with HIV or who are 'high infectivity' (HBeAg) carriers of HBV should not perform exposure-prone invasive procedures (UK Health Departments 1993, 1994). Exposure-prone procedures are defined as:

Those where there is a risk that injury to the worker may result in the exposure of the patient's open tissues to the blood of the worker. These procedures include those where the worker's gloved hands may be in contact with sharp instruments, needle tips or sharp tissues (spicules of bone or teeth) inside a patient's body cavity, wound or confined anatomical space where the hands or fingertips may not be visible at all times.

In the UK, until recently and according to the above guidelines, there were no practice restrictions to HBV carriers without detectable HBeAg, unless transmission to patients had been demonstrated. In the light of accumulated evidence of transmission of HBV from HBeAg-negative carrier surgeons (harbouring precore variants of HBV) to their patients and better knowledge of levels of viraemia associated with such transmission events (The Incident Investigation Teams 1997), new guidelines became available in 2000. The Department of Health now recommends additional molecular-based tests for HBeAg-negative carriers who perform exposure-prone procedures (UK Health Departments 2000). Healthcare workers whose HBV viral load exceeds 10^3 genome equivalents per millilitre should not perform exposure-prone procedures. Those with viral loads below 10^3 are not restricted from any areas of work but should be retested at 12 monthly intervals.

For some surgeons and other healthcare workers, confidential discussion between the person concerned and his or her health adviser may lead to minor changes in practice that would allow work to continue with the avoidance of exposure-prone procedures. If there is any doubt, advice should be sought from a specialist occupational health physician, who may, in turn, wish to present the situation anonymously to the UK Advisory Panel for Health Care Workers Infected with Bloodborne Viruses (UKAP).

Some specialities, e.g. dentistry, are concerned almost totally with activities that are, by definition, exposure prone. For HIV, HbeAg-positive and HBeAg-negative carriers with high viral load (as defined above) working in such specialities, the only option in the UK is for retraining in another speciality which does not require the use of exposure-prone procedures.

No recommendations have yet been issued in the UK for healthcare workers found to be carriers of HCV unless they have been demonstrated to have transmitted their virus to a patient, in which case exclusion from exposure-prone procedures has been advised. Nevertheless, following several reports of transmission of HCV from healthcare workers to patients, the Advisory Group on Hepatitis has proposed new guidelines. One of the likely upcoming recommendations is that healthcare workers who are found to have been infected with HCV and who are involved in exposure-prone procedures will have to be tested for HCV RNA. Demonstration of viraemia (detectable RNA) will preclude the individual from performing exposure-prone procedures, until sustained response to antiviral therapy is

documented. A consultation exercise has recently taken place and implementation of the new guidelines is awaited.

CONCLUSIONS

You will continue to be at risk, albeit small, of acquiring blood-borne viruses from your patients. The level of risk varies depending on the prevalence of viruses in the local population. Adoption of universal precautions and careful attention to operative technique reduces the risks to the operator and other staff to a minimum. There is considerable cause for concern if you are expected to operate in situations where, for lack of resources, there is inadequate provision of protective clothing, such as impermeable gowns and disposable gloves, and hepatitis B vaccine. A significant exposure to the blood of a patient causes considerable anxiety for a period of up to 6 months and until laboratory tests confirm negativity. There is no reason for you to avoid exposure-prone procedures during this period, providing you are aware that there is a possibility of infection developing and provided that you practise a high standard of infection control. It may be necessary, however, for your medical adviser to recommend lifestyle changes, such as condom usage for sexual intercourse, and avoidance of donating blood, semen, etc. to prevent transmission to others by non-occupational routes. In the UK, as described earlier, guidelines for HIV- and HBV (HBeAg-positive, HBeAg-negative with high viral load)-infected healthcare workers advise strongly against participation in exposure-prone procedures. This is likely to be extended, in the very near future, to HCV-infected individuals who are shown to be viraemic. This approach is not adopted in many other countries where either no restriction is placed on clinical practice or exposure-prone procedures can continue providing the patient is informed of the situation.

Summary

- Do you recognize the procedures that raise the risks of viral transmission?
- Will you determine to take precautions on behalf of yourself, your patients and your colleagues?
- Will you resolve not to abandon universal precautions in emergency circumstances?
- Do you know what to do if an incident has exposed you or anyone else to the risk of contamination?

References

Advisory Committee on Dangerous Pathogens (ACDP) 1995 Protection against bloodborne viruses in the workplace: HIV and hepatitis. HMSO, London

Breuer J, Jeffries DJ 1990 Control of viral infections in hospital. Journal of Hospital Infection 16: 191–221

Brough SJ, Hunt TM, Barrie WM 1988 Surgical glove perforation. British Journal of Surgery 75: 317

Centers for Disease Control 1987 Recommendations for prevention of HIV transmission in health care settings. Morbidity and Mortality Weekly Report 36(2S): 1S–18S

Centers for Disease Control 1988 Update: universal precautions for prevention of transmission of human immunodeficiency virus, hepatitis B virus, and other bloodborne pathogens in health care settings. Morbidity and Mortality Weekly Report 37: 377–388

Centers for Disease Control 1991. Recommendations for preventing transmission of human immunodeficiency virus and hepatitis B virus to patients during exposure prone invasive procedures. Morbidity and Mortality Weekly Report 40(RR–8): 1–9

Church J, Sanderson P 1980 Surgical glove punctures. Journal of Hospital Infection 1: 84

Jaeckel E, Cornberg M, Wedemeyer H et al 2001 Treatment of acute hepatitis C with interferon alpha 2b. New England Journal of Medicine 345: 1452–1457

Jeffries DJ 1995a Viral hazards to and from health care workers. Journal of Hospital Infection 30(suppl.): 140–155

Jeffries DJ 1995b Surgery and bloodborne viruses. PHLS Microbiology Digest 12: 150–154

Jeffries DJ 1997 Viral agents of bloodborne infections. In: Collins CH, Kennedy DA (eds) Occupational bloodborne infections. CAB International, Wellingford, pp 1–16

Maffulli N, Capasso G, Testa V 1989 Glove perforation in elective orthopaedic surgery. Acta Orthopaedica Scandinavica 60: 565–566

Mast ST, Woolwine JD, Gerberding JL 1993 Efficacy of gloves in reducing blood volumes transferred during simulated needlestick injury. Journal of Infectious Diseases 168: 1589–1592

Matta H, Thompson AM, Rainey JB 1988 Does wearing two pairs of gloves protect operating theatre staff from skin contamination? BMJ 297: 597–598

Palmer JD, Rickett JWS 1992 The mechanisms and risks of surgical glove perforation. Journal of Hospital Infection 22: 279–286

Smith JR, Grant JM 1990 The incidence of glove puncture during caesarean section. Journal of Obstetrics and Gynaecology 10: 317–318

The Incident Investigation Teams and Others 1997 Transmission of hepatitis B to patients from four infected surgeons without hepatitis B e antigen. New England Journal of Medicine 336: 178–185

Tokars JL, Bell DM, Culver DH et al 1992 Percutaneous injuries during surgical procedures. JAMA 267: 2899–2904

UK Health Departments 1990 Guidance for clinical health care workers. Protection against infection with HIV and hepatitis viruses. Recommendations of the Expert Advisory Group on AIDS. HMSO, London

UK Health Departments 1993 Protecting health care workers and patients from hepatitis B. Department of Health, London

UK Health Departments 1994 AIDS/HIV-infected health care workers: guidance on the management of infected health care workers. Department of Health, London

UK Health Departments 1997 Guidelines on post-exposure prophylaxis for health care workers exposed to HIV. Department of Health, London

UK Health Departments 1998 Guidance for clinical health care workers. Protection against infection with bloodborne viruses. Department of Health, London

UK Health Departments 2000 Hepatitis B infected health care workers. HSC 2000/020. Department of Health, London

OPERATION

21 Good surgical practice

R. M. Kirk, J. Dawson

Objectives

- **Understand and accept your responsibilities.**
- **Commit yourself to the care and well-being of your patients and preserve their confidentiality.**
- **Work within your capabilities.**
- **Allocate your time sensibly.**
- **Keep good notes.**
- **Be a good team player.**
- **Preserve your integrity.**

Try not to be a man of success, but try to be a man of value.
Albert Einstein

If you are going to worry about this in bed tonight, Doc, get it right now.'

The peerless London surgeon Norman Tanner never said this; his every action proclaimed it. This chapter was previously contributed by the late John Dawson, a good friend, dedicated teacher, setter of high standards, and, like me, privileged to train with Norman Tanner.

INTRODUCTION

You must behave competently and honourably towards your patients, colleagues and society, and maintain openness to inspection. Aim to achieve high standards in all aspects of your life. Incompetence or dishonesty detected in one area implies similar failings in other areas.

In the past we were privileged to satisfy only our own consciences. At the end of each day we hoped to be able to say, 'I may have made errors but not from want of trying to achieve the best for my patients and those with whom I have worked.' Most of us relied on this and resolved ourselves, without the need to be exhorted by others, to do better when we fell below the standards to

which we aspired. However, because our profession sometimes failed to weed out the few identified as incompetent, lazy or dishonest, we have lost some of the trust we formerly commanded. Society regards us more critically than formerly, and we need to help restore our former high reputation.

CLINICAL COMPETENCE

1. This is the foundation of all your professionalism. You need knowledge, and skill in taking a history, examining patients, making decisions and acting upon them. You constantly need to improve them by following your results to assess the outcomes, in the hope of learning how to improve them.

2. Your competence is most under strain in emergency circumstances. When performing electively you can obey the rules. In an emergency you often need to decide in an instant whether you should or should not conform. There are circumstances when you need to interpret rules sensibly, as they are made to cover most but not all situations. The heroic, legless, Second World War airman, Douglas Bader, declared, 'Rules are for the guidance of wise men, and the blind obedience of fools.' But remember that you may be called upon to justify your actions.

3. Competence is not a 'once-and-for-all' achievement. It is a continuous process of critically noting your performance in all aspects, identifying your failures and learning from them. It depends upon meeting, watching and listening to your colleagues, attending courses and critically reading the literature.

Key points

- **Surgical improvement does not develop by merely working hard.**
- **Stand back, identify weaknesses, search for improvements and implement them.**

PATIENT TRUST

A vital characteristic for a medical attendant is to be trust-worthy. If we are trusted, our patients are open with us, allow us to examine them and perform procedures that may be difficult or impossible without their cooperation. They will not tell us the often private information we need to know, unless they trust us.

To gain patients' trust we need to:

1. Communicate with them (see Ch. 47). This implies not just giving them information but also being receptive to the verbal and non-verbal information they transmit.
2. Involve them in the decision making (see Ch. 13) so they can give informed consent to what is agreed upon (see Ch. 14). Accede to a request for a second opinion; it is not a blow to your dignity.
3. Be open with them in admitting ignorance, in admitting that there has been a failure in managing them, in admitting our own error of judgement or practice. Whenever we admit to a failure we should always clearly state, and be prepared to discuss, what we intend to do to correct it.
4. Respond to the patients' anxieties regarding their outlook, discomfort or pain, complications, loss of function and loss of dignity. Saying 'Sorry,' is not an admission of guilt but an expression of sympathy.
5. Provided the patients agree, inform and discuss with relatives at all stages what is happening, what is proposed and what is the likely outlook. Relatives often exert great influence in supporting and reassuring your patients. Conversely, they may undermine patients' trust in their recovery and in your management.
6. Protect patients' confidentiality and preserve their dignity. Illness attacks not only their bodies but also their morale; they may wish to keep their health problems private.

PROFESSIONALISM

1. Strictly speaking surgeons (Greek *cheir* = hand + *ergon* = work; hence, manual workers) are not professionals – but we now consider ourselves to be 'physicians who perform operations'. This is not strictly correct; many medical specialists perform skilful manipulations (Latin *manus* = hand + *plere* = to fill). 'Professionalism' carries the connotation of performing competently and autonomously without the need to be directed, in order to produce a satisfactory result.

2. The four most important qualities of a professional surgeon, which are often overlooked because they are not subject to objective assessment, are the four 'Cs' – common sense, competence, commitment and compassion. When you take up a task, ensure that you apply these qualities to achieve the best possible result.

3. Maintain your professionalism in whatever circumstances you practise:

a. Respect the fact that some patients have different beliefs from you and may reject aspects of your proffered treatment for religious or other reasons. Jehovah's Witnesses, for example, may reject blood transfusion. Because many beliefs are subject to personal interpretation, make sure you know what exactly are the implications when patients declare their adherence to a particular sect.

b. In an emergency your professional judgement is put under increased strain (see Ch. 13). You may be called on to carry out procedures at the edge of, or beyond, your capabilities. As you make your decision and act upon it, recognize that you will need to justify it to your patient, your peers and to your own conscience.

c. If you participate in specialist procedures, such as organ transplantation, adhere strictly to the legal and ethical requirements.

d. If you are present at an armed conflict, be aware that your actions may be under intense scrutiny to detect whether you are favouring one side over the other. Treat all patients who are presented to you on an equal basis and to the highest possible standard.

e. Treat prisoners as you would anyone else. Refuse to participate in any action that may cause physical or mental suffering.

f. If you work in another country, avoid offending against local laws and customs. Do not, however, allow your standards to fall, even though you may not have all the facilities you would normally have at your command.

g. Do not perform any operations that conflict with your own moral values.

4. We are all in part the products of our teachers. One of the privileges of being in the profession of surgery is that we are always trainees and at the same time we can all be teachers. Pass on to your juniors the ideas, the wisdom, the skills that you have acquired. With permission from your seniors, delegate procedures in which you are skilled, while you teach and supervise your juniors. In the past, too much unsupervised responsibility was delegated to trainees, summed up in the aphorism, 'See one, do one, teach one.' This is no longer tolerated.

5. Preparing to teach forces you to be ready to justify statements that you make, and actions you take. It is one of the most effective ways of learning for yourself and honing your skills. Many procedures are best taught by example, copied – often unconsciously – by the trainee, not by reading or listening.

RECORDS

1. We like to be considered as people of action, rather than reporters of action. If we are to be accountable, however, we must keep accurate records (see Ch. 48). It is not enough that you have acted correctly. Others, wishing to inspect your actions, must be able to confirm them.

2. Write or dictate records as soon as possible after the event. Ensure they are comprehensive, comprehensible, dated and signed so they are attributable to you. Record not only the positive findings but also the negative ones: if you do not mention these it could be assumed that you did not examine for them. Do not use abbreviations that can be misconstrued: spell out 'Left,' 'Right.' Jargon that you use may be incomprehensible or misconstrued by others.

3. There are no more important records than those describing surgical operations. Detail what you found, what you sought but did not find. Describe all the procedures, any difficulties and the situation at the end of the operation. It is vital to recount what must be done in the immediate postoperative period regarding monitoring, circulatory and respiratory management, pain control, drug treatment, and any special instructions you wish to be followed. Make sure you inform those who look after the patient under what circumstances you wish to be informed.

HUBRIS

1. I have deliberately used this unusual word (Greek = excessive pride). Although it is reasonable to take pride in accomplishment, overweening pride is a dangerous emotion. We are all fallible. No one can claim to make the right decisions and perform perfectly every time. Protecting your pride is a dangerous path on which to embark; each step racks up the likelihood of disaster.

2. Do not be too proud to call for – and accept – help or advice, or the taking over of your patient by someone who is more capable than you are.

3. Do not be too proud to admit error to your patients, your peers and, particularly, yourself.

TIME MANAGEMENT

1. This is often self-management. You rarely have but a single commitment. More frequently you have many. You must rank your commitments and review the ranking at intervals, as a previously non-urgent problem may suddenly become urgent.

2. Except in an emergency, ensure that you fully complete one task before leaving it to start another. It is ineffective and unprofessional to leave a trail of almost completed tasks. However, be aware that acute situations develop so that you are called urgently. Although there is a temptation to complete the present task, in some cases you must abandon whatever you are doing and return to it later.

 Key point

- **React to changed circumstances. Compare the urgency of competing demands, decide the correct action and carry it out.**

3. Some people apply pressure on you for immediate action, against your better judgement. If other problems are more urgent, you may need to refuse. Be as diplomatic as possible but do not make undeliverable promises.

TEAM MEMBERSHIP

1. In the past, surgeons were undisputed team leaders and decision makers. We were depicted as the courageous pioneers, sometimes succeeding, sometimes failing to cure or relieve our patients.

2. The mores (Latin *moris* = custom) have changed dramatically. No one is immune from criticism or from comparison of their results with those of their peers (Latin *par, paris* = equal). We no longer work as individuals. For example, anaesthetists who initially worked under orders from surgeons now unequivocally take charge of the patient's well-being, freeing us to concentrate on the decisions and technical problems of the operation. The specialists in imaging and other diagnostic aids, assistants, specialist and general nurses, physiotherapists, technicians and many others form part of the team, each one having an input into the general decisions and necessary actions. The best teams work in harmony, with each member feeling important, respected and therefore loyal to the team.

3. The change in attitude is fundamental. In the past an opinion carried weight according to the distinction and seniority of the proposer. Now each opinion is, or should be, judged on the merits of its logic and the evidence offered to support it.

4. Being a good team member offers you many benefits. Your colleagues will celebrate your successes and sympathize with your failures. When you need help they will respond. If you are a poor team member you may not always rely on these important supports, or they may be

given reluctantly. We all need encouragement when our self-esteem is reduced, as inevitably happens from time to time when a series of things go wrong.

5. Team membership, however, places you in circumstances of conflicting loyalties. Although you wish to support and protect your colleagues, this must not take precedence over your responsibilities to patients and society. If any of your colleagues fail in their duties, or are physically or mentally sick and present a risk to patients, you must encourage them to take appropriate treatment and inform appropriate authorities if they do not.

TEACHING AND TRAINING

1. Take every opportunity to pass on your knowledge to your trainees. Of course, it is not your own knowledge. It is mainly acquired from your own trainers and you are an intermediary. It is not just the facts that you transmit but the unconscious influence you have on their attitude, if your behaviour and performance are to the highest standards you can achieve.

2. Always try to give those junior to you time to express their opinions first, to give them the opportunity and challenge of making and preparing to act on decisions, as they will need to do when they become autonomous consultants.

3. It is often difficult to delegate responsibility to others, but monitored, progressive delegation is a vital process of preparing for tomorrow's consultants.

Key point

- **As a surgeon in training, always seek your chief's approval before delegating responsibility or practical procedures.**

4. You may find it even more difficult to delegate practical procedures that require skilful accomplishment. Again, first delegate simple procedures under direct observation and progress to more complex ones with less obvious – more discreet – monitoring.

INTEGRITY

1. Place a high value on your probity and integrity. Patients, colleagues and the general public will usually forgive you for mistakes. We all, inevitably, make them from time to time, as we work in a field in which we do not, and cannot, know all the facts in the present state of

our knowledge. They will not so easily forgive deceit, dishonesty or duplicity.

2. Moreover, once you have been found guilty of discreditable behaviour you have forfeited your good character and will never again be fully trusted.

3. As a professional, be honest in publishing your clinical results, your research techniques and the findings.

4. You cannot separate your professional from your private reputation. A surgeon who unfairly blames a colleague for his or her own mistake, falsifies a legal report, claims money illegally or is corrupt in any matter has a stained character.

5. Avoid conflicts of interest. Avoid accepting gifts, favours, hospitality or anything that puts pressure on you. You must be able to make decisions on clinical necessity, not for any other reasons.

6. Financial dishonesty arouses particular scorn. Take exceptional care not to take or accept any money to which you are not entitled or which puts you under an obligation, which will undoubtedly subsequently be called in.

HEALTH

1. In addition to the other qualities required, the practice of surgery demands outstanding stamina. It is necessary to respond to a sudden emergency at the end of a long and busy routine day, or to a sudden disaster near the end of an arduous major operation.

2. Avoid risking your health from accidents and infections, including from needlestick injuries (see Ch. 20); if you sustain a needlestick injury, report it – do not hope for the best. In emergency circumstances do not unnecessarily place yourself at risk.

3. Alcoholism and drug taking impair your judgement, put your patients at risk and also risk your career.

4. If you develop any condition that places your patients at risk, either because it impairs your performance or because you may pass on an infection, you must immediately seek a medical opinion

5. If one of your colleagues develops a condition that threatens the welfare of patients you must exhort him or her to seek medical care. If your advice is rejected, remember that your first loyalty must be to the patients. In the past we have placed loyalty to our colleagues above our responsibility to our patients.

ERRORS

1. There are errors of judgement. Such errors arise from the complexity of weighing the multiple factors to be taken into account.

Key points

- Errors of judgement are inevitable in medicine and surgery. The problems are too complex, rarely black and white, often affected by unknown and unknowable factors. Accept that you will inevitably make judgements that prove wrong in retrospect.
- Success is not always a sign of good judgement; robust patients survive poor management. Equally, failure may result from factors you could not have anticipated.

2. We all make them. Often we recognize errors in retrospect because we have more information, especially the outcome of our earlier decisions. As we gain experience we hope to reduce the number of errors we make in the future. We hope to learn from our own errors and from the errors of others.

3. A different type of error is sometimes called a 'systems' error, perhaps because it could be prevented by changes in the way in which the system works. Examples are the administration of a harmful substance, or administration by an incorrect route. The first of these could be prevented by placing the harmful substance out of easy access; the second could be prevented by making the connection of a type that can be made only to the correct acceptor. Comparisons are often made between medical errors and those that occur in aeroplanes. In the former there is a tendency to apportion blame and label it, 'human error'. This makes no contribution to preventing repeated errors but it dissuades those who make errors from declaring them. If an airline pilot makes an error and admits it, attempts are made to study it and consider whether some change in the system could prevent it from occurring again. Be prepared to report when things go wrong but should have gone right – these are sometimes pompously called 'adverse incident reports[3]' (AIR)s. In bringing them to attention you may be saving future patients and colleagues from disaster.

4. As a trainee, report any error to your chief without delay. Do not attempt to deal with it beyond your competence, hide it or blame it on others. Honestly admitted errors are excusable; failure to admit to them loses the trust of your chief.

Key point

- Gain and retain the trust of your chief. The greatest compliment your chief can pay you is to say, 'If that person is on call for me at night, I sleep well.'

COMPLAINTS AND CLAIMS

1. Make every effort to avoid patient dissatisfaction by adhering to good surgical practice and maintaining good, open relations with your patients.
2. Keep complete, up-to-date, comprehensive, comprehensible records of what you have done, what is happening, what your plans are, what you have discussed with your patients.
3. If, in spite of your best efforts, there are complications, or patients are disappointed with the results, openly declare the situation and state what you intend to do.
4. Do not hesitate to express your compassion if something has gone wrong. Do not hesitate to declare your responsibility if you have made an error.
5. Make a written record of what passes between you and the patients.
6. Continue your normal careful comprehensive treatment.
7. Cooperate with any investigation.

Further reading

1997 The surgeon's duty of care: guidance for surgeons on ethical and legal issues. Senate of Surgery of Great Britain and Ireland, London
2001 Good medical practice. General Medical Council, London
2002 Good surgical practice. Royal College of Surgeons of England, London

Useful link
www.rcseng.ac.uk   Code of practice for the surgical management of Jehovah's Witnesses. Royal College of Surgeons of England 1996 (available on line only)

22 Surgical access: incisions, and the management of wounds

D. J. Leaper, L. Low

Objectives

- **Be aware of the technical factors contributing to wound infection.**
- **Understand the principles underlying choice and techniques of wound access.**
- **Accept the need for aftercare of surgical wounds.**

INTRODUCTION

There are records which describe successful wound management from as long ago as the time of the Assyrians and the ancient Egyptian Empire. Techniques using sutures and threads, linen adhesive strips, and even soldier ant heads as skin clips, have all been described historically. The management of wounds, their classification, surgical dressings and subsequent healing is an ever-evolving field based upon a better understanding of the pathophysiological principles behind them. From the time of Hippocrates and Galen, who recognized that infection impaired wound healing, to the development of antiseptic and aseptic technique through the work of Semmelweis, Pasteur and Lister, research continues into the factors that affect the quality of healing, cosmetic outcomes and the functional recovery of the damaged tissue.

The development of operative surgery and anaesthesia seems to know no bounds, yet the fundamental process of wound healing must not be forgotten. The aphorism of 'cut well, sew well, get well' depends on a knowledge of wound healing mechanisms and the adverse effects that may influence them.

SURGICAL ACCESS AND INCISIONS

1. Before you even consider placing a knife to skin, there are general steps to consider before each and every case. These include correct positioning of the patient, hair removal, sterile skin preparation and wash, and sterile draping.

2. Should you give antibiotic prophylaxis, and deep venous thrombosis prophylaxis (see Chs 8, 15, 19)?

3. Carefully position the patient for most advantageous surgical access and patient safety. Take care to avoid pressure, particularly on the skin over bony prominences, and on superficial arteries and nerves. Depending on the operation, changing body position will enhance exposure of the area involved. Examples are the modified Lloyd-Davis position for approach to the perineum, a lateral position for a retroperitoneal approach to the kidney, the prone jack-knife position for access to the rectum and anus, the Trendelenburg position for varicose vein surgery. Operator preference may also influence patient position.

4. Hair removal was conventionally performed the day before surgery. However, it has been shown that in clean operations, shaving body hair more than 12 h before the operation doubles the rate of wound infection. If it is necessary, undertake shaving shortly before surgery; supervise and check it. Clipping of hair reduces infection rates to a tenth of those following shaving, and avoids the risk of minor skin abrasions and cuts due to inexpert or unsupervised shaving. Remove hair for aesthetic reasons and to allow painless removal of dressings. Leaving it in situ does not increase wound infection rates.

5. The most popular sterile skin preparation in the United Kingdom is 10% povidone–iodine (1% available iodine) in 70% alcohol. This helps by staining the skin to demonstrate any areas that have been missed. If the patient is allergic to iodine, use 0.5% chlorhexidine in alcohol.

6. Now delineate the operative field with sterile drapes. Conventionally these are resterilized double-thickness linen sheets that are held in place with towel clips. Take care, as they are designed for multiple use. A drawback is that they allow permeation by body fluids and, once soaked, can desterilize the operative field. Use waterproof disposable fabrics which do not allow this permeation, especially in cases of contamination, or when there is a risk of hepatitis or human immunodeficiency

viral contamination. They are expensive. Incise drapes of adhesive polyurethane film were introduced over 30 years ago. They are most commonly used in prosthetic orthopaedic and vascular surgery, when there is a risk of opportunistic infections by skin organisms such as *Staphylococcus epidermidis*. Newer versions of antibiotic-impregnated drapes significantly reduce bacterial skin counts, but there is no definite indication that they reduce infection rates. In general surgery they are useful in isolating stomas or other infected areas, such as a separate infected wound that is close to the planned incision. Wound guards may also be used to reduce wound contamination during open viscus surgery, but they do not reduce the risk of wound infection.

Principles of access incisions

1. In conventional open surgery, the purpose of the incision is to allow adequate exposure of the affected area or organ. Careful organization and planning is essential. If the operation is unfamiliar to you, revise the anatomy or obtain help from a more senior colleague. In order to perform any procedure competently, you must have good access, with a long enough incision to avoid excessive retraction. Plan the incision using surface landmarks as a guide, then perform the incision as a single movement. This leaves a better cosmetic result than one that has been extended. The exposed area then allows viewing, manipulation of tissues and control of other structures. In some cases, linear incisions may not provide this and angled incisions may offer better exposure, the side within the angle being widely retractable; for example, the roof-top abdominal incision used for pancreatic operations.

2. When operating on limbs, do not make the incision cross a joint perpendicular to the flexure line, as subsequent scarring and contracture may limit the function of the joint on recovery. Wrinkles and contour lines (Langer's lines) are useful to disguise resultant scars. With a good knowledge of the anatomy, and gentle tissue handling, damage to important structures will be minimized. An assistant can also warn of potential trouble. Nerves, tendons and vessels often lie in the most direct path to the area affected and damage to them can impair future function and healing; for example, vascular supply to a skin flap and subsequent necrosis.

3. *Vascular supply and wound healing*. Linear incisions rarely fail to heal because of injury to the vascular supply, but angled incisions may do so. When an incision is made parallel to a previous scar, for example a paramedian incision next to a midline incision, the intervening tissue is rendered ischaemic and healing will be prejudiced. Avoid this by reopening the old scar or excising it if there will not be any undue tension on subsequent closure. There is danger to underlying structures if you use an old scar

with, for example, bowel adherent to the base of an old abdominal wound.

4. *Tissue planes*. Acquire an intimate knowledge of tissue planes to obtain correct exposure. Normal anatomy is often distorted in the presence of disease. If you dissect in the wrong plane, you may cause inadvertent damage and also fail to encompass diseased tissue completely, as in cancer clearance.

5. *Cosmetic aspects*. The resulting scar is the only part of the operation seen by the patient. This is particularly important in facial surgery, but an ugly scar in any area of the body can make the patient feel self-conscious. A young woman may feel permanently embarrassed by an ill-planned and distorted breast scar.

6. *Infection*. Do not allow an initially clean operation to become contaminated as a result of operation. In potentially clean-contaminated procedures, for example elective large bowel resection, minimize and isolate any faeculent contamination by placing clean packs around the bowel and wound before entering the bowel. Discard swabs or instruments once they have been soiled, change to sterile gloves, and make use of peritoneal lavage to wash out dirty and infected material. Antibiotic prophylaxis has been unequivocally shown to reduce wound infections. In clean procedures their use is controversial. Frequently, an operation is carried out for established infection, or you encounter infection unexpectedly. Be willing to limit the procedure to drainage of pus and excision of necrotic tissue. Once the wound is clean and granulating you may then explore the wound and close it at a later date. This is delayed primary or secondary closure.

Key points

- **Acquire an intimate knowledge of the anatomy to reach your objective safely, and in the right plane.**
- **Remember that disease processes distort the anatomy and may weaken the tissues.**

Closure

1. The ability of a wound to heal is based upon several factors: both local and systemic. Locally, ensure that there is an adequate blood supply to the tissues, avoid tension, dead space and haematoma formation. Deal adequately with infection. Systemic factors include comorbidity such as diabetes, jaundice or renal failure, low serum albumin below 30 g l^{-1}, and trace element deficiencies. Ask about medications such as corticosteroids, immunosuppressives and cytotoxics, and enquire about previous irradiation (see Ch. 6).

2. Take care to achieve the best appearance of the scar, as the patient's perception of success is often based on the resulting appearance, not on the speed of healing or its ultimate tensile strength. Appose the tissues on either side of the incision and prevent them from separating. Inflammatory cells and fibroblasts can then bridge the defect. Healing cannot take place if differing tissues are opposed or other structures interposed.

3. Avoid tension when closing, particularly when tissues are excised and the margins of excision are brought together. This may demand a simple relieving incision, or a more complicated flap. There are circumstances when tension is inevitable and you must accept and allow for it.

4. As a general rule, repair each layer of tissue separately to restore the tissue planes. You thus avoid leaving a potential dead space where fluid, blood or infection may accumulate. If this is unavoidable, consider inserting a drain tube, preferably a closed system, under vacuum; remove it as soon as possible to avoid an ascending infection.

5. Control bleeding. If you do not, you risk haematoma formation, thereby separating the tissues. This prevents healing and becomes a nidus for infection.

6. The opposing edges are most frequently united using sutures. Choose materials that provide maximum strength and minimum tissue reaction. Historically, natural substances were popular, such as silk and catgut, which is now avoided for fear of transmitting prion diseases. 'Prions', coined from 'proteins', are transmissible 'rogue' proteins postulated to cause diseases. They are now replaced by synthetics that behave reliably, whether they are intended to be absorbed or to remain relatively unchanged.

 Key point

- **The need to restore tissue planes is vital when structures move against each other; tendons adhere and become fixed if they are not resheathed in flexible areolar tissue.**

Laparotomy incisions

1. Opening the abdomen has some special aspects. The choice of incision depends on the purpose of the intended operation. When it is performed to carry out a specific procedure, place the incision to provide maximum exposure (Fig. 22.1). If you are exploring the abdomen, use a midline vertical incision or paramedian approach in adults. The paramedian (Greek *para* = beside + Latin *medius* = middle) incision passes through the

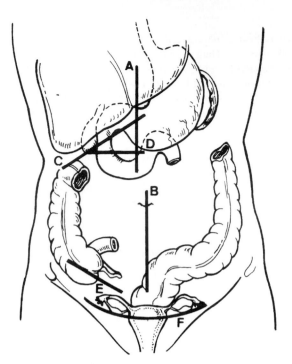

Fig. 22.1 Favoured laparotomy incisions: **A**, paramedian; **B**, midline; **C**, Kocher; **D**, transverse; **E**, Lanz; **F**, Pfannenstiel.

rectus sheath but you can draw aside the medial part of the intact rectus muscle. It acts as a shutter on closure (Fig. 22.2). In infants, transverse incisions may be more appropriate.

2. Intra-abdominal pressure is unavoidable in closure of the abdomen, therefore tension is inevitable. If the abdomen is distended, this increases tension. Avoid the factors that increase the risks of wound dehiscence and incisional hernias.

3. Delay closing the abdomen if this will so increase tension that it creates abdominal compartment syndrome, risking respiratory complications, sepsis and organ failure.

4. Upper abdominal incisions are more likely to dehisce (Latin *de* = intensive + *hiare* = to gape) than lower incisions; it is rare for Pfannenstiel, transverse or appendix wounds to dehisce. The lateral paramedian incision is virtually free of risk of dehiscence, and has a very small risk of hernia formation. Hernias through laparoscopic ports are now well recognized and various techniques have been described to close them.

5. The value of layered closure or mass closure has also been debated. The wound dehiscence rate following layered closure with catgut sutures fell from approximately 10% to less than 1% when using a mass closure

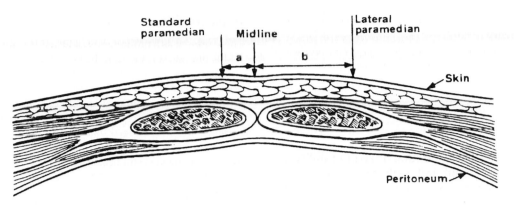

Fig. 22.2 Lateral and standard paramedian incisions: *a* = 2 cm; *b* = two-thirds from midline to lateral rectus sheath.

with a non-absorbable suture. As a result of the work of Jenkins (1976), a surgeon at Guildford in Surrey, wound dehiscence occurred in only 1 in 1505 cases using a non-absorbable, continuous mass suture. He hypothesized that the suture used should be at least four times the length of the incision, placed 1 cm from the wound edge and not more than 1 cm apart. The suture tension should be just sufficient to oppose the edges. Do not draw sutures too tightly, rendering the edges ischaemic or causing the sutures to cut through, allowing buttonhole hernias to form through the lateral suture line.

6. Use of an absorbable thread may avoid 'cutting through' of a suture. Polydioxanone (PDS), polyglactin (Vicryl), and polyglycolic acid (Dexon) are predictably absorbed and their tensile strength is long lasting.

7. Prevention of intra-abdominal adhesions has gained interest, in the hope of avoiding the morbidity associated with subsequent small bowel obstruction. Minimize tissue trauma and irritation, handle the tissues gently, use non-reactive suture materials, avoid drying and cooling the tissues by using frequent, warmed sterile saline lavage. Steroids, non-steroidal anti-inflammatory drugs and dextran have all been used but their efficacy is unknown. Newer techniques involve using a sodium hyaluronate-based bioresorbable membrane or 0.5% ferric hyaluronate gel (Intergel) solution, which have been shown to be efficacious at a second look laparoscopy 6–12 weeks later. Whether they have a long-term prophylactic effect has not been proven.

Key point

- **Avoid complications by correctly siting the incision, choosing the correct materials to close, and employing impeccable technique throughout.**

Chest incisions

There are three principal routes into the chest. The lateral thoracotomy follows the line of the upper edge of a rib, avoiding the neurovascular bundle under the rib. It allows exploration of the hemithorax for trauma or pulmonary surgery. In some cases a combined thoracoabdominal incision is used. This usually continues the line of an incision along one of the lower ribs and is carried through the costal margin into the abdomen. Endoscopic procedures can be undertaken for cervical sympathectomy. It gives outstanding exposure of the lower third of the oesophagus and fundus. Access to the pericardium, heart and great vessels is achieved through a median sternotomy.

PRECAUTIONS AGAINST LOSS OF INSTRUMENTS OR SWABS

1. Correctly organize instrument trays, limiting the number of individually packed instruments as far as possible.
2. Arrange swabs and packs in 'fives' bound together with red cotton, or, if small, carefully packaged, for example on a safety pin.
3. Check the number of instruments on trays against printed lists incorporated in each pack.
4. Record all sutures, packs, swabs, needles and extras clearly and legibly on a board in the theatre.
5. Use special swab racks, including the modern disposable wallets, which facilitate counting at the end of the operation.
6. Mark radio-opaque, non-implantable, non-metallic equipment such as drains and the laparomat.
7. Sign the theatre record book and have it countersigned by the scrubbed and assistant nurses.

8. Ensure the count is complete and correct before you commence closure.
9. Record and sign that the count was correct at the end of the operation note in the patient's record.

Key points

- **Establish a simple routine of accountability, and a permanent and accurate record.**
- **Precautions are like a chain – every link must be intact or it fails.**

SKIN CLOSURE

1. Close skin perfectly, avoiding tension and inversion of the edges. Several techniques are available: continuous or interrupted, simple or mattress and subcuticular. All are acceptable but the last gives the best results.
2. Skin clips give a good cosmetic result, are easy to apply and remove, and are associated with a low infection rate.
3. Tape closure using Steri-strips also gives good results, and does not disrupt the blood supply to the tissues, as sutures might. They do, however, require a dry surface for adhesion. They act as an adjunct to sutures and spread wound tension to provide the best cosmetic effect.
4. Cyanoacrylate skin adhesives are expensive and demand near perfect haemostasis. They may be most appropriate in children for closing lacerations.
5. Remove sutures at, as a working rule, 3–5 days in head and neck, 7 days inguinal and upper limb, 10 days abdominal and lower limb, and up to 14 days for dorsal incisions. Place knots well to the side of the incision to facilitate removal.

Langer's lines

The lines described by the Viennese Carl von Langer in 1861 mainly correspond with the skin tension lines and natural skin creases. An incision across them risks an unacceptable hypertrophic scar. Whenever possible, incise along the tension lines. If you have to cross them for surgical access, as in operations on small joints, cross the skin creases obliquely or employ Z-plasties, or plan an S-shaped incision.

Hypertrophic skin scars

These present as a proliferation of heaped-up and red scar tissue, but this stays within the boundaries of the wound and do not extend beyond it, as do keloids. They tend to occur in scars around joints and in areas of skin tension. With the passage of time, at least 6 months, they become avascular, and may regress to form a white, stretched, widened scar. It is alleged that covering these scars with a silicone gel produces a clinical improvement but the exact mechanism is still unknown.

Contractures

Do not confuse these with the normal process of wound contraction. Contractures follow delayed wound healing and occur after infection and inadequate treatment of deep burns in particular. Established contractures can be released by excising them and covering the raw area with split-thickness grafts or with transposition flaps.

Keloids

Formed by abnormal collagen metabolism, keloids (Greek *chele* = claw) result in a proliferation of scar tissue beyond the boundaries of the original wound. They occur in dorsal areas of the body and over the face and delto-pectoral region. Keloids occur most frequently in dark-skinned people and may be encouraged to form as a cultural body decoration.

Simple excision is almost always followed by a more exuberant recurrence. X-rays have been used but topical steroid creams or steroid injections are more effective. Pressure on an excised keloid scar may also prevent recurrence. Experimental work is in progress, using calcium antagonists and manipulating the effects of transforming growth factor β.

SURGICAL DRESSINGS

The ideal surgical dressing does not exist, but should:

1. Be absorbent and able to remove excess exudate
2. Maintain a moist environment, aid tissues to remove necrotic material, and promote healing
3. Prevent trauma to underlying healing granulation tissue and exclude foreign particles from the wound
4. Be leak-proof, preventing 'strike through' (passage of organisms through soaked dressings) causing secondary infection
5. Maintain temperature and gaseous exchange

6. Allow easy, pain-free, simple dressing changes, with less frequent application and removal
7. Be odourless, cosmetically acceptable and comfortable
8. Be inexpensive.

The last 30 years have seen an increasing depth of understanding of wound healing processes. Many dressings are now manufactured to provide the requirements of the ideal wound environment. There is no clear-cut evidence, however, as to whether wounds should be left open, with a dry surface of fibrinous coagulum which seals the wound, or whether they should be covered and hidden from view. Exuding wounds are at risk of secondary infection and may not be protected by a dressing. Pathogenic organisms can track through a soiled wet dressing from its surface. Only some of the requirements listed above are based on sound experimental evidence. The armamentarium of modern surgical dressings is intended for managing chronic open wounds such as venous leg ulcers.

Polyurethane incise drapes have become popular as a primary wound dressing for sutured wound and skin donor sites. They retain moisture, which enhances epithelial closure, and allow easy inspection and aspiration of excessive exudate. They are claimed to relieve pain at donor sites. They are gas and water-vapour permeable but if the wound becomes macerated (Latin *macerare* = to soak) there is a risk of secondary infection. However, the dressings are impermeable to organisms. More traditional wound dressings include perforated absorbent plastic film, such as Melolin, or non-adherent sheet dressings, which require a secondary pad dressing if there is excessive exudate.

A wide choice exists for managing open wounds such as a healing pilonidal sinus cavity or a superficially ruptured, infected abdominal wound. Moulded polymeric silicone gel foam dressing is ideal, allowing pain-free wound care. The patient may be able to perform this. Bead and powder dressings, such as the exudate-absorbent Iodosorb and the sterile hydrogel Intrasite, may be useful. Some incorporate antibiotics or antiseptics. They absorb exudate and maintain a moist environment. Reserve sheet polymeric hydrocolloid or hydrogel dressings for more superficial open wounds. They may be occlusive, such as Comfeel ulcer dressing and Granuflex, or semiocclusive, such as Geliperm. Some are biological alginates, such as Kaltostat and Sorbsan, and may be interactive, promoting granulations. The list of dressings increases, and satisfactory trials are required to show their merit and comparative worth. Biologically active dressings and living skin equivalents are examples of these.

Key point

- **Choose wound dressings of proven cost-effectiveness, not for novelty value.**

PRINCIPLES OF WOUND MANAGEMENT

1. An operation is a responsibility undertaken with informed consent (see Ch. 14), performed in optimal circumstances. Surgery is based on ritual and it is difficult to measure the quality of operative surgery, although we achieve much through audit and morbidity and mortality meetings.

2. Lord Moynihan (1865–1936) taught that an operation should start with a clean sweep of the knife. William Halsted (1852–1922) preached gentleness, haemostasis, asepsis and accurate apposition of tissues. While aseptic procedures and swab and instrument counts are easy to teach, gentle handling of tissues is more difficult to learn. Some trainee surgeons acquire it naturally, others take time to be able to oppose cut tissues perfectly without undue suture tension. It is logical to secure haemostasis in surgical wounds. These principles were directed to the whole of surgery but apply particularly to the creation and management of surgical wounds.

Summary

- Do you understand the complex influences acting on incidental and surgical wounds?
- How will you select appropriate incisions, particularly in the abdomen, the chest and near joints?
- What principles underlie surgical closure of wounds?
- Can you justify your selection of wound dressings based on evidence or experience?

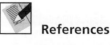

References

Jenkins TPN 1976 The burst abdominal wound: a mechanical approach. British Journal of Surgery 63: 873–876

Further reading

Anonymous 1986 Dressings for ulcers. Drug and Therapeutics Bulletin 24: 9–12

Cox PJ, Ausobsky JR, Ellis H, Pollack AV 1986 Towards no incisional hernias: lateral paramedian versus midline incisions. Journal of the Royal Society of Medicine 79: 711–712

Harland RNL, Irving MH 1988 Surgical drains. Surgery 1: 1360–1362

Leaper DJ 1985 Laparotomy closure. British Journal of Hospital Medicine 33: 317–322

Leaper DJ 1992 Local effects of trauma and wound healing. In: Burnand KG, Young AE (eds) Ian Aird's companion to surgical studies. Churchill Livingstone, Edinburgh, ch. 2, pp 27–35

Leaper DJ 1992 Surgical factors influencing infection. In: Taylor EW (ed.) Infection in surgical practice. Oxford University Press, Oxford, ch. 3, pp 18–27

Leaper DJ, Foster ME 1990 Wound healing and abdominal wound closure. In: Taylor I (ed.) Progress in surgery. Churchill Livingstone, Edinburgh, vol. 3, ch. 2, pp 19–31

Lucarotti ME, Billings PJ, Leaper DJ 1991 Laparotomy, wound closure and repair of incisional hernia. Surgery 10: 1–6

Wadstrom J, Gerdin B 1990 Closure of the abdominal wall: how and why. Acta Chirurgica Scandinavica 156: 75–82

23 Minimal access surgery

A. Darzi

Objectives

- **Understand the nomenclature and boundaries of minimal access surgery.**
- **Recognize that minimal access surgery aims to accomplish surgical therapeutic goals with minimal physical and psychological trauma.**
- **Recognize the limitations of minimal access surgery in its current state, considering future improvement in training and technology.**

Diseases that harm call for treatments that harm less.
William Osler

INTRODUCTION

Minimal access surgery aims to accomplish surgical therapeutic goals with minimal physical trauma. The properly controlled performance of minimal access surgery with well-considered pre- and postoperative management offers benefits, including cost benefits, without sacrificing the quality of care of the patient. Minimal access techniques are less invasive, less disabling and less disfiguring. With increasing experience, they offer cost effectiveness to both health services and employers by shortening operating times, shortening hospital stays and allowing faster recuperation. State-of-the-art video recording can help communication, bring the patient and family closer to the process, improve clinical decision making and enhance rapport.

The urologists Wickham and Fitzpatrick (1990), who were instrumental in highlighting the need for techniques which reduced therapeutic and surgical trauma, advocated the term 'minimally invasive therapy'. Cuschieri (1992) argues that this inaccurately implies increased safety but there is no correlation between invasiveness and risk. He suggests minimal access surgery (MAS), as

the essential attribute is the reduction of surgical trauma. Other terms include endoscopic, keyhole and laparoscopic surgery.

Technology has effectively miniaturized our eyes and extended our hands to perform microscopic and macroscopic operations in places that formerly could be reached only through large incisions. It has also provided new ways to look at tissues, using light, sound waves and magnetic fields which can detect disease and guide therapy (Darzi et al 1993). These same technologies, more highly focused and used at much higher power, can also be used to give highly controlled resection and tissue destruction. You must understand the principles of these devices so that you can help to shape the future development of minimal access surgery and not become the servants of the machines you use.

BOUNDARIES OF MINIMAL ACCESS SURGERY

Techniques

Minimal access surgery has crossed all traditional boundaries of specialities and disciplines. Shared, borrowed and overlapping technologies and information are encouraging a multidisciplinary approach that serves the whole patient rather than a specific organ system. Broadly speaking, minimal access techniques can be categorized as follows.

1. *Laparoscopy*. A rigid endoscope is introduced through a port in the abdominal wall into the peritoneal cavity, which has been inflated with carbon dioxide (pneumoperitoneum). Further ports are then placed in the abdominal wall, through which operating instruments can be introduced. Laparoscopic cholecystectomy has revolutionized the surgical management of cholelithiasis and is now the mainstay in its management. As a result of improved instruments and increasing experience, Nissen fundoplication, hiatal and inguinal hernia repair, appendicectomy, and colorectal surgery are now performed laparoscopically.

2. *Thoracoscopy.* A rigid endoscope is introduced through an incision in the chest to gain access to the thoracic contents. The lung is deflated, producing a natural cavity without the need for gas insufflation. A common thoracoscopic procedure is sympathectomy for hyperhydrosis.

3. *Endoluminal endoscopy.* Flexible or rigid endoscopes can be introduced into hollow organs or systems for diagnosis and therapy. Examples are the urinary tract (cystoscopy), upper (oesophagogastroduodenoscopy) or lower gastrointestinal tract (colonoscopy), respiratory tract (bronchoscopy) and vascular systems.

4. *Perivisceral endoscopy.* Body planes can be accessed even in the absence of a natural cavity. Examples are mediastinoscopy, retroperitoneoscopy, and retroperitoneal approaches to the kidney, aorta and lumbar sympathetic chain. A recent example is subfascial ligation of incompetent perforators in varicose vein surgery.

5. *Arthroscopy and intra-articular joint surgery.* Orthopaedic surgeons have long used arthroscopic access to the knee and have now extended the techniques to other joints, including the shoulder, wrist, elbow, hip and ankle. Apart from diagnosis, therapeutic procedures include meniscectomy.

6. Neurosurgeons employ minimal access procedures within the cranial cavity and the spinal canal.

7. *Combined approaches.* A diseased organ may be visualized and treated using a combination of endoluminal and extraluminal endoscopes and other imaging devices.

 Key point

- **Endoscopic techniques for diagnosis and therapy can be adapted wherever a space exists or can be created.**

COMPARISON OF SURGICAL TRAUMA FROM OPEN AND LAPAROSCOPIC SURGERY

1. Most of the trauma of an open procedure stems from the need for a wound large enough to give exposure for safe dissection at the target site. The wound is often the cause of morbidity, including infection, dehiscence, bleeding, herniation and nerve entrapment. Wound pain prolongs recovery time and, by reducing mobility, contributes to increased incidence of pulmonary collapse, chest infection and deep venous thrombosis.

2. Mechanical and human retractors exert additional trauma. Body wall retractors tend to inflict localized

damage, which may be as painful as the wound itself. By contrast, during laparoscopy the body wall is retracted by the low pressure pneumoperitoneum, giving a diffuse force applied gently and evenly over the whole body wall, causing minimal trauma.

3. Exposure of any body cavity to the atmosphere is harmful because of loss of heat and loss of body fluid by evaporation. There is evidence from the surgical literature that the incidence of postsurgical adhesions is reduced in laparoscopic compared with open procedures because there is less damage to the delicate serosal coverings. Handling of intestinal loops reduces peristaltic activity and provokes adynamic ileus; this is reduced following laparoscopic surgery.

 Key points

- **Compared with laparoscopy, open laparotomy produces more trauma, exposure, heat loss and fluid evaporation.**
- **Postoperative pain, immobility, the risk of pulmonary and deep vein complications and of adynamic ileus are more frequent following open procedures.**
- **There is probably a lower incidence of postoperative adhesions following laparoscopy.**

LIMITATIONS OF MINIMAL ACCESS SURGERY

1. When performing minimal access surgery you are remote from the operative field, using a two-dimensional imaging system to represent the operative site. You must learn to navigate the anatomical landscape without the usual clues by which you judge depth.

2. The instruments are longer and sometimes more complex than those used in open operations.

3. These two factors combine to create significant problems of hand–eye coordination, but with experience these difficulties can be overcome.

4. Three-dimensional imaging is available, using two cameras side by side, delivering a stereoscopic image. It can be used to perform robotically assisted minimally invasive surgery. This confers benefits in the ability to perform complex laparoscopic tasks, such as intracorporeal suturing. In the future, continuing cost reduction will make elaborate image-processing techniques available for a wide range of transformed presentations. Ultimately it will be possible to call up any view of the operative region

that is accessible to a camera presented stereoscopically in any size or orientation, superimposed on past images taken in other modalities. We shall need to decide which of these many imaginative possibilities will contribute most effectively.

5. Intraoperative bleeding may be very difficult to control endoscopically because blood obscures the field of vision and there is a significant reduction in the image quality due to light absorption.

6. Some of the new procedures are more technically demanding and are slower to perform. Indeed, on occasions a minimally invasive operation is so technically demanding that both you and patient are better served by conversion to an open procedure. Do not feel a sense of embarrassment or humiliation, which is quite unjustified. It is vital for you and your patients to appreciate that the decision to convert to open operation is not a complication but rather implies sound surgical judgement.

7. Loss of tactile feedback is a disadvantage. Laparoscopic ultrasonography might provide a substitute for the need to 'feel' in intraoperative decision making. Although ultrasonography has progressed significantly, laparoscopic ultrasound is still in its infancy. The rapid progress in advanced laparoscopic techniques, including biliary tract exploration and surgery for malignancy, provides a strong impetus for the development of laparoscopic ultrasound, which already offers advantages that far outweigh its disadvantages:

a. It offers a safe, easily performed and economic substitute for a sense of touch, allowing visualization through tubular fluid-filled and solid organs as well as vascular structures.

b. It differentiates between solid and cystic masses.

c. The wall layers of hollow viscera can be evaluated.

d. Better staging of tumours is possible because the dimensions, infiltration and dissemination can be detected.

e. Guided biopsies can be obtained.

f. It does not involve the use of ionizing radiations or contrast media.

g. It has no contraindications, can be used during pregnancy and can be employed at any time during the operation.

8. In more advanced techniques, the large piece of resected tissue, such as the lung or colon, must be extracted from the body cavity (Monson et al 1992). Occasionally it can be removed through a nearby natural orifice, such as the rectum or mouth. At other times a novel route can be used, such as extraction of a benign colonic specimen through an incision in the vault of the vagina. Tissue mincers, morcellators and liquidizers can be used but have the disadvantage of reducing the amount of information available to the pathologist.

9. Minimal access techniques are applied to staging and resection of gastrointestinal, urological, gynaecological and thoracic malignant tumours. Reports of tumour implantation in port sites, particularly early on, are being studied in a prospective controlled trial (CLASICC) of laparoscopic colorectal resections for malignancy in the UK.

10. There is a growing need for improved dissection techniques in laparoscopic surgery, specifically the safe use of electrocautery and lasers. Ultrasonic dissection and tissue removal is utilized in a growing number of specialities. Adaptation of the technology to laparoscopic surgery grew from the search for alternative and possibly safer methods of dissection. Current units combine the functions of three or four separate instruments, reducing the need for instrument exchanges. This flexibility, combined with the ability to provide a clean, smoke-free field, saves time and improves safety.

11. Dramatic cost savings are possible with laparoscopic cholecystectomy, particularly as some can be performed as day cases, but the position is less clear for other procedures. In contrast, there has been a rise in the cholecystectomy rate, resulting from a lower threshold for referral, following the introduction of the laparoscopic approach – increasing the overall cost of treating symptomatic gallstones.

TRAINING FOR MINIMAL ACCESS SURGERY

It is probably true to say that no previous surgical innovation has aroused so much public questioning of how surgeons are trained. While the pioneers of a new technique are inevitably self-trained, patients then rightly demand that their successors are properly trained to perform it safely and effectively. This is particularly so in laparoscopic surgery, which employs skills not commonly used in everyday life.

The importance of training in minimal access surgery has been recognized with the establishment of several centres dedicated to teaching the fundamentals of safe minimal access surgery. These centres, including the Minimal Access Therapy Training Unit (MATTU) at the Royal College of Surgeons of England, are working to develop training methods using various methods of simulation, allowing surgeons to complete a significant part of their skills training before operating on patients. Virtual reality training simulators are now in use and the technology will improve further, to generate an artificial environment in which surgeons can practise in complete safety.

Key points

- The skills you require to undertake minimal access surgery are exceptional. Take every opportunity to acquire and practise them.
- The principles of good surgery still apply: case selection, exposure, retraction, haemostasis, technical expertise.
- Minimal access has changed practice but not the nature of disease. A conventional procedure that does not make sense does not make sense performed by minimal access techniques.

Summary

Do you understand:

- The scope and limits of minimal access surgery?
- The potential benefits for the patients?
- The need for careful selection and for conversion to open surgery in response to difficulties?
- The imperative need to train yourself before embarking into a field requiring exceptional skills?

THE FUTURE

Improvements in instrumentation and the development of structured training programmes are the key to the future of minimal access surgery. There is much that is new in minimal access surgery; time will tell how much of what is new is better.

The cleaner and gentler the act of operation, the less the patient suffers, the smoother and quicker his convalescence, the more exquisite his healed wound.

Lord Moynihan of Leeds

References

Cuschieri A 1992 A rose by any other name: minimal access or minimal invasive surgery. Surgical Endoscopy 6: 214

Darzi A, Goldin R, Guillou PJ, Monson JRT 1993 Extracorporeal shock wave thermotherapy: new antitumour option. Surgical Oncology 2: 197–204

Monson JRT, Darzi A, Carey PD, Guillou PJ 1992 Prospective evaluation of laparoscopic assisted colectomy in an unselected group of patients. Lancet 340: 831–833

Wickham J, Fitzpatrick JM 1990 Minimally invasive surgery [editorial]. British Journal of Surgery 77: 721

24 Principles of skin cover

P. E. M. Butler, J. L. Atkins

> **Objectives**
>
> - **Understand the pathophysiological changes accompanying, and resulting from, different types of skin loss.**
> - **Recognize the importance of pre-existing conditions in the skin and contiguous tissues before the skin loss.**
> - **Differentiate between the special features of skin in different parts of the body.**
> - **Identify circumstances in which primary closure is possible, better deferred, and contraindicated.**
> - **Recognize the available methods of achieving closure and their indications.**

INTRODUCTION

The skin is the largest organ of the body, forming just under a sixth of the total body weight. Skin function varies in different parts of the body and this is reflected in its qualities. Although the basic structure of skin is constant, thickness and elasticity, pigmentation, and the presence or absence of specialized skin appendages, such as exocrine glands, nails, hair and sensory apparatus, differ.

Skin provides a number of diverse but vital functions to the body. Most obviously, it provides a physical barrier to the outside world, giving limited protection against mechanical, chemical and thermal damage as well as preventing invasion by microorganisms, including viruses. Its integrity is critical for homeostasis, maintaining the internal milieu by providing a relatively impermeable barrier to the passage of water, proteins or electrolytes in either direction. Similarly, a vital role in thermoregulation is manifest by the controlled release of sweat and variability of blood flow to the body surface, leading to heat loss or conservation as required. Melanin pigment within the dermis protects the skin by absorbing ultraviolet rays of long (UVA) and medium (UVB) wavelength. Sensory information received from sensory appendages located within the dermis is both vast and subtle, while the synthesis of vitamin D and deposition of fat in the subcutaneous layer are functions of metabolic importance. The appearance and feel of our skin is critical; abnormalities are readily visible to the world at large, can be socially stigmatizing and are a source of psychological distress as well as physical discomfort to the affected individual.

Skin loss through disease or trauma exposes an individual to the risk of bacterial and viral infections, uncontrolled loss of serous fluid, proteins and electrolytes, and loss of mechanical protection to vulnerable underlying tissue. When skin wounds are very extensive they can be painful, disabling and life threatening, as is seen in burn injuries. Smaller wounds also deserve careful attention as they provide a defect through which serious infections may enter and produce life threatening conditions such as gas gangrene, toxic shock syndrome and necrotizing fasciitis. Chronic skin wounds can undergo malignant transformation, as seen in Bowen's disease (intradermal precancerous skin lesion described by the Harvard dermatologist in 1912), which may progress to squamous cell carcinoma.

Poorly managed wounds heal slowly, and form ugly, weak scars with a poor functional result. Your primary aims in restoring skin cover are to provide optimal function and form in a timely fashion. Understanding how certain injury types affect tissue viability and lead to skin loss is paramount. Undertake a systematic and thorough assessment of the patient in general, and the wound in particular, before instituting an appropriate course of treatment and rehabilitation.

SKIN CHARACTERISTICS

1. You are not dealing with a homogeneous body covering but with a varied, dynamic, responsive complex surface overlying varying supportive tissues.
2. Skin varies in different parts of the body in thickness, vascularity, nerve supply, ability to tolerate trauma,

mobility, and also in special attributes; for example, palmar skin of the hands, and especially of the fingertips of the index finger and thumb, are irreplaceable. Although it is tough and able to withstand and respond to hard usage, it is richly supplied with a variety of afferent nerve endings, enabling us to utilize our fingers as important sensory organs.

3. The elasticity of the skin varies with age and the individual, producing tension lines. These tend to run circumferentially around joints and the trunk, at least in early life. They are often named Langer's lines after Carl von Langer, the Austrian anatomist. By puncturing cadaveric skin with round spikes, he observed, in 1832, how the circular defects deformed as a result of skin tension. Incisions orientated parallel to tension lines heal with superior scars.

4. Fetal skin heals without scar formation; at birth skin is extremely elastic but with increasing age it becomes less so. In old age, following loss of fat and muscle bulk, the inelastic skin hangs in folds, especially on the abdomen and neck.

5. Viability is reduced by defective nutrition (such as vitamin C, zinc, protein), ischaemia, denervation, vascular congestion, inflammation and infection. The skin is friable overlying an abscess and also in an area of cellulitis or erysipelas (Greek *erythros* = red + *pella* = skin).

6. Pathological changes may develop as a result of exposure to solar or ionizing radiation, cancer chemotherapy and various drug treatments. A variety of drugs, such as sulphonamides, barbiturates and non-steroidal anti-inflammatory substances (NSAIDs), may induce toxic epidermal necrolysis (TEN or Lyell's syndrome), in which fluid-filled bullae develop, separating sheets of epithelium from the underlying dermis.

WOUND ASSESSMENT

Key point

- **The history is as important as the appearance when assessing wounds.**

1. Ascertain the timing, nature and force of the injury sustained. Accurately describe the appearance of a wound, and recognize how this changes over time; time elapsed since injury influences how you manage the wound. Ascertain exactly what tissue has been lost and what remains; are tendons, bones or neurovascular structures exposed? These may need urgent soft tissue cover to preserve function and prevent infection, and may require a more complex reconstruction. Wounds present-ing early (<48 h) exhibit features of an acute inflammatory response. Following this acute phase, observe signs of healing in an untreated wound with some or all of the features of the acute inflammatory response having dispersed. Identify slough and granulation tissue in the wound base, with an advancing epithelial edge at the wound margin. Chronic inflammation occurs with continuing tissue damage; the wound exhibits features of ongoing tissue necrosis, acute inflammation, granulation tissue and fibrous scarring.

2. If you are inexperienced you may be distracted by the presence of an obvious or dramatic wound from other pathology. Carry out a full, careful examination of traumatized patients. Give priority to potentially life-threatening injuries; they require urgent treatment.

3. Different mechanisms of injury compromise tissue in different ways. Recognize and understand the effects of patterns of injury. The severity of the wound is affected by a number of factors. Elderly patients have thin, delicate skin, easily lost with relatively minor trauma compared with the skin of children or young adults. Take note of the anatomical area; pretibial skin is thin, vulnerable to trauma and slow to heal; skin on the back is thick and robust, while facial skin is delicate but heals quickly because it has a rich blood supply. Chronic systemic steroid use produces thin, atrophic skin, easily lost following minor trauma. Diabetics may develop peripheral neuropathy leading to chronic or recurrent ulceration of the lower limb; combined with microvascular disease and an impaired immune response, the ulcers heal reluctantly.

SKIN LOSS

Mechanical trauma

1. *Contusion* (Latin *tundere* = to bruise) results from blunt trauma. This is not usually a serious skin injury, but if it produces a haematoma, the swelling may cause pressure necrosis of the overlying skin. In elderly or anticoagulated patients large haematomas may develop following a minor blow, leading to the formation of very large haematomas. Incise and evacuate these urgently to prevent loss of the overlying skin. Blood loss may be great enough to require transfusion.

2. *Abrasion* (Latin *ab* = from + *radere* = to scrape) is a superficial epidermal friction injury, often patchy. The epidermis regenerates by advancement of epithelium remaining within the skin appendages deep within the dermis. Healing is usually complete and can be encouraged by gently and thoroughly cleaning the wound with a mild antiseptic to remove dirt or debris, and applying a moist, non-adherent occlusive dressing. Unless you

remove the dirt ground into the wound, permanent skin tattooing (Tahitian ta'tau) will develop.

3. *Retraction* (Latin *re* = back + *trahere* = to draw) of skin edges occurs when it is lacerated (Latin *lacerare* = to tear). Skin is innately elastic, the extent varying with age, race, familial trait, the use of systemic steroids, smoking and nutrition. If you are inexperienced you may mistake skin-edge retraction for skin loss, most commonly seen in children whose greater skin elasticity may lead to dramatic opening up of the wound. Avoid this mistake by carefully examining the wound and recognizing the pattern and markings of one edge that match those of the opposite edge if the skin has merely retracted.

4. *Degloving* results from severe shearing of the skin, for example, a pneumatic tyre running over a limb, detaching the skin from the underlying tissue. This separation may occur superficially, or beneath the layer of deep investing fascia, causing skin loss over a large area. The skin may tear, or remain intact initially, disguising the severity of this injury. Rupture of the vessels connecting the deeper tissues to the skin commonly produces ischaemic necrosis of the skin and other tissues superficial to the plane of separation. Prejudiced skin perfusion may be apparent from an absence of dermal bleeding at the skin edges, as may the absence of blanching followed by capillary refill, when you apply then release pressure. Subsequently the area of injury becomes more defined as the skin becomes mottled, then necrotic. You may be able to resurface the underlying tissue using a split thickness skin graft.

5. *Avulsion* (Latin *ab* = from + *vellere* = to pull) is the partial or complete tearing away of tissue and may involve skin, deeper structures such as bone, tendon, muscle and nerve, including digits, limbs or scalp. The force required to do this is considerable and creates a zone of injury around the point at which the tissue separates. Tissue is usually stretched, twisted and torn, leading to irreversible damage, in particular of neurovascular structures. It may be possible, when you have appropriate experience, to reattach or replant avulsed tissue using microvascular techniques. Completely avulsed tissue can be temporarily stored in moistened sterile gauze, sealed in a plastic bag and placed in ice, or stored in a refrigerator at 4°C. Vascular tissue such as muscle cannot be safely replanted if it has been ischaemic for more than 6 h. Tendon, skin and bone are more tolerant of ischaemia. Make every effort to salvage an avulsed or amputated upper limb, thumb, multiple lost digits, or digits in children. They are important for restoration of function, and especially in children they offer greater potential for recovery. Loss of individual digits is relatively less important in terms of benefit. An avulsed toe or foot is rarely suitable for microvascular replantation because sensory and functional recovery is poor and therefore unlikely to be satisfactory. If the patient has other significant life threatening injuries you may decide against attempting to reimplant divided tissues

Key point

- **Remember that even trivial skin loss may offer entry to strains of *Staphylococcus aureus* that may cause toxic shock syndrome, especially in vulnerable patients such as children, the elderly and the sick.**

Thermal injury

1. A scald (Latin *ex* = from + *calidus* = warm, hot) is caused by contact with hot liquids. A variety of agents may cause burns, such as flames, contact with hot objects, radiant heat and corrosive (Latin *rodere* = to gnaw) chemicals.

2. Through and through electrical injuries differ from other burns in that the passage of the electrical current through the body causes injury to deep tissue that may not be immediately apparent. A small entrance and exit burn of the skin may be the only visible manifestation of the injury. The electrolyte-rich blood acts as a conduit for the current flow and the vascular endothelium is damaged so that the vessels subsequently undergo thrombosis. Deep-seated tissue necrosis becomes apparent as the patient becomes increasingly unwell over hours or days. High voltage injuries are the most destructive, and alternating current is more likely to cause myocardial fibrillation than direct current.

Surgical diathermy heats the tissues as a result of intense vibration of the ions caused by the low amperage high frequency, high voltage, alternating current (see Ch. 17). Faulty equipment and inexpert use may result in skin burns.

3. Exposure to cold air may cause frostbite. Excessive exposure to cold causes peripheral vascular spasm, with ischaemia and anoxia of the extremities, affecting a localized area of soft tissue. The extent of the injury is affected by temperature, duration of contact and pre-existing hypoperfusion of tissues. Four phases of injury have been described. These are;

a. Pre-freeze (3–10°C): increased vascular permeability

b. Freeze–thaw (–6 to –14°C): formation of intra- and extracellular ice crystal.

c. Vascular stasis: blood is shunted away from the damaged area

d. Late ischaemic phase: cell death, gangrene.

Thawing, with restoration of the circulation, liberates inflammatory mediators. Microemboli form on the damaged endothelium and these increase the ischaemia and tissue loss. Treatment includes rewarming by immersion of the affected part in circulating warm water, elevation and splinting. Ischaemic areas are allowed to demarcate prior to amputation of the necrotic parts.

Cryosurgery (Greek *kryon* = frost) offers a method of destroying skin lesions almost painlessly (see Ch. 17).

A lesser result of exposure to cold is chilblains (Old English *blain* = a boil or blister).

Contact with very cold objects can result in adherence of the skin, which is pulled off on separation.

4. Assess burns, in terms of site, percentage of the body surface damaged and depth of damage, to determine the prognosis and as a guide to treatment. Depth is superficial (1st degree), partial skin thickness including the dermis (2nd degree) and full thickness of all the layers of the skin (3rd degree). Burn depth is difficult to assess. White, insensate areas are generally full thickness. Partial thickness burns usually blanch on pressure and refill when the pressure is released; it remains sensate and may be blistered. Superficial burns are often erythematous, perfused, painful and tender to touch.

5. Generally, full thickness burns are managed by excision and skin grafting of the underlying tissue bed; partial thickness burns may be suitable for conservative treatment, allowing epidermal regeneration from remaining epithelial elements within the skin appendages of the dermis.

Ulceration

'Ulcer' (Greek *elkos*, Latin *ulcus* = sore) usually has a connotation of chronicity. An acute loss of skin is not called an ulcer unless it fails to heal.

1. *Pressure sores* develop from unrelieved pressure on the tissues in a debilitated patient, especially if there is neurological impairment. Other factors include nutritional deficit, diabetes mellitus, immunosuppression, incontinence and an inappropriate physical environment. The commonest affected areas are on the lower body within tissue overlying bony prominences. The sore develops as the tissue becomes compressed and oedematous; the pressure within the tissue exceeds the capillary perfusion pressure, leading to ischaemia and tissue necrosis. The tissue adjacent to the bony prominence suffers the most extensive injury, with the least at the level of the skin; the visible skin wound belies the reality of a much more extensive tissue loss.

Key point

• **Development of pressure sores represents a failure to protect skin at risk from continuing pressure or contact with damaging substances, including body secretions and excretions.**

Treatment is predominantly conservative. Institute measures to relieve pressure, such as the use of specially adapted wheelchairs, beds and other padding, correct any nutritional deficiency, eliminate infection, control incontinence and apply appropriate dressings. A minority require surgical intervention, such as wound debridement, excision of the bony prominence to encourage closure, or covering the area with a soft tissue flap. Use flaps cautiously in the presence of chronic predisposing illness such as multiple sclerosis.

2. *Other common causes of ulceration* include diabetes, autoimmune disorders, infection, ischaemia, venous disease and neoplastic lesions. Identify the underlying cause, if necessary by obtaining an incisional or punch biopsy of the margin, and treat the underlying cause. Any chronic ulcer may undergo malignant change, with the formation of Bowen's disease prior to malignant invasion as squamous cell carcinoma.

3. *Raynaud's disease*, described by the Parisian physician in 1862, is an excessive arteriolar sensitivity to cold of the extremities. In Raynaud's phenomenon the spasm is secondary to vascular or connective tissue disease, or occupations in which vibrating tools need to be used. The spasm causes necrosis and ulceration of the extremities.

Key point

• **Record the progress by keeping serial photographs of wound size, extent and healing.**

BIOLOGY OF SKIN HEALING (see also Ch. 33)

1. Wound healing is a multistep overlapping process involving an inflammatory response, granulation tissue formation, new blood vessel formation, wound closure and tissue remodelling. Tissue damage causes extravasation of blood and its constituents. Platelets and macrophages release a number of chemical mediators including transforming growth factors (TGF), fibroblast growth factor (FGF), vascular endothelial growth factor (VEGF), platelet-derived growth factor (PDGF), insulin-like growth factor (IGF) and keratinocyte growth factor (KGF).

2. The injured cells and other cells and platelets generate vasoactive and chemotactic (Arabic *al kimiea*, Greek *chemeia + tassein* = to arrange; cell movement in response to a chemical stimulus) substances that attract inflammatory neutrophils. Monocytes are also attracted and convert to macrophages. These phagocytes remove

dead tissue and foreign material, including bacteria. As inflammatory exudate accumulates, there is a cascade of events leading to oedema, erythema, pain, heat and impaired function. Macrophages and factors derived from them are essential in stimulating repair (Singer & Clark 1999).

3. Epidermal cells from skin appendages break desmosomal contact with each other and also with the basement membrane; they migrate in the plane between the viable and necrotic tissues by producing collagenase, which degrades the intercellular substance (matrix) reinforced by matrix metalloproteinase. Epithelial cells behind the migrating ones proliferate after 1 or 2 days, probably from the release of growth factors. As re-epithelialization proceeds, the epithelial cells reattach themselves to the basement membrane and underlying dermis.

4. As a result of hypoxia, growth and angiogenesis factors are released by macrophages and activated epithelial cells. The wound is invaded by blood capillaries, macrophages, fibroblasts after 3–4 days, bringing nutrients and oxygen. The crests of the capillary loops appear like small cobblestones, hence the name of 'granulation' tissue. Blood capillaries require the presence of perivascular fibronectins (Latin *nectere* = to bind, tie) in order to move into the wound. Vascular growth is a delicate balance of positive regulators such as VEGF and PDGF, and negative regulators such as angiopoietin-2, endostatin and angiostatin. Once the wound is covered with granulation tissue angiogenesis stops. The fibroblasts synthesize extracellular matrix, which is later replaced with acellular collagen, when cells in the wound undergo apoptosis (Greek *apo* = from + *piptein* = to fall; programmed cell death). During the second week following injury, fibroblasts become myofibroblasts, acquiring actin-containing microfilaments (Greek *aktinos* = ray) and cell-to-cell and cell-to-matrix linkages. Probably under the influence of TGF and PDGF, the fibroblasts attach to the collagen matrix through integrin receptors and form cross-links. Myofibroblast contraction draws together the attachments at each end of the cell. However, in animal experiments the evidence for the role of myofibroblasts has been questioned (Berry et al 1998).

5. The contribution of epithelial migration and wound contraction to healing is not fully resolved. There are also differences in the factors involved between humans and in animal experiments. One suggestion is that wound contraction in granulation tissue results from the compaction of collagen fibres influenced by cellular forces, not directly from contraction of cells pulling on the surrounding tissues.

6. When closure of large raw areas has failed or is unavailable, healing and scar formation continues for weeks, months or years. This is often termed scar contracture. Powerful forces draw in skin and scar tissue is laid down, often causing severe limitation of function. A classical example is that of a young child who pulls over a pan of scalding water, burning the face, neck, shoulder, chest, axilla and upper arm. The head is permanently drawn to the side of the burn, the neck is webbed, the shoulder is drawn upwards and fixed; the shoulder cannot be abducted and the deltoid muscle atrophies, while the anterior axillary fold and skin over the chest circumference is tight, restricting inspiration.

7. Collagen degradation proceeds in step with wound contraction. The wound gains only 20% of its final strength in the first 3 weeks, and the maximum strength it achieves is only 70% of that of normal skin.

8. Healing is prejudiced in diabetes, especially in the presence of neuropathy and ischaemia. Wounds are prone to infection because of impaired granulocyte function and chemotaxis.

9. Abnormal accumulation of collagen causes hypertrophic scarring and keloid formation. Normal mature scars and keloids display no scar contraction and they do not contain any myofibroblasts. Increased levels of TGFβ, PDGF, interleukin 1 (IL-1) and IGF-I are present in both, with TGFβ appearing to predominate.

10. Growth factors have proved disappointing in accelerating wound healing, possibly because they need to be administered in carefully graded doses and sequence.

11. Fetal skin wounds heal rapidly without scarring; the epithelial cells are drawn across the wound by contraction of actin fibres. Scarring does not occur because there is a reduced level of TGFβ1. *PRX-2*, a member of the Paired Related Homeobox gene family, is upregulated in dermal fibroblasts during scarless fetal wound healing.

DEBRIDEMENT

1. Debris, foreign material, devitalized tissue, slough, pus or heavy contamination with pathological bacteria form a focus for infection, irritate the wound, prevent the formation of granulation tissue and obstruct epithelial migration.

2. Excise all non-viable skin under anaesthesia and, if you are in doubt regarding viability, return the patient to the operating theatre for a second inspection and debridement after 24–48 h. Debridement (French *de* = from + bridle; unbridle = release from constriction) was originally used for releasing tension but has been extended to mean the removal of dead tissue.

3. It can often be achieved non-surgically using saline irrigation, topical agents to lift slough or with dressings

or sharp dissection under anaesthesia. Debride areas with specialized and precious tissue, such as the fingertips, palm and face, adequately but minimally. If there is uncertainty at the time of surgery as to the viability of tissue or adequacy of debridement, be willing to redress the wound with an occlusive non-adherent dressing and return the patient to the operating theatre for a second inspection after 24–48 h.

ACHIEVING WOUND CLOSURE AND SKIN COVER

No skin loss

1. Clean incised wounds vary, depending on where and how the wound is made. If it is made parallel to the lines of tension the edges remain closely apposed, if made across the tension lines they gape. There is virtually no damage to contiguous tissues so that, apart from the almost singular layer of cells along the line of division, the remainder of the tissues are viable. Such a wound, once closed, is said to heal by primary intention, and should heal with a fine linear scar.

2. If the incision is only partial thickness the deeper intact parts maintain the edges in good apposition. If the wound extends through the full thickness this support is partially lost, depending on the strength and attachment of the deeper tissues.

3. Abraded skin has intact deeper layers and will heal spontaneously. Torn skin dragged as a flap may initially appear viable; a triangular flap attached distally over the subcutaneous face of the tibia notoriously fails to survive.

4. In wounds with very irregular margins, it is helpful to close the most obvious matching points first and then to close the other points in between. Do not be afraid to remove and reposition sutures until the edges are perfectly matched. Small bridges of skin separating lacerations are best excised to achieve a cosmetic result.

Skin loss

1. When a skin or other superficial lesion has been excised, the surviving edges and the base are normally left healthy, dry and free of bacterial contamination, foreign material or dead tissue.

2. Closure can usually be performed immediately (primary closure); indeed the excision is usually planned with this in mind, except in the presence of malignant disease, when total clearance of the tumour is paramount. Primary closure allows more rapid healing and an earlier return to normal function.

3. In elective surgical procedures, the closure can be planned before operation and discussed with the patient. It may be possible to close the defect directly, reconstruct or resurface it.

4. As far as possible, replace large defects with skin and tissue giving the closest possible match to the surrounding tissues with regard to colour, thickness and texture.

5. To achieve the best results the wound edges must be accurately opposed. If the wound is irregular, perfect apposition can be aided by first identifying and apposing landmarks with key sutures before inserting intervening sutures.

6. Perfect closure is prejudiced by unevenness, inversion of the edges and tension, as inevitable postoperative oedema increases the tension.

7. Many small wounds of 1 cm in diameter or less, including many fingertip injuries, usually heal with a satisfactory result by secondary intention within 2–3 weeks. Treat larger wounds conservatively in ill, frail patients, and those likely to heal within a reasonable time. This may include pressure sores.

 Key point

- **Assess the nature of the skin at the margins of the defect that you intend to close.**

Complicating factors

1. The skin may be atrophic or stretched, especially in elderly people, or affected by eczema, solar or ionizing radiation, hypertrophy or the scar of a previous operation. Neonatal and infant skin usually heals well.

2. Inflammation, neoplasm, ischaemia, oedema, infection, congestion or injury – possibly with the presence of foreign material – of contiguous tissues such as bones, muscles, tendons, nerves or vessels may force a change of strategy.

3. Repair is prejudiced if the patient is very old, undernourished, immunosuppressed is undergoing chemotherapy, or has general infection, neoplasia or organ failure.

4. The wound may be too large to close.

Achieving closure

1. Grafting (Greek *graphein* = to write; from the Roman use of tree grafting using shoots sharpened like a pencil), may allow transfer of completely detached partial or full thickness skin from a donor site to a

wound that cannot be closed directly. The graft adheres by fibrinous bonds, initially gaining nourishment by serum imbibition – metabolites diffusing through the thin film of intervening serum. Capillaries connect from the recipient site and are functioning by the second day, but the connection is fragile and susceptible to shear stress for 2–3 weeks. The best recipient sites for skin grafts are clean, granulating and well vascularized; unsuitable sites include bone lacking periosteum, tendons stripped of paratenon, denuded cartilage, irradiated or avascular wounds and those covered in blood clot. Gross contamination with microorganisms prejudice graft survival and *Streptococcus pyogenes* is an absolute contraindication because it produces fibrinolysin, destroying the fibrin bond between the bed and the graft. The likelihood of graft movement can be reduced by applying moderate pressure with a conforming, tie-over dressing, which will also inhibit the development of a seroma or haematoma.

2. A split thickness skin graft consists of epidermis and a variable proportion of dermis, harvested in sheets using a handheld knife or electronic dermatome. Retained epidermal components, such as pilosebaceous follicles, provide foci for epidermal regeneration. The thinner the graft harvested, the more epidermal elements left behind, the quicker the epidermis regenerates. If the volume of donor skin is inadequate, split skin grafts can be expanded by the use of a meshing machine; this creates fenestrations throughout the graft, allowing it to expand and cover a larger area, with a net-like appearance. Split skin grafts can be harvested, wrapped in sterile saline-soaked gauze and stored in a refrigerator at 4°C, with up to 3 weeks viability. The commonest donor site for these grafts is the thigh or buttock area. The donor site often heals with altered pigmentation, and occasionally with a hypertrophic scar. Split thickness grafts, especially thin ones, tend to contract during the healing process, limiting movement across flexor surfaces. The application of compression garments when the graft is healed improves the appearance, flattens the scar and minimizes contraction, aided by daily massage with moisturizing cream.

3. Full thickness skin grafts comprise the epidermis and full thickness of the dermis. It is harvested using a template to plan the size and shape, and subcutaneous fat is removed. The donor site, such as post- or preauricular, supraclavicular or groin, is closed directly. It generally provides good colour match on the face and contracts minimally. Such grafts are inevitably limited in size and must be placed on a healthy, vascular base.

4. Flaps are detached tissue, containing a network of arterial, venous and capillary vessels, transferred from one site to another. They can retain their intact circulation on the original vascular pedicle. Random pattern flaps do not have an anatomically recognized vascular supply and as a general rule the length of the flap should not exceed twice the length of the attached base. Some flaps have identified vessels supplying them – axial pattern flaps, including the forehead, groin and deltopectoral region; these may be raised on a narrow pedicle and disconnected completely, for the vessels to be joined to vessels at the recipient site – a free flap. This is achievable as a result of microsurgical techniques. They may include other tissues, including deep fascia, muscle or bone. Useful sites include the forehead, groin and deltopectoral region.

5. Myocutaneous flaps provide a robust vascularized wound cover over exposed bone, tendon or areas subjected to high mechanical demands. Skin in many areas is supplied by perforating vessels from the underlying muscle and an island of skin can be transferred with the muscle to provide simultaneous skin cover. The muscle is isolated onto its vascular pedicle alone and rotated into the defect. Commonly used myocutaneous flaps include the latissimus dorsi, rectus abdominis, pectoralis major and gastrocnemius.

6. Deep fascia included with overlying layers of skin improves vascularity and safety; they can also be transferred as vascularized free flaps.

7. Tissue expansion allows the skin and subcutaneous tissue to be stretched in order to fill a defect nearby. An expandable silicone (Silastic) bag is inserted beneath the skin and subcutaneous fat. When the wound is healed, the sac can be filled percutaneously with increasing volumes of saline though a special subcutaneous port. Once the overlying skin is sufficiently stretched, the implant is removed and the stretched excess skin can be advanced into the defect.

SKIN SUBSTITUTES

Wound coverage is vitally important. If sufficient skin is not available it may be possible to apply a substitute. The main need for these substitutes is in the management of extensive burns.

1. Autologous (derived from the same individual) cultured epidermal cells provide permanent coverage but they require 3 weeks in order to grow sufficient cells.

2. Allografts (Greek *allos* = other; from another individual) cultured epidermal cells from living persons or cadavers do not appear to be rejected, possibly because they do not express major histocompatability complex

class II antigens and are not contaminated with Langerhans cells, which are the antigen-presenting cells of the epidermis. They are eventually replaced by host cells, so they offer temporary coverage.

3. Neonatal epidermal cells, for example from excised foreskins, release growth factors. Cultured cells accelerate healing and relieve painful chronic ulcers.

4. A composite collagen-based dermal lattice in a silicone covering may be valuable in the treatment of burns. The dermal cells are gradually degraded but after 3 weeks the Silastic sheet cover can be removed and replaced by cultured autologous cells. Human epidermal cells and viable fibroblasts may be included in the composite. Viable fibroblasts may also be included in a nylon net cover overlaid with Silastic to reduce evaporation.

5. In order to provide substitute dermal as well as epidermal cells, bovine collagen and allogeneic human cells may be combined.

Summary

- Are you aware of the multiplicity of factors to which the skin is exposed?
- Do you recognize the varied causes of skin damage and loss?
- Do you understand the complex biology of skin healing?
- Can you discuss the methods of skin closure?

References

Berry DP, Harding K, Stanton MR, Tasani B, Ehrlich HP 1998. Human wound contraction: collagen organization, fibroblasts and myofibroblasts. Plastic and Reconstructive Surgery 102: 124–131

Singer AJ, Clark RA 1999. Mechanisms of disease: cutaneous wound healing. New England Journal of Medicine 341: 738–746

Further reading

Brough M 2000. Plastic surgery in general surgical operations, 4th edn. Churchill Livingstone Edinburgh, pp 727–773

Kirk RM 2002 Basic surgical techniques, 5th edn. Churchill Livingstone, Edinburgh

McGregor IA, McGregor AD 1995 Fundamental techniques in plastic surgery and their surgical applications. Churchill Livingstone, Edinburgh

Nedelec B, Ghahary A, Scott PG, Tredget EE 2000. Control of wound contraction. Basic and clinical features. Hand Clinics 16: 289–302

Richard R, DerSarkisian D, Miller SF, Johnson RM, Staley M 1999. Directional variance in skin movement. Journal of Burn Care and Rehabilitation 20: 259–264

Saba AA, Freedman BM, Gaffield JW, Mackay DR, Ehrlich HP 2002. Topical platelet-derived growth factor enhances wound closure in the absence of wound contraction: an experimental study. Annals of Plastic Surgery 49: 62–66

Witte MB, Barbul A 2002. Role of nitric oxide in wound repair. American Journal of Surgery 183: 406–412

Younai S, Venters G, Vu G, Nichter L, Nimni E, Tuan TL 1996. Role of growth factors in scar contraction: an in vitro analysis. Annals of Plastic Surgery 36: 495–501

25 Transplantation

P. McMaster, L. J. Buist

Objectives

- **Appreciate the causes of organ rejection.**
- **Understand the principles of transplantation and immunosuppression.**
- **Be aware of the source of transplanted organs, and the associated ethical and legal considerations.**

Table 25.1   Forms of tissue transfer

- *Transfer of tissue*
  Blood
  Bone marrow

- *Transfer of solid organ*
  Skin
  Cornea
  Kidney
  Heart
  Liver
  Pancreas

BASIC PRINCIPLES

Early Christian legends attest to the attempts to replace diseased or destroyed organs or tissues by the transfer from another individual. The father of modern surgery, John Hunter, carried out extensive experiments on the transposition of tissues and concluded what he thought were successful experiments on the transposition of teeth! However, it was not until the dawn of the 20th century that the practical technical realities of organ transfer were combined with sufficient understanding of the immunological mechanisms involved to allow transplantation to become a practical reality.

While it had long been recognized that successful blood transfusion was in large measure dependent on matching donor and recipient cells, it was only in the 1950s that Mitchison (1953) demonstrated that, while cell-mediated immunity was responsible for early destruction and rejection, it was the humeral mechanism with cytotoxic antibodies that was primarily involved in the host response to foreign tissue. It became increasingly recognized that all tissue and fluid transfer was governed by basic immunomechanisms (Table 25.1).

The need in the Second World War to find improved ways of treating badly burned pilots led Gibson & Medawar (1943) to carry out a series of classic experiments on skin transplantation. They were able to conclude that the transfer of skin from one part of the body to another in the same individual (an *autograft*), survived indefinitely, whereas the transfer of skin from another individual (an *allograft*) was in due course destroyed and that the recipient retained memory of the donor tissue and further transfers or allografts were destroyed in an accelerated mechanism. Thus the wider recognition of the universal acceptance of autografts became realized, whereas the failure of an allograft was recognized as part of an immune response. An alternative source of organs is, of course, the animal world, and the transfer from another species is known as a *xenograft*.

FIRST CLINICAL PROGRAMMES

The recognition that an autograft would be universally acceptable led to the first successful attempts at organ grafting in humans. In the early 1950s, Murray et al (1955) at the Peter Bent Brigham Hospital in Boston, were able to demonstrate the successful transfer of a kidney graft from an identical twin, with acceptance and successful function, and to develop a programme of renal transplantation between monozygotic twins.

Some of the recipients of kidney transplants from identical twins remain well more than 40 years after grafting; however, grafts between unrelated living individuals performed by this same group invariably failed, although not as quickly as experimental studies might have suggested.

RESPONSE

The other major human source of organs, other than from living relatives, is from individuals who have died as a result of road traffic accidents or cerebral injuries. Cadaveric organ grafting from non-related individuals is now the major source of organs. Within Europe, more than 80% of all organs transplanted are from brain-dead donors.

Thus, although technical considerations presented the initial formidable barrier to organ transfer, it was increasingly the understanding of the immune response causing organ destruction by rejection, which led to clinical schedules permitting practical transplantation services to be established. The body's immune response to destroy the invading organ we now recognize as *rejection*.

REJECTION

Early experimental studies involving tissue transfer suggested genetic regulation of the rejection process. It was suggested in the 1930s that rejection was a response to specific foreign antigens (alloantigens) and that they were similar to blood groups of other species. The development of inbred lines of experimental animal models allowed the demonstration of antigens present on red blood cells and the concept of histocompatibility. This suggestion of an immunological theory of tissue transplantation stimulated Medawar's (1944) work in rabbits and later in mice, and led to similar studies in humans, with the discovery of the human leucocyte antigen (HLA) system.

Further experimental studies defined the concept of rejection into three primary categories: *hyperacute rejection*, which can occur in a matter of hours due to pre-formed antibodies in a sensitized recipient; *acute rejection*, which takes place in a few days or weeks and is usually caused by cellular mechanisms; and *chronic rejection*, which occurs over months or years and remains largely undefined, but involves primarily humeral antibodies. A detailed review of experimental and modern transplantation biology is quite beyond the scope of this chapter, but increasing understanding of this area will allow more refined changes in rejection management and increasingly successful organ grafting.

AVOIDING REJECTION

The degree of disparity between donor and recipient is an important key element in the severity of the immune rejection response. In xenografting (transfer between species) the presence of preformed antibodies leads to rapid endothelial damage, causing vascular thrombosis, gross interstitial swelling and necrosis of the graft, all within a matter, usually, of hours.

Similarly, when transfer occurs between human beings, the degree of compatibility between donor and recipient is important to the success, or otherwise, of the graft.

As indicated earlier, transfer between identical twins is associated with universal success, without the need to modulate the immune mechanism. However, transfer between non-identical relatives or using cadaveric organs produces the recognition of non-self by the recipient and the mounting of an immune response. It is the avoidance or modification of this immune response that has been the main target over the last 25 years, and the avoidance of overwhelming rejection has been a prime goal.

Two approaches have been taken to the problem: tissue typing and reduction of immune response.

Tissue typing

In the attempt to match the donor and recipient more closely, the concept of typing has become widely developed. Early work demonstrating that blood transfusion was dependent on matching between donor and recipient was extended into experimental and then clinical transplantation studies in the 1960s and 1970s.

The human chromosome 6 contains the genetically determined major histocompatibility complex (MHC), i.e. the HLA-A, HLA-B, HLA-C (class I) and HLA-DR (D-related; class II) loci. A whole series of additional genetic regions have been linked to the HLA complex, although in clinical terms these are probably less significant.

Thus it has become increasingly possible, using serological studies, to map genetically an individual on the basis of the HLA region of this chromosome. Since one chromosome is inherited from each parent and each individual has two HLA haplotypes, there is a 25% chance that two siblings will share both haplotypes (i.e. identical) and, by standard and mendelian inheritance, a 50% chance that they will share one haplotype. Thus in first-degree relatives when the donor and recipient are matched for HLA-A and -B antigens there is an excellent likelihood of graft success, whereas because of the complexity of the MHC allele, the wide divergence of antigens and random cadaveric donors, even if matched for one or two antigens, there may still be very substantial disparity.

Thus, in order to avoid rejection, the concept of tissue typing trying to match more accurately the donor and the recipient has gained wide acceptance. Serological methods allow class I HLA antigens to be defined using typed serum obtained from nulliparous women. Using a microcytotoxicity assay, multiple antisera against HLA-A, -B, -C and -DR antigens are provided on Terasaki trays and then frozen until required. When needed, the trays are thawed and the donor lymphocyte cells are added to the wells containing complement and the antisera against specific HLA types. If the antibody causes the cells to lyse, acridine orange (a dye) enters the damaged cell and appears orange under fluorescence microscopy. Thus, by using microcytotoxicity tests it is possible to identify quite rapidly the HLA class I antigens present in a donor.

Until recently, class II antigen typing required a mixed leucocyte reaction to determine individual constituents, but more recent techniques have avoided this laborious investigation. From the clinical standpoint the practical importance of identification of the degree of compatibility between donor and recipient is clearly defined in many organ-grafting systems. Cadaveric grafting can only achieve this level when beneficially matched donor and recipient pairs, in which all major class I and class II antigens are identical, are grafted. This so-called 'full house' HLA match can give 1 year cadaveric graft survival approaching 90%. However, this is only when combined with chemical non-specific immunosuppression.

When grafts are transferred between cadaveric donor and recipient with a complete mismatch an additional 20–25% of grafts will be lost over the ensuing 5 years. Thus, in cadaveric grafting the degree of matching has an important role in determining the severity of the immune response and the ultimate success, or otherwise, of the graft.

Nevertheless, no matter how good the matching is in cadaveric situations, modulation of the immune response continues to be necessary to ensure graft survival.

Reduction of immune response

Reduction in the immune response occurs frequently in clinical practice in such situations as uraemia, profound jaundice and in patients with advanced malignancy and acquired immunodeficiency syndrome (AIDS). The controlled reduction of an immune response to foreign antigen on the graft requires careful clinical judgement. Initial attempts using widespread radiation produced severe depletion of not just lymphocytes but also a pancytopenia, and although the recipients readily accepted skin grafts and other organs immunologically, the majority of patients quickly died from overwhelming infection. A refinement of this technique, in which partial lymphocyte irradiation was used, has been successful both experimentally and in clinical practice, depleting the immune response so that grafts can be accepted.

Chemical immunosuppression

Since the mid-1950s the primary mode of immunomodulation has been the administration of chemical agents. A demonstration by Hitchings & Elion (1959), over 40 years ago, that 6-mercaptopurine had immunosuppressive potential, allowed Schwartz & Dameschek (1959) to treat rabbits stimulated by foreign antigen. The treated animals did not produce antibodies to the antigen stimulation, and work by Calne in 1960 showed that 6-mercaptopurine could also inhibit the immune response in dogs. A number of other agents were studied at that time and those found to be of clear benefit were steroids, reducing the cellular response, and eventually azathioprine, which showed improved results when compared to 6-mercaptopurine.

For more than 20 years chemical immunomodulation with the combination of steroids (prednisolone) and azathioprine was to be the main non-specific immunosuppressant used. They inhibited the immune response largely by depressing circulating T cells.

The production of antilymphocytic globulin by sensitization in animals was also demonstrated to inhibit the immune response, although variability and efficacy limited its clinical use.

Ciclosporin. Clearly the ultimate goal of selectively inhibiting the recipient's immune response remains a long way off, and in clinical practice non-specific agents continue to be used. In 1976, Borel and colleagues working in Sandoz laboratories assessed the potent immunosuppressive properties of ciclosporin A, a cyclical peptide with 11 amino acids. The demonstration of both the in vitro and in vivo immunosuppressive activity was quickly followed by extended clinical studies. It was clearly demonstrated that ciclosporin could suppress both antibody production and cell-mediated immunity, exhibiting a selective inhibitory effect on T cell-dependent responses. Of critical importance was the observation that the drug was neither profoundly lympho- nor myelotoxic and had no influence on the viability of the mature T cells or the antibody-producing B cells. Further agents have recently been introduced to clinical practice, perhaps resulting in less rejection still (FK506 or tacrolimus, mycofenolate and monoclonal antibodies).

CURRENT CLINICAL IMMUNOSUPPRESSIVE USE

For nearly 30 years the mainstay of clinical immunosuppression was the combined use of steroids and azathioprine. With increasing clinical experience it became possible to adjust the dosage of these agents so that in many individuals it was possible to maintain immunosuppression and thus prevent rejection, while minimizing the risk to the recipient of over immunomodulation, a delicate balance that requires considerable clinical skill.

Patients receiving steroids and azathioprine required careful monitoring for signs of early infection and the presence of organ rejection. Progressive reduction in haemopoietic production leads to thrombocytopenia and leucopenia, with the attendant risk of infection (bacterial, fungal and viral). The major complications of long-term steroid and azathioprine immunosuppression are outlined in Table 25.2.

Thus, considerable clinical skill was needed to avoid the risks of infection, and in cadaveric grafting, when the degree of matching between donor and recipient was often less than optimal, death from infection was the commonest cause of death in the first 3 months after grafting. In addition, the need to administer steroids continually became a major limiting factor, particularly in children, where the complications of steroids can be so crippling (Table 25.3).

The results of organ grafting using prednisolone and azathioprine left much to be desired, and so the introduction of ciclosporin into clinical trials in the early 1980s was an important step forward in the more selective use of immunomodulation. Not only could steroids be minimized or avoided in some individuals, but also pancytopenia was rarely encountered. Nevertheless, ciclosporin was rapidly found to have its own attendant problems and difficulties and nephrotoxicity remains a persistent problem (Table 25.4).

Table 25.2 Side-effects of steroids and azathioprine
• *Steroids*   Avascular necrosis of bones   Diabetes   Obesity   Cushing's syndrome   Pancreatitis   Cataract   Skin problems   Psychosis   • *Azathioprine*   Bone marrow suppression   Polycythaemia   Hepatotoxicity

Table 25.3 Side-effects of steroids in children
• Growth retardation   • Cushingoid appearance   • Diabetes   • Obesity

Table 25.4 Side-effects of ciclosporin
• Nephrotoxicity   • Hepatotoxicity   • Tremors, convulsions   • Skin problems   • Gingival hypertrophy   • Haemolytic anaemia   • Hypertension   • Malignant change

With increasing clinical experience, however, many of these toxic effects can now be minimized, such that excellent rehabilitation can be achieved and organs can now be grafted which previously would have been unsuccessful in the prednisolone and azathioprine era. The overall results of ciclosporin will be outlined in the individual sections, but there have been no clinical series in which the results of ciclosporin have been inferior to the treatment with azathioprine and prednisolone, and for the most part an improved benefit of between 15 and 20% of graft survival at 1 year has been reported.

Postoperative monitoring of all patients with transplanted organs involves regulation of the immunosuppressive regimen, detection of the development of organ rejection and constant vigilance for signs of infection.

CADAVERIC ORGAN DONATION

The concept of the diagnosis of brain death and increased awareness by both the public and doctors alike of the need for organ donation have improved the supply of cadaveric organs for grafting. In the UK, about half of patients who become organ donors have died from spontaneous intracranial haemorrhage, although head injuries and road traffic accidents also provide donors.

SPECIFIC ORGAN TRANSPLANTATION

Kidney

Kidney transplantation is now well established as the most effective way of helping patients with end-stage renal failure. Despite a significant expansion in the number of kidney transplants, long waiting lists exist for those on dialysis awaiting treatment. In the UK an integrated approach has shown a steady increase in the proportion of patients treated by transplantation, such that nearly 50% of patients now have a functioning transplant.

Patient selection

With kidney transplantation affording the optimal quality of rehabilitation, few patients will be denied the prospect, although the patient's age and underlying renal condition may need to be taken into account.

Age. In general, children do very well after transplantation, although infants below the age of 5 years present a more controversial issue because of the difficulty of management of immunosuppressive agents. The newer immunosuppressive regimens, however, allow adequate growth and physical development. The goal for children must be the establishment of normal renal function before maturity and to take full advantage of the growth spurt that occurs at puberty.

While in the early days patients over the age of 55 years were frequently denied transplantation, many centres now offer renal transplantation to patients over 65 or 70 years. Patient and graft survival has been very satisfactory in this group, but immunosuppressive schedules frequently need to be reduced in the elderly to ensure that overwhelming infection does not occur.

Renal disease. Renal transplantation is now offered for many primary and secondary renal conditions resulting in chronic renal failure, including glomerulonephritis, pyelonephritis and polycystic disease. Some types of autoimmune glomerulonephritis antibodies have been demonstrated to cause damage to the transplanted kidney, but this is not a contraindication to transplantation, as probably less than 10% of grafts will be seriously injured.

Assessment of potential recipient

Careful review of both the physical and psychological status of the patient is needed before transplantation, and factors that may increase the hazards of surgery or immunosuppressive management require evaluation. Patients in renal failure frequently suffer from cardiovascular problems (hypertension with left ventricular hypertrophy, and coronary artery disease) and the symptoms are increased by anaemia. There is a high incidence of peptic ulceration in uraemic patients, and of metabolic bone disease, causing renal osteodystrophy. All these associated conditions must be optimally treated or controlled before transplantation surgery. Sources of underlying or potential infection, such as an infected urinary tract or peritoneal cavity from peritoneal dialysis, must be eradicated or treated and the patient's status for viruses such as hepatitis B, HIV and cytomegalovirus must be known to minimize activation following immunosuppression. Careful surgical review related to previous abdominal operations, peripheral vascular ischaemia or the presence of ileal conduits following previous urogenital surgery needs also to be carefully taken into account and a surgical plan initiated.

Careful counselling and support are also needed to ensure that the patient understands and is prepared for transplantation.

Surgical technique

The technique of renal implantation has remained unchanged now for nearly 40 years, with the donor kidney being implanted extraperitoneally in one of the iliac fossae. The renal artery is anastomosed to either the internal or the external iliac artery, and the renal vein to the recipient's external iliac vein. The donor ureter is then implanted into the recipient's bladder. Over 150 000 kidney grafts have been performed around the world, but total transplantation rates vary significantly from one country to another.

Postoperative problems

Monitoring of the kidney allograft is required to detect signs of rejection, suggested by a reduction in urinary output and an elevation in serum creatinine, and then confirmed by biopsy or aspiration cytology. This allows the prompt recognition of an acute rejection crisis and its treatment by steroids.

With increased clinical experience the hurdles of acute rejection and infectious complications can usually be overcome, and patient survival at 1 year is in excess of 95% in many programmes, with over 85% of kidney grafts functioning well; however, a steady attrition of renal grafts will occur over the next 10 years, so that only just half of all renal transplants will be functioning well at 10 years, with many having been lost from the slow process of chronic rejection.

Rehabilitation can be spectacular, allowing patients the freedom to eat without restriction on salt, protein or potassium, the resolution of anaemia and infertility and an improvement in their overall sense of well-being.

Renal transplantation in the diabetic patient can be combined with pancreas transplantation, with implantation of the whole organ and drainage of the pancreatic duct into the gastrointestinal tract or the urinary bladder. Transplantation of isolated pancreatic islets is in its infancy.

Heart

While the patient afflicted by renal disease has the benefit of chronic haemodialysis, the individual with progressive cardiac problems has no life support system and death invariably ensues unless cardiac transplantation is undertaken. Initial efforts in the late 1960s by Barnard (1967) led to a progressive expansion of increasingly successful programmes. The majority of patients will suffer from cardiomyopathy, terminal ischaemic cardiac disease or, more rarely, some congenital form of cardiac disease. Donor selection must be rigorous because immediate life-sustaining function is required of the graft.

Orthotopic replacement of the diseased heart has been the most frequently undertaken procedure, although the heterotopic placement of auxiliary cardiac implants has been undertaken. The donor atria are anastomosed to the posterior walls of the corresponding chambers of the recipient prior to joining the pulmonary artery and the aorta.

Postoperative cardiac function is monitored and endomyocardial biopsy allows histological examination of heart muscle for ventricular cellular infiltration indicative of acute rejection. While the early attempts at cardiac grafting resulted in poor overall survival, the situation has improved remarkably. A 1 year survival of over 85% and a 5 year survival of 60% of patients with excellent quality of rehabilitation are most encouraging.

This solid foundation of cardiac grafting inevitably led to an extension to combined heart and lung transplantation, primarily for those suffering from pulmonary hypertension, or for some terminal lung diseases, such as cystic fibrosis or emphysema. If the recipient has lung disease but a good functioning heart on receipt of a combined heart–lung graft, the heart from the first recipient can be implanted into a second cardiac patient – the domino procedure. As a result of technical advances, transplantation of single lung is now possible. Because of the risk of infection in the implanted lungs, immunosuppressive management is critical. Sputum cytology and even lung biopsy may be needed to differentiate infection from rejection. In spite of this, the Stanford University Series now reports 2-year survival of over 60% in heart–lung recipients.

Liver

Although the first attempts at liver transplantation were made in the early 1960s, the formidable technical, preservation, immunological and organ availability difficulties meant that it was only in the early 1980s that successful programmes were established. The majority of adult patients coming to liver grafting have extensive cirrhosis (primary biliary cirrhosis, chronic active hepatitis and hepatitis B) or, less frequently, primary liver cancer. In the paediatric group the most common indication for liver transplantation is biliary atresia.

The liver is particularly susceptible to ischaemic injury and the ability to harvest and store livers for only a few hours led to an extremely complex surgical procedure, undertaken often in the most difficult emergency situations.

The liver is placed orthotopically after removal of the diseased organ, and venovenous bypass is employed to reduce the physiological changes during the anhepatic phase. Improvements in organ preservation (principally the introduction of the University of Wisconsin solution) mean that livers can now be stored for 12–14 h and transferred from one country to another. The evidence that tissue matching is important in liver grafting has yet to be fully established, but, as in other forms of transplantation, this may prove to be the case.

Patients coming to liver grafting are frequently critically ill with multisystem failure, and the complexity of the operation has inevitably meant that technical failures have been frequent. In spite of this, results have continued to improve, and with nearly 30 000 liver transplants performed in Europe and 1 year survival of over 85%, liver transplantation is increasingly being established as one of the most effective modalities of treatment for liver disease. In some groups the results have shown even more impressive improvement. Infants and children with biliary atresia undergoing grafting stand a greater than 90% chance of 1-year survival, with more than 75% well at 5 years. The longest survivor is now over 25 years after transplantation.

The major limiting factor in liver grafting now is donor availability and, while in the UK some 650 grafts were performed in 2001, the need is probably double that. The most acute shortage is of paediatric organs, and often a larger liver has to be divided and only part transplanted into a child. Recently partial lobe donation has become possible from live donors, usually a parent, especially in countries where cadaveric programmes are not available, such as Japan. This same approach is also being explored in adults.

Other organs

Pancreas transplantation is increasingly being undertaken in diabetics, often in kidney failure who need a kidney transplant. The techniques developed allow the pancreas to drain through the bladder and >85% of patients are insulin free at 1 year. It remains to be confirmed that the improvement in carbohydrate control will improve the diabetic complications, but sugar control is excellent.

In children, programmes of intestinal transplantation are also developing with encouraging results, allowing the children to come off total parentral nutrition and resume normal feeding.

ETHICAL ISSUES

The development of transplantation in the 1950s and 1960s caught not just the imagination of the medical profession but that of the public as well, and led to the reappraisal of fundamental beliefs in many areas. The concept of death was challenged, from the traditional one of the cessation of the heart beat to that of the concept of brainstem death, and wide public and professional debates ensued. Death, the great taboo of the 20th century, was addressed in a new, fundamental way. The majority of countries enacted legislation or medical guidelines identifying new criteria which would allow more effective recognition of an individual's incapacity to regain essential and vital functions. Some of these issues were challenged in courts of law and were often widely reported in the media.

Thus ethical and moral issues were raised from the very outset of organ grafting. With the increasing success of organ transplantation these pressures have grown. The rights of the individual to dispose of his or her own organs as they wish has been a matter of debate, and the profession has loudly condemned the commercialism which is in danger of entering clinical practice. The purchase or sale of organs is now condemned by almost all international transplantation organizations.

Should a living individual during his or her lifetime voluntarily donate an organ to another? The first successful grafts between identical twins from within a family were clearly perceived to be an act of great charity and compassion. Living-kidney grafting in the USA accounts for more than a third of all grafts, but should such altruism be permitted between non-family members, or those in whom a loving and caring bond does not exist? These new issues continue to be addressed by society.

One other issue has particularly focused on cardiac and liver transplantation and this relates to the consumption of economic resources for an individual. In the UK the cost of renal transplantation in total is approximately £8000–10 000, whereas the cost of dialysis per year per patient approaches £15 000. While renal transplantation is clearly the most cost-effective way of dealing with renal failure, compared with some other forms of medical and surgical treatment and perhaps healthcare initiative, it is seen as being expensive.

Cardiac and liver transplantation can equally be seen to consume a large amount of health resources and may be given a low priority in some health systems.

The development of live related liver lobe donation is also giving rise to some concerns because of the potential risk of such major surgery to the donor.

Each new development in science and clinical medicine raises its own issues, which need to be addressed, and, as these modalities of treatment spread to other countries, different cultural approaches may be required. It will be for the individual community to decide whether such treatments are appropriate for its members and to what extent resources can be made available.

Clinical organ transplantation has evolved rapidly over the last 25 years, affording treatment to many thousands of patients who would otherwise be dead or enduring an existence of chronic illness. Further advances are sought in the fight against the recipient immune response and to procure donor organs of the highest quality, thus enabling even more patients to experience the increasing benefits of transplantation.

Summary

- Successful whole organ transplantation has depended on a number of advances in understanding of infection and immunosuppression.
- Awareness of the public and of doctors has increased the supply of cadaveric organs but a severe shortage remains so that many patients who could benefit will die while awaiting a donor organ.
- Results have improved because of better monitoring and management, rather than from any technical changes.

References

Barnard CN 1967 The operation. A human cardiac transplant: an interim report of a successful operation performed at Groote Schuur Hospital, Cape Town. South African Medical Journal 41: 1271–1274

Borel JF, Feurer C, Gubler HU, Stahelin A 1976 Biological effects of cyclosporin A: a new antilymphocytic agent. Agents and Actions 6: 468–475

Calne RY 1960 The rejection of renal homografts: inhibition in dogs by 6-mercaptopurine. Lancet i: 417–418

Gibson T, Medawar PB 1943 The fate of skin homografts in man. Journal of Anatomy 77: 299–309

Hitchings GH, Elion GB 1959 Activity of heterocyclic derivatives of 6-mercaptopurine and 6-thioguanine in adenocarcinoma 755. Proceedings of the American Association for Cancer Research 3: 27

Medawar PB 1944 Behaviour and fate of skin autografts and skin homografts in rabbits. Journal of Anatomy 78: 176–199

Mitchison NA 1953 Passive transfer of transplantation immunity. Nature 171: 267–268

Murray JE, Merrill JP, Harrison JH 1955 Renal homotransplantation in identical twins. Surgery Forum 6: 423–426

Schwartz R, Dameschek W 1959 Drug induced immunological tolerance. Nature 183: 1682–1683

MALIGNANT DISEASE

26 Pathogenesis of cancer

P. D. Nathan, D. Hochhauser

Objectives

- **Recognize that gene defects cause cancer.**
- **Understand the processes involved in normal cell cycle control.**
- **Understand the genetic events leading to loss of cell cycle control.**
- **Appreciate the genetic background to invasion, metastasis and angiogenesis.**
- **Recognize that this understanding is leading to new therapeutic approaches.**

INTRODUCTION

Cellular processes are controlled by the products of gene expression. A gene is a unit of inheritance that carries information representing a protein; it is a genetic storehouse, a stable information packet, transmitted from one generation to the next. Information flows from DNA to RNA (transcription) to proteins (translation). Some genes have key functions controlling cell growth and, if these are damaged, abnormal cell proliferation may result. Deregulation (freedom from control) of genes, either inherited or acquired, may result from mutations (Latin *mutare* = to change), deletions and other mechanisms of gene 'silencing'. This may result in a breakdown of normal cell cycle control, including the avoidance of programmed cell death – apoptosis (Greek *apo-* = from + *piptein* = to fall).

Cancer (Latin = crab, German = krebs; possibly from the appearance of the distended veins extending outwards in all direction, like crab's legs) is now a major cause of death in the United Kingdom. Cancers develop because of genetic alterations, including the acquisition of power to invade normal structures and to metastasize (Greek *meta* = often implies change + *stasis* = a standing).

As our understanding of these processes develops, we can identify novel therapeutic targets, improving anti-cancer treatment.

CELL CYCLE CONTROL

1. Successful cell cycle control is critically important. Fortunately, a number of key regulatory elements have evolved that reduce the likelihood of uncontrolled cell growth. Regulatory signals may be positive or negative. The normal cell cycle is controlled by a balance of positive and negative signals from both outside and inside the cell.

2. A normal gene that exerts a positive growth signal is a proto-oncogene (Greek *protos* = first, primitive; *onkos* = tumour). If it is damaged, it gives an abnormally increased 'on' drive to cell growth and is termed an oncogene if such an alteration results in development of a cancer cell.

3. A normal gene that exerts a restraining effect on cell growth is a tumour suppressor gene. If it is damaged or lost, the cell is deprived of the 'off' signal.

4. The activation of oncogenes and absence of tumour suppressor genes deregulates (frees from restraint) cell cycle control.

5. Under normal circumstances, environmental information from outside the cell is relayed to the cell via cell surface receptors which may bind growth factors such as epidermal growth factor (EGF), inhibitory factors or components of the extracellular matrix (ground substance). When a molecule such as a growth factor (a ligand, from Latin *ligare* = to bind) unites with its receptor, this receptor–ligand binding induces a change of form in the receptor. This in turn activates an enzyme, for example a tyrosine kinase. Tyrosine kinases function within cells to attach phosphate groups to the amino acid tyrosine – phosphorylation. This triggers an intracellular signalling cascade, mediated via protein–protein interactions, inducing enzyme activity. The result is a change in gene expression, producing an increased cellular proliferation. Tyrosine phosphorylation is thus an early event in a complex signalling system. Depending upon the incoming information, the cell may respond in a variety of ways. If the ligand is a growth factor, the cell enters into the S phase of the cell cycle (Fig. 26.1).

6. Once a resting cell is in G_0 it can remain quiescent and viable, yet it can reinitiate growth after latent periods of months or years. When a resting cell enters the late G_1

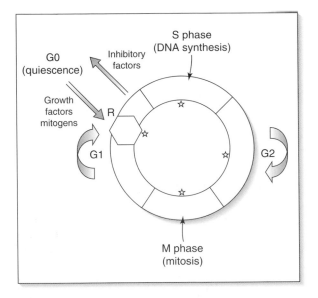

Fig. 26.1 Resting or quiescent cells (G$_0$) can pass into the cell cycle by the action of growth factors. Once past the restriction point R, they are committed to progress through S phase where DNA synthesis occurs. The stars indicate checkpoints that allow the fidelity of the process to be monitored and errors dealt with.

phase it passes a restrictive checkpoint, where any damage to DNA is detected. If no abnormality is detected, the cell is committed to DNA synthesis (Fig. 26.1). There are further checkpoints at S (synthesis), G$_2$ (second gap) and M (mitosis) phases to ensure the fidelity of the DNA synthetic process.

 Key point

- **Checkpoint controls ensure that, if an error is detected, further replication is prevented.**

7. Repair of an abnormality in the DNA may be possible but, if not, the cell undergoes programmed cell death. Apoptosis is the final common pathway for a large number of cellular insults and allows cells to avoid passing damaged DNA sequences on to the next generation. Under normal circumstances apoptosis is avoided by a combination of the presence of antiapoptotic signals and the absence of proapoptotic signals.

ABNORMAL CELL CYCLE CONTROL

1. Oncogenes and suppressor genes have been identified at many of those stages of cell cycle control described above.

2. Cancer cells escape reliance on exogenously produced growth factors to stimulate their growth. They may do this by (Fig. 26.2):

a. Overproducing growth factors which are released into the cellular microenvironment and which auto-stimulate the cancer cells

b. Overexpressing growth factor receptors

c. Expressing mutated or truncated receptors that give constant 'on' signals

d. Expressing altered components of the downstream signalling pathway.

3. Cancer cells also avoid normal antiproliferative signals. For example, the effects of the antigrowth signal, transforming growth factor beta (TGFβ), can be downregulated at the receptor level or within its signal transduction pathway (Latin *trans* = across, beyond + *ducere* = to lead; the path followed by the signal) in a

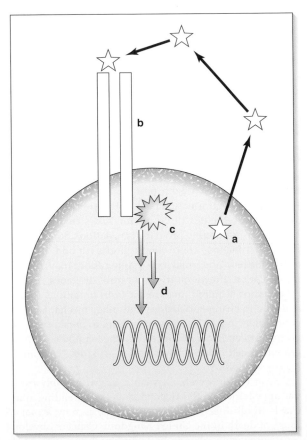

Fig. 26.2 How cells escape reliance on external growth factors: a, overproduction of growth factors; b, upregulation of growth factor receptors; c, constitutive signalling by mutated receptor; d, constitutive signalling by mutated components of signal cascade.

similar way to those growth factors described above. Many antiproliferative signals ultimately appear to exert their action through the retinoblastoma protein (Rb) which inhibits E2F transcription factors; these are proteins with DNA-binding motifs. They bind to specific nucleotide sequences – promoters close to the initiating codon of each gene, thus controlling transcription. They control the expression of many genes involved in cell cycle progression and DNA synthesis. Mutations in the *Rb* gene, the archetypal tumour suppressor gene, deregulate this pathway, allowing E2F transcription factors to exert their effect by stimulating the release of genes involved in proliferation.

4. Avoidance of apoptosis is a central feature of most, if not all, cancers. A variety of pro- and antiapoptotic signals converge on a final common pathway of mitochondrial release of cytochrome *c*, the pigment that transfers electrons in aerobic respiration. Mitochondria (Greek *mitos* = thread + *chondros* = granule) are cytoplasmic organelles involved in cellular respiration. Apoptosis is regulated by members of the *bcl-2* gene family, an oncogene, described initially in B-cell lymphoma, which prevents cell death by apoptosis. The effect of increased expression of *bcl-2* may in part explain resistance to the effect of chemotherapy in cancer cells that express high levels. The most common proapoptotic signal lost in carcinogenesis is the *p53* suppressor gene, which is mutated in over 50% of human common solid tumours. Under normal circumstances, *p53* plays a key role in detecting DNA damage, and initiating cell cycle arrest and DNA repair.

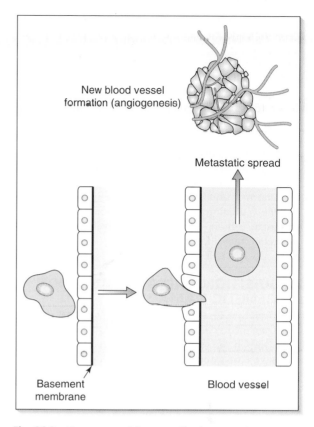

Fig. 26.3 Cancers must traverse the basement membrane before infiltrating blood vessels, metastasizing to distant sites and stimulating new blood vessel growth if they are to spread and grow.

Key point

- **Loss of cell cycle regulatory control is a critical factor in the development of cancer cells and resistance to treatment.**

ANGIOGENESIS AND METASTASIS

1. The features that differentiate benign from malignant growth are invasion and metastasis. Cells must traverse the basement membrane and other extracellular boundaries and then attract a blood supply to support tumour growth (Fig. 26.3). Changes in expression of cell–cell adhesion molecules (CAMs) and cell–matrix adhesion molecules (integrins) are thought to be pivotal. Loss of E-cadherin function, a CAM facilitating epithelial cell–cell interaction, occurs in many epithelial tumours. Integrin expression is switched on to allow movement through local extracellular matrix and adhesion to distant matrix, and enzymes which digest matrix components, matrix metalloproteinases (MMPs), are expressed and digest local stroma (connective tissue framework), facilitating movement of the cell through the extracellular matrix.

2. In addition to loss of adhesion, previously static, specialized cells may lose their special function, their ability to differentiate, and migrate. Many solid tumour cells attract fibroblasts, which lay down collagen around them. It is the appearance of the resulting radiating strands of fibrous tissue that makes cancers resemble a crab's body – the primary tumour, with claws – the result of cancer cell migration, hence the name of cancer.

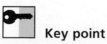

Key point

- **Angiogenesis is a key factor in development of tumours.**

3. Control of new blood vessel formation, angiogenesis, is dependent upon the interaction of pro- and anti-angiogenic stimuli. Vascular endothelial growth factor (VEGF) is upregulated in some tumours, and in animal models VEGF inhibitors have antitumour activity. The angiogenesis inhibitor thrombospondin has also been shown to be downregulated. Other components of this process are being identified and may offer future therapeutic targets.

4. Although cancer cells are thought of as being rapidly dividing cells, the rate of division of many cancers is not as high as in many normal tissues such as the gut mucosa, bone marrow and skin. However, the loss of apoptosis and the reduction of telomeric erosion mean that the malignant cells have increased survival, provided that they retain their blood supply.

ACQUISITION AND ACCUMULATION OF GENETIC DAMAGE

1. Damaged genes may be inherited through germline DNA (see Ch. 40). This is responsible for cancer families that have a preponderance of cancer often presenting at an early age. A variety of genes have been identified that are associated with an inherited high risk of cancer. For example, mutations, and consequent loss of function of the tumour suppressor genes BRCA-1 and BRCA-2, occur in breast and ovarian cancer, and of the familial adenomatous polyposis (FAP) gene in some forms of inherited colon cancer.

2. The majority of cancers are sporadic – scattered, occurring casually and caused by derangement of somatic (Greek *soma* = body) genes. It is now well recognized that there is a latent period, sometimes of many years, between the time of the initiating influence and the development of the cancer. Cancers do not result from a single mutation but from a stepwise accumulation of abnormalities. The fact that cancers arise more commonly as age increases is in keeping with the accumulation of mutations with time. Those who inherit a germline risk factor that affects every cell in their bodies are already primed, awaiting further stepwise mutations.

3. Environmental factors are recognized as important, as the incidence of cancer arises between different stable populations and between stable populations and members who migrate elsewhere. For example, when Japanese migrate to Hawaii the incidence of gastric carcinoma is reduced, and is even further reduced if they move to the USA. The best known environmental cause of bronchial cancer is cigarette smoking. Gastric cancer is associated with a diet rich in smoked foods; mesothelioma is closely linked to contact with asbestos; aflatoxins released by the fungus *Aspergillus flavus* are implicated in hepatocellular carcinoma.

4. Electromagnetic and particulate radiation act by increasing mutations. X-rays initiate them, especially in the bone marrow; ultraviolet light from solar radiation affects the skin.

5. DNA oncogenic viruses act by encoding proteins that interfere with growth regulation (Table 26.1). Epstein–Barr virus (EBV), may promote cancers, including Burkitt's lymphoma and nasopharyngeal cancer. Hepatitis B virus (HBV) is associated with hepatocellular cancer. Human papillomavirus (HPV) is associated with cervical carcinoma.

Table 26.1 **Carcinogenic agents**	
Agent	Tumour type
Viruses	
Human papilloma virus (HPV)	Cervical cancer
Hepatitis B and C viruses (HBV, HCV)	Hepatocellular carcinoma
Epstein–Barr virus (EBV)	Burkitt's lymphoma, nasopharyngeal cancer
Human T-lymphocyte virus 1 (HTLV-1)	Adult T-cell leukaemia and lymphoma
Chemical carcinogens	
Cigarette smoke	Lung, laryngeal and bladder cancer; some increased risk of many others
Asbestos	Mesothelioma
Nickel, chromates, arsenic	Lung
Aromatic amines	Bladder
Polyvinyl chloride	Angiosarcoma of liver
Aflatoxin	Hepatocellular carcinoma
Radiation	
Ionizing radiation	Leukaemia, breast cancer, thyroid cancer
Ultraviolet radiation	Melanoma, basal cell and squamous cell cancers of skin

6. RNA retroviruses, single-stranded viruses, initiate copies into DNA proviruses. They do not appear to cause human cancers directly but human immunodeficiency viruses (HIV) are associated with Kaposi's sarcoma.

7. Some substances are believed to initiate cancers not by causing mutations directly but by increasing cell growth and turnover, thus increasing the opportunities for mutations to occur. Alcohol abuse may act by causing chronic liver inflammation, producing high liver cell turnover. Oestrogen is a stimulant for breast and endometrial cell multiplication.

8. Some substances do not initiate cancer if given first, but if given repeatedly following mutation from an initiator they induce cancer development. They are called promoters.

9. Parasites may be involved in the development of cancer, notably the liver fluke (*Schistosoma* spp) and *Clonorchis sinensis*, which causes bladder cancer.

Key point

- **Most cancers are generated by factors in the environment, not by inherited gene mutations.**

10. Point mutations, deletions (a portion of a chromosome is lost) and translocations (a chromosome segment is transposed to a new site) all occur and they are all capable of interfering with normal gene function.

11. Every gene exists as two copies or alleles (a shortened form of allelomorph: Greek *allelon* = of one another + *morphe* = form; one of two or more alternative forms of a gene). Mutation of only one allele of a proto-oncogene may result in oncogenesis if it produces much variation of the patient's oncogenic phenotype. The phenotype (Greek *phainein* = to show + *typtein* = to strike) is a structural or functional characteristic resulting from combined genetic and environmental activity. Damage is required to both alleles of a protosuppressor gene if a tumour suppressant effect is to be overcome. This was described by Knudson in his 'two-hit hypothesis' (Fig. 26.4).

12. Given the complexity of the biological processes that must be overcome for a cell to exert a malignant phenotype, it can be seen that damage to a number of critical genes is required. This 'multi-hit hypothesis' was

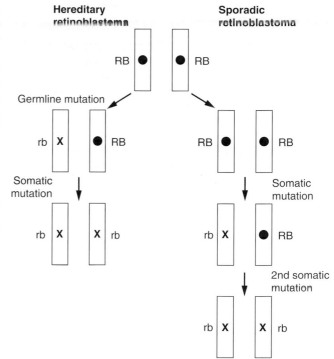

Fig. 26.4 Knudson's two-hit hypothesis. RB, normal retinoblastoma gene; rb, mutated gene. Patients who inherit (i.e. in the germline) one defective (mutated) copy of the gene have a high chance of acquiring a somatic mutation at an early age, resulting in loss of RB function. Patients who inherit two normal genes require two somatic mutations, resulting in sporadic disease occurring at a later age.

described by Vogelstein, who argued that the progression from premalignant to malignant lesions seen in colorectal carcinoma is associated with the accumulation of key mutations in oncogenes and suppressor genes (Fig 26.5). This model is now generally accepted as occurring in many cancers.

13. It would be unlikely for a normal cell with intact DNA repair machinery to accumulate the significant amounts of genetic damage required to exert a malignant phenotype. The fact that cancer cells accumulate extensive DNA damage may be a reflection of their damaged DNA repair mechanisms and genomic instability.

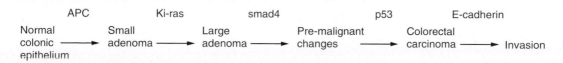
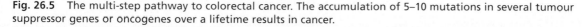

Fig. 26.5 The multi-step pathway to colorectal cancer. The accumulation of 5–10 mutations in several tumour suppressor genes or oncogenes over a lifetime results in cancer.

Summary

- Do you understand the genetic damage to those genes responsible for normal cell cycle control and cell behaviour that result in cancer?
- Do you realize that multiple events, in a number of oncogene and suppressor gene activities, are required for carcinogenesis?
- Can you understand why therapies are targeted to gene products responsible for carcinogenesis?

Further reading

Hanahan D, Weinberg RA 2000 The hallmarks of cancer. Cell 100: 57–70

Kinzler KW, Vogelstein B 1996 Lessons from hereditary colorectal cancer. Cell 87: 159–170

Sporn MB 1991 The war on cancer. Lancet 347: 1377–1381

27 Principles of surgery for malignant disease

P. J. Guillou, I. A. Hunter

> **Objectives**
>
> - **Appreciate the importance of histological diagnosis.**
> - **Realize the multidisciplinary implications of management.**
> - **Accept that surgery may be valuable even when cure is no longer possible.**

INTRODUCTION

In 2000 malignant disease was responsible for 151 200 deaths in the UK, a figure that accounts for 25% of all registered deaths (Cancer Research UK). Tables 27.1 and 27.2 indicate the contribution of different types of malignant disease to both cancer incidence and cancer-related mortality. Over the last 50 years there have been major improvements in the survival rates of some solid tumours, but for many the prognoses remain poor and largely unchanged (Fig. 27.1).

Despite recent advances in the use of adjuvant therapies (Latin *ad* = to + *juvare* = to help) such as chemotherapy and radiotherapy, surgery remains the main modality of treatment for many solid organ tumours, including cancer of the breast, lung, urogenital tract and gastrointestinal tract. You must fully assess the tumour and the patient before deciding on surgical intervention. This demands detection, histological diagnosis, staging and consideration of the role of other adjuvant interventions. The process is best planned, carried out, monitored and followed up in cooperation with a multidisciplinary team including radiologists, pathologists, radiotherapists and medical oncologists.

ASSESSMENT

Patient assessment is a vital part of operative planning. Establish a pathological diagnosis and the extent of

Table 27.1	The most common cancers in 1997	
	Males	Females
Lung	24 440 (19)	14 430 (11)
Prostate	21 770 (17)	
Breast		38 000 (29)
Colorectal	18 130 (14)	16 180 (12)

Values in parentheses are percentages of total malignancies registered.

Table 27.2	Gastrointestinal cancer deaths, 2000	
	Males	Females
Oesophagus	4300	2620
Stomach	4060	2530
Large bowel	8540	7730
Pancreas	3370	3530

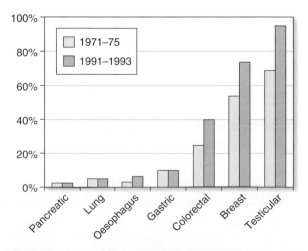

Fig. 27.1 Changes in 5 year survival rates from 1971–1975 to 1991–1993 according to cancer type. (Source Office for National Statistics, Cancer Trends in England and Wales 1950–1999).

spread of the disease prior to operative intervention, as these factors have a major influence on the treatment you can offer an individual patient. Assess the patient's physiological and psychological status; as in all surgery, they impact on the extent of the operative intervention that you can safely consider.

Pathological diagnosis and tumour grading

Before considering operative intervention obtain a biopsy specimen for histological analysis to confirm the presence of malignant disease and indicate its expected behaviour. Biopsies of gastrointestinal and urogenital tumours can usually be obtained by luminal endoscopy. For most solid organs, biopsy specimens can be obtained using needle core biopsy or fine needle aspiration cytology, if necessary under ultrasound or radiological guidance or at laparoscopy.

Histological grading helps predict the behaviour of a neoplasm based on its histological appearance. Grading systems focus on the apparent differentiation status of the tumour. Simple histological grading has poor prognostic value and is an unreliable guide to treatment. Advances in molecular biology now allow specific molecules to be identified that more accurately predict tumour behaviour and response to available treatment.

Immunohistochemical detection of oestrogen receptors in breast cancer tissue is a good example of the predictive value of identifying a molecular marker, as it gives the probable response of the tumour to oestrogen antagonists such as tamoxifen. In the future, molecular grading will increase in value.

Tumour staging

Staging often has a direct impact on the extent of surgery that must be performed to eradicate malignant disease, or may indicate that curative resection is not possible and that only palliative (Latin *palliare* = to cloak) procedures are worth considering.

Key point

- **In planning surgical intervention, the staging of tumours is of greater relevance than grading.**

The tumour, node, metastases (TNM) system describes the extent of spread and generally correlates well with prognosis. It is based on the size and local spread of the primary tumour (T), the presence of lymph node metastasis (N) and distant metastasis (M). Imaging modalities such as computed tomography (CT), magnetic resonance

imaging (MRI), conventional and intraluminal ultrasound and [^{18}F]-fluorodeoxyglucose-linked positron emission tomography (FDGPET) have greatly improved the quality of preoperative staging (see Ch. 5). Despite these advances, preoperative staging is by no means 100% sensitive or specific and accurate staging may still be possible only at, or after, operative intervention. In many cases true staging is determined by the histological examination of resection specimens. Although preoperative assessment is essential, you must be prepared to alter your planned interventions in the light of the findings at operation.

SURGICAL MANAGEMENT

The aims of surgery in malignant disease are:

- To remove all malignant cells from the patient to achieve a complete cure. The complete removal of tumour is termed an R_0 resection.
- To maintain or restore the integrity of tissues in order to preserve function following tumour removal.

Curative resection may be impossible or unsuccessful because:

- The tumour has invaded vital, unresectable, local structures.
- An intra-abdominal tumour has seeded into the peritoneal cavity.
- Tumour cells have metastasized into distant organs and still be undetectable (micrometastasis).
- Tumour cells have metastasized into distant organs and these deposits cannot be safely removed.

R_0 resection usually involves removing the tissue containing the tumour with an intact covering of unaffected tissue to leave the resection margins free of disease, to avoid exposing and shedding viable tumour cells. Imaging techniques cannot yet detect individual tumour cells, therefore you must expect undetected local spread.

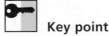

Key point

- **Learn how tumours spread, in order to obtain clear resection margins and avoid local recurrences (see Ch. 26).**

Local invasion

Tumours spread locally into the surrounding tissues.

1. Epithelial gastrointestinal tract tumours often spread longitudinally in the submucosal layer or laterally

through the muscular layers towards the serosa; for example, oesophageal tumours tend to spread longitudinally in the submucosa beyond the visible luminal limits, so the longitudinal resection must be extensive to avoid local recurrence at the resection margins. In contrast, rectal carcinoma spreads a relatively short distance longitudinally, so resection margins 3 cm from the tumour are considered safe.

2. If surrounding tissues are invaded, consider these for resection, based on the principles outlined in this chapter. For instance, if gastric carcinoma invades the body and tail of the pancreas, transverse colon, or retroperitoneal nodes and spleen, resect them en bloc (French = in one piece) with the stomach.

Lymphatic spread

Tumour cells also spread within draining lymphatics to regional nodes and may develop into metastatic foci. Anticipate this and, where possible, remove local nodal groups in continuity with the lymphatic connections to the primary tumour.

1. Colonic lymphatic drainage is initially via the paracolic nodes, then through the nodes lying alongside the supplying arteries and on into the preaortic nodes at the origin of the superior or inferior mesenteric arteries. The supplying vessels are removed at their origins in order to excise as many draining lymph nodes as possible. Therefore the full extent of colon that is dependent on those arteries for blood supply must be resected. Rectal cancers tend to spread laterally in lymphatic vessels within the pelvic mesorectum. Recognition of this has led to total mesorectal excision, resulting in a lowering of local recurrence rate.

2. Lymphatic drainage of the testis is to the para-aortic lymph nodes (due to their embryological origin within the abdomen). Testicular tumours are treated surgically by orchiectomy, an approach that does not address potential lymphatic involvement; however, surgical treatment of anticipated lymphatic involvement is usually not required due to the sensitivity of seminomas to radiotherapy. Following orchiectomy for seminoma it is standard practice to give adjuvant radiotherapy to the para-aortic nodes, even in stage I disease (where no lymphatic metastasis are clinically or radiologically evident). Such approaches have resulted in 5 year survival rates approaching 100% in stage I disease.

3. The main route of lymphatic drainage of breast tumours is to the ipsilateral (Latin *ipse* = same) axillary nodes.

a. The great American surgeon William Halsted (1852–1922) described in 1882 the principle of radical

(Latin *radix* = root; hence, by the roots) mastectomy. The primary tumour should be removed together with the draining lymphatics and a wide margin of intervening tissue in one block.

b. The psychological consequences of radical mastectomy and the development of adjuvant therapies have introduced alternative treatments. In wide local excision, the breast tumour is excised with a surrounding cuff of unaffected tissue. This risks leaving residual undetected disease in the axilliary nodes and in the breast. It is therefore combined with adjuvant radiotherapy to the breast, and either a sampling, or partial clearance, of the ipsilateral axilliary nodes. This is potentially curative, but can also be considered as a form of staging surgery; later examination of the resected breast tissue and nodes may reveal the presence of residual disease or nodal involvement. On the basis of postoperative staging, further radical surgery or systemic chemotherapy can be planned if necessary.

c. Sentinel lymph node biopsy (SLNB) offers a further option instead of axilliary clearance or nodal sampling. It is based on the principle that the lymphatics will initially drain to a single node before progressing to further nodal groups. A tracer molecule such as patent blue V dye, or radiolabelled technetium, can be injected into the vicinity of the primary tumour at operation, allowing it to enter local lymphatics and become concentrated in the sentinel node. Once the sentinel node has been identified it is removed and subjected to histological examination. If the node is free of metastatic deposits then the axilla can be considered free of disease, as it is unlikely that more distant nodes are involved. A positive sentinel node indicates axilliary spread, demanding further operation or adjuvant therapy. Its role is currently under investigation in a number of UK randomized clinical trials.

4. Cutaneous malignant melanoma is another tumour that commonly spreads to local lymph nodes. Treatment of the primary tumour again follows oncological principles and aims to remove the melanoma together with a clear margin of uninvolved tissue; however, this approach fails to address possible involvement of local lymph nodes.

a. Elective lymph node dissection (ELND) of regional nodes has been advocated in an attempt to reduce recurrence in the draining nodal basin. However, in stage I disease only 20% of patients are found to have histologically positive nodes, and ELND is associated with increased postoperative morbidity and cost. The practice of ELND has also failed to emerge as a statistically significant predictor of improved survival in several prospective randomized trials.

b. SLNB can also be considered in the management of malignant melanoma. As with breast cancer its role is still controversial, although it has been declared as standard care for patients with melanoma by the World Health Organization.

Transcoelomic spread

Tumours within intra-abdominal organs can breach the serosal covering to reach the peritoneal cavity – transcoelomic (Latin *trans* = across + Greek *koilos* = hollow) spread – and may there form multiple deposits. Clearance of all tumour cells is now practically impossible. This accounts for the poor prognosis associated with serosal involvement in gastric carcinoma. Bear this in mind when removing tumours so that you do not spread or encourage the seeding of primary tumour cells within the peritoneal cavity.

Haematogenous spread

Tumour cells can gain direct access to the vascular system through the endothelium of their supplying vessels, or through lymphatics to major ducts draining into the bloodstream. They may then form metastatic (Greek *meta*, signifying change + *stasis* = a placing; a change of situation) tumour deposits, typically in the liver, lung and bone marrow. These are often undetectable at the time of surgery and become clinically apparent months or years after the primary resection. Although metastatic deposits threaten survival, some are suitable for resection. Of the 50–60% of patients with colorectal cancer who develop liver metastases, around 25% are suitable for attempted curative resection, with 5 year survival rates of 27–37%. Likewise, in selected cases, pulmonary metastases may also be considered for surgical treatment using solitary wedge resection, multiple wedge resections or lobectomy. Five year survival rates of 21–43% have been achieved, although a high preoperative carcinoembryonic antigen (CEA) level or lymph node metastases are both predictors of a poor outcome in these patients.

Palliative procedures

Curative (R_0) resection involves the removal of the tumour and a large amount of unaffected tissue. Extensive resections increase the short- and long-term risks of complications; therefore, such resections are warranted only with the prospect of achieving a cure. If removal of all malignant tissue is not possible, tumour recurrence is inevitable unless adjuvant therapy, such as chemotherapy or radiotherapy, is given to destroy residual tumour. If this is ineffective, consider a palliative (Latin *palliare* = to cloak) procedure if it offers symptomatic benefit.

1. Oesophageal, gastric, small bowel or colonic obstruction can often be relieved by palliative resection, bypass or construction of an external stoma. Malignant oesophageal or colonic obstruction is often amenable to endoscopic insertion of a stenting tube, or a self-expanding stent introduced under radiological control, avoiding open operation. Intraluminal tumour incursion can be temporarily destroyed with a laser beam controlled endoscopically.

2. Despite modern imaging methods it is often difficult to decide, preoperatively, whether malignant biliary obstruction is amenable to curative surgery. Potentially, 25% of pancreatic cancer patients and 35% of those with ampullary carcinoma may survive 5 years following resection. Alternatively, a plastic stent may be inserted percutaneously or endoscopically, but it tends to block and then needs to be replaced. Metal stents are less likely to block but are more expensive. Consequently, there is considerable controversy about the management of malignant biliary obstruction.

3. In some cases surgery may alleviate symptoms or reduce the need for treatment, even though it does not affect the outcome. For example, patients with incurable carcinoma of the stomach or colon may bleed chronically and require regular blood transfusions. Resection of the affected tissue stops the bleeding and mitigates the symptoms of anaemia.

4. Apart from relieving obstruction-related colic, resecting locally invasive bowel tumours rarely reduces pain. Neurectomy occasionally helps but often results in motor loss. Coeliac axis block is usually more effective than systemic analgesia in relieving the deep infiltrating pain of, for example, unresectable pancreatic cancer.

Curative surgery for secondary malignant disease

Local or locoregional malignant recurrences are not always irrecoverable.

1. Regional nodal metastases from malignant melanoma may follow excision from a limb or trunk. If there are no detectable distant secondaries, block dissection may produce 20–25% 5 year survival.

2. Recurrent colorectal cancer suspected clinically, or through regular monitoring of plasma CEA (see Ch. 30) and liver ultrasound, may be indications for 'second look' surgery. Locally recurrent colorectal cancer is rarely cured by further resection but valuable palliation can often be provided.

Reconstructive surgery for malignant disease

Radical excision of malignant disease often demands subsequent reconstruction, restoration or replacement:

1. Stomach mobilized and supplied only by the right gastric and gastroepiploic arteries can be drawn up to the neck to replace the resected pharynx or oesophagus.
2. Following mastectomy, a myocutaneous flap of rectus abdominis or of latissimus dorsi can be used for reconstruction.
3. Free tissue transfer may be employed, with anastomosis of the divided supplying vessels to local vessels, using microvascular surgical techniques.
4. Lost skin and tissue can sometimes be replaced by inserting an inflatable tissue expander to stretch the skin or develop a space. This is then removed, allowing the skin to be closed. Following mastectomy a silicone implant can be inserted as a substitute for the breast.

ADJUVANT THERAPY

Adjuvant treatment is an extra remedy added to the treatment to increase its effectiveness (see Chs 28, 29). When applied before surgery it is called neoadjuvant (Greek *neos* = new – perhaps revived in a new form) therapy. Examples are preoperative radiotherapy for rectal cancer, chemoradiotherapy for oesophageal cancer and some stages of breast cancer. In these cases the intention is to 'down stage' the primary tumour.

Adjuvant therapy may be administered after surgery, when the histological staging is available. Patients at high risk of postoperative recurrence can now be identified and given additional therapy. An example of this is the administration of 5-fluorouracil and folinic acid to patients undergoing resection of Dukes' stage C colonic cancer (Cuthbert Dukes, pathologist at the famous St Mark's Hospital in London, classified rectal cancers as 'A' if the tumour was limited to the rectal wall, 'B' if it extended through the wall but without involving adjacent lymph nodes, and 'C' when regional nodes were invaded). This adjuvant therapy provides a 30% improvement in 5 year survival compared with surgery alone.

Postoperative chemotherapy has also proved to be highly effective in the management of testicular cancer. Recurrence rates for men with high risk (those with vascular invasion within the resection specimen) non-seminomatous germ cell tumours are reduced from 50% to around 2% after two courses of adjuvant chemotherapy containing cisplatin.

THE MULTIDISCIPLINARY APPROACH

The multidisciplinary approach to cancer management combines the expertise of pathologists, radiologists, oncologists, radiotherapists and surgeons. This has resulted in the development of new treatment protocols that in the case of some tumours have seen a great improvement in survival and functional outcome. The advances in the treatment of osteosarcoma provide a good example of how different disciplines can work together in the management of malignant disease.

1. Osteosarcoma is classically a disease of young adults; it exhibits aggressive local invasion and a propensity to metastasize early. Historically, treatment involved amputation of the affected limb and achieved survival rates of only 10–20%. Osteosarcomas are usually contained within a pseudocapsule of reactive tissue around the primary tumour. Although well-defined anatomical compartments initially limit their spread, these tumours do have a tendency to metastasize via the haematogenous route, mainly to the lungs and other bones. As well as forming distant metastatic deposits, more local metastases also occur in the form of intramedullary 'skip lesions' within the same bone.

2. The surgical principles applied to the treatment of osteosarcoma are in keeping with those outlined within this chapter. Ideally a tumour is removed in its entirety with a margin of unaffected tissue. This may have to include joints and other local soft tissue structures. Such an approach often necessitated amputation, due to bone loss or the removal of neurovascular bundles; however, advances in reconstructive surgery and neoadjuvant therapies have resulted in the increased success of limb-sparing surgery and a reduction in the occurrence of distant disease.

3. A biopsy specimen is usually obtained at open biopsy by the surgeon planning the definitive operation. This allows the biopsy incision to be incorporated in the final resection specimen. Histological examination confirms the diagnosis and also grades the tumour. Osteosarcoma is one example in which grade is a part of the staging system and therefore has an influence on treatment protocols.

4. Initial assessment using combined imaging modalities such as CT, MRI and scintigraphic bone scanning allow accurate assessment of local and distal spread. This is essential in the planning of surgical intervention. The

degree of surrounding soft tissue involvement, the identification of skip lesions and intramedullary spread will dictate the extent of the resection margin required for potentially curative surgery. The feasibility of limb salvage can also be assessed. Although bone and soft tissue will be lost in order to achieve local control, function may be restored by the utilization of prosthetic implants, cadaveric bone allografts, bone autografts and rotationplasty. In some cases a 'down staging' of the primary tumour can be achieved by using neoadjuvant chemotherapy. A good response to such therapy may induce necrosis in the tumour and reduce surrounding inflammation. This may make a surgeon more inclined to attempt limb salvage surgery. The use of preoperative chemotherapy in non-metastatic high grade resectable osteosarcoma is now standard.

5. Postoperative chemotherapy is employed, even after a successful resection of the primary tumour, in an attempt to target micrometastases to distant organs. Following resection and reconstruction, histological examination of the resection specimen is used to establish the tumour's response to neoadjuvant chemotherapy. The degree of induced tumour necrosis has been shown to be a good predictor of clinical outcome. A poor histological response after neoadjuvant therapy is often addressed by modification of the postoperative chemotherapy regimen.

6. This combined approach to the treatment of osteosarcoma has resulted in a reduced amputation rate and an improvement in long term survival rates to over 60%.

Summary

- Do you recognize that clinical assessment of patients with suspected malignant disease is still paramount?
- Why does early diagnosis improve the prognosis?
- Can you reason why emergency intervention carries a poorer outlook than elective surgery?
- Why is it inappropriate to plan operative treatment of malignant disease in isolation from other modalities?
- Why is it imperative to make a tissue diagnosis before embarking on ablative operation for suspected cancer?
- What can surgical operation offer patients when malignant disease has extended beyond curative resection?
- Have you made a decision with the patient, or for the patient? (see Ch. 14).
- Can you offer palliation if you cannot cure cancer, or if it recurs following resection?

 Further reading

Taylor I, Cooke TG, Guillou PJ 1996 Essential general surgical oncology. Churchill Livingstone, Edinburgh

28 Principles of radiotherapy

R. A. Huddart

Objectives

- **Understand the physics and biology of radiation, determining how radiotherapy is used.**
- **Understand the process of delivering a course of radiation.**
- **Recognize the role of radiotherapy treatment in modern oncology, with emphasis on its interaction with surgical oncology.**
- **Understand the basis of radiation side-effects and how they may interact with surgical treatment.**

SOURCES OF IONIZING RADIATION

Radiotherapy is the therapeutic use of ionizing radiation for the treatment of malignant disorders. Natural sources of radiation include radioactive isotopes which decay with the production of β-particles (electrons) and γ-rays (a form of electromagnetic radiation). Originally radium was used, but over the last 20 years this has been replaced by safer artificial isotopes such as cobalt-60, caesium-137 and iridium-192, which are generated in nuclear reactors. Isotopes are used mainly as sources implanted directly into tissues, such as iridium needles in the treatment of carcinoma of the tongue, or inserted into a cavity, for example caesium sources inserted into the uterus and vagina for the treatment of carcinoma of the cervix. Radioactive isotopes may also be given systemically, such as iodine-131 in the treatment of thyroid cancer.

External beam radiotherapy was revolutionized in the 1950s by the advent of megavoltage treatment machines; initially cobalt machines and later linear accelerators. The linear accelerator generates a stream of electrons which is accelerated to high speed by microwave energy before hitting a tungsten target. This interaction results in the emission of high energy X-rays. The high energy X-ray beam produced by a linear accelerator has several properties that make it well suited for present day radiotherapy:

1. The greater penetration of the γ-rays means that a high proportion of the dose applied to the body surface reaches the tumour.

2. All X-ray beams have a fuzzy edge (the *penumbra*) due to the reflection and scattering of the beam by tissues. High energy X-rays suffer relatively little sideways scatter as they pass through tissues, and this helps to keep the edge of the beam sharp.

3. The forward scattering effect is also indirectly responsible for the point of maximum dose being 1–2 cm below the skin surface (Fig. 28.1). The skin therefore receives a low dose and is spared from radiation reactions. It was the high skin doses associated with low

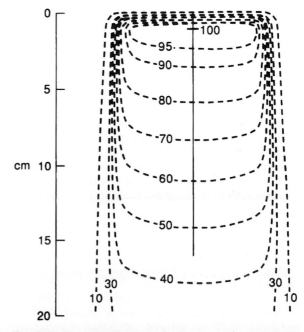

Fig. 28.1 Dose distribution of a linear accelerator. Note the maximum dose is below the skin surface and 65% of the applied dose is present at 10 cm.

energy X-ray machines that in the past caused the uncomfortable skin reactions and limited treatments of deep-seated tumours.

In addition, cyclotrons can be used to produce ionizing beams of heavier particles such as neutrons or protons; however, these machines are yet to find a place in routine clinical practice.

ACTIONS OF IONIZING RADIATION

X-rays (from linear accelerators) and γ-rays (from isotopes) are both forms of electromagnetic radiation and are biologically indistinguishable. High energy X-rays consist of packets of energy (photons) which interact with the molecules of body tissues to cause ionization and release electrons of high kinetic energy. These electrons cause secondary damage to adjacent molecules, including DNA, via an oxygen-dependent mechanism. The resultant DNA damage is mostly repaired by enzymes in a matter of hours, but certain DNA lesions are irreparable. In some normal cell lineages (e.g. lymphoid, myeloid, germ cells) the DNA damage triggers immediate programmed cell death (apoptosis). Non-repairable DNA damage causes a variety of chromosomal abnormalities. This DNA damage does not stop most cells from performing their normal physiological functions effectively, but when the cell tries to divide it dies in the attempt. Thus damage is expressed when the cell undergoes mitosis, and in fully differentiated cells incapable of further division (e.g. muscle cells) this damage may never be expressed.

Key points

- **Tissues may be severely damaged by irradiation but appear essentially normal; damage is expressed only if they are stimulated to divide.**
- **Response to radiotherapy by tumours may be delayed, especially in tumours with slow rates of growth (e.g. pituitary tumours).**

There are many data on the respective effects of radiotherapy on normal tissues and tumours. It appears that tumour cells may not differ greatly from the cell of origin in response to single doses of radiotherapy, although there may be differences in the ability of tumours and normal tissues to recover from the effects of cell damage. For example, normal tissues have a greater ability to respond to radiation-induced cell depletion by accelerated repopulation, an ability which seems to be less developed in tumours. To eradicate a tumour within the limits

of tolerance of surrounding normal tissues, radiotherapy must exploit these and other subtle differences in DNA repair and regrowth of normal tissues.

In external beam treatments, therapeutic advantage is generally achieved by dividing the total dose of radiotherapy into small parts over several weeks, a practice called *fractionation*. A full discussion of the effects of fractionation is not possible in this chapter, but generally:

1. Reducing the dose per fraction allows certain critical normal tissues, such as the nervous system, the lungs and other slowly proliferating tissues, to repair damage more effectively than tumours.

2. Fractionation over a period of several days or weeks gives rapidly proliferating normal tissues, such as skin and gut, a chance to repopulate and hence recover from radiotherapy-induced damage faster than tumours.

3. Many tumours contain hypoxic areas. As the major effect of radiotherapy is by an oxygen-dependent mechanism, these areas are relatively resistant to radiotherapy. Each fraction of radiotherapy reduces the number of tumour cells and allows some hypoxic areas to become better oxygenated. Fractionation allows this process of reoxygenation, which may take hours or days to occur and is thought to make tumours more radiocurable.

The above comments help to explain the empirical finding that radiotherapy is most effective when given daily over several weeks. A comparable effect to fractionation is seen with interstitial and intracavity treatments where a continuous low exposure over several days is biologically equivalent to multiple small fractions.

The ability to cure a tumour probably depends on being able to eliminate every clonogenic tumour cell from the target volume. This is influenced by a variety of factors, as discussed below.

Size of tumour

A number of factors means that the larger the tumour the less successful radiotherapy tends to be:

- The larger the tumour the greater the number of cells present and hence a larger number of fractions will be necessary to have a high probability of eliminating the last clonogenic tumour cell. For example, the majority of 2 cm carcinomas can be controlled by 60 Gy, whereas a 4 cm carcinoma needs 80 Gy for similar control rates.
- Large tumours may contain large hypoxic areas which are relatively radioresistant and thus reduce the chance of cure.
- Large tumours usually need a larger treatment volume than small tumours. This generally increases the volume of normal tissue irradiated; the greater the volume of normal tissue, the higher the chance that a part of that

tissue is damaged by the radiotherapy, and hence the normal tissue complication rate rises. To reduce this complication rate a dose reduction is often necessary, with a corresponding reduction in the chance of cure.

Radiosensitivity of tumour cells

The commonest histological types of tumour have cells of similar radiosensitivities (e.g. squamous carcinoma cells and adenocarcinoma cells). Differences in tumour cure between these common histological types probably relate more to differences in tumour bulk, oxygenation and proliferation. There are exceptions, with the cells of some tumours being more radiosensitive, such as seminoma and lymphoma, and others being more radioresistant, such as melanoma, glioma and sarcoma. The reasons for these differences are not clear. Radiosensitive tumours may be more sensitive due to a greater tendency to undergo apoptosis in response to DNA damage, but there is evidence, at least in vitro, that a variety of other mechanisms may have a role; for example, melanoma seems to be more resistant to radiotherapy due to an increased ability to repair DNA damage.

Tolerance of normal tissues

The total dose that can be applied to a tumour is limited by the tolerance of the surrounding normal tissue. This varies greatly between tissues. If the tumour lies close to a sensitive organ, such as the spinal cord, then the total dose that can be safely delivered is much less than if the tumour lies within muscle or bone, for example. Hence the chance of cure may be reduced. The dose that can be applied will also depend on the volume that needs to be irradiated. A good example of this is the lung. The tolerance dose for whole lung to be able to function after treatment is in the region of 20 Gy in 10 fractions of 2 Gy. Therefore, if the whole lung or large sections need to be treated, as in selected cases of Hodgkin's disease, this is the maximal fractionated tolerated dose. However, doses as high as 60 Gy can be given to portions of a lung, such as a lobe, because small areas of permanent damage are acceptable and have little overall effect on lung function.

RADIOTHERAPY PLANNING

Key point

- **The major principle of radiotherapy is to give the maximum possible dose to the smallest volume that will encompass all the tumour.**

This volume, termed the *treatment volume*, consists of:

1. The macroscopic tumour volume determined from clinical findings, imaging by, for example, X-rays, computed tomography (CT) scans and radioisotope scans, and operative findings, termed the *gross tumour volume* (GTV)
2. A biological margin (often 0.5–1 cm) which allows for microscopic tumour spread beyond the visible tumour: the *clinical target volume* (CTV)
3. A technical margin, usually 0.5 cm to allow for errors and variability in daily set-up such as that due to respiratory movements of the patient: the *planning target volume* (PTV).

Minimizing these errors and improving quality assurance is an area of active research. Techniques such as megavoltage imaging may enter clinical practice in the future; in this, an X-ray image of the patient is produced as the treatment beam passes through the tumour, showing how well the area actually treated corresponds to the treatment plan.

Accurately localizing the tumour in the patient is essential to the success of radiotherapy. In most cases the tumour cannot be visualized directly and localization depends on physical examination, imaging and operative notes. The importance of accurate and detailed operative records cannot be overemphasized. An operation is a unique opportunity to visualize the tumour directly. Take full advantage of this opportunity to describe the extent of disease and acquire as much additional information as possible about local pathology. Limited information invariably leads to larger target volumes, increased radiotherapy morbidity and reduced cure rates.

Once the radiotherapist has determined the exact size, shape and location of the target volume the aim is to encompass the target volume with a radiation dose distributed as homogeneously as possible. A variation of under 10% is aimed for and achieved. Single fields are usually inadequate in this respect, except for superficial tumours. Opposing two fields at 180° to each other treats intervening tissue homogeneously. This arrangement is very simple to plan and is suitable for most low dose palliative and a few radical treatments. Two opposed fields usually include more normal tissue in the high dose volume than is strictly necessary (Fig. 28.2). Therefore, more complex multifield arrangements are normal for curative treatments to confine the high dose volume more closely to the target. These arrangements are usually planned by the cross-sectional target volume from CT scans of the patient in the treatment position.

Conventional therapy uses rectangular fields to encompass the target volume. As tumours are not cubes, an unnecessary amount of normal tissue is included in the

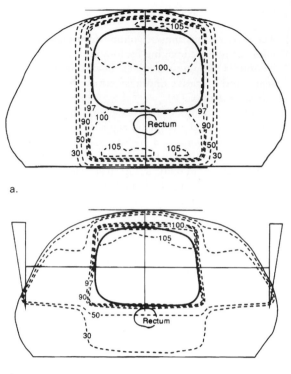

a.

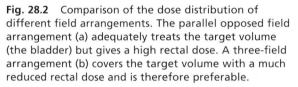

b.

Fig. 28.2 Comparison of the dose distribution of different field arrangements. The parallel opposed field arrangement (a) adequately treats the target volume (the bladder) but gives a high rectal dose. A three-field arrangement (b) covers the target volume with a much reduced rectal dose and is therefore preferable.

treated volume. This causes increased morbidity and limits the doses that can be given (e.g. for pelvic tumours the dose given is limited by the amount of small bowel included in the target volume). Conformal therapy uses new engineering and computer technology to generate irregularly shaped fields so that tumours can be encompassed by high dose volumes that correspond more precisely to the tumour's shape. A recent randomized trial in prostate cancer at the Royal Marsden NHS Trust has demonstrated a reduction in the risk of late side-effects and has allowed dose escalation which should improve cure rates (Dearnaley et al 1999).

Directing several beams of radiation accurately to intersect across the target volume does not necessarily guarantee an even dose distribution because the X-rays have to pass through different amounts of tissue on the way from the entry point on the skin to the target volume. In addition, lung absorbs less energy than other tissues because of the air it contains. These potential sources of dose inhomogeneity (Greek *in* = not + *homos* + *genos* = kind; not having the same constituent elements

throughout) within the target volume must be calculated and compensated for using a number of measures that alter the beam shape and profile, for example different weightings on each X-ray beam and the introduction of wedge-shaped filters which absorb different amounts of energy across the beam (Fig. 28.3). Production of homogeneous dose distributions has been greatly facilitated by the introduction of planning computers and CT planning which can visualize and allow for tissue inhomogeneities directly. This area continues to develop rapidly, and in the future more sophisticated means of compensating for potential sources of uneven dose distribution will come into routine practice, as will more advanced beam-defining devices.

Once satisfactory dose distribution and treatment plans have been produced and checked, treatment of the patient can begin. It is important that treatment is applied in a reproducible fashion. The patient must be positioned, lying in a recorded position, with appropriate supports to maintain stability. Lasers are frequently used to help establish and monitor patient alignment. If extra accuracy is desirable, especially in the head and neck region, a light

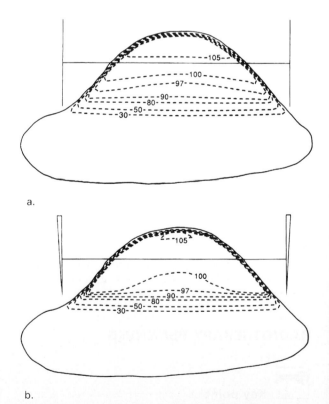

a.

b.

Fig. 28.3 Treating the breast without compensation for breast curvature produces an inhomogeneous dose distribution (a). When this is compensated for by a wedge filter (b) the dose distribution is improved.

plastic shell may be used to immobilize the patient. The machine is then positioned according to skin markings and recorded settings determined during planning, and treatment is commenced.

Planning radiotherapy

The radiotherapist:

- **Defines the volume to be treated.**
- **Designs radiation fields to encompass the volume to be treated. Complex 3 or 4 beam field arrangements are used for radical treatment to minimize the volume of normal tissue irradiated. Irregularly shaped ('conformal') fields are now being used to further reduce the volume of normal tissue treatment.**
- **Produces a radiotherapy plan which allows for dose inhomogeneity to produce a uniform dose distribution across the volume to be treated.**

RADIOTHERAPY: THE FUTURE

In recent years several new techniques have improved the therapeutic ratio in selected circumstances.

Accelerated radiotherapy

This involves giving multiple daily treatments of the same size as used in conventional fractionation but given to shorten the overall treatment time from 6 weeks to less than 3 weeks. Recent research suggests that clonogenic tumour cells can proliferate significantly during a treatment course of 6 weeks and this could, theoretically, reduce the chance of tumour control. Reducing the overall treatment time could make an important difference, allowing less time for proliferation and leaving fewer tumour cells to kill; however, reducing treatment time also gives normal tissues less time to recover. Enhanced early skin and mucosal reactions may limit this approach.

Hyperfractionation

This delivers two or three smaller fractions a day over the conventional treatment period; the number of treatment days remains the same but the number of fractions is increased. Reducing fraction size reduces late tissue damage, with relatively less effect on tumour control. This has allowed dose escalation, with an increased

chance of cure, especially in head and neck cancer (Horiot et al 1992).

CHART (continuous hyperfractionated accelerated radiotherapy)

This new regimen aims to combine the advantages of accelerated and hyperfractionated radiotherapy by giving three treatments a day over a 12 day period with no gaps – including no breaks for weekends and bank holidays. Results from a multicentre trial have shown that CHART improved survival in patients with localized lung cancer and, to a lesser extent, local control and survival in patients with head and neck cancer (Dische et al 1997).

Stereotactic radiosurgery

This technique utilizes fixation devices adopted for neurosurgical practice to localize tumours precisely in three dimensions, using fiducial (Latin *fidere* = to trust; trustworthy) markers. By using arcing radiation beams, conformally shaped fixed fields or multiheaded cobalt units (gamma knives), radiation beams can be delivered to a concentrated area with a high degree of precision.

Particularly applicable to cranial radiotherapy, this allows a high dose to be delivered to the target but a very low dose to surrounding tissue. This technique can be used as a boost after a conventional treatment course, retreatment of recurrences, or as a sole ablative treatment, as for arteriovenous (AV) malformations not suitable for surgery (Brada & Ross 1995).

Conformal radiotherapy

Conformal radiotherapy (see above) is now entering routine clinical practice. Further technical advances, including the use of multileaf collimators (Latin *col* = together + *linea* = a line; to make parallel: beam defining devices allowing irregular shaping of fields), which can vary during treatment administration, and 'inverse planning' where the radiotherapist determines what he or she wishes to achieve and the computer determines optimum field size, shape, direction and weighting, are likely to lead to further sophistication in treatment administration, including treatment of concave or annular shapes. This should further reduce radiation morbidity, particularly near sensitive structures such as the spinal cord, optic chiasm and eye.

ROLE OF RADIOTHERAPY

Radiotherapy may be used in the management of malignant disorders in the following ways:

- As primary treatment
- As adjuvant treatment before or after primary surgery or chemotherapy
- For palliation of symptoms
- As a systemic treatment, either in the form of external beam total body irradiation or of systemic administration of a radioactive isotope.

Radiotherapy as primary treatment

When radiotherapy is used as the primary treatment the aim is to effect cure with the minimum of side-effects. It is an alternative modality (method) of local control to surgery (Table 28.1). Radiotherapy, like surgery, is most effective at controlling small, well-localized and defined tumours, but has the advantage of preserving normal function. For many cancers, surgery and radiotherapy are equally effective modes of treatment and close liaison between surgeons and radiotherapists is essential if the appropriate modality of treatment is to be chosen for any given patient. This choice may vary between patients and depends on a variety of factors, such as tumour site, stage and histology, and patient age and performance status. Choice of treatment is not restricted to either surgery alone or radiotherapy alone; the patient may be best served by a policy of initial radiotherapy followed by planned salvage surgery if this fails, as in many head and neck tumours, or initial combination therapy.

Radiotherapy may be indicated as the initial treatment by a variety of circumstances, including:

1. Sites where surgery and radiotherapy are equally effective but radiotherapy gives better functional or cosmetic results, as in bladder cancer where radical radiotherapy gives good results and avoids the necessity for cystectomy and ileal conduit, or laryngeal cancer where radiotherapy gives equal results to surgery but allows preservation of the voice.
2. Very radiosensitive tumours, such as lymph node metastases from testicular cancers or early Hodgkin's disease.
3. Inoperable tumours; occasionally radiotherapy can be used for attempted cure of brainstem gliomas or pelvic sarcomas.
4. At sites where operations carry a high morbidity/mortality and equivalent results are gained by radiotherapy, as for carcinoma of the upper or mid-oesophagus.
5. In patients unfit for the radical surgery that would otherwise be the treatment of choice; for example, patients with bronchial cancer and chronic airways disease.

All cases, however, need to be carefully assessed to decide the appropriate treatment option. In some cases where radiotherapy would normally be indicated, other factors

Table 28.1 Results of curative radiotherapy

Site	Stage	Five year survival (%)	Comments
Skin	All	90–95	Equivalent to surgery. Choice depends on site
Head and neck			
Tongue	T1	91	50–60% for all stages
Glottis	T1	90	
Other sites	All	30–80	Local control rates with salvage surgery used for local relapse
Lung			
Conventional	T1	30	40% 2 year survival
Gastrointestinal tract			
Oesophagus	All	9	Equivalent to surgery
Anal canal	All	66	Better results than anoperineal resection
Urology			
Bladder	T2/3	34	Salvage cystectomy for local relapse. Surgery only 28% 5 year survival
Prostate	T1/2	80	Equivalent to surgery
	T3	60	
Penile	All	75	Over 90% cure for stage 1 tumours
Gynaecology			
Cervix	1B	85–90	Equivalent to surgery in randomized studies
	2A/B	61–85	
Endometrium	All	60–65	For patients unfit for surgery only
Vagina	Stage 1	75	

may make surgery preferable for that patient. For instance, it may not be possible to apply a radical dose because of an adjacent sensitive structure; cystectomy may be indicated if small bowel is adherent to the affected bladder, precluding a full radical dose without a risk of severe morbidity. Operation may be preferred, especially in head and neck cancer, as the tumour may involve bone or cartilage, risking osteoradionecrosis following radical radiotherapy.

Key points

- Radiotherapy is an effective alternative modality to surgery to obtain local control.

- The choice of radiotherapy versus surgery often depends on tumour- and patient-related factors.
- Closely cooperate with the radiotherapist to achieve an optimum treatment strategy for each patient.

Adjuvant radiotherapy

For some tumours, preoperative or postoperative radiotherapy may improve local control. Adjuvant (Latin *ad* = to + *juvare* = to assist) radiotherapy (Table 28.2) achieves this by controlling microscopic spread beyond resection margins, tumour spilled at operation or lymph node metastases. The low tumour burden means that lower doses than those normally used in radical treatments can

Table 28.2   Effect of adjuvant radiotherapy (RT) on local control and/or survival

Site	Stage	Criteria	Results (%)		Comment
			No RT	RT	
Breast	T1/2 N0	LC	63	88	NSABP randomized trial of conservative surgery
	T1/2 N+	LC	57	94	Radiotherapy
Central nervous system					
Astrocytoma	Gd1	S	25	58	
Oligodendroglioma	All	10 year S	27	50	
Pituitary	All	10 year LC	10	90	RMNHST data
Craniopharyngioma	Incomplete excision	S	35	90	70% survival for complete excision
Lung small cell					
Thoracic	Limited stage	2 year LC	23	48	} Overview of nine randomized trials*
		2 year S	16	22	
Cranial RT	Limited stage	2 year LC	45	84	} Danish trial†
		2 year S	16	25	
Gastrointestinal tract					
Pancreas	Operable tumour	2 year S	15	42	GITSG trial (NO RT versus RT with 5-fluorouracil)
Rectum	Dukes' C	LC	65	90	MRC 3rd trial survival advantage in some series
Gynaecology					
Endometrium	Stage 1	LC	88	99	
	Stage 1	S	64	81	
	Stage 2	S	20	56	
Parotid					
Carcinomas	All	LC	62	87	
Pleomorphic adenomas	Incomplete excision	LC	76	98	
Bladder	T2/T3B	S	28	45	Non-randomized data
Soft tissue sarcoma	Limited stage	LC	60	75	Review of French experience‡

LC, local control; S, survival; NSABP, National Surgical Adjuvant Breast and Bowel Project; RMNHST, Royal Marsden NHS Trust.
*Warde & Payne (1992).
†Work et al (1996).
‡Coindre et al (1996).

be employed, with a resultant reduced morbidity, while obtaining a high rate of local control. If local control is an important determinant of survival, then this may equate with an improvement in overall survival. Even if metastases limit survival, adjuvant radiotherapy often has a valuable role in improving locoregional control and quality of life. This may be especially important if symptoms of relapse cannot be easily controlled, for example in rectal cancer.

Adjuvant treatment may be given to (1) the site of primary disease to reduce local recurrence or (2) sites of potential metastatic spread.

Postoperative radiotherapy gives the radiotherapist the advantage of having details of the surgical and pathological findings in addition to the clinical and radiological assessments. This allows for accurate staging, and selection of those patients who will most benefit from radiotherapy. However, the planning of postoperative radiotherapy can be more difficult, as the radiotherapist can no longer directly image the tumour. Accurate operation notes greatly aid localization of treatment, as does marking the tumour bed with clips. If it is likely that postoperative radiotherapy will be given, invite the radiotherapist to see the patient preoperatively, for example, before wide local excision of a small breast cancer. Postoperative radiotherapy is of proven value in reducing local recurrence at many sites, some of which are discussed below. At most sites postoperative radiotherapy is of no proven benefit in prolonging survival after complete resection of the primary tumour.

In selected circumstances, *preoperative radiotherapy* may be of value. This has the potential advantage of 'downstaging' the tumour, potentially allowing an easier or less extensive operation to be performed, for example in rectal cancer or limb sarcomas. It may also reduce the risk of seeding at the time of operation and control microscopic disease at the edges of the tumour. Certain problems have limited the usefulness of this approach; foremost is the fear that radiotherapy increases the surgical morbidity. However, it is now thought that, as long as the operation is performed within 4 weeks of radiotherapy, this increase is minimal with doses of radiotherapy up to 40 Gy. A further problem is that the downstaging effect of the radiotherapy makes interpretation of the subsequent surgical specimen and pathological staging difficult. This also causes difficulties in comparing different series of patients, assessing prognosis and giving advice on further treatment. It is therefore a less established form of treatment, but has been used in bladder cancer, rectal cancer and sarcomas and, less often, in the treatment of oesophageal and endometrial cancers (Pollack & Zagars 1996, Graf et al 1997).

Radiotherapy to sites of lymph node spread has been used in the treatment of many cancers, especially when it was thought that blood-borne spread followed lymph node invasion. Increasingly, studies suggest that lymph node metastasis may be a marker of synchronous blood-borne metastasis, and at several sites prophylactic lymph node irradiation has been shown to be of little value in survival terms, such as in bladder and prostate cancer (Asbell et al 1988). Despite this, in a variety of cancers, lymph node irradiation is of value when initial spread is to lymph nodes and is an important determinant of survival, as in head and neck cancers, or relapse-free survival, as in seminoma. Prophylactic lymph node irradiation is also justified in reducing the risk of macroscopic nodal disease when symptomatic relapse is difficult to salvage. An example of this is supraclavicular fossa irradiation in axillary lymph node-positive breast cancer. Node relapse at this site is difficult to salvage and has a high morbidity in terms of lymphoedema and brachial plexus neuropathy. The risk of such relapse is markedly reduced by applying adjuvant radiotherapy.

In a similar fashion, craniospinal irradiation improves prognosis when central nervous system (CNS) spread is common, for example, in medulloblastoma and ependymomas. Chemotherapy only poorly penetrates the CNS, and for some otherwise chemosensitive tumours the CNS may act as a sanctuary site, such as in acute lymphoblastic leukaemia (ALL) and small cell lung cancer. If cerebrospinal fluid (CSF) metastases are common, cranial or craniospinal irradiation is a highly successful form of prophylaxis. For example, following the introduction of irradiation, the incidence of CNS relapse in patients with acute lymphoblastic leukaemia has been dramatically reduced and it has had a major impact on the chances of cure in this illness.

 Key points

- **Adjuvant radiotherapy may significantly reduce the risk of locoregional recurrence, especially if the tumour is larger or excision is marginal.**
- **Accurate preoperative staging and operation records improve the effectiveness of radiotherapy.**

Palliation

Of all modalities used to treat advanced cancer, radiotherapy is the most useful for the palliation of symptoms either from advanced primary or metastatic disease. The criteria of success must be in terms of quality of life rather than survival. The aim is therefore to give sufficient treatment to relieve symptoms without short-term side-effects for as long as the patient is expected to survive. The trend is towards short courses delivering a few large fractions of radiotherapy, thereby achieving maximum symptom relief with minimal interference in the patient's life. Frequently, a single large fraction of radiotherapy is all that is necessary to palliate symptoms. For example, most patients with lung cancer present with disease too advanced for any radical treatment. Such patients are frequently symptomatic with, for example haemoptysis, dyspnoea, pain or cough. These are usually well controlled with one or two fractions of radiotherapy (Bleehen et al 1991). In certain circumstances in pelvic tumours, or recurrent chest wall breast cancer, longer fractionated courses to higher doses are necessary to offer a good chance of sustained symptom relief. In addition, palliative radiotherapy may be used for relief of symptoms due to metastases. The treatments of different types of metastasis are considered below.

Bone metastasis

Symptomatic bone metastases affect approximately 20% of patients at some stage during their illness. Radiotherapy is a highly effective means of controlling local pain due to such bone involvement. Recent work has shown that a single 8 Gy fraction of radiotherapy will relieve pain partially or completely in 80% of patients 4 weeks after treatment (Price et al 1986). Orthopaedic fixation followed by radiotherapy should be used to prevent fracture for lesions with substantial cortical bone erosion. Patients with extensive bone metastases, as are frequently seen in prostate cancer, obtain good palliation from wide-field hemibody irradiation given as a single treatment. The other half-body can be treated 4–6 weeks later. Approximately two-thirds of patients will obtain good pain relief from such treatments. An alternative approach is to use a radioactive isotope (strontium-89) which is taken up by bone metastases. It is given as a simple intravenous injection and may be repeated. In randomized studies in prostate cancer, strontium-89 produced pain relief equivalent to local or hemibody irradiation, with the advantage of lower toxicity and the appearance of fewer new sites of pain on subsequent follow-up (Quilty et al 1994).

Spinal cord compression

This is an emergency which can cause devastating motor, sensory and sphincter disturbances. Metastatic disease can cause cord compression by direct extension from vertebral disease, epidural deposits or, rarely, intramedullary disease.

There has been no large trial of radiotherapy versus surgery in the treatment of this disorder, but most series suggest radiotherapy alone, in most instances, is as effective as surgical decompression followed by radiotherapy. Surgical treatment should be considered when there is no diagnosis, in radioresistant tumours such as melanoma and sarcomas, where there is evidence of spinal instability or progression through radiotherapy. Over 70% of patients will achieve good pain relief and 50% a useful response if treated before a major neurological deficit develops. Some patients will regain the ability to walk, but only 10% of total paraplegics regain useful function (Huddart et al 1997).

Brain metastases

This is a frequent complication of advanced cancer and is associated with a high morbidity. They are especially common in lung cancer, breast cancer (10% of all patients at some stage), melanoma, kidney and colon carcinomas. They are usually multiple and the prognosis is poor, with the median survival if untreated being 6 weeks. A 50% symptomatic response rate to radiotherapy and dexamethasone is expected, the radiosensitive tumours such as small cell lung, breast and colon cancers responding better than average. A good response to dexamethasone and good performance status also predict for good outcome. Frail patients with poor performance status tend to gain little and treatment may not be indicated in such patients. Short courses of treatment seem to be as effective as longer courses (Priestman et al 1996). Patients with a single metastasis have a better outlook, with a median survival of 4–6 months, and 30% of patients with breast cancer survive over 1 year. There is some evidence that surgical resection followed by whole-brain irradiation is better than whole-brain irradiation only, in selected patients fit for surgery. Recent work with stereotactic boost (see above) suggests that similar results may be obtained with radiosurgery (Wurm et al 1994).

Superior venal caval obstruction (SVCO)

SVCO is caused by enlarged right-sided mediastinal lymph nodes or tumours, especially lung cancers. It causes engorgement of veins to the neck, cyanosis, facial oedema and dyspnoea. Following mediastinal radiotherapy, 70% of patients gain relief within 14 days.

Other indications

Some other indications for palliative radiotherapy are retinal metastases, skin metastases and lymph node metastases.

Key points

- Radiotherapy is effective at relieving symptoms of advanced local or metastatic disease.
- Short courses of treatment are usually sufficient to palliate symptoms.
- Longer courses of treatment are sometimes justified, especially to obtain locoregional control.

Radiotherapy for the treatment of systemic disease

Radiotherapy is generally used to treat local disease. There are, however, two areas where radiotherapy is used to treat systemic disease: total body irradiation and radioactive isotopes.

Total body irradiation

A total body dose of >4 Gy will result in bone marrow failure. This has limited the usefulness of the technique for the treatment of malignant disease until the onset of bone marrow transplantation. Total body irradiation using a dose of 8–10 Gy as a single dose or a higher fractionated dose is a highly effective conditioning regimen for the treatment of leukaemias. It is also being examined in trials in the treatment of other radiosensitive tumours such as lymphomas.

Radioactive isotopes

This technique uses radioactive isotopes which emit short-range β-particles and/or γ-rays. If the tumour concentrates the isotope compared to the surrounding tissues it will be preferentially irradiated. The best example is the use of iodine-131 in the treatment of follicular and papillary thyroid cancer. The malignant tissue takes up and concentrates iodine, and hence residual tumour is irradiated to a high dose. Using this technique, lung and sometimes bone metastases can be eliminated. Other examples are the use of phosphorus-32 in polycythaemia rubra vera, strontium-89 in metastatic prostate cancer (see above) and *m*-iodo-benzylguanidine (MIBG) in neuroblastoma.

COMPLICATIONS

Normal tissue side-effects are due to cellular damage inflicted at the time of irradiation. This damage is largely expressed at the time of mitosis, so the sensitivity to and the expression of this damage depend on the proliferative characteristics of each tissue.

Acute effects

In some tissues, such as the epidermal layers of the skin, the small intestine and bone marrow stem cells, turnover is rapid and damage is expressed early. Skin is the classic example of such a tissue. Stem cells in the basal layers of the skin divide; the daughter cells differentiate and move to the surface over a 2 week period to replace shed cells. After irradiation, production of replacement cells is reduced or halted. The epidermis gradually thins and, if sufficient damage has occurred, epidermal integrity is lost and desquamation occurs. Recovery will occur over a period of days or weeks after the end of treatment by surviving stem cells producing enough daughter cells to cover the deficient area. It can be seen that:

- The time to onset of side-effects is determined by the skin turnover time: 2 weeks for skin but 5 days for small intestine
- The severity and length of time to recovery depend on the amount of damage to the stem cells and hence on radiation dose
- Provided there is a certain number of clonogenic cells surviving, recovery is likely to be complete.

Although this mechanism is responsible for most acute reactions, the clinical effect varies from site to site. For example, in the upper gastrointestinal tract acute reactions cause inflammation and discomfort with mucositis and oesophagitis; small or large bowel damage by similar mechanisms causes vomiting, diarrhoea or, more rarely, ulceration and bleeding.

Other acute reactions, however, may operate by different mechanisms and are less well understood, such as somnolence after cranial irradiation.

Late irradiation effects

Although acute effects are important for the tolerance of radiotherapy, the dose of radiotherapy applied is usually limited by long-term, late radiation effects.

Stem cell effects

Stem cell damage usually recovers completely but, if it is severe, long-lasting effects can occur. The most important example of this is gonadal damage. Oocytes are particularly radiosensitive and even moderate doses of a few grays of radiation precipitate premature menopause. Spermatogenesis is also sensitive to radiotherapy. Doses in the region of 3 Gy cause oligospermia or azoospermia that may last 6 months to 1 year, but higher doses, more than 6 Gy, cause permanent sterility.

Depletion of parenchymal or connective tissues

In many tissues the parenchymal cells turn over very slowly. As radiation damage is expressed at mitosis, lethal damage will not be expressed until cells divide, weeks, months or even years later. Irradiation of the thyroid gland, for example, leads to gradual depletion of thyroid follicular cells and can cause hypothyroidism over a period of many years.

Vascular damage

Damage to the vasculature is a common mechanism of damage, especially in tissues that never replicate, such as neurons or cardiac muscle, or which replicate only very slowly, such as fibroblasts. Radiation has a wide range of pathological effects on the vasculature, due to damage to both endothelial cells and connective tissue. This leads to impairment of the fine vasculature, often in a patchy fashion. The damage can result in poor wound healing, tissue atrophy, ulceration, strictures and formation of telangectasia.

The precise clinical effect depends on the organ involved. For example, in the bladder the telangiectasia can cause haematuria, while fibrosis, ulceration and tissue atrophy can cause a constricted fibrotic bladder resulting in frequency and nocturia. Similar changes in the gastrointestinal tract may cause bowel obstruction by stricturing of the viscus or by peritoneal adhesions.

At other sites vascular damage manifests differently. In the central nervous system, glial tissues are depleted as a direct effect of radiation and via vascular effects, causing secondary demyelination and neuronal loss. Damage to the cardiac vasculature may result in early ischaemic heart disease if the dose is high enough, with myocardial infarction being an increasingly recognized cause of late morbidity and mortality in a minority of patients 15 years after internal mammary irradiation for breast cancer.

Lymphatic damage

High-dose radiotherapy can also damage lymphatic vessels, leading to reduced drainage and limb lymph-oedema. The risk is increased if there has been previous or successive surgery. For example, radiotherapy to the axilla after complete axillary dissection for early-stage breast cancer carries a much higher risk of arm lymph-oedema than either modality alone.

Late effects are usually irrecoverable and show a dose response. Low doses are less likely to cause damage, while progressively higher doses have a greater chance of causing complications and this damage becomes clinically relevant at an earlier stage. The radiation dose there-fore has to be chosen carefully, taking into account normal tissue tolerance as well as predicted tumour cure dose and, as long as this is done, organs will function normally for the remainder of the patient's life. The actual dose chosen depends on a variety of factors. For each site an acceptable level of damage must first be decided and balanced against the chance of tumour control (Fig. 28.4). Damage to the spinal cord has such disastrous consequences that no morbidity can be accepted. A lower dose than that used at many other sites has to be accepted, even at the expense of tumour cure probability. Damage to other soft tissues, such as muscle and fat, is undesirable but of lesser importance and a higher dose and higher risk are accepted. As mentioned previously, the volume treated is important: the larger the volume, the greater the risk of damage and the lower the tolerable dose; for example, for the spinal cord a short length of cord can be treated to 50 Gy, but long segments, over 10 cm, will not tolerate more than 40 Gy. Other factors affecting tolerance include age, children and the elderly being less tolerant, or pre-existing vascular disease and previous surgery.

Second malignancy

In addition to specific organ complications the problem of secondary malignancies is being increasingly recognized. This has been best studied in Hodgkin's disease, where an increased incidence of acute leukaemias are seen 3–10 years after irradiation, with a smaller increased risk of solid tumours following (Swerdlow et al 1992).

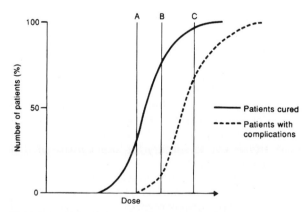

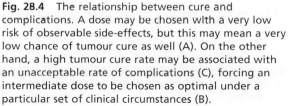

Fig. 28.4 The relationship between cure and complications. A dose may be chosen with a very low risk of observable side-effects, but this may mean a very low chance of tumour cure as well (A). On the other hand, a high tumour cure rate may be associated with an unacceptable rate of complications (C), forcing an intermediate dose to be chosen as optimal under a particular set of clinical circumstances (B).

The precise risk is difficult to quantify, but data give an overall risk of leukaemia of approximately 1–2% at 15 years. The risk is greatest if radiotherapy is given in conjunction with, or is followed by, chemotherapy – especially chemotherapy with alkylating agents such as cyclophosphamide or chlormethine (mustine); in one series it was 0.2% if no chemotherapy was used and 8.1% if the patient received multiple courses. Similar increased incidence of leukaemia has been seen in other cohorts of patients, including those with ankylosing spondylitis who have received spinal irradiation (Weiss et al 1994). Of perhaps more concern is the risk of solid malignancy, which is increasingly recognized, estimates rising to 10% of patients surviving Hodgkin's disease 15–20 years following radiotherapy, although a disease-related phenomenon could also be responsible (Swerdlow et al 1992). This risk of secondary malignancy has to be balanced against the risks of dying from the primary disease in most cancer sufferers.

In conclusion, radiotherapy is set to remain the chief curative modality in patients with non-surgical cancer. As screening and other early detection methods diagnose an increasing percentage of individuals with truly localized disease, its importance is likely to increase. This continued role in the curative treatment of cancer patients continues to stimulate research into the technical and biological basis of radiotherapy. In future years, further improvements in the efficacy and safety of radiotherapy should be expected to result from this research.

Summary

- Do you recognize that treatment with multiple beams of high energy X-rays given daily over several weeks is the optimal method? This is because of the physical and biological attributes of radiotherapy.
- Can you identify circumstances when radiotherapy offers an effective alternative to surgery for local control of many cancers?
- Do you understand what adjuvant radiotherapy is and its frequent value in improving local control?
- In advanced cancer do you appreciate the value of short courses of palliative radiotherapy?
- Will you remember the limitations on radiation dose because of possible late effects that may develop after months or years?

References

Asbell SO, Krall JM, Pilepich MV et al 1988 Elective pelvic irradiation in stage A-2, B carcinoma of the prostate: analysis of RTOG 77–06. International Journal of Radiation Oncology Biology Physics 15(6): 1307–1316

Bleehen NM, Girling DJ, Fayers PM, Aber VR, Stephens RJ 1991 Inoperable non-small-cell lung cancer (NSCLC): a Medical Research Council randomised trial of palliative radiotherapy with two fractions or ten fractions. British Journal of Cancer 63(2): 265–270

Brada M, Ross G 1995 Radiotherapy for primary and secondary brain tumors. Current Opinion in Oncology 7(3): 214–219

Coindre JM, Terrier P, Nguyen-Binh B et al 1996 Prognostic factors in adult patients with locally controlled soft tissue sarcoma: a study of 546 patients from the French Federation of Cancer Centers sarcoma group. Journal of Clinical Oncology 14(3): 869–877

Dearnaley DP, Khoo VS, Norman A et al (1999) Comparison of radiation side-effects of conformal and conventional radiotherapy in prostate cancer: a randomized trial. Lancet 353: 267–272.

Dische S, Saunders M, Barrett A, Harvey A, Gibson D, Parmar M 1997 A randomised multicentre trial of CHART versus conventional radiotherapy in head and neck cancer. Radiotherapy and Oncology 44(2): 123–136

Graf W, Dahlberg M, Osman MM, Holmberg L, Pahlman L, Glimelius B 1997 Short-term preoperative radiotherapy results in down-staging of rectal cancer: a study of 1316 patients. Radiotherapy and Oncology 43(2): 133–137

Horiot JC, Le Fur R, N'Guyen T et al 1992 Hyperfractionation versus conventional fractionation in oropharyngeal carcinoma: final analysis of a randomized trial of the EORTC cooperative group of radiotherapy. Radiotherapy and Oncology 25(4): 231–241

Huddart RA, Rajan B, Law M, Meyer L, Dearnaley DP 1997 Spinal cord compression in prostate cancer: treatment outcome and prognostic factors. Radiotherapy and Oncology 44(3): 229–236

Pollack A, Zagars GZ 1996 Radiotherapy for stage T3b transitional cell carcinoma of the bladder. Seminars in Urology and Oncology 14(2): 86–95

Price P, Hoskin PJ, Easton D, Austin D, Palmer SG, Yarnold JR 1986 Prospective randomised trial of single and multifraction radiotherapy schedules in the treatment of painful bony metastases. Radiotherapy and Oncology 6(4): 247–255

Priestman TJ, Dunn J, Brada M, Rampling R, Baker PG 1996 Final results of the Royal College of Radiologists' trial comparing two different radiotherapy schedules in the treatment of cerebral metastases. Clinical Oncology 8(5): 308–315

Quilty PM, Kirk D, Bolger JJ, Dearnaley DP et al 1994 A comparison of the palliative effects of strontium-89 and external beam radiotherapy in metastatic prostate cancer. Radiotherapy and Oncology 31(1): 33–40

Swerdlow AJ, Douglas AJ, Vaughan Hudson G, Bennett MH, MacLennan KA 1992 Risk of second primary cancers after Hodgkin's disease by type of treatment: analysis of 2846 patients in the British National Lymphoma Investigation. BMJ 304(6835): 1137–1143

Warde P, Payne D 1992 Does thoracic irradiation improve survival and local control in limited-stage small cell carcinoma of the lung? A meta-analysis. Journal of Clinical Oncology 10(6): 890–895

Weiss HA, Darby SC, Doll R 1994 Cancer mortality following x-ray treatment for ankylosing spondylitis. International Journal of Cancer 59(3): 327–338

Work E, Bentzen SM, Nielsen OS et al 1996 Prophylactic cranial irradiation in limited stage small cell lung cancer: survival benefit in patients with favourable characteristics. European Journal of Cancer 32A(5): 772–778

Wurm R, Warrington AP, Laing RW et al 1994 Stereotactic radiotherapy for solitary brain metastases as alternative to surgery (Meeting abstract 050). British Journal of Cancer 70(suppl 22): 21

Further reading

Dobbs J, Barrett A 1985 Practical radiotherapy planning. Edward Arnold, London

Horwich A 1995 Oncology: a multidisciplinary textbook. Chapman & Hall, London

Steel GG 1993 Basic clinical radiobiology for radiation oncologists. Edward Arnold, London

29 Cancer chemotherapy

V. M. Macaulay, C. Coulter

Objectives

- **Understand the actions of cytotoxic drugs, endocrine therapy and the new biologicals.**
- **Recognize the indications for, and timing and administration of, chemotherapy by multidisciplinary teams.**
- **Understand objective clinical response, and adjuvant, neoadjuvant and palliative chemotherapy.**
- **Appreciate the importance and design of new drug trials.**

INTRODUCTION

Localized tumours can be cured by surgery and/or radiotherapy. Primary tumours are rarely the cause of death unless they are in critical sites such as the brain. Most cancer deaths are attributable to direct or indirect effects of metastatic disease, and this requires systemic treatment. There are three main types of systemic anticancer therapy: chemotherapy, endocrine therapy and biological therapy.

Paul Ehrlich was the first to use the term 'chemotherapy', in the early 1900s. Chemotherapy was initially shown to be effective in the 1940s and 1950s when nitrogen mustard, aminopterin and actinomycin were used to treat lymphoma, leukaemia and Wilms' tumour. Subsequent work has confirmed that cytotoxic drugs can indeed cure disseminated disease in a significant proportion of patients with germ cell tumours, lymphomas, leukaemias and a few with small cell lung cancer and ovarian cancer. Unfortunately, most metastatic common solid tumours remain incurable, although cytotoxic and endocrine therapies undoubtedly have useful anticancer activity that can effectively palliate symptoms. The last 10–20 years have seen many advances in our knowledge of the cellular and molecular processes that characterize cancer cells. The challenge now for oncologists is to translate these advances into new therapeutic approaches that will improve the outlook for patients with common cancers.

BASIC PRINCIPLES

Growth characteristics of tumours

1. Cancers are caused by mutations in genes that influence critical aspects of normal growth regulation (see Ch. 26). A common early event is the loss of ability to replicate (copy) faithfully deoxyribonucleic acid (DNA). This so-called genomic instability (genome = the full set of genes) leads in turn to mutations in other genes, including those that regulate growth and survival, drug resistance, cell–cell interactions, invasion, angiogenesis (formation of new blood vessels) and the ability to evade immune recognition. These changes give the cell a growth advantage, leading to tumour formation.

2. Within an individual tumour only a subset of cells is proliferating – the 'growth fraction'. In general, small tumours have high growth fractions, but as the tumour enlarges the growth fraction often falls. Chemotherapy tends to be less effective in larger tumours because the growth fraction is smaller, and there has been a longer time for mutation to occur in genes that determine drug resistance. In addition, central regions of large tumours are often poorly perfused, reducing drug access, and the hypoxic cells are usually chemoresistant. This is why early diagnosis is so important.

3. The smallest tumours currently detectable are well advanced in their natural history: a tumour of ~1 cm³ weighs ~1 g, contains 10^9 cells, and has gone through 30 doublings. In only 10 more doublings it will reach 10^{12} cells, representing ~1 kg of tumour, which is usually lethal. This problem of the threshold of detectability applies not only in the diagnosis of a primary tumour, but also in patient management after apparently curative resection of a localized cancer. Many such patients harbour tiny tumour deposits, so-called micrometastases. These can be found by examining bone marrow using specialized immunostaining or molecular techniques, but cannot be detected by currently available clinical scans. Little is understood about how tumour cells can remain viable but quiescent, presumably in the G_0 phase of the cell cycle, and how or why they can reinitiate growth after latent periods of months or years.

Principles of cytotoxic chemotherapy

Cytotoxic drugs damage DNA, inhibit DNA synthesis or block cell division

Many standard cytotoxic (Greek *kytos* = vessel, hollow, cell + *toxon* = bow, *toxikos* = for the bow, *toxikon* = arrow poison) drugs kill rapidly-growing cells by damaging their DNA. DNA double-strand breaks are highly toxic, and if not repaired will lead to cell death. Other drugs act by interfering with DNA synthesis or cell division (Fig. 29.1). Cytotoxic drugs show no intrinsic specificity for cancer cells versus normal tissues; in addition to killing tumour cells, they damage normal tissues that are rapidly dividing, including the normal bone marrow, gut lining and hair follicles. An element of selectivity can be introduced by careful adjustment of dose and schedule to maximize damage to the tumour while allowing recovery of normal tissues (Fig. 29.2).

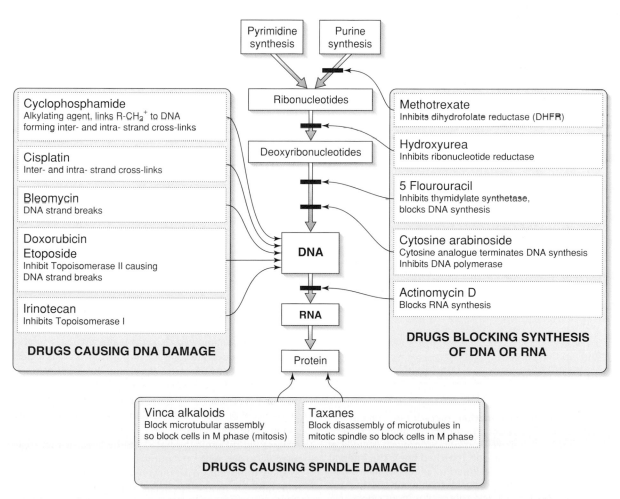

Fig. 29.1   Actions of cytotoxic drugs at the molecular level. Pathways involved in DNA synthesis and gene expression, the process whereby information encoded in DNA is transcribed (copied into RNA) and translated into protein. Cytotoxic drugs in the box on the left-hand side act primarily by causing DNA damage. This may be a direct effect (e.g. due to bleomycin) or may occur indirectly, e.g. via inhibition of topoisomerases, enzymes that bind to DNA and induce and reseal strand breaks. These breaks are important for relieving torsional stress as the DNA double helix unwinds prior to DNA synthesis. Drugs in the box on the right-hand side block specific steps in DNA or RNA synthesis, and drugs in the lower box interfere with the function of tubulin, the protein in the mitotic spindle. Modified with permission from Grahame-Smith DG, Aronson JK 2002 Oxford textbook of clinical pharmacology and drug therapy, 3rd edn. Oxford University Press, Oxford.

Classification of cytotoxic drugs

The mechanism of cell kill dictates when cytotoxic drugs are effective, and how cell kill varies with increasing dose (Table 29.1 and Figs 29.2 and 29.3):

- Non-phase-dependent drugs:
  Are equally toxic to cycling cells and those that are non-cycling (i.e. G_0)
  Kill by damaging DNA directly
  Kill exponentially with increasing dose.
- Phase-dependent drugs:
  Kill cells only in a specific part of the cell cycle, usually S (DNA synthesis) or M (mitosis)
  Linear cell kill up to a plateau, limited by proportion of cells in target phase.

Some drugs have multiple mechanisms of action. For example doxorubicin intercalates between the DNA strands, generating free radicals, and also inhibits the enzyme topoisomerase II (see Fig. 29.1). It is toxic

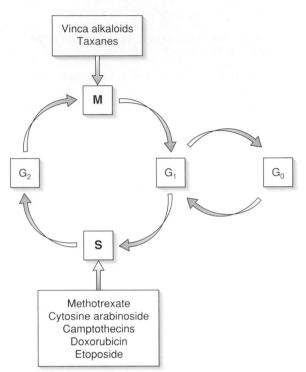

Fig. 29.3 Actions of cytotoxic drugs within the cell cycle. M, mitosis; S, DNA synthesis; G_1, first gap phase; G_2, second gap phase; G_0, quiescent non-cycling cells.

during all phases of the cell cycle but particularly in S phase.

'Fractional cell killing'

In 1964, Skipper showed that survival is inversely related to tumour burden and that for most drugs there is a clear relationship between drug dose and the eradication of tumour cells. A given dose of a drug kills a constant proportion of cells, not a constant number. The implication of this concept of 'fractional cell killing' is that tumour eradication requires either a sufficiently high dose of the drug(s) within limits tolerated by the host, or that treatment is started when the number of cells is small enough to allow tumour destruction at reasonably tolerated doses. Standard chemotherapy uses doses that often cause mild/moderate side-effects, most of which can be controlled by simple symptomatic treatments such as antiemetics (see below). In contrast, high dose chemotherapy, used for example in the treatment of leukaemias and lymphomas, causes severe and sometimes life-threatening toxicity, including profound myelotoxicity (Greek *myelos* = marrow; bone marrow).

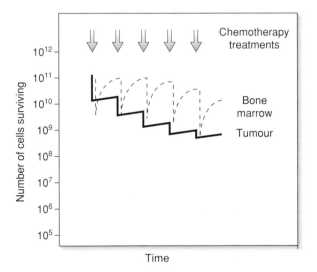

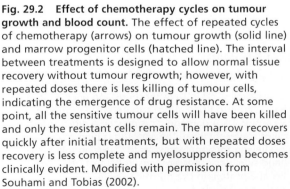

Fig. 29.2 Effect of chemotherapy cycles on tumour growth and blood count. The effect of repeated cycles of chemotherapy (arrows) on tumour growth (solid line) and marrow progenitor cells (hatched line). The interval between treatments is designed to allow normal tissue recovery without tumour regrowth; however, with repeated doses there is less killing of tumour cells, indicating the emergence of drug resistance. At some point, all the sensitive tumour cells will have been killed and only the resistant cells remain. The marrow recovers quickly after initial treatments, but with repeated doses recovery is less complete and myelosuppression becomes clinically evident. Modified with permission from Souhami and Tobias (2002).

Table 29.1 Cytotoxic drugs

Class of agent	Mode of action	Examples	Uses (examples)	Main toxicities
Alkylating agents	Link alkyl group (R–CH–) to chemical groups in proteins and nucleic acids	Cyclophosphamide	Breast, SCLC, NHL, Hodgkin's, sarcomas	Marrow, cystitis
		Cisplatin	Ovary, teratoma, seminoma, bladder, lung, head and neck	Neuropathy, renal (irreversible), deafness (irreversible)
		Carboplatin	Ovary	Marrow
		Gemcitabine	Pancreatic, NSCLC	Flu-like symptoms, skin rash
		Dacarbazine (DTIC)	Melanoma	Marrow, flu-like symptoms, arm pain
		Chlorambucil	Low grade NHL	Marrow, leukaemia
Antimetabolites	Resemble DNA precursors, block DNA synthesis or replication	Methotrexate	Breast, sarcomas, NHL	Mucositis (eyes, mouth), renal, liver
		5-Fluorouracil (5FU)	Colorectal, breast	Gut toxicity, hand–foot syndrome
		Capecitabine	Colorectal	As 5FU
Antitumour antibiotics	Bind to DNA, intercalate between base pairs. Inhibit topoisomerase II	Doxorubicin,	Breast, lymphomas, SCLC, ovary, bladder	Marrow, cardiotoxic
		Epirubicin	Breast	Marrow, mild cardiotoxicity
		Mitoxantrone	NHL, breast	Mild cardiotoxicity
	Single-and double-strand DNA breaks	Bleomycin	Teratoma, seminoma, head and neck, lymphomas	Pulmonary toxicity
Vinca alkaloids	Bind to tubulin, prevent assembly of mitotic spindle	Vincristine	NHL, SCLC	Neuropathy, constipation
		Vinblastine	Testicular, NHL	Marrow, mucositis
		Vindesine	Melanoma	Neuropathy
		Vinorelbine	NSCLC, breast, ovary	Neuropathy, constipation
Taxanes	Bind to tubulin, stop disassembly of mitotic spindle	Paclitaxel (Taxol)	Ovary, breast	Neuropathy, rash
		Docetaxel (Taxotere)	Breast, ovary	Neuropathy, rash
Epipodophylotoxins	Inhibit topoisomerase II	Etoposide	Lung, testicular	Bone marrow
Camptothecins	Inhibit topoisomerase I	Irinotecan	Colorectal	Gut, bone marrow
		Topotecan	Lung, ovary	Marrow

NHL, non-Hodgkin's lymphoma; NSCLC, non-small cell lung cancer; SCLC, small cell lung cancer.

Mechanisms of drug resistance

Resistance to specific drugs can be conferred by:

- Drug efflux, i.e. the cancer cell is able to pump the drug out. The product of the multidrug resistance (MDR) gene, a transmembrane protein (P-glycoprotein), acts as a drug efflux pump. Unfortunately clinical trials of efflux pump inhibitors have so far been disappointing.
- Increased synthesis within the cell of:
  Cytoplasmic enzymes that detoxify the drug, e.g. overexpression of certain glutathione-S-transferases confers resistance to cyclophosphamide
  The drug target, e.g. amplification (increased copy number) of the dihydrofolate reductase (DHFR) gene confers resistance to methotrexate.
- Reduced expression of:
  Enzymes that activate the drug, e.g. enzymes that convert 5-fluorouracil (5FU) to its active metabolite
  Proteins targeted by the cytotoxic drug, e.g. reduction in levels of the enzyme topoisomerase II confers resistance to topoisomerase II inhibitors e.g. anthracyclines, etoposide.
  In addition, cancer cells may become generally resistant to killing via mutation or altered expression of proteins that regulate cell survival and susceptibility to apoptosis (Greek *apo* = from + *ptosis* = a falling), such as Bcl-2, p53.

Likelihood of cell killing

This depends on:

- Whether the cell is intrinsically sensitive or resistant to the action of the drug.
- The cycling of the tumour cell (for phase-specific agents).
- The concentration of drug delivered to the tumour. This is a function of dose and schedule. There is evidence of a dose–response relationship for some cytotoxic drugs, and in breast cancer doxorubicin has been shown to confer greater therapeutic benefit at high dose. Very high dose chemotherapy, with autologous bone marrow or stem cell support, is a technique used for treatment in acute leukaemia or as second-line therapy in lymphomas. So far no benefit has been shown for trials of this approach as treatment for women with high risk early breast cancer or metastatic breast cancer.

Combination chemotherapy

To maximize the chance that a tumour will respond to therapy, cytotoxic drugs are often used in combination.

The principles of combination chemotherapy are that the selected drugs should:

- Be active against the tumour when used alone
- Have different mechanisms of action, to maximize tumour cell kill
- Have a different spectrum of side-effects, to minimize toxicity to the patient.

Timing of chemotherapy

- Primary therapy for chemosensitive tumours such as lymphomas, leukaemias and teratomas. Here chemotherapy is the main treatment modality and can achieve cures.
- Palliative chemotherapy (Latin *palliare* = to cloak; hence mitigate, extenuate). Most common cancers are less chemosensitive, and patients with metastatic disease cannot hope to be cured, but they may obtain useful symptomatic benefit. It is important to monitor tumour response and stop or change treatment if there is no evidence of objective response (see point 11 below).
- Adjuvant chemotherapy (Latin *ad* = to + *juvare* = to help). Many patients with early cancer can be cured by surgery. Certain features suggest a high risk of recurrence; these vary with tumour type but often include size of the primary, grade (i.e. degree of differentiation), involvement of local lymph nodes, and vascular invasion. Current imaging techniques are unable to detect tumour deposits smaller than 2–3 mm, so it is impossible to know with certainty which patients have been cured by surgery and which have micrometastatic disease that will later cause overt recurrence and death. In cancers of the breast and colon, patients at high risk of recurrence should be offered adjuvant chemotherapy and/or endocrine therapy, in an attempt to kill residual tumour cells remaining after apparently complete local resection. There is no way to judge the efficacy of this approach in individual patients other than to await relapse. Therefore, in designing adjuvant therapy, use only those agents shown to be active in advanced disease.
- Neoadjuvant chemotherapy describes the use of cytotoxic drugs as initial (presurgery) treatment for patients who present with localized but extensive cancer, such as large primary breast cancers. The aim is to shrink the primary tumour to permit a more conservative operation, and to control micrometastatic disease. The effect can be monitored by serial measurement of the size of the primary tumour. In patients with breast cancer this is most accurately done by serial magnetic resonance imaging (MRI) scans, or failing that by ultrasound; clinical measurements are notoriously inaccurate.

Manage cancer patients within multidisciplinary teams

- Work closely with pathologists, clinical oncologists (radiotherapists), medical oncologists, clinical nurse specialists, radiologists and palliative care physicians.
- Unit policies for cancer treatment should be based on the results of published studies including randomized trials.
- Make management decisions after joint consultation with other members of the team.
- Offer patients treatment options appropriate for their age, health, tumour type and stage.

Practicalities of administration

- It is essential that cytotoxic drugs be given by a trained doctor or nurse.
- Most standard chemotherapy regimens are given on an outpatient basis every 3–4 weeks.
- The dose is usually calculated on the basis of milligrams per square metre of body surface area.
- Dose and schedule may need to be adjusted according to the function of:
  Liver: principal site for metabolism/excretion of doxorubicin, mitozantrone and vinca alkaloids. If the serum bilirubin is elevated use these agents with caution, at reduced dose.
  Kidneys: drugs that are cleared by the kidney may cause increased toxicity if the patient has impaired renal function. Check the renal function before each course of chemotherapy when giving certain drugs, especially cisplatin, cyclophosphamide, ifosfamide and procarbazine, and any high dose chemotherapy. Ensure that the patient is well hydrated before, during and after drug administration. Carboplatin has similar activity to cisplatin and may be given to patients with renal impairment, tailoring the dose to creatinine clearance.

Key points

- **A given dose of chemotherapy kills a constant proportion of cells, not a constant number of cells.**
- **Cytotoxic drugs are used in combination to maximize tumour cell kill.**
- **Cancer patients should be managed by multidisciplinary teams.**
- **It is essential that cytotoxic drugs are given by a trained doctor or nurse.**

- **Tumour responses are defined by objective criteria.**
- **Chemotherapy works better in fit patients.**

Routes of administration

- Intravenous injection/infusion: the commonest route for cytotoxic drugs, usually via a temporary venous cannula (drip). Long term venous access devices may be required for convenience, because of poor veins or for infusional chemotherapy. Long term catheters are inserted so that the tip lies in a large central vein. Various catheters are available, including those suitable for insertion into the subclavian or internal jugular veins, such as Hickman or Groshong, and others for insertion into a peripheral (e.g. antecubital) vein.
- Oral administration, e.g. cyclophosphamide, methotrexate, etoposide, capecitabine.
- Subcutaneous administration: commonly used for interferon or interleukin-2 administration.
- Intra-arterial: an implanted pump may be placed into the common hepatic artery to infuse chemotherapy continuously into the liver. This technique is being evaluated in patients with liver metastases from the colon and rectum.
- Intrathecal chemotherapy with methotrexate or cytosine arabinoside is used for brain/meningeal involvement by leukaemias, lymphomas, teratomas, choriocarcinomas and occasionally for central nervous system (CNS) involvement by common solid tumours such as breast cancer. As with all chemotherapy, this should be administered only by trained personnel, to avoid the catastrophic and invariably fatal consequences of intrathecal administration of vincristine.

Clinical assessment of response

So that oncologists around the world can compare the efficacy of different agents, it is important to define what is meant by a response. One or more tumour deposits (marker lesions) are selected for measurement in two dimensions, on plain X-ray, ultrasound, computed tomography (CT) or MRI scan. This enables calculation of the cross-sectional area (product of the two dimensions) of each deposit. These measurements are made immediately before the start of treatment and again during/after treatment, and responses are defined as shown below. It is worth remembering that tumour shrinkage need last for only 4 weeks to count as a response. These are the World Health Organization criteria:

- Complete response (CR): no evidence of disease remains after treatment

- Partial response (PR): marker lesion(s) shrink by 50%, no new lesions have appeared
- Stable disease (SD): marker lesions remain at 50% to 125% of pretreatment size (to allow for observer error in measurement)
- Progressive disease (PD): marker lesions have increased to ≥125% of pretreatment size or appearance of new lesions
- Response rate: CR plus PR.

There has recently been a move to replace these criteria, emphasizing the role of CT and MRI imaging of marker lesions and formalizing the monitoring and analysis of response. Time will tell whether these new 'RECIST' criteria (response evaluation criteria in solid tumours) will replace the WHO criteria listed above.

Fit patients do better with chemotherapy

In general, chemotherapy has greater benefit in patients who have 'good performance status', that is, they are fit and able to walk about. In patients with 'poor performance status', that is, confined by their illness or by concomitant disease to a bed or chair for most of the day, chemotherapy often has more severe side-effects and less benefit than in fit patients. This should not deter you from offering chemotherapy to a patient with a potentially curable tumour. However, in a patient with a cancer that can only be palliated by chemotherapy, it may be better to face the reality that such treatment may do more harm than good. In either case, make full use of simple measures such as analgesics and laxatives, which palliate symptoms without severe toxicity.

TOXICITY OF CHEMOTHERAPY

The dose of an anticancer drug is limited by its toxic effects on normal tissues. Some of these effects are manifest acutely, within minutes to weeks of administration, and may necessitate adjustment of dose or schedule. Some effects may be delayed for months or years, in some cases long after completion of the therapy that caused them, that is, when it is too late for dose modification or cessation of treatment.

 Neutropenic sepsis:

- **Can cause collapse and death within a few hours.**
- **Can occur any time after chemotherapy.**
- **Greatest risk 7–14 days after most drugs.**

- **Always check blood count if the patient is unwell.**
- **Requires urgent admission and intravenous antibiotics.**

Acute toxicity

Extravasation

Doxorubicin and vinca alkaloids are vesicant (Latin *vesica* = blister) drugs; they cause tissue destruction when extravasated. This leads to severe pain, burning and scarring and can be avoided by ensuring that the needle is within the vein and that the vein is tested using a non-vesicant substance before starting injection of the vesicant drugs. If extravasation does occur, stop drug administration immediately. Tissue damage can be limited by promptly administering corticosteroids by local injection or topical application.

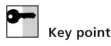 **Key point**

- **Every chemotherapy unit should display clear protocols outlining action to be taken in the event of extravasation.**

Bone marrow toxicity

For many cytotoxic drugs, bone marrow toxicity is dose limiting. It is mandatory that a full blood count is taken on the day of the treatment; most treatments can go ahead with a white blood count of $>1.5–2 \times 10^9$ l^{-1}, and platelets of $>100 \times 10^9$ l^{-1}, although this varies with different protocols. Delay or modify treatment, that is reduce the dose, if the blood count is inadequate. The risk of myelosuppression is greatest approximately 10–14 days after cycles of most sorts of chemotherapy. Warn patients to alert the oncology department if they have a fever above 37.5°C. Act promptly, because patients can die from neutropenic sepsis within a few hours. Manage fever in a patient with an absolute neutrophil count of less than 1.0×10^9 by urgent admission and treatment with intravenous broad-spectrum antibiotics. Include in the investigations cultures of blood, urine and from any indwelling line. It is unusual to isolate a pathogen, although patients with indwelling lines are at particular risk of staphylococcal infection, which may necessitate line removal if it cannot be eradicated with antibiotics. Spontaneous bleeding does not usually occur until the platelet count falls to 20×10^9, but check patients with low counts for signs of haemorrhage. Give platelet support if bleeding occurs – typically on the shins but you should check all over, including the mouth and ocular fundi, and prophylactically if the count falls below 10–20×10^9 per litre.

Key points

- **Chemotherapeutic agents are dangerous. They must be administered only by skilled, trained people.**
- **Monitor the white cell count assiduously and respond to falls by delaying or modifying treatment.**
- **Keep neutropenic sepsis in mind – always.**

Gastrointestinal toxicity

Nausea and vomiting are caused by many drugs and can be severe with cisplatin, cyclophosphamide, doxorubicin and actinomycin C. This is probably the result of a combination of stimuli from the chemoreceptor trigger zone, the gut and the cerebral cortex. Patients receiving mildly emetic chemotherapy, such as cyclophosphamide, methotrexate, fluorouracil (CMF) for breast cancer, respond to metoclopramide or domperidone and dexamethasone. For patients receiving highly emetogenic drugs such as cisplatin, give a 5-hydroxytryptamine antagonist such as ondansetron or tropisetron prophylactically, together with dexamethasone. Oral premedication with lorazepam may help the patient to relax before treatment. Uncontrolled vomiting is not only extremely unpleasant, but also dangerous, as dehydration can increase toxicity, for example, the nephrotoxicity of cisplatin. You may need to admit a patient for intravenous rehydration if vomiting cannot be controlled by oral medication. Standard dose methotrexate can cause mucositis, manifest as soreness of the mouth and eyes. If this is severe, give calcium leucovorin (folinic acid) for 48 h, starting 24 h after subsequent courses of chemotherapy. Folinic acid is an alternative intermediary metabolite that bypasses the block in DHFR activity, terminating the cytotoxic effect of methotrexate (note that folinic acid enhances the activity of 5-fluorouracil). High dose methotrexate requires prophylactic folinic acid, at doses that depend on the results of methotrexate drug level monitoring. Vincristine may cause constipation and paralytic ileus, which may respond to laxatives. 5-Fluorouracil and its oral analogue capecitabine can cause severe gut toxicity. Loperamide can be used prophylactically or for mild diarrhoea, but stop treatment of patients with severe diarrhoea – that is, 4–6 times a day or at night, or bloody.

Alopecia (Greek alopex = fox; fox-like, patchy baldness)

This results from treatment with doxorubicin, cyclophosphamide, etoposide, vincristine, paclitaxel and docetaxel. Hair loss usually starts 18–21 days after the first injection of these drugs, but is temporary and patients can be reassured that the hair will regrow after treatment has been completed. Wigs are available on the National Health Service (NHS) and should be provided for patients before hair loss occurs. Alopecia due to doxorubicin and docetaxel may be avoided or reduced by scalp cooling, which limits blood flow and hence drug access to the scalp. This carries a theoretical risk of scalp recurrence, but in practice this is very rare.

Neuropathy

Irreversible peripheral neuropathy and ototoxicity can be a serious problem with cisplatin. Vinca alkaloids and taxanes inhibit, respectively, the assembly and disassembly of microtubules; as well as blocking mitosis, this also interferes with nerve conduction. Peripheral neuropathy causes paraesthesia and numbness, which improve on stopping taxanes but can be severe and irreversible with pain and muscle weakness with the vinca alkaloids. Vincas also cause autonomic neuropathy, manifest as paralytic ileus and constipation.

Long-term toxicity
Cardiotoxicity

This is the most important chronic and dose-limiting side-effect of doxorubicin, and causes arrythmias and cardiac failure. The risk of cardiotoxicity is dose-related (so total dose should not exceed 450 mg m^{-2}) and is increased in patients with pre-existing heart disease, previous treatment with trastuzumab (Herceptin), or radiotherapy to the mediastinum or left chest, for example postmastectomy. The risk of cardiotoxicity appears to be less with the related drugs mitoxantrone and epirubicin. Herceptin itself causes cardiac dysfunction in approximately 5% of patients and should not be administered in combination with anthracyclines.

Pulmonary toxicity

Bleomycin can cause acute pulmonary infiltrates that may disappear when the drug is stopped, but which often heal leaving chronic fibrosis. This is a dose-related effect, commonly occurring at total doses over 300 000 units, but it can occur after lower doses in patients with renal impairment. Remember to alert the anaesthetist if a patient previously treated with bleomycin is being prepared for operation.

An example is a young man with a teratoma undergoing excision of a residual tumour mass; high concentrations of oxygen can acutely damage lungs exposed to bleomycin. Mitomycin C can also cause pulmonary infiltrates and fibrosis, and busulphan and other alkylating agents can cause fibrosis.

Carcinogenesis

After long-term treatment with alkylating agents such as chlorambucil and melphalan, patients are at risk of developing acute leukaemia. Leukaemia with specific chromosomal characteristics can develop after treatment with etoposide. The risk is directly related to the total dose of the drugs given. This is an important reason for reducing the length of treatment and, therefore, the cumulative dose of these agents. There is negligible risk of developing a second solid tumour after chemotherapy alone, although the risk increases if chemotherapy is combined with local irradiation.

Gonadal damage

This can follow treatment with alkylating agents, especially when used in combination. Ensure that patients receiving chemotherapy receive counselling about the risk of long-term infertility and the inadvisability of pregnancy during chemotherapy. After combination chemotherapy (e.g. MOPP; mustine, oncovin, procarbazine, prednisolone) for Hodgkin's disease, the majority of men are azoospermic, although the risk of this effect is reduced by using alternative regimens such as ABVD (adriamycin, bleomycin, vinblastine, dacarbazine). Offer all male patients sperm banking before starting chemotherapy. With modern assisted reproductive techniques it is possible to achieve ovum fertilization with a very low sperm count. Men do not need hormone replacement therapy. For women aged over 30 years there is a very high risk of permanent amenorrhoea when they have received combination chemotherapy for Hodgkin's disease. It is now possible, but time-consuming and expensive, to hyperstimulate the ovaries before chemotherapy to obtain ova which can be fertilized and frozen. Female patients will need hormone replacement therapy. Men who receive treatment with cisplatin for germ cell tumours usually retain fertility, as do women who have received chemotherapy for choriocarcinoma.

HORMONE THERAPY

Hormone therapies (= endocrine therapies) are used in the management of patients with cancers of the breast, prostate and endometrium. Historically this was the first form of systemic treatment offered to patients with cancer, when in 1896 Beatson performed oophorectomy for metastatic breast cancer. Surgical approaches have now been almost completely replaced by medical treatments designed to manipulate the levels or activity of key hormones (Fig. 29.4).

Breast cancer

Breast cancer cell growth is stimulated by oestrogens, and hormone responsiveness is likely if the tumour cells express the nuclear hormone receptors oestrogen receptor (ER, for US spelling, estrogen) and progesterone receptor (PgR). Approximately one-third of all breast cancer patients respond to hormonal measures; response rates are ~70% in patients with ER+, PgR+ tumours, and 30-40% in tumours positive for ER or PgR. Active agents include:

- *Tamoxifen (Nolvadex):* a drug that acts as an antioestrogen in tumour cells, blocking activation of the ER by endogenous oestrogens. In the rest of the body, tamoxifen acts as an oestrogen, protecting against osteoporosis and cardiovascular disease but also causing a slightly increased incidence of endometrial cancer. Tamoxifen is used both in the adjuvant setting and in metastatic disease, and trials indicate that it can significantly reduce the incidence of breast cancer in women whose family history puts them at high risk of the disease. In recent years, pure antioestrogens have become available, and these are currently being assessed in advanced disease.
- *Anastrozole (Arimidex)*: an aromatase inhibitor that blocks the conversion of androgens to oestrogens. Aromatase inhibitors are effective in postmenopausal patients but not in premenopausal women where the intact hypothalamic–pituitary–gonadal axis is able to overcome the drug-induced enzyme block.
- *Goserelin (Zoladex)*: a leutinising hormone releasing hormone (LHRH) analogue that prevents pituitary LH release, leading to a fall in gonadal steroid production in premenopausal women.
- *Megestrol acetate (Megace)* and *medroxyprogesterone acetate (Provera)*: synthetic progestins that antagonize the cellular effects of oestrogens. These drugs are less active than the above and they are usually used as third-line therapy, for example after tamoxifen and an aromatase inhibitor.

Prostate cancer

Prostate cancer cell growth is stimulated by androgens, and treatment here aims to reduce circulating levels or to block androgen effects at the cellular level. Since Huggins

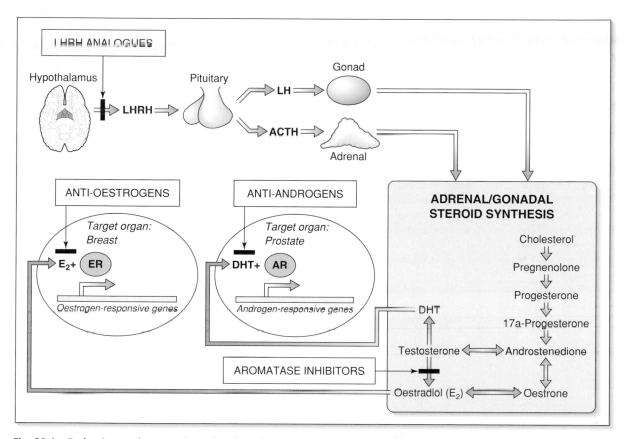

Fig. 29.4 **Endocrine pathways, sites of action of main hormonal agents.** The main pathways involved in synthesis of adrenal and gonadal hormones (shaded box) are shown. Dihydrotestosterone (DHT) binds to and activates the androgen receptor (AR), which drives expression of androgen-responsive genes. Similarly, the expression of estradiol-responsive genes is activated by binding of oestradiol (E_2) to the oestrogen receptor (ER). Hormonal anticancer agents act either by blocking hormone production, e.g. aromatase inhibitors (note that luteinizing hormone releasing hormone (LHRH) analogues first stimulate then suppress luteinizing hormone (LH) release, leading to a fall in production of testosterone from the testis or oestrogen from the ovary). Other agents block the effect of the steroid hormone at the molecular level, e.g. antiandrogens, antioestrogens. ACTH, adrenocorticotrophin.

discovered, in 1941, that metastatic prostate cancer is almost always androgen-dependent, orchidectomy and oestrogen therapy have been standard treatments. Nowadays hormonal control can be achieved with fewer side-effects using LHRH analogues such as goserelin, and antiandrogens such as flutamide (Drogenil) and bicalutamide (Casodex), which block the binding of dihydrotestosterone to the androgen receptor.

Endometrial cancer

Progestogens such as medroxyprogesterone acetate are useful in the treatment of patients with locally recurrent or metastatic endometrial cancer. Approximately one-third of patients respond, and responders live longer than non-responders.

BIOLOGICAL THERAPY

Biological therapy produces antitumour effects through the action of natural substances, or the use of agents that block key biological processes in tumour cells.

Cytokines

Recombinant cytokines are agents that have roles in normal physiology, and can now be made by recombinant technology. This means that the cytokine gene is put into bacteria or yeast, expression of the gene is induced, that is the gene is 'switched on', leading to production of messenger ribonucleic acid (RNA) and hence protein, and the protein is purified from the culture in sufficient quantities to be used as therapy.

- *Interleukin 2 (IL-2)* is a T-cell growth factor that is central to T-cell-mediated immune responses. IL-2 has been approved for treatment of metastatic renal cell carcinoma. Response rates of 20% have been observed, and 50% of responding patients remain progression free 4–7 years following therapy. IL-2 also has activity against malignant melanoma, but again the response rate is only ~20%.
- *Colony stimulating factors (CSFs)* such as *erythropoietin* and *granulocyte CSF (filograstin)* stimulate haematopoiesis and immune functions. They do not have antitumour effects but reduce chemotherapy-induced haematological toxicity and are useful in the context of high dose chemotherapy and bone marrow transplantation.
- *α-Interferon (IFNα)*. Interferons are made by the body in response to viral infection. It is they, rather than the virus per se, that are responsible for the malaise and myalgia characteristic of influenza. IFNα has demonstrated activity against many solid and haematogenous

malignancies. A response rate of 80–90% has been observed among patients with hairy cell leukaemia, with apparent prolongation of survival. IFNα has been approved for use in chronic myeloid leukaemia, Kaposi's sarcoma, malignant melanoma and renal cancer, with response rates of 20–30%. As might be expected from their physiological role, interferons are toxic, causing influenza-like symptoms which can be intolerable.

Inhibitors of key biological processes

Current research is generating many new agents of potential therapeutic value that interfere with tumour growth by blocking the function of key pathways in cancer cells (Fig. 29.5 and see Ch. 26).

- *Antibodies*. Herceptin is a monoclonal antibody directed against the HER2 protein, a growth factor receptor

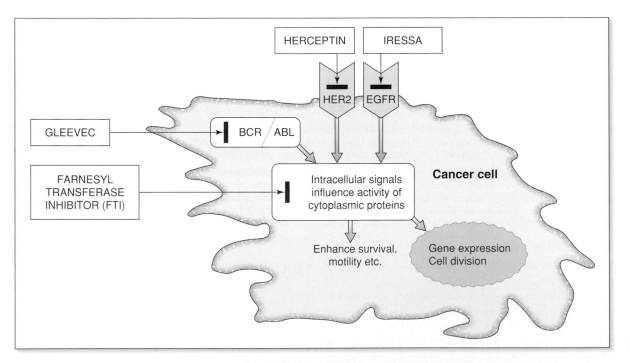

Fig. 29.5 Simple growth pathways with sites of action of selected novel biological anticancer agents. A growth factor binds to a specific cell surface receptor, generating intracellular signals that activate cytoplasmic proteins. Depending on the signal, this may lead directly to increased resistance to killing, increased motility, changes in attachment to other cells or substratum. Activation of cytoplasmic signalling cascades also leads to changes in gene expression (i.e. switching on/off protein production from specific genes) and changes in the rate of progression through the cell cycle (i.e. faster/slower growth). The sites of action of Herceptin, a monoclonal antibody to HER2 (a growth factor receptor), and of Iressa and Gleevec, small molecule inhibitors of the enzyme activity of the epidermal growth factor receptor (EGFR) and BCR-ABL, respectively, are shown. Farnesyl transferase inhibitors are agents that block the attachment to the cell membrane of ras protein, a specific signalling intermediate, so inhibiting ras activation and thus blocking ras-mediated proliferation.

expressed by ~20% of breast cancers but not by normal cells. The antibody is generated in mice but has been 'humanized' to avoid triggering immune responses to mouse proteins. Herceptin has been in clinical use for several years and has significant anticancer activity in patients whose breast tumours are strongly HER2 positive. It can enhance response to cytotoxic drugs such as taxanes, and is now being assessed as adjuvant therapy. Like most new treatments, it is very expensive, and it can cause cardiotoxicity, but it is an extremely valuable new drug in the treatment of aggressive breast cancer. Several other antibodies have been shown to have objective anticancer activity, including anti-CD20 for B-cell lymphomas and edrecolomab (Panorex) for colorectal cancer.

- *Small molecule inhibitors.* Chemical inhibitors are generally more successful drugs than antibodies; the latter are large molecules that require administration by intravenous infusion, and generally penetrate poorly into tumours. In contrast, chemical inhibitors are small molecules that penetrate well, they can be modified to improve characteristics of specificity, stability, solubility, etc., and they can often be administered orally. A recent success story is Gleevec (STI-571), rationally designed as a small molecule inhibitor of the enzyme activity of the BCR-ABL fusion protein that is produced as a result of the chromosomal translocation characteristic of chronic myeloid leukaemia (CML). Gleevec has recently been shown to have dramatic anticancer activity in patients with CML. Iressa is a small molecule inhibitor of the epidermal growth factor receptor (EGFR); it has anticancer activity in cancers of the lung and colon that express high levels of the EGFR. Many other small molecule inhibitors are currently being developed, including those that influence the activity of cytoplasmic signalling pathways and regulation of gene expression (Fig. 29.5).

- *Gene therapy.* Although cancer often results from defects in multiple genes, it may be possible to influence its course by altering the expression of individual genes. Strategies include replacement of a missing tumour suppressor gene, inhibition of production of an oncogene (see Ch. 26), introduction of genes that cause the cancer cell to convert a prodrug to a toxic product, and production of proteins that enhance the host immune response. Many trials are currently evaluating such approaches, and some trials are reporting clinical activity, but at present these remain in the realms of research.

NON-SURGICAL TREATMENT OF COMMON CANCERS

Anticancer treatments are particularly demanding and have potentially serious side-effects. You must confirm the diagnosis histologically before treatment begins, and ensure that patients understand why each treatment is offered and what it is intended to achieve. In the treatment of early, curable cancers, ensure that patients understand what sort of survival benefit may accrue from the multiple treatment modalities on offer. In the management of metastatic common cancers, you must unfortunately explain that chemotherapy cannot cure, nor with certainty prolong life, but may shrink tumours temporarily and so give symptom relief. See Chapters 27 and 28 for more information on cancer surgery and radiotherapy.

Breast cancer

Early breast cancer is treated surgically (see Ch. 27). Analysis of the resected specimen indicates the main prognostic factors: tumour size, grade, nodal involvement and tumour expression of oestrogen receptor (ER) and progesterone receptor (PgR). Patients at risk of micrometastatic disease include those with large or high grade tumours and/or involved axillary lymph nodes. These patients should be offered adjuvant or neoadjuvant chemotherapy (Fig. 29.6). For patients aged <50 with involved nodes, adjuvant chemotherapy leads to a 12% improvement in 10 year survival, from 41% to 53%. The benefit is less in patients with node-negative tumours and those aged over 50. Patients should have radiotherapy after breast-conserving surgery to reduce the risk of local recurrence. If the tumour was ER positive, patients should be offered tamoxifen 20 mg daily for 5 years. Tamoxifen should not be used in patients with ER-negative tumours. The timing of these treatments is shown in Figure 29.6, and the magnitude of the benefit is summarized in Table 29.2. You will need to explain the plan to patients during admission for surgery. Reassure them that they will be given effective antiemetics to combat nausea, that they may temporarily lose their hair (depending on the chemotherapy offered), and that radiotherapy can cause local skin soreness. The whole treatment plan is long, tiring and daunting, especially if reasons for giving each component are not clearly understood.

Metastatic breast cancer can be treated with endocrine therapy and/or chemotherapy. Patients may work their way through a range of different regimens and agents, depending on the pattern of disease. Radiotherapy is useful for controlling local symptoms, for instance due to bone or brain metastases. Endocrine therapy such as tamoxifen or anastrozole is a good option for patients with slow tempo ER-positive disease involving the skin, lymph nodes and/or bones. Rapid tempo disease, especially involving the viscera, for example lungs or liver, should be treated with chemotherapy. Many single agents

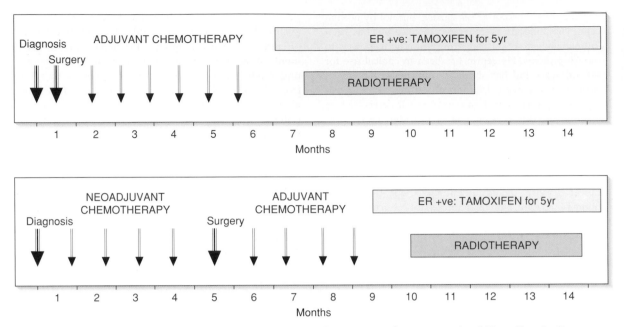

Fig. 29.6   Treatment of early breast cancer. Patients at risk of recurrence after surgery should be offered adjuvant chemotherapy (upper panel), usually 4–6 cycles of an anthracycline-containing combination (e.g. doxorubicin plus cyclophosphamide) or CMF (cyclophosphamide, methotrexate, 5FU). Patients with large tumours or those at very high risk of recurrence (e.g. high grade tumour) may be offered neoadjuvant chemotherapy (lower panel). This is given before surgery, with the aim of controlling micrometastatic disease and shrinking the tumour, enabling more conservative surgery. The timing of endocrine therapy and radiotherapy is also shown. ER, oestrogen receptor.

and combinations have activity in breast cancer but the objective response rates are often no more than 20–50%. In general, as with many tumour types, responders live longer than non-responders, but responses are often short-lived, so weigh these benefits against the adverse effects in non-responders.

Lung cancer

A small proportion of patients with non-small cell lung cancer (NSCLC) may be cured by operation, and occasionally by radical radiotherapy if surgery is inappropriate or is refused by the patient. However, 35–65% of patients suffer recurrent disease within 5 years of apparently curative resection. Meta-analysis of many trials suggests a small but significant benefit from chemotherapy given before or after surgery or radiotherapy. Fit patients with metastatic disease can be offered combination chemotherapy; responses occur in 20–60% and are associated with symptomatic improvement and modest survival benefit.

Small cell lung cancer (SCLC) has usually metastasized at the time of presentation. Even in patients with limited disease, such as a tumour confined to one hemithorax, there is a high risk of micrometastases, and so all patients

who are fit enough should be offered combination chemotherapy. Unlike most common solid tumours, SCLC is highly chemosensitive and 70–85% of patients respond to combination chemotherapy; however, most relapse with drug-resistant disease, and only a very few (~8% with limited disease, 2% with extensive disease) survive 5 years.

Cancers of the gastrointestinal tract

Localized carcinomas arising in the oesophagus and stomach are treated surgically (see Ch. 27); however only 40% of patients are eligible for potentially curative resection, and recurrence rates are high. Recent evidence suggests that the survival of high risk gastric cancer patients can be significantly improved with postoperative irradiation and concurrent 5FU. Fit patients with advanced or recurrent adenocarcinoma should be offered chemotherapy. Compared with intermittent conventional dose 5FU, response rates are significantly better with continuous low dose infusional 5FU combined with cisplatin and epirubicin. Pancreatic cancer is unfortunately highly chemoresistant, and most patients are too unfit for systemic treatment because of advanced disease at presentation.

Table 29.2   Benefits of adjuvant therapy for early breast cancer

Subgroup	treatment	Relapse-free(%)	Risk reduction	Survival (%)	Risk reduction
Node –ve	Tamoxifen*	79.2	14.9	78.9	5.6
	Control	64.3		73.3	
Node +ve	Tamoxifen*	59.7	15.2	61.4	10.9
	Control	44.5		50.6	
<50 years					
Node –ve	Chemotherapy[†]	68.3	10.3	77.6	5.7
	Control	58.0		71.9	
Node +ve	Chemotherapy[†]	47.6	15.4	53.8	12.4
	Control	32.2		41.4	
50–69 years					
Node –ve	Chemotherapy[†]	65.6	5.7	71.2	6.4
	Control	59.9		64.8	
Node +ve	Chemotherapy[†]	43.4	5.4	48.6	2.3
	Control	38.0		46.3	

Table shows figures at 10 years for: percent of patients free of relapse; percent surviving (including mortality from any cause); and reduction in risk of relapse and death.
*Data for ~5 years tamoxifen treatment in patients with tumours that were oestrogen receptor-positive or unknown.
[†]Data for patients involved in trials of polychemotherapy, including CMF (cyclophosphamide, methotrexate, 5FU) and anthracycline-containing regimens. There was clear benefit from chemotherapy in young women (<50 years) especially those with node-positive tumours (Early Breast Cancer Trialists' Collaborative Group, 1998a, b). A more recent analysis suggested that young women (<50 years) gained an average of approximately 10 months of relapse-free survival, and 5 months of overall survival, compared with patients receiving no adjuvant chemotherapy. These benefits significantly outweighed the toxicity of chemotherapy. Benefits in older women (50–69 years) were also significant, though smaller, and outweighed the toxicity burden to a lesser degree (Cole et al 2001).

Adjuvant 5FU-based chemotherapy has been shown to improve survival after surgery for localized colorectal cancer, and is now standard treatment for patients with Dukes' C colon cancer (see Ch. 27). In metastatic disease, 20% of patients respond to 5FU, with improvement in tumour-associated symptoms; several studies have shown survival benefit. Newer drugs with activity in colorectal cancer include capecitabine, an orally active prodrug which is converted in the body to 5FU, irinotecan, a topoisomerase I inhibitor, and oxaliplatin, a cisplatin analogue.

Urological tumours

Renal cancer can be cured only by complete resection. If technically feasible, nephrectomy may also confer survival benefit and symptom relief in fit patients with low volume metastatic disease. Metastatic renal cancer is resistant to hormone therapy and cytotoxic drugs. Biological therapy with IL-2 or IFNα offers a chance of inducing response, but only in 15–20% of patients.

Superficial bladder cancer is treated surgically, and localized invasive bladder cancer is managed by surgery and/or radiotherapy. In approximately 50% of patients with advanced bladder cancer a response can be induced with combination chemotherapy, usually including cisplatin, although this may be problematic if renal function is compromised.

Organ-confined prostate cancer can be cured by radical surgery or radiotherapy, either external beam or brachytherapy, but metastatic disease is incurable. Most patients (80%) respond to endocrine therapy, using an LHRH analogue or an antiandrogen, or the two combined – 'total androgen blockade'. Tumour responses are associated with improvement in symptoms such as bone pain, and a fall in the tumour marker prostate-specific antigen (PSA, see Ch. 30). Unfortunately, all tumours become androgen-resistant, usually after 12–18 months of endocrine therapy. At this point there may be minor symptomatic improvement with oral steroids or mitoxantrone, but metastatic prostate cancer is essentially chemoresistant.

Gynaecological cancers

Early stage cervical cancer can be treated with radical surgery or radical chemoradiation. There is a high risk of recurrence in those with positive lymph nodes, parametrial invasion or positive resection margins. If these patients are fit enough they should be offered postoperative radiotherapy and concurrent cisplatin chemotherapy, which have recently been shown to significantly prolong survival. Advanced cervical cancer is treated with irradiation, and recurrent disease may respond temporarily to chemotherapy.

Patients with ovarian cancer often present with advanced disease that has spread within the peritoneal cavity. This is optimally treated by maximal cytoreductive surgery – removing all visible tumour, and platinum-based chemotherapy.

Malignant melanoma

Patients with localized melanoma may be cured by surgery, and thickness of the primary lesion is the most important prognostic factor. Patients who experience skin recurrence near the primary site may be salvaged by further resection. In the 1960s and 1970s there was a vogue for regional limb perfusion, usually with melphalan, in patients with skin metastases confined to one limb. Responses occurred in 40% but were generally short-lived, with no convincing survival benefit. Many trials have assessed the role of IFNα as adjuvant treatment in high risk patients. Recent analyses suggest that low dose adjuvant interferon confers no survival benefit. High dose adjuvant interferon does, however, appear to be of benefit but has significant toxicity. The outlook for patients with metastatic disease is grim; only ~20% of patients respond to chemotherapy, usually with DTIC (dacarbazine), or to immunotherapy with IFNα, but these responses are usually brief and without survival benefit. A small percentage of patients obtain durable complete remissions, most often those with a small tumour burden.

Sarcomas

The outlook for patients with osteosarcoma is significantly improved if surgery is followed by immediate adjuvant chemotherapy, typically using cisplatin, doxorubicin and high dose methotrexate. This cures approximately 60% of patients. Neoadjuvant chemotherapy is increasingly used as well, to gain control of micrometastatic disease and to shrink the primary tumour to facilitate limb-sparing surgery. Pulmonary metastases are not necessarily incurable; patients with fewer than six metastases may be salvaged with

second-line chemotherapy, thoracotomy and excision of metastases. The prognosis of adults with soft tissue sarcomas is less good: tumours often recur after surgery, and are relatively resistant to both chemotherapy and radiotherapy.

Myeloma

In ~75% of cases, patients with myeloma respond to oral melphalan and prednisolone. Younger, fitter patients may derive greater benefit from more complex or intensive chemotherapy regimens, such as intravenous combination chemotherapy or high dose melphalan with bone marrow transplantation.

NON-SURGICAL TREATMENT OF HIGHLY CHEMOSENSITIVE CANCERS

Approximately 12% of cancer patients have tumours that are highly responsive to chemotherapy. These patients are often young, and even those with advanced disease may stand a good chance of being completely cured. Therefore it is essential that they should be managed in specialist centres by experienced multidisciplinary teams, as this has been shown to lead to improved survival.

Lymphoma

Hodgkin's disease can now be cured in most patients. The best chance of cure is when the patient first presents, and disease recurrence worsens the outlook. Patients with localized disease are treated with radiotherapy (see Ch. 28), and those with advanced disease are offered combination chemotherapy. Both chemotherapy and irradiation are used in defined situations such as a large mediastinal mass.

Non-Hodgkin's lymphomas (NHLs) are a heterogenous group of conditions for which there is a plethora of classifications based on cellular, immunological and molecular criteria. In essence the prognosis is better when the cellular infiltrate is comprised mainly of small rather than large cells, and shows evidence of organization into a follicular pattern rather than diffuse infiltration. 'Low grade' lymphomas are generally treated with intermittent oral chlorambucil plus prednisolone. These lymphomas often pursue an indolent course with a long median survival, but cannot be cured. Approximately 30–40% of patients with 'high grade' NHL can be cured with intravenous chemotherapy, typically with CHOP (cyclophosphamide, doxorubicin (= hydroxydaunorubicin), vincristine (= Oncovin), prednisolone).

Germer cell and trophoblastic tumours

Key point

Germ cell tumours are highly curable.

Teratomas limited to the testis can be cured in 80% of cases by orchidectomy. Combination chemotherapy is required in those that relapse, and in patients presenting with poor risk features. Most regimens are intensive, incorporating cisplatin, etoposide and bleomycin, and are often highly toxic to the gut, bone marrow, kidneys and lungs. Surgery may be required after chemotherapy to excise residual lymph node masses or pulmonary metastases. Modern combination chemotherapy can achieve cures in 80–90% of patients, although survival rates fall to ~50–60% in poor prognosis patients with liver, bone or brain metastases, extreme elevation of tumour markers α-fetoprotein, human chorionic gonadotrophin or lactate dehydrogenase, or primary mediastinal mass.

Seminomas are highly curable. Patients with stage 1 disease can be treated with prophylactic para-aortic irradiation or a single dose of carboplatin. Alternatively they can be managed by surveillance; many will be cured by surgery alone, and virtually all the 10–15% that relapse can be cured by chemotherapy or irradiation. Patients with stage 2–4 disease are treated with chemotherapy, and the majority are cured.

Choriocarcinoma is a rare tumour which usually follows a pregnancy resulting in a hydatidiform mole. Choriocarcinomas are extremely sensitive to chemotherapy, which can cure virtually 100% of patients with localized disease and over 70% with advanced disease. See Chapter 30 for more details on the clinical monitoring and treatment of patients with these tumours.

TALKING TO PATIENTS ABOUT CANCER

It does not need to be said that a diagnosis of cancer is a devastating and extremely frightening situation for any family. You should be aware that the way you talk to patients and their families can have a huge bearing on how they view the situation and try to come to terms with it. Clear, sympathetic and sensitive explanations can help to minimize the fear, anger and confusion that patients and their families experience. If people ask direct questions about their anticancer treatments and prospects of survival, it usually means that they are ready to hear straight answers. If you need to talk to patients about such issues and you are not sure how much they know or want to know, start by asking what they understand about the situation. This will let you know what they have been told (or what they remember – not always the same thing), and what terminology they are comfortable with (e.g. lump/tumour/cancer/adenocarcinoma). Then explain what the situation is as you see it, using and expanding on the terms they are already familiar with. Don't use words like 'lesion' or 'neoplasm' which are meaningless to a non-medic. Then go on to explain what can be done about the situation.

In patients embarking on complex treatments for early stage, potentially curable cancer, it is important to be encouraging and to explain the role of each component of therapy. If the prospects of long-term survival are poor, it is best not to be too brutally accurate. For example, the meta-analyses may suggest that a woman with high grade breast cancer and more than four positive nodes has only a 20–30% chance of survival. Knowing this would inevitably cause severe anxiety that may be hard to live with, and it may be reasonable in such a case to be vague about the long-term outlook.

When discussing the prognosis with patients who have advanced and incurable disease, it is generally better to be honest. There is never 'nothing that can be done', and it is important to explain sympathetically what support and treatments are available. For each treatment you should highlight the main advantages and disadvantages, but keep it simple and avoid giving too much information at once. Outline the chances of response, and the main side-effects, and be realistic about the overall benefit. You could say, for example: 'This treatment has a 40% chance of shrinking the tumour and helping you to feel better. But I am afraid it is not going to cure you, and the cancer will catch up with you in the end.' This will give the patient the opportunity to ask, if they wish, the $64 000 question 'How long have I got?' Explain that this is impossible to answer with accuracy. You could reply 'Months, perhaps many months or a few years' to a fit patient with metastatic cancer, but an ill patient may expect only a few weeks or months. If a patient is clearly terminally ill and could die within a few days or weeks, assess whether the patient can cope with this information, and gain his/her permission to tell the family. Many relatives feel a lasting sense of bitterness if they were unaware up to the last moment that death was imminent. Patients and their families usually give fairly clear verbal and non-verbal clues to indicate how much of this sort of information they can take at any one time. See Chapter 47 for a discussion of the principles of palliative care and the effective use of analgesia.

EVALUATION OF NEW ANTICANCER DRUGS

There is intensive laboratory-based effort to address the urgent need for more effective anticancer therapy. These may be derivatives of standard cytotoxic drugs, such as oxaliplatin and capecitabine, which are related to cisplatin and 5FU, respectively. Increasingly, research is generating new biological agents. Drugs that block key biological processes can be sought by large scale screening, such as that conducted at the National Cancer Institute in the USA using assays suitable for processing large numbers of compounds. Alternatively, the first step can be the identification of a biological target, which could be a process or a specific protein, and a drug is designed that is capable of inhibiting the function of that target. Potential treatment targets include not only the genes that regulate growth but also those that influence motility, invasion, cell–cell interaction, the formation of new blood vessels (angiogenesis), resistance to killing, and the ability to evade immune recognition (see Ch. 26). If a drug is shown to be effective in animal models of cancer, the next step is to assess its effect in clinical trials (Table 29.3).

Table 29.3   Organization of new drug trials

Phase I	Phase II	Phase III
Conducted in a range of tumour types. Assess: • Maximum tolerated dose • Toxicity • Pharmacology • Therapeutic effect	Assess: • Therapeutic effect in specific tumour types • Dose–response relationship	Controlled clinical trials: • Compare with existing standard therapy

New drug trials are conducted in distinct phases to assess toxicity and efficacy. It can take up to 10–15 years for a promising new agent to complete preclinical evaluation and the standard phase I, II and III clinical trials.

Summary

- Chemotherapy and radiotherapy should be used only in patients with confirmed histological diagnosis of malignancy.
- Adjuvant chemotherapy definitely increases the proportion of patients cured after surgery for cancers of the breast, colon and osteosarcoma, and may have a similar effect in cancers of the stomach, lung and cervix.
- Chemotherapy can cure patients with advanced teratoma, lymphoma, and some patients with SCLC and ovarian cancer.
- Chemotherapy and endocrine therapy are only palliative for most patients with metastatic disease.
- New biological therapies hold promise for the future.

References

Cole BF, Gelber RD, Gelber S, Coates AS, Goldhirsch A 2001 Polychemotherapy for early breast cancer: an overview of the randomised clinical trials with quality-adjusted survival analysis. Lancet 358: 277–286

Early Breast Cancer Trialists' Collaborative Group 1998a Tamoxifen for early breast cancer: an overview of the randomised trials. Lancet 351: 1451–1467

Early Breast Cancer Trialists' Collaborative Group 1998b Polychemotherapy for early breast cancer: an overview of the randomised trials. Lancet 352: 930–942

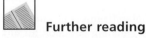

Further reading

Nature Reviews Cancer has regular reviews on new therapeutics, for example:

Greenwood E 2002 Therapeutics: stop signals. Nature Reviews Cancer 2: 640

Hurley LH 2002 DNA and its associated processes as targets for cancer therapy. Nature Reviews Cancer 2: 188–200

McCormick F 2001 Cancer gene therapy: fringe or cutting edge? Nature Reviews Cancer 1: 130–141

De Vita V, Hellman S, Rosenberg S (eds) 2001 Cancer: principles and practice of oncology, 6th edn. Lippincott Williams and Wilkins, Philadelphia. *Extremely comprehensive textbook with good references to primary sources.*

Souhami R, Tobias J (eds) 2002 Cancer and its management, 3rd edn. Blackwell Science, Oxford. *Medium length textbook, excellent general read.*

Therasse P, Arbuck SG, Eisenhauer EA et al 2000 New guidelines to evaluate the response to treatment in solid tumors. Journal of the National Cancer Institute 92(3):205–216

Useful links

www.cancerbacup.org.uk *This is an extremely useful resource to pass on to patients for information, practical advice and support.*

www.cancer.gov/cancer_information/pdq *The National Cancer Institute's 'Physicians Data Query' site, with pages for medical staff and patients. Very detailed information on management of all types of cancer including all relevant references, levels of proof, updated monthly.*

www.cancerresearchuk.org *Informative UK site for health care professionals and patients, includes general and tumour site specific information on incidence, diagnosis and treatment, downloadable leaflets, etc.*

30 Tumour markers

G. J. S. Rustin, A. E. Guppy

> **Objectives**
>
> - Appreciate the potential uses of circulating tumour markers.
> - Recognize which tumour markers are most commonly elevated in particular tumours.
> - Understand how tumour markers can be used to affect management of certain tumours.
> - Lead to more appropriate requesting of tumour marker measurements.

INTRODUCTION

Tumour markers are substances present in the body in a concentration that is related to the presence of a tumour. A tumour marker does not have to be tumour specific. It may be secreted or shed into blood and other body fluids or expressed at the cell surface in larger quantities by malignant cells than by non-malignant cells. Tumour markers can be detected either by measuring the concentration of the marker in body fluids (usually by immunoassay) or by detecting the presence of the marker on the cell surface in paraffin sections or fresh biopsies (by immunohistochemistry). This chapter examines critically those situations where estimation of circulating tumour marker levels may be of clinical value.

DEFINITIONS

The terms most commonly used to describe the usefulness of a tumour marker are defined in Table 30.1. Sensitivity is a measure of how commonly a tumour marker level is elevated in the presence of that particular tumour. Specificity measures the proportion of patients without tumour who have normal marker levels, and are therefore the true negatives. The positive predictive value is the percentage of positive results (i.e. elevated marker levels) which are true positives. An ideal tumour marker would have 100% sensitivity, thus detecting all cases of a particular tumour, and 100% specificity, being elevated only in the presence of that tumour and not in any other situation.

POTENTIAL USES OF TUMOUR MARKERS

The potential clinical uses of tumour marker estimation are:

- Screening
- Diagnosis
- Prognostic indicator
- Monitoring therapy
- Early diagnosis of relapse.

Examples of these uses will be given for the cancers where tumour markers are currently of greatest value. Although they will not be discussed in any further detail

Table 30.1 Terms used to describe tumour markers

	Tumour	
	Present	Absent
Assay positive	TP	FP
Assay negative	FN	TN
Sensitivity	$= \dfrac{TP}{TP + FN} \times 100$	
Specificity	$= \dfrac{TN}{FP + FN} \times 100$	
Positive predictive value	$= \dfrac{TP}{TP + FP} \times 100$	
Negative predictive value	$= \dfrac{TN}{FN + TN} \times 100$	

TP, true positive; FP, false positive; FN, false negative; TN, true negative.

in this chapter, the existence of cell surface tumour markers is being exploited to localize a tumour either for imaging purposes, using a radiolabelled antibody, or as a treatment modality, using antibodies to carry radioactivity or toxins selectively to the tumour.

REVIEW OF THE USE OF TUMOUR MARKER ESTIMATION IN THE MANAGEMENT OF PARTICULAR TUMOURS

Gestational trophoblastic tumours (GTT)

The role of human chorionic gonadotrophin (hCG) in the management of GTT comes closest to the ideal use of a tumour marker. hCG is a glycoprotein produced by trophoblast cells. The α-subunit is identical to that of follicle-stimulating hormone (FSH), luteinizing hormone (LH) and thyroid-stimulating hormone (TSH), but the C-terminal end of the β-subunit is unique to hCG and provides the basis of the specific immunoassay. There are many different assays for hCG available. It is essential to know whether the assay in use locally recognizes just the β-subunit or the intact complete hCG molecule, as they can give quite different results.

Diagnosis and screening

Elevated levels of hCG are found with as few as 10^5 trophoblast cells, but elevated serum hCG levels are also found in normal pregnancy, in ectopic pregnancy, in patients with germ cell tumours and, occasionally, in patients with non-germ-cell tumours. Pelvic ultrasound examination therefore remains the best method for diagnosing hydatidiform mole. The great sensitivity of hCG, however, allows it to be used to screen a high risk population. The first national screening programme for any cancer was set up in 1972 so that, following a diagnosis of hydatidiform mole, all patients are centrally registered. Patients are then followed using serial hCG measurements in blood or urine. This screening allows those patients with persistent trophoblastic disease after evacuation of hydatidiform mole to be detected on the basis of plateauing or rising tumour markers before any clinical evidence of disease develops (Bagshawe et al 1986).

Prognosis and monitoring response to treatment

Since hCG levels in patients with GTT reflect the total body burden of viable tumour, the level is a major factor in deciding whether a patient fits into a good or poor prognostic group. In patients with GTT, serial hCG estimation is used to monitor response to chemotherapy and to detect the development of drug resistance. The hCG value may initially increase after starting treatment, possibly due to tumour lysis or to increased syncytial differentiation induced by the therapy. The hCG level then falls at a rate which is a function of metabolic clearance and the rate of synthesis. Plateauing of hCG values or rising values during the course of chemotherapy indicate the development of drug resistance, and need to change chemotherapy.

Detection of recurrence

Serial measurement of hCG will detect any recurrence of GTT with 100% sensitivity. The accurate measurement of hCG in urine, which is stable in the post, increases the ease of monitoring and obviates the need for frequent hospital visits. A rise in hCG is not, however, diagnostic of recurrent disease, and a new pregnancy must always be considered and ruled out by ultrasound examination. Patients who have had a hydatidiform mole have a slightly increased risk of choriocarcinoma after any subsequent pregnancy and should have further hCG estimations at 4 and 12 weeks postpartum.

Germ cell tumours

α-Fetoprotein (AFP) and hCG are elevated, either singly or in combination, in more than 80% of patients with disseminated non-seminomatous germ cell tumours (NSGCT) and in approximately 60% of patients with localized, stage I disease (Bower & Rustin 1996). Other markers of use in patients with germ cell tumours include lactate dehydrogenase (LDH), but many laboratories only measure hydroxybutyrate dehydrogenase (HBD), which is mostly isoenzyme 1 and 2 of LDH. Placental alkaline phosphatase (PLAP), although elevated in about 50% of patients with seminomas and in smokers, adds little to clinical management, as it is rarely greatly elevated and usually falls to normal so quickly on therapy that it adds little to monitoring (Nielsen et al 1990).

Diagnosis and staging

All patients who are suspected of having a germ cell tumour should have serum sent for tumour marker estimation before excision of the primary tumour. Patients whose clinical status could be compromised by a biopsy (e.g. a patient with severe dyspnoea due to extensive lung metastases) should be considered to have an NSGCT if the distribution of the disease is compatible with such a tumour and there is gross elevation of either hCG or AFP. Elevated hCG is associated with the presence of trophoblastic elements in an NSGCT, and can be produced by syncytial giant cells in a pure seminoma. AFP, a glycoprotein with a molecular weight of 63–70 kDa, is secreted by the yolk sac element of an NSGCT, and a patient with an elevated AFP should never be considered to have a pure seminoma, regardless of the histological findings.

Failure of tumour marker levels to fall to normal postoperatively indicates the presence of occult metastatic disease, even if all other staging investigations are normal. One further situation in which hCG estimation may be of diagnostic value is in the detection of brain metastases. A pretreatment cerebrospinal fluid hCG level that is more than one-sixtieth the serum hCG level indicates the presence of brain metastases; the normal ratio, however, does not exclude brain metastases (Bagshawe & Harland 1976).

Prognosis and staging

Initial tumour marker levels are now recognized as the single best predictor of failure to achieve complete response following chemotherapy. An international collaborative group has recently proposed a prognostic classification (Table 30.2) based on an analysis of 5202 patients that found tumour marker levels and the presence or absence of mediastinal and non-pulmonary, non-nodal visceral metastases as the important risk factors (International Germ Cell Collaborative Group 1997).

Monitoring response to treatment

In patients with elevated hCG or AFP, these markers are the most sensitive method for assessing response to treatment. Although, in general, successful chemotherapy is invariably accompanied by a fall in serial hCG and AFP levels, there are two situations in which this may not occur. Firstly, an initial rise in tumour marker levels may occur soon after starting the first course of chemotherapy due to tumour lysis. The second situation is a plateau or even a rise in AFP levels, despite evidence of response

from all other investigations. This is thought to be due to AFP production by the liver in response to toxicity and appears to be more common in those patients receiving hepatotoxic drugs such as methotrexate and ifosfamide. The only situation where falling marker levels are not associated with a decreasing germ cell tumour mass is when there is enlargement of cystic differentiated teratoma. These masses require resection before they become inoperable.

Early detection of recurrence

All patients with germ cell tumours should continue to have serial tumour marker estimation after completion of chemotherapy to detect relapse early. The other situation in which serial marker estimation is invaluable is in surveillance of patients with stage I disease following orchidectomy. Close follow-up by clinical examination, tumour markers, chest X-rays and CT scans will detect relapse early in the 25–30% of those in whom the disease is destined to recur and, with adequate treatment, virtually all patients will be cured. In view of the potential for tumour markers to double rapidly, it is important that markers are measured at least monthly, and more frequently if raised.

Gastrointestinal tumours

There are a number of antibodies currently available which detect antigens expressed by gastrointestinal tumours. The most widely used are the antibodies which react with carcinoembryonic antigen (CEA), a 200 kDa glycoprotein. Assays dependent on monoclonal antibodies include CA 19.9, an antigen derived from a human colon adenocarcinoma cell line with an epitope (the portion of an antigen which combines with the antibody binding site) structurally identical to the sialylated Lewis A antigen, and CA 50, which is similar but not identical to CA 19.9. Elevated levels of several other markers such as CA 72-4 have also been found.

Table 30.2 Tumour markers in prognostic classification of germ cell tumours

	Marker		
	AFP (ng ml^{-1})	hCG* (ng ml^{-1})	LDH† ($\times N$)
Good	<1000	and <1000	and <1.5
Intermediate	1000–10 000	or 1000–10 000	or 1.5–10
Poor	>10 000	or >10 000	or >10

*For hCG, 1 ng ml^{-1} is approximately equal to 5 iu l^{-1}.
$^\dagger N$, upper limit of normal.

Diagnosis and screening

Serum CEA is elevated in fewer than 5% of patients with Dukes' grade A colorectal cancer, about 25% of Dukes' grade B, 44% of Dukes' grade C and about 65% of patients with distant metastases (Begent & Rustin 1989). CEA can be elevated not only in cancers of the gastrointestinal tract but also in a variety of other conditions, including: severe benign liver disease; inflammatory lesions, especially of the gastrointestinal tract; trauma; infection; collagen disease; renal impairment; and smoking. The low incidence of high serum CEA levels in early disease and its poor specificity explain its lack of value in screening normal populations for colorectal cancer. The low sensitivity precludes it being useful even for screening patients with ulcerative colitis or familial polyposis coli; although these patients are at high risk of developing colorectal cancer, both conditions may cause raised serum CEA in the absence of malignancy.

Prognosis and monitoring treatment

A raised preoperative CEA level has been shown to be associated with a poorer prognosis, but the value of preoperative CEA as an independent prognostic factor is unclear. Serum CEA levels should fall to normal within 4–6 weeks of complete resection of a colorectal carcinoma, the mean half-life being about 10 days. Levels usually rise with disease and fall with response to chemotherapy or radiotherapy. Failure of CEA to fall during radiotherapy usually indicates the presence of tumour outside the radiation field. Several studies have shown that survival is longer in patients who have a fall in serum CEA level during chemotherapy than in those in whom there is no change or an increased level (Allen-Mersh et al 1987). CA 19.9 is elevated in 75–90% of patients with pancreatic carcinomas and is increasingly used to monitor palliative chemotherapy.

Follow-up and detection of relapse

In approximately two-thirds of patients with recurrent colorectal cancer, a rise in serial serum CEA values predicts recurrence on average 11 months before it becomes clinically apparent (Begent & Rustin 1989). Surgical resection of isolated metastases of colorectal cancer has been advocated. Unfortunately, a randomized, multicentre trial under the auspices of the Cancer Research Campaign has failed to show any survival benefit from surgery after early detection of recurrence by rising CEA levels (Lennon et al 1994); however, further work is required to determine whether such patients would benefit from chemotherapy.

Ovarian cancer

The site and pattern of spread of ovarian cancer make it very difficult to detect and monitor using conventional clinical and radiological techniques, so a circulating tumour marker is potentially very valuable. CA 125 is the most commonly used tumour marker for ovarian cancer. CA 125 is found in derivatives of coelomic epithelium, including pleura, pericardium and peritoneum, but is not detected in normal ovarian tissue.

Diagnosis

CA 125 is elevated in over 95% of patients with advanced (stage III or IV) ovarian cancer, but in less than 50% of patients with stage I disease (Bast et al 1983). However, an elevated CA 125 is not diagnostic of ovarian cancer. Levels above 30 iu ml^{-1} are frequently seen during the first trimester of pregnancy, in patients with endometriosis or with cirrhosis, especially if ascites is present, and in 1% of healthy controls. In addition, over 40% of patients with advanced non-ovarian intra-abdominal malignancies have elevated CA 125 levels. None the less, in a patient suspected of having ovarian cancer, the presence of an elevated CA 125 should prompt you either to refer the patient to a gynaecological oncologist or to perform the surgery through a more extensive midline incision to allow adequate debulking of tumour.

Screening

Despite the low sensitivity of CA 125 for potentially curable stage I tumours, large screening studies have been performed. One study at the Royal London Hospital measured serum CA 125 in 22 000 postmenopausal well women. Those women who had CA 125 levels above 30 iu ml^{-1} underwent pelvic ultrasound, and if that was positive a laparotomy was performed. In all, there were 11 confirmed cases of epithelial ovarian cancer (true positives) and 11 cases in whom laparotomy did not reveal an ovarian tumour (false positives). Of note, however, is the fact that only 3 of the 11 patients with screen-detected ovarian cancers had stage I disease (Jacobs et al 1993). A large randomized trial is currently investigating whether serial CA 125 screening with ultrasound in patients with elevated or rising levels leads to improved survival. New research tools such as the use of proteomic (the protein profile) patterns in serum of patients with ovarian cancer which have both an increased specificity and sensitivity may have a future role in screening (Petricoin et al 2002). However until further work has been conducted, screening for ovarian cancer should not be offered to women outside a clinical trial unless there is a high risk of familial ovarian cancer.

Assessing completeness of excision

In order to decide optimum postoperative management, it is important to know whether one is dealing with a patient with completely excised stage I disease, or whether the patient has residual tumour after surgery. A persistently elevated CA 125 after oophorectomy for suspected stage I disease is definite evidence of residual tumour.

Prognosis and response to treatment

Very high CA 125 levels prior to surgery are associated with a worse prognosis, but knowledge of this is unlikely to lead to any alteration in management. The exception is in women with stage I disease where a preoperative level > 65 iu ml^{-1} has been shown to be a powerful adverse prognostic indicator (Nagele et al 1995). Such patients are candidates for chemotherapy rather than surveillance. Several groups have shown that the CA 125 level after one, two or three courses of chemotherapy, a long half-life or greater than seven-fold fall are the most important prognostic factors for survival. Prognostic information based on CA 125 should not be used to decide therapy, as in nearly 20% of cases where CA 125 predicts a poor prognosis the patient has no cancer progression in the next 12 months (Fayers et al 1993).

Definitions for response based on serial CA 125 estimations have been proposed (Rustin et al 1995) and appear more accurate than scans for monitoring therapy. For use in clinical trials they have to be very precise and use mathematical logic in a computer program. Put simply, response according to CA 125 has occurred if either of the following criteria are applicable:

- *Either* 50% response has occurred if there is a 50% decrease in serum CA 125 levels. There must be two initial elevated samples. The sample showing a 50% fall must be confirmed by a fourth sample (requires four CA 125 levels).
- *Or* 75% response has occurred if there has been a serial decrease in serum CA 125 levels of more than 75% over three samples (requires three CA 125 levels).

(In each the final sample has to be at least 28 days after the previous sample.) These definitions are particularly useful for clinical trials, where they indicate which new treatments are active more easily and cheaply than the use of standard response criteria.

Detection of progression or relapse

A serial rise of CA 125 of more than 25% appears the most accurate method of predicting progression of ovarian cancer during therapy and could lead to ineffective, toxic and expensive therapy being withheld. A confirmed doubling from the upper limit of normal during follow-up predicts relapse with almost 100% specificity. There is controversy about the role of serial CA 125 measurements during follow-up in asymptomatic patients, with the anxiety from knowing CA 125 levels often inducing CA 125 *psychosis*. Although the use of CA 125 estimation to define progression may reduce the number of radiological investigations performed, there is no evidence at present that early reintroduction of chemotherapy or searching for a resectable site of relapse produces any survival benefit. A large Medical Research Council (MRC) and European Organization for Research and Treatment of Cancer (EORTC) trial is currently witholding all serial CA 125 results from clinicians and patients during follow-up until the levels double. Patients are then randomized between immediate therapy or the clinician not being informed of the result so the patient continues on observation. Until the results of this trial are available, monitoring by CA 125 during follow-up should be discouraged.

Prostate cancer

Prostate-specific antigen (PSA) is the most useful tumour marker in patients with prostate cancer. PSA is a serine protease, produced by prostate epithelium, with the function of liquefying the gel which surrounds spermatazoa to enable them to become fully mobile. In serum, PSA is found either free or complexed to proteins. PSA estimation has superseded that of prostatic acid phosphatase as it is elevated in a higher proportion of men with prostate cancer.

Diagnosis, screening and staging

Elevated levels of PSA (>4 ng ml^{-1}) occur in about 53% of men with intracapsular microscopic prostatic cancer, and 77% of men with intracapsular macroscopic prostatic cancer, but can also occur in 30–50% of men with benign prostatic hypertrophy (BPH), a condition common in men of similar age group to those who develop prostate cancer (Dorr et al 1993). The combination of PSA and digital rectal examination, followed by prostatic ultrasound in patients with abnormal findings, is commonly used for screening in the USA but is not recommended in the UK as there is so far no evidence of survival benefit from early detection of prostate cancer. There is a vocal debate raging, with those who advocate screening stating that an individual with early prostate cancer may be cured by radical surgery or radiotherapy. Those against screening point out that, despite a 9% chance of developing clinical prostate cancer, there is only a 1% chance of dying from it and we cannot predict which cancers will be aggressive, so most patients will suffer the side-effects of therapy without any benefit. Furthermore, about 40% of those patients with PSA levels of 4.0–9.9 ng ml^{-1} at screening will already have tumour spread outside the prostate (Catalona et al 1991).

Several methods are being used to improve diagnostic specificity. The best appears to be the measurement of the ratio of free to total PSA, as more of the PSA is protein bound in patients with prostate cancer than in those with BPH. The ratio of free to total PSA is low (about 10%) in prostate cancer, compared with >16% in BPH and prostatitis. Using this ratio increases the specificity for diagnosing prostate cancer from 30% to 61% (Froschermaier et al 1996). PSA density and PSA density of the transition zone rely on ultrasound size estimations leading to lack of precision, but some centres have shown this measurement to improve specificity. Another method is based on the observation that PSA levels generally rise by more than 20% per annum in cases of malignancy. The PSA velocity calculated from serial levels can improve specificity but at the expense of delaying diagnosis.

PSA is less reliable than transurethral ultrasound in the detection of capsular invasion. A recently studied research tool is the use of the ultrasensitive reverse transcriptase polymerase chain reaction to detect PSA gene expression on circulating prostate cells. This technique might improve staging by detecting preoperatively those patients with extracapsular extension who do not benefit from radical surgery. Patients with PSA levels of <20 ng ml^{-1} can be assumed to have no bone metastases and do not necessarily need bone scans. However, not all patients with a PSA of >20 ng ml^{-1} will have distant metastases. Lymph node metastases are usually associated with elevated PSA.

Prognosis, monitoring response and detection of recurrence

As the PSA level correlates with prostatic volume and tumour differentiation, it is not surprising that a high pre-treatment PSA is associated with a poor prognosis. PSA levels fall rapidly to normal after complete removal of tumour by radical prostatectomy, although the rate of fall is slower after successful radiotherapy or endocrine therapy. A serial rise in PSA frequently precedes other evidence of disease progression in the patient with a past history of prostate cancer. The development of back pain in the presence of an elevated PSA level suggests the development of bone metastases.

Hepatocellular carcinoma

Serum AFP is elevated at presentation in 50–80% of UK patients with hepatocellular carcinoma (HCC). Although HCC is one of the most common malignant tumours in the world today, the relatively low incidence in the UK does not justify general population screening, although such screening may be justified in areas, such as China, with high incidence populations. In the UK, serial AFP estimation and ultrasound examination can be justified, however, for selective screening of high risk populations (i.e. patients with cirrhosis, chronic hepatitis B or haemochromatosis) because patients who have successful resection of a solitary, screen-detected tumour have a higher chance of long-term survival. Modest elevations of AFP occur in about 20% of patients with hepatitis, cirrhosis, biliary tract obstruction and alcoholic liver disease and in up to 10% of patients with hepatic metastases. Despite these caveats, a massively elevated AFP in a patient with known cirrhosis is virtually diagnostic of HCC.

Breast cancer

A variety of tumour markers have been studied in patients with breast cancer, including CEA and tissue polypeptide antigen (TPA) and several polymorphic epithelial mucin markers (HMFG1, HMFG2, MSA, MCA, CAM-26, CAM-29 and CA 15-3). The most widely investigated mucin marker in breast cancer is CA 15-3. The commercially available CA 15-3 kit utilizes a sandwich technique which employs two monoclonal antibodies: the 115D8 antibody as the capture antibody and the DF3 antibody as the tracer antibody.

Diagnosis and screening

Although elevated levels of CA 15-3 are found in 55–100% of patients with advanced breast cancer, serum CA 15-3 is raised in only 10–46% of patients with primary breast cancer and in about 10% of patients with early (T1/2N0M0) operable disease. As 2–20% of patients with benign breast disease have elevated levels, it is clear that mucin assays such as CA 15-3 are lacking in both specificity and sensitivity as a screening tool. No other tumour marker or combination of markers contribute to the diagnosis of breast cancer (Nicolini et al 1991).

Prognosis and monitoring response to treatment

Elevated preoperative levels of CA 15-3 have been shown to be associated with a poorer prognosis

(Kallioniemi et al 1988). However, this may well be due to the association between CA 15-3 and tumour burden, and there is no convincing evidence to date that measurement of CA 15-3, or any other tumour marker, provides significant independent prognostic information. Although tumour marker levels can fall with reduction in tumour burden following systemic therapy, the variation between patients makes tumour markers unreliable for assessing response.

Early detection of relapse

The observation that over 60% of patients who develop recurrent breast cancer have raised levels of CA 15-3 suggests a potential value in early detection of recurrence. The use of a panel of tumour markers might further increase the pick-up of recurrent disease. However, it is questionable whether such early detection of relapse will alter survival and thus whether the patient will benefit.

Other cancers

- Neuron-specific enolase is elevated in many patients with advanced small cell lung cancers and in children with neuroblastoma, where it is used for screening.
- Paraprotein levels are very important in the management of patients with myeloma, where β_2-microglobulin may be of prognostic value.
- Carcinoid tumours can be monitored by urine levels of 5-hydroxyindoleacetic acid (5HIAA), and polypeptides such as gastrin or glucagon are useful in the management of rare gastrointestinal tumours.
- Squamous cell carcinomas are associated with elevated levels of squamous cell carcinoma antigen (SCC) as well as cytokeratin fragments. SCC and CA 125 give valuable prognostic information in patients with cervical carcinoma, and may indicate relapse before scans.
- Calcitonin and calcitonin-gene-related peptide are used in the diagnosis and screening for medullary thyroid carcinoma.
- Serum S-100 and reverse transcriptase polymerase chain reaction to detect mRNA of tyrosinase on circulating melanoma cells are being studied for staging and following patients with melanoma.

There are many other markers not mentioned, either because they are not considered to be of clinical value or because information related to value is inadequate. Many cytokines, growth factors, oncogenes and oncogene products are being investigated as tumour markers, and some may well prove to be useful. Despite many claims, there are no markers that are of use as general cancer screens.

Summary

- Tumour markers may have a high sensitivity in patients with advanced cancer but most have a low sensitivity in patients with early stage cancer.
- When using a tumour marker to help in diagnosis it is essential to know its specificity.
- The potential uses of tumour markers are best demonstrated by hCG, where it is used for screening, diagnosis, determining prognosis, monitoring therapy and in follow-up of patients with gestational trophoblastic disease.
- The most commonly used tumour markers are PSA for prostate cancer, CA 125 for ovarian cancer, CEA for colorectal cancer, and hCG and AFP for germ cell tumours.
- Before requesting detection of a tumour marker, always consider whether the result would alter your management.

References

Allen-Mersh TG, Kemeny N, Niedzwiecki D et al 1987 Significance of a fall in serum CEA concentration in patients treated with cytotoxic chemotherapy for disseminated colorectal cancer. Gut 12: 1625–1629

Bagshawe KD, Harland S 1976 Immunodiagnosis and monitoring of gonadotrophin producing metastases in the central nervous system. Cancer 38: 112–118

Bagshawe KD, Dent J, Webb J 1986 Hydatidiform mole in England and Wales, 1973–1983. Lancet ii: 673–677

Bast RC, Klug TL, St John E et al 1983 A radioimmunoassay using a monoclonal antibody to monitor the course of epithelial ovarian cancer. New England Journal of Medicine 308: 883–887

Begent RJ, Rustin GJS 1989 Tumour markers: from carcinoembryonic antigen to products of hybridoma technology. Cancer Surveys 8: 107–121

Bower M, Rustin GJS 1996 Serum tumor markers and their role in monitoring germ cell cancers of the testis. In: Vogelzang NJ et al (eds) Comprehensive textbook of genitourinary oncology. Williams & Wilkins, Baltimore, pp 968–980

Catalona WJ, Smith DS, Ratliff T L et al 1991 Measurement of prostate specific antigen in serum as a screening test for prostate cancer. New England Journal of Medicine 324: 1156–1161

Dorr VJ, Williamson SK, Stephens RL 1993 An evaluation of prostate-specific antigen as a screening test for prostate cancer. Archives of Internal Medicine 153: 2529–2537

Fayers PM, Rustin GJS, Wood R et al 1993 The prognostic value of serum CA 125 in patients with advanced ovarian cancer: an analysis of 570 patients by the Medical Research Council Working Party on Gynaecological Cancer. International Journal of Gynaecological Cancer 3: 285–292

Froschermaier SE, Pilarsky CP, Wirth MP 1996 Clinical significance of the determination of noncomplexed prostate-specific antigen as a marker for prostate carcinoma. Urology 47: 525–528

International Germ Cell Collaborative Group 1997 International germ cell consensus classification: a prognostic factor-based staging system for metastatic germ cell cancers. Journal of Clinical Oncology 15: 594–603

Jacobs I, Prys Davies A, Bridges J et al 1993 Prevalence for screening for ovarian cancer in postmenopausal women by CA 125 measurement and ultrasonography. BMJ 306: 1030–1034

Kallioniemi OP, Oksa H, Aaran R et al 1988 Serum CA 15-3 assay in the diagnosis and follow up of breast cancer. British Journal of Cancer 58: 213–215

Lennon T, Houghton J, Northover J on behalf of the CRC/NIH CEA Trial Working Party 1994 Post-operative CEA monitoring and second-look surgery in colorectal cancer: trial results. British Journal of Cancer 70: 16

Nagele F, Petru E, Medl M et al 1995 Preoperative CA 125: an independent prognostic factor in patients with stage 1 epithelial ovarian cancer. Obstetrics and Gynecology 86: 259–264

Nicolini A, Colombini C, Luciani L et al 1991 Evaluation of serum CA 15-3 determination with CEA and TPA in the postoperative follow up of breast cancer patients. British Journal of Cancer 64: 154–158

Nielsen OS, Munro AJ, Duncan W et al 1990 Is placental alkaline phosphatase (PLAP) a useful marker for seminoma? European Journal of Cancer 26: 1049–1054

Petricoin EF, Ardekani AM, Hitt BA et al 2002 Use of proteomic patterns in serum to identify ovarian cancer. Lancet 359: 572–577

Rustin GJS, Nelstrop AE, McClean P et al 1995 Defining response of ovarian carcinoma to initial chemotherapy according to serum CA 125. Journal of Clinical Oncology 14: 1545–1551

POSTOPERATIVE

31 The body's response to surgery

J. P. S. Cochrane, C. G. Hargreaves

Objectives

- Understand the multisystem nature of the impact of surgery on the body.
- Recognize the clinical features resulting from the body's response.
- Appreciate that these responses can be modified, resulting in improved clinical outcomes.

INTRODUCTION

The body responds to trauma with local and systemic reactions that attempt to contain and heal the tissue damage, and to protect the body while it is injured. The response is remarkably similar whether the trauma is a fracture, burn, sepsis or a planned surgical operation, and the extent of the response is usually proportional to the severity of the trauma.

The response, with neuroendocrine and inflammatory cytokine components, increases the metabolic rate, mobilizes carbohydrate, protein and fat stores, conserves salt and water and diverts blood preferentially to vital organs. It also stimulates important protective mechanisms such as the immunological and blood clotting systems. However, the overall result is one of immunosuppression leading to increased vulnerability to infection.

The interplay between the many inflammatory mediators and cellular responses is very complex and events at a molecular level are only slowly being unravelled. New signalling systems and feedback mechanisms continue to be discovered. These will provide opportunities for future therapies aimed at blocking the unwanted aspects of what can be an exaggerated, detrimental systemic inflammatory response.

Remember also that major surgery has other inevitable consequences (such as hypothermia and immobility) which predispose to postoperative morbidity. With optimal perioperative management, however, their impact can be minimized. Another common sequel, anaemia, appears to be well tolerated and physiologically less significant for most patients than previously assumed.

Key point

- Surgical operation is a controlled form of trauma in which many aggravating factors can be manipulated.

INITIATION OF THE RESPONSE

Various noxious stimuli produce the response but they rarely occur alone, and multiple stimuli often produce greater effects than the sum of single responses. The response is modified by the severity of the stimulus, the patient's age, nutritional status, coexisting medical conditions, medication and if the trauma or operation has affected the function of any particular organ. Recent trauma or sepsis will also modify the response to a subsequent surgical operation.

Pain. Stimuli from the skin, the musculoskeletal system, the visceral stretch receptors and, especially, pulling on the mesentery stimulate the sympathetic nervous system, adrenocorticotrophic hormone (ACTH) and arginine vasopressin (AVP).

Tissue injury. Tissue disruption causes local cytokine release with capillary endothelial damage and leak. This in turn leads to the migration of inflammatory cells, amplifying the release of mediators, which can develop into a systemic inflammatory response. Another mechanism of tissue injury is ischaemia followed by reperfusion, leading to production of oxygen free radicals (reactive oxygen species, ROS).

Infection. This is often the underlying reason for presentation in surgical patients, especially emergencies, and so the effects of sepsis are often present. Endotoxin from the cell walls of Gram-negative bacteria is the most powerful stimulus for release of one of the cytokines, tumour necrosis factor (TNF), from macrophages. Infection can also enter the circulation from the bowel if the mucosal barrier is impaired.

Hypovolaemia. Most injuries lead to hypovolaemia, either from haemorrhage, plasma loss in burns or third-space losses. This stimulates baroreceptors, releasing vasopressin (AVP), catecholamines, renin–angiotensin and aldosterone, and leads to impaired excretion of sodium and water, manifesting clinically as oliguria. Hypoperfusion, especially in the presence of hypotension, can also initiate endothelial damage and progress to organ dysfunction. Recent evidence suggests that maintaining optimal circulating volume throughout the perioperative period can avoid these consequences and reduce mortality after major surgery.

Starvation. If starvation accompanies trauma it causes the body to use muscle protein as a source of energy, leading to muscle wasting and weakness, which slows recovery. Failure to provide nutritional support can also impair the immune response, resulting in poorer healing and more postoperative infections, especially in those malnourished prior to surgery.

Hypoxia, hypercarbia or pH changes. Chemoreceptors in the carotid and aortic bodies react to these changes and stimulate the sympathetic nervous systems, ACTH and AVP.

Energy substrates. Hypoglycaemia stimulates ACTH, growth hormone, β-endorphin, AVP and catecholamines. This catabolic state also favours muscle breakdown. Certain amino acids also have particular effects.

Fear, anxiety and emotion. These stimulate the sympathetic nervous system, AVP and ACTH.

Temperature. Hypothermia, which is difficult to avoid in lengthy major surgery, stimulates the hypothalamus and leads to increased secretion of AVP, ACTH, growth hormone, thyroxine and catecholamines. Studies have shown improved recovery times with fewer infections when normothermia is maintained intraoperatively.

SYSTEMS CONTROLLING THE RESPONSE

The response to surgery is modulated both by the neuroendocrine system and the inflammatory mediators, and the cells controlling their release. The effects are closely intertwined, with locally produced cytokines having systemic effects proportional to the extent and severity of tissue injury. There are multiple feedback loops which prevent excessive activation of the inflammatory cascades.

Sympathetic nervous system. The immediate fight and flight reaction may help the injured person avoid further injury, but it has short-lasting effects on metabolism. Activation of the sympathetic pathways also stimulates the adrenal glands.

Endocrine response. This includes not only the hypothalamic–pituitary–adrenal (HPA) axis but also growth hormone, AVP, thyroxine, insulin and glucagon, causing some metabolic effects, particularly changes in carbohydrate and fat metabolism. This response appears to protect not so much against the stress but more against the body's acute phase response from overreacting.

Acute phase response. The wound becomes a 'cytokine organ' whose metabolism and local healing responses are controlled by cytokines and other mediators that are produced locally and also released from activated inflammatory cells, including neutrophils and monocytes. In severe trauma, proinflammatory cytokines produce a systemic 'acute phase' response, with profound changes in protein metabolism, and immunological activation; these effects are mostly beneficial but in severe trauma can be lethal.

Vascular endothelial cell response. This affects vasomotor tone and vessel permeability, so it affects perfusion, circulating volume and blood pressure and can lead to the clinical picture of shock and lung injury. There are close interactions between the endothelium, acute phase mediators and leucocytes (neutrophils and monocytes). Endothelial damage also activates the coagulation cascades and can result in microvascular clotting despite a generalized abnormal bleeding tendency.

Sympathetic nervous system

The central and peripheral sympathetic systems are stimulated particularly by pain and hypovolaemia and this has direct actions and indirect effects, by releasing adrenaline (epinephrine) from the adrenal medulla and noradrenaline (norepinephrine) predominately from peripheral ganglia. These catecholamines have both α and β effects on sympathetic receptors that prepare the body rapidly for fight or flight by cardiovascular, visceral and metabolic actions. These effects begin when the operation starts and continue for several days into the postoperative period for all but minor procedures.

Cardiovascular effects

Blood is redistributed from the viscera and skin (α effects) to the heart, brain and skeletal muscles ($β_2$ effects), and there is an increase in heart rate and contractility ($β_1$ effects).

Visceral effects

Non-essential visceral functions such as intestinal motility are inhibited, resulting in paralytic ileus, and bladder sphincter tone is increased; other actions are: bronchodilatation (β_2); mydriasis – dilatation of the pupil (α_1); uterine contraction (α_1); and relaxation (β_2); visual field increases.

Metabolic and hormonal effects

Blood glucose rises due to increased breakdown of liver and muscle glycogen and by gluconeogenesis (α_1), and indirectly by suppression of insulin secretion (α_2) and stimulation of glucagon secretion (β). Other hormonal actions are stimulation of growth hormone (α) and renin (β_1). Lipolysis is stimulated in adipose cells, and ketogenesis is stimulated in the liver.

Endocrine response

The HPA axis is stimulated mainly by the injury itself, but probably its most important function is to control the effects of systemically released cytokines.

ACTH. This is released from the anterior pituitary by neurological stimuli reaching the hypothalamus, or by hormones such as AVP, angiotensin II or catecholamines. The ACTH response to stress is not inhibited by administered steroids. ACTH stimulates the adrenal cortex to release glucocorticoids and also potentiates the action of catecholamines on cardiac contractility.

Glucocorticoids. These usually have only a 'permissive' action (allowing other hormones to function) but the increased levels after trauma have important metabolic, cardiovascular and immunological actions proportional to the severity of the trauma. *Cortisol* is the main glucocorticoid and its serum level usually returns to normal 24 h after uncomplicated major surgery but may remain elevated for many days in extensive burns or if infection supervenes. It stimulates the conversion of protein to glucose (catabolic action); it stimulates the storage of glucose as glycogen; it is an antagonist of insulin and this assists gluconeogenesis to increase plasma glucose (diabetogenic action); it helps to maintain blood volume by decreasing the permeability of the vascular endothelium and enhancing vasoconstriction by catecholamines and suppressing synthesis of prostaglandins and leucotrienes (anti-inflammatory action); it also inhibits secretion of interleukin 1 (IL-1) and IL-2 antibody production and mobilization of lymphocytes (immunosuppressant action).

The normal glucocorticoid response can be reduced or absent (due to previous long-term administration of steroids, adrenalectomy or adrenal infarction). This presents with hypoglycaemia, hyponatraemia and refractory hypotension.

Key point

- **Adrenal failure is often fatal if you fail to recognize it at an early stage; it requires immediate steroid replacement.**

Aldosterone. The inevitable release of ACTH after trauma stimulates a short-term release of aldosterone from the adrenal cortex, but the rise may be prolonged if other stimuli such as hypovolaemia or vasomotor changes (which activate the renin–angiotensin system in the kidney) occur. A rise in plasma potassium concentration can also stimulate aldosterone release. Aldosterone causes increased reabsorption of sodium and potassium secretion in the distal convoluted tubules and collecting ducts, and hence a reduced urine volume.

Arginine vasopressin (AVP). Also referred to as antidiuretic hormone (ADH), this is released from the posterior pituitary by pain, a rise in plasma osmolality (via osmoreceptors in the hypothalamus), hypovolaemia (via baroreceptors and left atrial stretch receptors), anaesthetic agents or a rise in plasma glucose. Its actions on the distal tubules and collecting ducts in the kidney lead to increased reabsorption of solute-free water; it causes peripheral vasoconstriction, especially in the splanchnic bed, and it stimulates hepatic glycogenolysis and gluconeogenesis. Its secretion increases for about 24 h after operation, and during this time the kidney cannot excrete 'free' water (water that is not solute led), so the urine osmolality remains higher than plasma. After head injury, burns or prolonged hypoxia there may be continued secretion of AVP, resulting in oliguria and hyponatraemia.

Insulin. In the ebb phase after injury, plasma insulin concentration falls because catecholamines and cortisol make the β-islet cells of the pancreas less sensitive to glucose. Glucagon also inhibits insulin release and cortisol reduces the peripheral action of insulin; less carbohydrate is transported into cells and blood sugar rises. In the flow phase, plasma insulin rises but blood sugar remains elevated because various intracellular changes make the tissues resistant to insulin.

Glucagon. Secretion of glucagon from the α-islet cells of the pancreas increases after injury and this plays a small part in increasing blood sugar by stimulating hepatic glycogenolysis (Greek *lyein* = to loosen; hydrolysis of glycogen), and gluconeogenesis (Greek *glykos* = sweet + *neos* = new + *genesis* = origin; the formation of glucose from non-carbohydrate substances). It also stimulates hepatic ketogenesis and lipolysis in adipose tissue. Cortisol prolongs its actions.

Thyroxine. Total T_4 (but not usually free T_4) and total and free T_3 (tri-iodothyronine, the more active hormone) decrease after injury, because cortisol impairs conversion of T_4 to T_3.

Growth hormone. Growth hormone is released from the anterior pituitary as a result of neurological stimulation of the hypothalamus or by a rise in circulating levels of catecholamines, ACTH, AVP, thyroxine or glucagon. Its plasma levels increase after trauma, hypovolaemia, hypoglycaemia or a decrease in plasma fatty acids or increase in serum arginine. Its main effects are to promote protein synthesis and enhance breakdown of lipid and carbohydrate stores. It increases plasma fatty acids and ketone bodies through direct stimulation of lipolysis and potentiation of catecholamine effects on adipose tissue and by stimulation of hepatic ketogenesis. It is also associated with a fall in insulin levels that allows plasma glucose to rise.

Acute-phase response

Local effects

Noxious stimuli such as infection, trauma, toxins, haemorrhage or malignancy attract granulocytes and mononuclear cells to the site of injury, and these cells, together with local fibroblasts and endothelial cells, release cytokines. *Cytokines* (Greek *kytos* = hollow, cell + *kineein* = to move) are peptides produced by a variety of cells (unlike true hormones) and produce mainly paracrine (direct cell-to-cell) effects. Interleukins (IL) 1, 2 and 6, TNF and the interferons are the main cytokines released early. Their actions help to contain tissue damage by contributing to the inflammatory reaction through vasodilatation, increased permeability of vessels, migration of neutrophils and monocytes to the wound, activation of the coagulation and complement cascades, and proliferation of endothelial cells and fibroblasts.

Systemic effects

If cytokine production is large enough, systemic (Greek *syn* = together + *histanai* = to set; affecting the body as a whole) effects occur, such as fever, malaise, headache, myalgia (Greek *mys* = muscle + *algos* = pain) as well as vasodilatation. They may also produce a leucocytosis, activation of immune function, release of ACTH and glucocorticoids, activation of clotting cascades, an increase in erythrocyte sedimentation rate (ESR), a decrease in circulating levels of zinc and iron (inhibiting the growth of microorganisms requiring iron). They also affect the serum levels of *acute phase reactants* (APRs) which are

host-defence proteins synthesized in the liver; most increase (such as C-reactive protein, fibrinogen, complement C3, α-antichymotrypsin, caeruloplasmin and haptoglobin), but the levels of albumin and transferrin decrease.

- *IL-6* is the main mediator of this altered hepatic protein synthesis.
- *TNF – tumour necrosis factor* (cachectin) released primarily from macrophages by bacterial endotoxin, causes anorexia, tachypnoea, fever and tachycardia, with proliferation of fibroblasts and widespread effects on neutrophils; it stimulates production of other cytokines, ACTH, APRs and amino acids from skeletal muscle, hepatic amino acid uptake, and elevation of plasma triglycerides and free fatty acids. High concentrations cause multiple organ dysfunction syndrome (MODS).
- *IL-2* enhances immune function by T-lymphocyte proliferation and by enhancing the activity of natural killer cells.
- *IL-1* in low dosage causes fever, neutrophilia, low serum zinc levels, increased APR synthesis, anorexia, malaise, release of ACTH, glucocorticoid and insulin, and, in high dose, the features of MODS.
- *Interferons*, such as γ-interferon are glycoproteins produced by T lymphocytes which activate macrophages, enhancing both antigen presenting and processing as well as cytocidal activity; γ-interferon is synergistic with TNF, inhibits viral replication, and inhibits prostaglandin release.
- *Prostaglandins* are important components of the inflammatory response. They can be produced by all nucleated cells except lymphocytes; they increase vascular permeability and cause vasodilatation and leucocyte migration.
- *Leucotrienes* are 1000 times as effective as histamine at increasing postcapillary leakage and they cause increased leucocyte adhesion, vasoconstriction and bronchoconstriction.
- *Kallikreins and kinins.* Bradykinin release is stimulated by hypoxia and it is a potent vasodilator that increases capillary permeability, producing oedema, pain and bronchoconstriction and affecting glucose metabolism.
- *Heat shock proteins* (HSPs). These are produced by virtually all cells in response to many stresses (not just heat), mainly via the stimulus of the HPA axis, and they are also elevated in certain tissues in chronic diseases. The ability to produce them declines with age and they appear to protect cells from the deleterious effects of stress and to inhibit synthesis of APRs.
- *5-Hydroxytryptamine* (5HT). This is a neurotransmitter produced from tryptophan and found in enterochromaffin cells of the intestine and platelets. It is released

when tissue is injured and it causes vasoconstriction and bronchoconstriction, increases platelet aggregation and increases heart rate and contractility.

- *Histamine.* Histamine is released from mast cells, platelets, neurons, and the epidermis by trauma, sepsis and hypotension. Its main action is to cause local vasodilatation and increased vascular permeability, so large concentrations may lead to hypotension. It acts on H_1 cell surface receptors to increase histamine precursor uptake and cause bronchoconstriction, and increased intestinal motility and cardiac contractility; it also acts on H_2 receptors that inhibit histamine release and produce changes in gastric secretion, heart rate and immunological function.
- *Endogenous opioids.* Endogenous opioids such as β-endorphin increase after trauma and produce analgesia, a rise in blood sugar, a lowering of blood pressure and effects on immune function.

Interactions between APRs and the endocrine response

IL-1 and IL-6 can activate the HPA axis by increasing ACTH secretion and also directly stimulating glucocorticoid release from the adrenal gland. Glucocorticoids initially help cytokines to regulate APRs, but if glucocorticoid levels remain elevated they inhibit cytokine production.

The vascular endothelial response

The scattered 'endothelial organ' weighs about 1.5 kg. After tissue injury it is activated locally, resulting in the appearance of glycoprotein selectins (adhesion molecules) on the endothelial cell surface along with intercellular adhesion molecules (ICAMs). Neutrophils recognize these surface molecules, begin to stick and then migrate out into the interstitium, with a concurrent increase in endothelial permeability, particularly in the postcapillary venules.

Nitric oxide is a powerful vasodilator produced mainly by endothelial cells but also by macrophages, neutrophils, Kupffer cells and renal cells. It is inactivated by haemoglobin and opposed by endothelins. Its other action is to increase production of APRs.

Endothelins are a family of potent vasoconstricting peptides with mainly paracrine actions. They are released by thrombin, catecholamines, hypoxia, cytokines and endotoxins. They counteract nitric oxide and prostacyclins to maintain vasomotor tone.

Platelet-activating factor (PAF) is released from endothelial cells by the action of TNF, IL-1, arginine vasopressin (AVP or antidiuretic hormone) and angiotensin II. When platelets come into contact with PAF they release

thromboxane which causes platelet aggregation and vasoconstriction. PAF also reduces the permeability of endothelial cells to albumin and may also affect glucose metabolism.

Prostaglandins cause vasodilatation and reduce platelet aggregation. Other arachidonic acid derivatives include thromboxanes, which are also produced by cyclooxygenase. An inducible form of this enzyme (COX-2) is activated.

Atrial natriuretic peptides (ANPs) are potent inhibitors of aldosterone secretion and are released by atrial tissue (which is specialized endothelium) in response to changes in chamber distension. They can also be released by the CNS. It is not yet clear what role they play in the response to injury.

Intracellular signalling processes and regulation of the acute stress response

- *Gene transcription:* stimulation of cells by cytokines and other products of inflammatory damage, such as oxygen free radicals, appears to be coupled to signalling systems that lead to upregulation of the genes coding for enzymes and cytokines by increasing RNA transcription. These inducible enzymes then greatly increase the production of mediators, sustaining the inflammatory response. Families of transcription factor proteins known as inhibitor of kappa B kinase/nuclear factor kappa B (IKK/NF kappa B) seem to be one of the central components. They appear to control inducible nitric oxide synthetase (iNOS) and COX-2, as well as transcription of the IL-6 and TNFα genes.
- *Apoptosis* (Greek *apo* = from + *piptein* = to fall) is the programmed death of cells which ensures turnover of short-lived immune cells. It increases after trauma and also in sepsis, contributing to immunosuppression by loss of lymphocytes. Apoptosis also appears to be under the control of complex intracellular signalling processes.

CLINICALLY APPARENT SYSTEMIC EFFECTS OF THE RESPONSE

Body temperature

Following correction of any intraoperative hypothermia in the immediate postoperative period, there is often a 1–2°C increase in body temperature because the increased metabolic rate is accompanied by an upward shift in the thermoregulatory set point of the hypothalamus. Pyrexia can be difficult to interpret when infection is suspected or already present. Some of the effects of fever are detrimental, but more are beneficial.

Cardiovascular system

A mild tachycardia is commonly seen, along with peripheral vasodilatation. Cardiac output can rise at least threefold provided intravascular volume is maintained. Hypovolaemia due to blood and other fluid losses can exaggerate the tachycardia and lead to hypotension and peripheral shutdown, indicating inadequate fluid replacement. The acute phase response of vasomotor changes and increased vessel permeability causes fluid loss into the 'third space', the name for a sequestered part of the extracellular fluid (ECF) which includes oedema fluid in the peripheral tissues, wound, peritoneal cavity or the lungs.

Pulmonary effects

Reduction in forced vital capacity and functional residual capacity lead to shunting of blood and a decreasing PaO_2 after major surgery. Hypoxaemia is more pronounced and prolonged after upper abdominal surgery. The changes are significantly lessened by laparoscopic compared with open operation and by good quality pain relief. If secretions obstruct bronchioles, basal collapse can progress to pneumonia after any operation, particularly in immobile patients recumbent in bed. Tachypnoea leads to a respiratory alkalosis and a fall in $PaCO_2$.

Acute lung injury is the inflammatory reaction due to pulmonary capillary endothelial damage and fluid leak into the alveoli and interstitium. This 'non-cardiogenic pulmonary oedema' leads to hypoxaemia due to ventilation–perfusion inequalities (i.e. shunt). This can be a component of systemic inflammation or directly triggered by specific factors, e.g. blood transfusion. There is a spectrum of severity, with the most extensive, acute respiratory distress syndrome (ARDS), leading to severe respiratory failure and widespread infiltrates on X-ray. The changes improve with resolution of the underlying inflammation but overall survival in ARDS is at best 60–70%.

Effects on the gastrointestinal tract

- Adynamic ileus. There is inhibition of gastric emptying and reduced colonic motility from increased sympathetic tone and the effects of opioid analgesics. Small intestine peristalsis is minimally affected. Usually, adynamic (Greek *a* = not + *dyasthai* = to be able) ileus is transient and enteral intake can restart early in the postoperative period.
- Gut mucosal barrier. Increased permeability is thought to allow translocation of bacterial toxins into the circulation, leading to escalation of the inflammatory response. It is still unclear whether this is a primary cause or secondary response.

Biochemical and fluid balance disturbance

1. *Salt and water retention*. This results from the mineralocorticoid effects of both aldosterone and cortisol. This is compounded by raised levels of AVP, further hindering excretion of free water and resulting in lower volumes of high osmolality urine. Any reduction in renal perfusion from hypotension secondary to hypovolaemia or from the administration of non-steroidal anti-inflammatory drugs also worsens oliguria and can lead to acute renal failure. Although the maintenance of intravascular volume by administered intravenous fluids offsets these effects, weight gain of several kilograms from retained fluid can be seen. A major but uncomplicated surgical operation with adequate fluid replacement is, therefore, usually followed by 24 h of impaired free water clearance and about 5 days of impaired sodium excretion. This can be more pronounced in the presence of systemic inflammation where 'third space' losses are greater (see Cardiovascular system above). The diuresis that occurs when this third space fluid mobilizes is a welcome sign of recovery.

2. *Hyponatraemia*. This often accompanies the above changes, partly a dilutional effect from retained water (due to AVP), and partly because sodium drifts into cells (impaired sodium pump); it does not indicate sodium deficiency, as it occurs at a time when the total body sodium is elevated. Serum potassium may rise due to cell death, liberation of potassium by protein catabolism and from impaired potassium excretion. However, it is more usual to see increased urine potassium excretion, which can lead to an overall potassium deficit.

3. *Acid–base abnormalities*. The commonest change is a metabolic alkalosis because intense reabsorption of sodium in the distal tubules of the kidney is accompanied by excretion of potassium and hydrogen ions; this impairs oxygen delivery to the tissues because it affects the oxygen–haemoglobin dissociation curve. In more severe injuries a metabolic acidosis supervenes due to poor tissue perfusion and anaerobic metabolism with accumulation of lactic acid. Acidosis may decrease myocardial contractility and produce arrhythmias, as well as decreasing the effect of catecholamines on the myocardium and peripheral vessels. Respiratory compensation with tachypnoea and reduced $PaCO_2$ then occurs.

Metabolism after injury

1. There is an initial 'ebb' phase (Fig. 31.1) of reduced energy expenditure after injury for up to 24 h. This changes to a catabolic 'flow' phase with increased metabolism, negative nitrogen balance, hyperglycaemia, increased heat production, increased oxygen consumption and lean bodyweight loss. The increase in metabolic rate ranges from about 10% in elective surgical operations

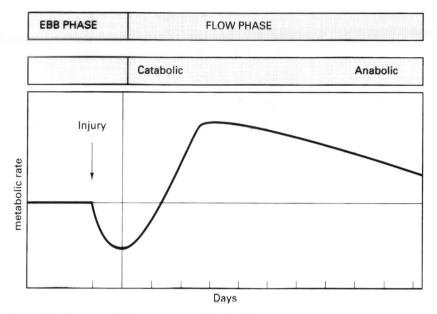

Fig. 31.1   Change in metabolic rate relative to preoperative level.

to 50% in multiple trauma and 200% in major burns. This may last for days or weeks, depending on the severity of the injury, previous health of the individual and medical intervention; it is less marked at the extremes of age or in previously malnourished individuals. Once started, it cannot be stopped rapidly by controlling infection, correcting hypovolaemia or blocking pain. If recovery occurs, it is followed by an anabolic phase in which weight gain is accompanied by restoration of protein and fat stores. This process is slow and prolonged.

2. Lipids are the principal source of energy following trauma. Lipolysis is produced mainly by catecholamines and increased sympathetic nervous system activity, and also by lower plasma insulin, a rise in ACTH, cortisol, glucagon, growth hormone and, probably, cytokines. Ketones are released into the circulation and are oxidized by all tissue except the blood cells and the CNS. Free fatty acids provide energy for all tissues and for hepatic gluconeogenesis.

3. Carbohydrates. Hyperglycaemia occurs immediately after injury because glucose is mobilized from stored glycogen in the liver by catecholamines and glucocorticoids, and because insulin resistance of peripheral tissues impairs their uptake of glucose (the 'diabetes of injury'). Glucose provides energy for obligate tissue such as the CNS, leucocytes in the wound and red cells (cells not requiring insulin for glucose transport). In major injuries the inflammatory cell infiltrate can account for 70% of glucose uptake.

4. Body glycogen stores can only maintain blood glucose for about 24 h. Subsequently it is maintained by gluconeogenesis, stimulated by corticosteroids and glucagon, and this is helped by the initially suppressed insulin levels encouraging the release of amino acids from muscle. Even when insulin levels rise, they do not suppress this increased hepatic gluconeogenesis because it is required for clearance of lactate and amino acids that are not used for protein synthesis.

5. Amino acids, protein and skeletal muscle. Shortly after injury, skeletal muscle protein breakdown supplies the three- to fourfold increased demand for amino acids (unless there is an exogenous protein source); this reaches a peak after 1 week and may continue for several weeks. The nitrogen loss is proportional to the severity of the trauma, the extent of sepsis and the muscle bulk (so it is greatest in fit young males). The mobilized amino acids are used for gluconeogenesis, oxidation in the liver and other tissues, and synthesis of APRs. Glutamine is a major energy source for the gastrointestinal tract, for lymphocytes and for fibroblasts during catabolism, and may become an 'essential' amino acid at this time. The negative nitrogen balance and skeletal muscle breakdown can be offset but not reversed by nutritional support. The catabolic phase is followed by an anabolic phase produced by growth hormone, androgens and 17-ketosteroids.

6. Other reasons for skeletal muscle loss include rhabdomyolysis in trauma and limb ischaemia, disuse

atrophy from prolonged immobility and denervation from the polyneuropathy of critical illness. These factors can all produce weakness which requires prolonged rehabilitation.

Haematological changes

Serum albumin falls after trauma because production by the liver decreases, and loss into damaged tissue increases due to the action of cytokines and prostaglandins on vessel permeability. The accompanying shift of fluid out of the intravascular compartment is a contributing cause of dysfunction in various organs.

The coagulation cascade and platelet activation leads to a state of hypercoagulability that may be beneficial at the site of injury but increases the risk of venous thrombi forming. If coagulation is triggered away from the wound, for example by sepsis or hypoxic damage to endothelial cells, then disseminated intravascular coagulation can result.

Leucocytosis occurs; it appears to be due mainly to cytokine-stimulated release of neutrophils from bone marrow.

Immunological responses

Trauma leads to impairment of the immune system, with defects in cell-mediated immunity, antigen presentation, neutrophil and macrophage function, complement activation and bacterial opsonization. This occurs at a time when the initial injury has usually breached mechanical defences, when catabolism impairs the mucosal barrier in the bowel and when many factors contribute to produce pneumonia and other infections.

Wound healing

The systemic responses give 'biological priority' to wound healing, but a wound still heals more slowly if there are other major injuries.

Systemic inflammatory response syndrome (SIRS)

This is defined by set criteria of fever, tachycardia, tachypnoea and leucocytosis. This cluster of clinical features is seen in a range of conditions where inflammation is present. These include those where infection is the cause, e.g. appendicitis, as well as those which can mimic sepsis but where infection is absent, e.g. pancreatitis or blunt trauma. SIRS features are often present in the postoperative surgical patient and reflect the extent of activation of the inflammatory cascades.

Multiple organ dysfunction syndrome

In some patients the inflammatory response may become so amplified that shock supervenes and support of failing organs is required. There may then be an irreversible progression to multiple organ failure and death. In this situation, inflammatory damage appears to be excessive and uncontrolled and not amenable to treatment. The clinical picture is the same as that in septic shock, even though infection is absent.

There is some evidence that an initial inflammatory stimulus, such as infection, trauma or surgery, 'primes' the cellular control of inflammation and that a second stimulus, e.g. sepsis, triggers an overwhelming response (two-hit theory). This may be linked to intracellular processes such as apoptosis.

WAYS OF AFFECTING THE RESPONSE

Although the local response to trauma is beneficial, the systemic response becomes less helpful as the degree of trauma increases, and in a hospital setting it is an advantage to suppress and control the response. In trauma and emergency surgery, pain, bleeding with hypovolaemia, hypoxia and anxiety have often been present for some hours before operation starts, whereas in elective surgery it is usually possible to control these stimuli and thereby reduce the systemic response.

Recent studies demonstrate that preoperative optimization of the circulation by the use of fluid loading and inotropes to increase cardiac output and oxygen delivery can improve the outcome of major surgery.

Beta blockers given through the perioperative period confer cardiac protection in vulnerable patients. There appears to be a prolonged survival advantage well beyond the duration of administration.

Reduce stimuli causing the response

- **Less trauma**
  - **care in handling tissues**
  - **minimally invasive surgery.**
- **Control of infection**
  - **remove source of toxins**
  - **debride wounds and drain pus**
  - **antibiotics (selective gut decontamination with antibiotic combinations is still being investigated).**
- **Nutritional support**
  - **enteral feeding to maintain the gut mucosal barrier integrity**

- 'immunonutrition' with added glutamine, arginine and omega-3 fatty acids may be of some additional benefit when delivered early.
- Control of pain
  - analgesics, local and regional blockade (given, if feasible, before the noxious stimuli occur).
- Correct hypovolaemia
  - prompt replacement of fluids and electrolytes lost
  - transfusion for haemorrhage only if anaemic with Hb < 80 g l^{-1} in fit patients
  - colloid for plasma losses.
- Correct metabolic alkalosis or metabolic acidosis.
- Correct hypoxaemia
  - attention to airway, breathing and administration of oxygen.
- Remove fear and stress
  - give explanations
  - administer analgesics or anxiolytics.

Metabolic manipulation

Protein administration to malnourished patients improves their immune function but has no immediate benefit on wound healing. *Enteral feeding* has particular benefits over the parenteral route because it helps to maintain the gut mucosal defence barrier. Increased intake of arginine (which improves weight gain, nitrogen balance, wound healing and immune function) and glutamine (which improves nitrogen balance and prevents the redistribution of body water) can be helpful.

Drug administration

Ways of manipulating the body's response to trauma are being sought but are still experimental. Many agents are only effective if given before the injury or sepsis occur, and it is difficult to block deleterious responses and still preserve beneficial ones.

Steroids, antiendotoxin antibodies, anti-TNF antibodies, IL-1 receptor antagonists and specific PAF receptor antagonists have increased survival in septic animals but have been disappointingly ineffective in humans. A recent study involving activated protein C in septic shock appears more promising; however, as bleeding tendency is increased it may not be suitable for septic patients

undergoing surgery. Other agents that have been used are adrenergic blockers (decrease the metabolic rate), aspirin (attenuates cytokine actions), growth hormone and anabolic steroids (stimulate protein synthesis), mannitol (hydroxyl radical scavenger), propranolol (improves postoperative nitrogen balance), allopurinol (inhibits free radical formation) and atrial natriuretic factor (natriuretic).

Summary

- Do you appreciate that multiple factors in the underlying disease, comorbidity, and the effects of the trauma of a surgical operation cause widespread effects in the body?
- Are you aware of the wide range of clinically detectable effects?
- Are you aware of your potential to reduce the stimuli, including trauma, in order to alleviate the effects of surgery?

Further reading

Beal AL, Cerra FB 1994 Multiple organ failure syndrome in the 1990s. JAMA 271(3): 226–233

Davies MG, Hagen PO 1997 Systemic inflammatory response syndrome. British Journal of Surgery 84: 920–935

Hill AG, Hill GL 1998 Metabolic response to severe injury. British Journal of Surgery 85: 884–890

Holte K, Kehlet H 2000 Post-operative ileus: a preventable event. British Journal of Surgery 87: 1480–1493

Huljamae H 1993 The pathophysiology of shock. Acta Anaesthesiologica Scandinavica 37(suppl. 98): 3–6

Le Quesne LP, Cochrane JPS, Fieldman NR 1985 Fluid and electrolyte disturbances after trauma: the role of adrenocortical and pituitary hormones. British Medical Bulletin 41(3): 212–217

Mainous MR, Block EFJ, Deitch EA 1994 Nutritional support of the gut: how and why. New Horizons 2(2): 193–201

Molloy RG et al 1993 Cytokines, sepsis and immunomodulation. British Journal of Surgery 80(3): 289–297

Schmidt H, Martindale R 2001 The gastrointestinal tract in critical illness. Current Opinion in Clinical Nutrition and Metabolic Care 4(6): 547–551

Senftleben U, Karin M 2002 The IKK/NF-κB pathway. Critical Care Medicine 30(1) (Suppl.): S18–S26

Treasure T, Bennett D 1999 Reducing the risk of major elective surgery. BMJ 318: 1087–1088

Woolf PD 1992 Hormonal responses to trauma. Critical Care Medicine 2(2): 216–226

32 Wound healing

S. R. Lakhani, A. Dogan

INTRODUCTION

The processes involved in wound healing are some of the most fascinating biological phenomena you are likely to encounter. In this chapter we shall examine the processes involved, and hopefully appreciate the complex interplay that allows the body to restore the integrity of its tissues. As a surgeon, you rely on the normal functioning of these processes on a daily basis.

Three fundamental things must happen if wound healing is to occur. First, the circulatory system must be able to control the bleeding (establish haemostasis; Greek *haima* = blood + *statikos* = causing to stand). Second, the inflammatory response must be effective and provide a defence against microbial infection as well as provide the necessary chemical environment for attracting and stimulating the cells needed for repair. Finally, the process of repair requires many different cell types to proliferate and to synthesize proteins necessary for restoring integrity and strength to the tissue. Although these three basic processes must occur in the healing of all wounds, you will be aware that not all your patients behave in exactly the same way. The process described above may be modified considerably by the size of the wound, the nutritional status of the patient, and hence his or her immune competence, the state of the vasculature at the site of injury, and the metabolic demands of the tissue that has been injured. It is not any one thing, but rather a complex and dynamic interplay between many factors within an intricate network, that determines the final outcome.

Wound healing requires:

- Haemostasis
- Inflammation
- Cell proliferation and repair.

THE PROCESS OF WOUND HEALING

The biological objectives of wound healing are twofold:

- To restore the integrity of epithelial surfaces if they have been lost, and hence protect the underlying tissues against infections and insults from the environment
- To restore the tensile strength of the subepithelial tissue.

Healing by 'primary' and 'secondary' intention

Although the basic mechanisms involved in wound healing are the same, by convention the healing of cleanly incised wounds, where the edges are in close apposition, is considered separately from those in which there is extensive loss of epithelium, a large subepithelial tissue defect that has to be filled in by scar tissue and where the edges cannot be brought together with sutures. These two circumstances are described as 'healing by primary intention' or 'healing by secondary intention'. These terms first appeared in a surgical treatise published in 1543, although Thomson (1813) in *Lectures on Inflammation*, gives the credit for introducing these terms to Galen.

THE HEALING OF AN INCISED WOUND: 'HEALING BY PRIMARY INTENTION'

Incision involves the division of:

- Epidermis
- Dermal connective tissue fibres and matrix

- Subcutaneous tissue
- Blood vessels.

The very first thing that must be established is haemostasis. Severing of blood vessels obviously leads to haemorrhage, with the resulting accumulation of blood within the tissue defect. Injury to blood vessels leads to arteriolar contraction, which helps to reduce the bleeding. Platelets and plasma proteins, particularly *fibrinogen* and *fibronectin*, also accumulate. Clotting occurs by both the 'intrinsic' and 'extrinsic' pathways. The former is due to exposure of the collagen and the latter due to release of 'tissue factors' from damaged cells. The platelet plug becomes converted to a clot consisting of polymerized fibrin, which is stabilized by fibronectin binding to it by means of a glutaminase bridge. 'Fibronectin' (Latin *nectere* = to bind, tie) is the term used for a set of large, extracellular matrix glycoproteins, and the gel formed by fibrin and fibronectin acts in the early stages of healing as a 'glue' which helps to keep the severed edges of the tissue apposed. Thrombin, which is involved in the generation of fibrin, also attracts macrophages and induces fibroblasts to divide. So here we have a molecule that not only has a role in haemostasis but also begins the process of repair. Platelet-derived growth factor (PDGF) released from degranulating platelets has a similar effect on fibroblasts. Transforming growth factor β and monocyte chemoattractant protein 1 are also responsible for pulling macrophages into the area, which in turn can release PDGF.

At the same time as haemostasis is being established, the process of inflammation is also kicking into action. This involves dilatation of capillaries and the formation of a fluid and cellular exudate. The polymorph leucocytes will attack and remove any bacteria and also scavenge any tissue debris from the cell death. The exudate is responsible for the tissue swelling that occurs. This not only splints and immobilizes the affected area but also the network of fibrin within the exudate forms an infrastructure that helps to localize the microorganisms, hence allowing the polymorphs easy access to them. As mentioned above, one of the biological objectives is to protect the tissues from infectious and environmental hazards and the exudate performs exactly this task by clotting and forming a scab over the wound.

The next important stage is one of cell proliferation and migration. Purely for convenience, the events are divided into those involving the epidermis and those involving the dermis.

Epidermal events

Within a few hours of wounding, a single layer of epidermal cells start to migrate from the wound edges to form a delicate covering over the raw area exposed by the loss of epidermis. This is a fascinating process. The epidermal cells have to undergo a phenotypic change that will allow them to detach from each other, from the basement membrane and hence dermal cells, and acquire properties that help them to move into the wound space. This is achieved by loss of intracellular tonofilaments, loss of desmosomes and formation of actin filaments, which allows cell movement. The cells express a family of *integrin receptors* that allows them to interact with extracellular proteins, in particular *fibronectin* and *vitronectin*. Epidermal cell migration across the area of epithelial loss depends on interaction between the keratinocytes at or near the wound edges, fibrin and fibronectin. Fibronectins are present both within plasma and within tissues. Originally they were thought to be cell surface proteins but it is now realized that they constitute part of the extracellular matrix and exert much of their effect by providing sites which act as ligands for receptors on a wide variety of cell types. This ligand–receptor binding mediates cell matrix adhesion. Keratinocytes from normal, unwounded skin do *not* possess receptors which bind to fibronectin, being tightly attached to basement membrane, which contains laminin and collagen type IV. Those derived from wounds, however, express a fibronectin receptor which is very similar to a fibronectin receptor expressed on fibroblasts. The cells migrate at a rate of approximately two cell diameters per hour.

 Key point

- **Recognize that static, adherent, epithelial cells have detached themselves and moved, like amoebae, to cover the wound.**

Epidermal cell movement can provide an initial covering for very small wounds, but in most instances epithelial recovering cannot be accomplished without proliferation of epidermal cells. The new cells are derived from the stem cell compartment of the epidermis. From about 12 h after wounding, there is a marked increase in mitotic activity in the basal cells about 3–5 cells from the cut edges. The exact biological mechanisms that lead to this proliferation are still unclear, although release of growth factors and expression of growth factor receptors must play a role. Candidates include epidermal growth factor, transforming growth factor α and keratinocyte growth factor. The new epidermal cells grow under the surface fibrin/fibronectin clot and for a little distance down the gap between the cut edges to form a small 'spur' of epithelium, which afterwards regresses. If the wound has been sutured, a similar downgrowth of new epidermis occurs in relation to the suture tracks and, on occasion, these may form the basis of keratin-forming cysts within the dermis – so-called 'implantation dermoid cysts'. This ability of epidermal cells to grow along tracts created by sutures or other foreign material is of course the basis for piercing of tissues for ear-rings, nose-rings, etc. Once re-epithelialization is complete, basement proteins will reappear and the epithelial cells revert to their normal non-migratory phenotype.

Dermal events

After the initial arrival of neutrophils to the site of injury, there is recruitment of macrophages into the area (1–2 days after wounding). This is a key event because it is these cells that orchestrate the complex interplay of chemical signs that now takes place. The macrophages are involved in:

- Demolition and removal of any inflammatory exudate and tissue debris.
- Restoring the tensile strength of the subepithelial connective tissue. This is accomplished by: (1) secretion of chemoattractants, which recruits cells that synthesize and secrete collagen and other connective tissue proteins (i.e. fibroblasts); (2) expansion of the existing small fibroblast population by stimulating the cells to proliferate; and (3) stimulation of these new fibroblasts to secrete extracellular connective tissue proteins.
- The ingrowth of new small blood vessels (angiogenesis) into the area undergoing repair; this is thought to be due to the secretion of vascular endothelial growth factor β, angiogenin, angiotropin, TNF-α (tumour necrosis factor), hypoxia and accumulation of lactate that occurs in anoxic tissues. The angiogenesis involves: (1) budding of new endothelial cells from small intact blood vessels at the edges of the wound; and (2) chemoattraction of these new endothelial cells into the fibrin/fibronectin gel within the wounded area.

In a surgical wound, fibroblasts and myofibroblasts appear in the wound between 2 and 4 days after wounding, and endothelial cells follow about 1 day later. The infiltration of macrophages and fibroblast proliferation are followed, as stated above, by the ingrowth of new capillary buds, which are derived from intact dermal vessels at the margins of the wound. Initially these buds consist of solid ingrowths of endothelial cells, but they soon acquire a lumen. An essential starting step for the ingrowth of new vessels is local degradation of the basement membrane of the existing capillary, this local defect permitting the budding of new endothelial cells. At this stage newly formed capillaries have little basement membrane substance and, compared with a normal capillary, are extremely leaky. This combination of a richly vascularized gel in which both inflammatory cells and collagen-producing fibroblasts are present is known as *granulation tissue*. The term, coined by the great German pathologist Rudolf Virchow (1821–1902), is derived from the observation that the raw surface of a wound shows a granular appearance rather like that seen on the surface of a strawberry. Each of these 'granules' contains a loop of capillaries and hence bleeds easily if traumatized.

 Key point

- **Granulation tissue formation is common to all forms of repair.**

The ultimate development of tensile strength in a wound depends on the production of adequate amounts of collagen and on the final orientation of that collagen. Collagen is the only protein that contains large amounts of the amino acids hydroxyproline and hydroxylysine. Within 24 h of wounding, protein-bound hydroxyproline appears within the damaged area, and within 2–3 days some fibrillar material may be seen, although at this time it lacks the dimensions and the typical 64 nm banding of polymerized collagen. Within a few weeks, the amount of collagen in the wounded area is normal, although preoperative tensile strength is not regained for some months. This suggests that replacement and remodelling of the collagen formed early in wound healing is an important part of the whole process. The final result is a scar composed of collagen fibres and very few cells or vessels. The scar therefore changes from pink to white, but this may take many months to occur. It will be apparent that abnormal regulation of this process is responsible for development of keloid scars.

HEALING OF WOUNDS ASSOCIATED WITH A LARGE TISSUE DEFECT: 'HEALING BY SECONDARY INTENTION'

A large volume of tissue loss can occur in cases of severe trauma or extensive burns, or, much less frequently, in relation to certain surgical procedures. Although qualitatively there are few differences between healing of an incised wound and healing of larger wounds, the most significant problem relates to filling the large defect. Clearly the formation of granulation tissue, and ultimately of scar tissue, occurs, albeit on a far larger scale. One feature, however, that helps to speed up the healing process, and which is not seen in relation to healing of incised wounds, is wound contraction.

Wound contraction

Two or three days after the formation of large open wounds, the area of raw tissue starts to decrease. This is the expression of a real movement of the wound margins and is quite independent of the rate at which covering by a new epithelial layer can take place. In some fur-bearing animals the raw area may decrease in size by as much as 80% in 2 weeks, and sometimes the degree of contraction may be so great as virtually to close the wound. The wound contraction occurs at a time when relatively little new collagen is being formed in the dermis and subcutaneous tissue, and it therefore seems unlikely that shortening of collagen fibres at the wound margins is responsible for the contraction. Indeed, inhibition of collagen formation does not interfere with the process of wound contraction. There appear to be two mechanisms by which wounds contract. Initially, the scab formed from coagulated exudate containing fibrin contracts. Later, contraction is brought about by the action of cells which appear at the margins of the wound in the first few days and which, on electron microscopy, show features suggesting both fibroblast and smooth muscle differentiation. These cells are called *myofibroblasts*. The cells contain actin, but no smooth muscle-type myosin within their cytoplasm. For a pulling force to be exerted there must be a connection between the object being pulled and whatever is applying the force. In wound contraction the connection is provided by fibronectin molecules which form bridges between collagen fibres on the one hand and receptors on the myofibroblasts on the other. Thus strips of granulation tissue from healing wounds can be made to shorten in vitro by any pharmacological agents that cause actin fibrils to contract. In vivo, it appears that transforming growth factors β1 and β2 may play a role. It has been postulated that a similar mechanism is responsible for the contracture of dermal connective tissue seen in such conditions as Dupuytren's contracture.

Key point

- **Wound contraction takes place before a significant amount of collagen has been laid down or matured, to contribute to it.**

Growth factors and cytokines in wound healing

It is clear from what has been said in the previous sections that the cellular events in wound healing must depend on a series of 'instructions' which:

- Facilitate *migration* of fibroblasts and endothelial cells
- Induce these cells, as well as the epithelial cells, to *proliferate*.

These instructions consist of a set of chemical signals derived from a number of sources. They fall into two principal types: growth factors and cytokines.

Growth factors

Growth factors are peptides which act via one or more of three pathways:

- The *endocrine pathway*, where the growth factors are synthesized at some considerable distance from their targets and are delivered via the bloodstream
- The *paracrine pathway*, where the growth factors are synthesized and released by cells which are in close proximity to their targets
- The *autocrine pathway*, in which the same cells both synthesize and stimulate their own growth.

The growth factors important in wound healing include platelet-derived growth factor, epidermal growth factor and transforming growth factors α and β. We will consider these briefly.

1. *Platelet-derived growth factor.* Platelet-derived growth factor is a basic protein which has a molecular weight of about 30 000. It consists of two peptides (an A chain and a B chain) which are bound by disulphide bridges. The name 'platelet-derived growth factor' is somewhat misleading in two senses. First, while it is certainly stored in the α granules of platelets and released from them when the platelets are activated, the growth factor is also synthesized and secreted from other cells. These include endothelial cells, macrophages, arterial smooth muscle cells and cells from certain tumours. Secondly, PDGF has a number of functions apart from its undoubted powerful mitogenic effect. It is chemotactic for the same cells for which it is a mitogen; it increases intracellular synthesis of cholesterol; and also increases binding of low density lipoprotein (LDL) by increasing the number of LDL receptors expressed on the plasma membrane of the target cell. It increases prostaglandin secretion, initially by making more of the starting material (arachidonic acid) available, and later by stimulating the synthesis of cyclooxygenase. It is able to induce changes in cell shape by a reorganization of actin filaments within the cells and it induces increased synthesis of RNA and protein. It is also a potent vasoconstrictor. Thus PDGF can carry out both tasks that were outlined at the beginning of this section. It can attract mesenchymal cells into the wound (with the exception of endothelial cells which do not possess the PDGF receptor) and it acts as a mitogen and stimulator of protein production. PDGF and other growth factors bind to receptors which, after ligand–receptor interaction, act as tyrosine kinases and hence activate the signal transduction pathways for mitogenesis.

2. *Epidermal growth factor and transforming growth factor α.* Epidermal growth factor (EGF) is a 53 amino acid polypeptide which is cleaved from a larger precursor protein. It was discovered by the Nobel laureate Cohen in the course of experiments in which he was engaged in a search for a nerve growth stimulating factor in the salivary glands of baby mice, such a factor having been discovered previously in the salivary glands of snakes. However, extracts of these glands, when injected into baby mice, caused their eyes to open prematurely and their incisor teeth to grow faster, these effects being due to a stimulation of epidermally derived tissues. The factor was purified and is now known as *epidermal growth factor*, although it stimulates mitogenesis in connective tissue as well as in epithelial cells. The salivary glands and the lacrimal glands are storage sites for EGF, which can be released in saliva and tears. Thus, licking one's wounds in the literal rather than in the metaphorical sense may be of definite biological advantage, as may be the irrigation of the cornea by tears in corneal abrasion or ulceration. EGF, or a molecule with considerable homology, is also produced in the Brunner's glands in the duodenum, and its metabolite, urogastrone, may be measured in the urine. In rodents, EGF may be found in the plasma but in humans, blood-borne EGF is concentrated within the α granules of platelets. Since EGF protein can also be found in the cytoplasm of megakaryocytes in the bone marrow, it seems almost certain that platelet EGF is derived from synthesis within the megakaryocytes rather than by uptake from the plasma. In experimental wounds the application of EGF has been found to significantly accelerate the rate of epidermal regeneration and it has also been shown to have a beneficial effect on the dermal component. In humans, topical application of EGF accelerates the healing of donor sites for skin grafts. There is no evidence that EGF is produced by any of the cells taking part in the healing process, although, as already stated, platelets store EGF. However, there is another factor, known as *transforming growth factor α* (TGF-α), which shows a considerable degree of homology with EGF and which can be produced by both epidermal cells and by macrophages in healing wounds. TGF-α binds to the same receptor on target cells as does EGF and has the same mitogenic effect. In this way TGF-α may be a direct mediator of wound healing.

3. *Transforming growth factor β.* Transforming growth factor β (TGF-β) is a polypeptide, first discovered in culture media conditioned by transformed cells, but produced by almost all cell lines in culture. In the presence of EGF it acts as a mitogen, but in some assays it has also been found to inhibit growth. It is possible that these contradictory actions may be a reflection of the different types of assay used and may not tell us much about what is happening in vivo. There is, however, good evidence that macrophages in healing wounds express mRNA for TGF-β as well as for TGF-α. TGF-β has also been shown to be a powerful chemoattractant for monocytes and its release from the first wave of inflammatory cells migrating into the wound may act as a mechanism for recruiting additional monocytes/macrophages. Studies from fetal wound healing suggest that TGF-β1 may be an important cytokine in scar formation. Fetal skin has very low levels of TGF-β1 and fetal wounds are able to heal without scarring. In animal models, antibodies to TGF-β1 and β2 are also able to reduce scarring.

Cytokines

'Cytokine' (Greek *kytos* = vessel, cell + *kineein* = to move) is the term used for a group of protein cell regulators that includes such members as lymphokines, monokines, interleukins and interferons. These are low molecular weight proteins (usually less than 80 kDa). They tend to be produced rapidly and locally and can act in either an autocrine or a paracrine fashion. They are produced by a wide range of cells and have many overlapping actions which are mediated by their binding to high affinity receptors on their target cells. The response of an individual cell to a given cytokine is dependent on the cell type, what other chemical signals are being received at the same time, and the local concentration of the cytokine. Two cytokines which play a significant role in wound healing are interleukin 1 (IL-1) and tumour necrosis factor α (TNF-α) (syn. cachectin).

1. IL-1 (formerly known as endogenous pyrogen) is a small (17 kDa) protein which is produced by a wide variety of cell types, including macrophages and epidermal cells. IL-1 has many biological actions which, in relation to healing, include a proliferative effect on dermal fibroblasts and upregulation of collagen synthesis by the fibroblasts. It also increases collagenase production and this may be one of the ways in which the collagen in wounds is remodelled so as to achieve maximal tensile strength.

2. TNF-α is another monocyte/macrophage product which is released following tissue injury or infection. It is the main factor responsible for macrophage-mediated tumour cell killing and is also responsible for the wasting (cachexia) which is seen in certain chronic bacterial and parasitic infections. Its biological activity has a remarkable overlap with that of IL-1, although it does not appear to have the immunoregulatory functions of that molecule. Its receptors, however, are quite distinct from those of IL-1 and presumably the similarities in their actions indicate that they stimulate the same 'second messenger' systems. The expression of TNF-α by monocytes and macrophages requires activation of these cells. This may

be brought about by interaction with fibrin (which is always present in wounds), binding of TGF-β, the action of α-interferon and the action of endotoxin.

3. TNF-α is a potent stimulus for the ingrowth of new blood vessels in healing wounds, being not only chemotactic for endothelial cells but also the agent responsible for the focal degradation of capillary basement membranes which precedes the migration of endothelial cells into a healing wound.

4. Both TNF-α and IL-1 play an important role in recruitment of inflammatory cells to the injury sites by regulating expression of adhesion molecules on the surface of endothelial cells.

 Important growth factors and cytokines in healing

- **PDGF, EGF, TGF-α and TGF-β (which appears to have a role in scarring).**
- **IL-1, TNF-α.**

REPAIR IN SOME SPECIALIZED TISSUES

Bone

The processes involved in the early stages of fracture healing are basically the same as those which have been described in the foregoing sections. Thus the tissue defect created by the fracture is, in the first instance, filled by granulation tissue similar to that in large open wounds. Later, more specific features peculiar to bone are imposed on the basic model of healing. These are necessary because bone, unlike soft tissues, has a mechanical and weight-bearing role. Two types of specialized cell play a central role:

- The *osteoblast*, which lays down seams of uncalcified new bone (osteoid)
- The *osteoclast*, a multinucleated cell, probably of macrophage lineage, which resorbs bone and which, therefore, remodels the new bone.

Stages of fracture healing

1. When a bone is fractured, tearing of blood vessels leads to *haemorrhage*, hence the defect between the fractured ends of the bone becomes filled with blood clot and other plasma-derived proteins. As in any other tissue, the injury elicits an *acute inflammatory reaction*, although the degree of neutrophil infiltration is mild. The combined effect of the haemorrhage and the inflammatory oedema causes loosening of the periosteum from the underlying

bone ends and this results in a fusiform swelling at the fracture site. Some degree of bone necrosis is almost inevitable and is due to the blood supply to some areas being cut off as a result of damage to blood vessels. It takes 24–48 h for the first morphological evidence of bone necrosis to become apparent, the marrow being the site of the first changes. Fat necrosis is seen and, if haemopoietic marrow is involved, the cells lose their nuclear staining. As far as the bony tissue itself is concerned, the extent of necrosis depends on the anatomy of the local blood supply, and some sites such as the talus, the carpal scaphoid and the head of the femur are particularly likely to show significant ischaemic necrosis after fracture. Empty lacunae, the dead osteocytes having disappeared, are a reliable indication of bone necrosis. *Macrophages* then invade the fracture site and commence the process of demolition. This is followed by the formation of granulation tissue, which also extends upwards and downwards within the marrow cavity for a considerable distance from the fracture site. Within the granulation tissue small groups of cartilage cells begin to differentiate from connective tissue stem cells.

2. *Provisional callus* is the term used to describe a cuff of woven bone admixed with islands of cartilage which serves to unite the severed portions of bone on their external aspect but not across the gap between the bone ends. The origin of the callus is from two sources, and the relative proportions of these vary depending on a number of factors. The first and more important is the *periosteum*. The cells on its inner aspects proliferate and begin to lay down woven bone (i.e. bone in which the collagenous osteoid tissue is not deposited in a lamellar or 'onion skin' fashion but in series of short bundles of parallel fibres, each bundle having a different orientation). Where the periosteum has been raised from the external surface of the bone, the new woven bone fills the gap so that there are two cuffs of new bone around the periosteal aspect of the separated fragments. These cuffs then extend upwards and downwards until they meet, although there is as yet no direct union across the gap between the separated bone ends. The degree of efficiency with which the external callus formation occurs depends on the adequacy or otherwise of the blood supply around the fracture site. Some of the new blood vessels are derived from the periosteum itself, while others come from the muscle and other soft tissues which abut onto the fractured bone. The amount of cartilage admixed with this periosteal new bone is small in human fractures which are healing well, but tends to be greater in cases where the local blood supply is poor or where the fractured bone ends have not been properly immobilized. The second source of provisional callus is the *medullary cavity*, where, following the formation of granulation tissue, fibroblasts and osteoblasts start to proliferate and lay down bone matrix.

Some of this is deposited on trabeculae of dead bone, while the remainder forms new trabeculae. Well after the provisional callus has been formed, the clot, which fills the gap between the fragments, is invaded, first by granulation tissue capillaries and then by osteoblasts. Ossification within this gap may occur as a primary event, the osteoblasts being derived from the provisional callus. In some cases the bone ends are united by fibrous tissue and over a period of time this is replaced by woven bone. This takes far longer than direct ossification and is more likely to occur if the fracture has not been properly immobilized or if there is any other factor present which is likely to inhibit healing (i.e. infection or extensive and severe periosteal damage). Occasionally the fibrous tissue filling the gap is not replaced by bone (non-union) and weight bearing by the affected limb is not possible. In cases of delayed or non-union some improvement may be brought about by electrical stimulation, which appears to accelerate ossification at fracture sites. Once union has occurred and the patient is bearing weight, the lumpy new cortical bone gradually becomes resorbed and smoothed out and the excess medullary new bone is similarly removed, with restoration of a normal medullary cavity. Woven bone, which is quite rapidly formed and which is much less efficient at weight bearing, is resorbed completely and is replaced by lamellar bone. This is a lengthy process of *remodelling* and restoration to normal may take up to a year.

Nervous tissue

Central nervous system

Most neurons cannot be replaced once they have been lost, although there is some evidence to suggest that a limited degree of regeneration can take place in the hypothalamic–neurohypophyseal system. In contrast to the peripheral nerves, where injury is not associated with any marked tendency towards scarring, necrosis within the central nervous system elicits the proliferation of glial cells, which, together with the ingrowths of capillaries, may constitute a physical barrier to the regeneration of new neuronal fibres. Recent work using bone marrow-derived stem cells is challenging these concepts and this area is likely to see major advances in the next 5 years.

Peripheral nerves

When an axon is severed, the nerve cell shows chromatolysis (i.e. it swells and the Nissl granules, which represent zones of the endoplasmic reticulum studded with many ribosomes, disappear). The axon swells and becomes irregular, and its lipid-rich myelin sheath splits and later breaks up. The surrounding Schwann cells proliferate and

accumulate some of the lipid released from the damaged myelin. Soon new neurofibrils start to sprout from the proximal end of the severed axon and these invaginate the Schwann cells, which act as a guide or template for the new fibrils. The neurofibrils push their way down through the Schwann cells at a rate of about 1 mm per day. Eventually they may reach the appropriate end organ and their myelin sheaths are reformed as a result of the secretory activity of the Schwann cells; in this way, a degree of functional recovery is attained. In some instances neurofibril sprouting takes place but the fibrils do not grow down existing endoneurial channels, and grow instead in a haphazard fashion. The end result may thus be a tangle of new nerve fibres embedded in a mass of scar tissue. This produces a 'traumatic' or 'stump' neuroma.

FACTORS AFFECTING WOUND HEALING

Failure to heal satisfactorily can be the result of either systemic or local factors.

Systemic factors

Nutrition

The state of nutrition of the patient is a potent factor in determining the success or failure of the healing process (see Ch. 10). Malnutrition causes depression of the immune system and hence wound infection, and the inflammatory response to this may delay healing. Deficient protein intake may inhibit collagen formation and so inhibit the regaining of tensile strength. In this regard, sulphur-containing amino acids such as methionine seem to be particularly important, and increasing the intake of this amino acid alone can partially offset the effects of a low protein intake on wound healing. Vitamin C has an important role in healing. It has been known since the seventeenth century that scurvy is associated with poor healing of wounds and fractures. Indeed, there are colourful descriptions of old wounds, acquired honourably or otherwise in combat, breaking down after the onset of scurvy. Lack of vitamin C has been found to inhibit the secretion of collagen fibres by fibroblasts; this is due to a failure of hydroxylation of proline in the endoplasmic reticulum of the fibroblast. In addition, vitamin C concentrations in biological fluids appear to affect the production of galactosamine and hence the deposition of chondroitin sulphate in the extracellular matrix of granulation tissue. Vitamin A has important functions in relation to morphogenesis, epithelial proliferation and epithelial differentiation, and the latter two are believed to be important in wound healing. A role for zinc in wound healing was discovered more or less by accident. In the course of a study on the effects of certain amino acids on wound healing, a phenylalanine analogue that had been expected to impair healing instead accelerated it. Careful study of this analogue revealed that the sample used had been contaminated by zinc. Further studies showed that zinc does indeed accelerate the healing of experimental wounds. Zinc deficiency, such as is found in patients who have been on parenteral nutrition for long periods and in patients with severe burns, is associated with poor healing and this is reversed by the administration of zinc.

Steroid hormones

Many studies show that glucocorticoids have an inhibitory effect on the healing process and on the production of fibrous tissue. Steroids are therefore administered in situations where inappropriate scarring is taking place, such as in interstitial fibrosis in the lung. It is still not clear whether steroids exert their effect indirectly by damping down the inflammatory process or whether they act directly on fibroblasts to alter collagen deposition.

Local factors

Presence of foreign bodies or infection

The presence of infection or of a foreign body increases the intensity and prolongs the duration of the inflammatory response to injury. It is worth remembering that fragments of dead tissue, such as bone, and other elements of the patient's own tissues that have become misplaced, such as hair or keratin, act as foreign bodies.

Excess mobility

The oedema that occurs following tissue injury may lead to immobilization of that part, hence the fifth cardinal sign of inflammation: 'loss of function'. Although this can be troublesome, it also has the benefit of aiding the healing process. It will be clear to everyone that a fractured bone is not going to heal unless it is immobilized. Excess mobility in any tissue will impair healing and prolong the time to full recovery.

Vascular supply

The degree of arterial perfusion and the efficacy of venous drainage play key roles in the healing of injured tissues. Where the arterial perfusion is compromised by stenosis or occlusion, a trivial injury may give rise to a disproportionate degree of tissue damage and healing may be delayed or even completely inhibited. A good example is diabetes mellitus. In patients with longstanding disease, trivial injuries develop into chronic, non-healing ulcers. Blood vessel disease affecting both the large muscular arteries of the lower limb (atherosclerosis and its complications) and changes in the walls of arterioles and capillaries probably make the major contribution to failures of healing. These patients are of course also susceptible to infection (particularly if their diabetes is badly controlled) and may also have a sensory neuropathy which makes them more liable to sustain injuries to their extremities.

Adequate venous drainage is also important, and impairment of this may play a part in the genesis of chronic ulcers, which often occur on the anterior surface of the legs in elderly patients. Histological examination of the margins of these lesions suggests that drainage is compromised by the presence of cuffs of polymerized fibrin round the venules. This can, in part, be prevented by administration of the synthetic steroid stanozolol. Suboxygenation of normally perfused tissue, such as may occur in the presence of severe anaemia, will also lead to defective healing.

 Factors modifying healing

- **Nutrition malnutrition, vitamin deficiency.**
- **Steroids.**
- **Systemic disorders, e.g. diabetes.**
- **Vascular supply.**
- **Mobility of affected tissues.**
- **Infection.**

COMPLICATIONS OF HEALING

Although the basic processes involved in healing are designed to be protective, they do occasionally go wrong. This occurs as a result of a loss of control in the complex interplay between the many varied cellular and chemical processes. Two complications worthy of mention are hypertrophic scar and keloid. Although these haunt all surgeons, they are a particular problem for the plastic surgeon. Hypertrophic scar is simply an overgrowth of scar tissue which causes a raised firm ridge. When the tissue overgrowth is so exuberant that it greatly exceeds the borders of the scar, it is called a keloid. Unfortunately, some patients have a tendency to form keloids (more common in black people) and hence excision of the keloid only results in more keloid.

It is worth remembering that, due to the contraction that occurs during wound healing, excessive tissue destruction, especially around joints, may result in contractures and joint deformity.

Summary

- Wound healing is a complex process relying on the integrated actions of the coagulation system, the inflammatory response and the chemical mediators required to stimulate cell proliferation and protein secretion.
- The processes are fundamentally the same in cleanly incised wounds and in large open wounds.
- A similar process also occurs in specialized tissues such as bone, with some changes related to functional demands of that tissue.
- The healing process can be modified by many factors, including nutritional status, steroids, infection and excess mobility of affected parts.
- Although designed to be protective, complications as a result of contractures and exuberant scar formation produce clinically significant morbidity.

Further reading

Kirsner RS, Eaglestein WH 1993 The wound healing process. Dermatology Clinics 11(4): 629–640

Lakhani SR, Dilly SA, Finlayson CJ 1998 Basic pathology: an introduction to the mechanisms of disease, 2nd edn. Edward Arnold, London, pp 78–86

Majno G, Joris I 1996 Wound healing. In: Cells, tissues and disease. Principles of general pathology. Blackwell Science, Oxford, pp 465–485

Singer AJ, Clark RAF 1999 Cutaneous wound healing. New England Journal of Medicine 341: 738–746

Waldorf H, Fewkes J 1995 Wound healing. Advances in Dermatology 10: 77–96

33 Responses of connective tissue and bone

W. J. Ribbans, M. Saleh

> **Objectives**
>
> - Appreciate that bone and connective tissues are not static but are living, dynamic and responsive to their changing environment.
> - Understand the responses of connective tissue and bone to trauma.
> - Be aware of the factors modifying the structure, strength, growth of bone and connective tissue.
> - Understand the response of bone to various surgical procedures.
> - Appreciate the inbuilt redundancy that often permits patients to overcome physical and functional defects.
> - Recognize the importance of restoring function following trauma and surgical intervention.

INTRODUCTION

We shall consider the responses of connective tissues and bone to their environment and stresses, including trauma and iatrogenic (Greek *iatros* = physician + *-gen* = to produce) interventions, which include operative surgery. There is a tendency to regard the skeleton and connective tissues as static but they are responsive and dynamic (Greek *dynasthai* = to be able). Do not regard any of these structural tissues as being simple; they are just as complex as any other parts of the body. Although bone is interspersed with inorganic calcium phosphate, it is largely composed of type I collagen. Collagen can be laid down by fibroblasts or reabsorbed, and in bone, calcium phosphate can be laid down, remoulded and reabsorbed.

The dynamic properties are well illustrated by the response to stress. Just as muscles undergo hypertrophy (Greek *hyper* = over + *trephein* = to nourish) when exercised, so do the tendons that transmit their tension. If bone is stressed, new bone is laid down to compensate; if

the direction of the stress changes, the architecture of the bone adjusts to meet it. In contrast, connective tissues and bones that are not stressed respond rapidly by undergoing atrophy, including bone decalcification. Striking examples are the changes that occur in the ligaments and bones of women during pregnancy, and in the muscles and skeleton of astronauts in space when the effects of gravity are removed.

None of the tissues works in isolation and all of them are involved in movements that require them to function in concert (Latin *com-* = with + *certare* = to strive). Fortunately we are constructed in a fashion that has inbuilt redundancy (Latin *re-* = again + *undare* = rise in waves; to overflow). If there is a failure of one part, there is 'spare' function available that can compensate. For example, if the hip is stiff, part of its function can be taken over by swinging the pelvis, using vertebral flexion and rotation, in order to swing the affected leg forward, using the other hip joint as a fulcrum. Animals can survive happily with severe disabilities; young humans are remarkably adaptable when born with congenital defects and functional incapacities. However, it is possible to overcome or alleviate many functional losses; a simple splint may provide lost support, an ankle foot orthosis (Greek *orthos* = straight; the straightening of a distorted part) can compensate for foot drop. An artificial limb (prosthesis; Greek *pros* = to + *thesis* = putting) provides effective replacement of a lost limb. Orthopaedic surgeons can aid fracture fixation using internal and external fixation, and repair or divert tendons to overcome paralysis or rupture. The field of activities constantly increases as joint replacement, limb lengthening, limb transplantation and minimal access procedures are developed and extended.

Make sure that you acquire a deep understanding of the connective tissues; they are fundamental to the success of surgical procedures.

Trauma

1. Damage can occur from sharp or blunt injury, or from a combination of the two. It may be direct or indirect,

open or closed (see Ch. 2). As a result of the injury, deep tissues may be distracted or misaligned and become incorporated within a large haematoma. Open, contaminated wounds are at increased risk of infection.

2. Operative surgery is a form of trauma but gentle handling of tissues, perfect haemostasis and meticulous technique, as advocated by the great American surgeon William Halsted (1852–1922), together with observance of sterile precautions minimize its effects. Injury may be increased by rough handling, thermal damage from using diathermy haemocoagulation, power-driven tools, and bone cement. Healing can be prejudiced by inserting unsuitable materials, such as excessive or irritating sutures.

3. The initial injury may be compounded by the effects of immobilization and disuse on bones, joints, muscles, tendons and ligaments, including those not directly involved within the surgical field.

CONNECTIVE TISSUE

Collagen

1. This is a family of proteins accounting for about one-third of the total body protein, comprising about 90% of the organic matrix of bone. The molecule is about 280 nm long. A number of polypeptide chains are involved. Type I is the most widely distributed in fascia, dermis, cornea and tendon, providing excellent tensile strength. Type II is the main component of hyaline (Greek *hyalos* = glass) cartilage and also occurs in the nucleus pulposus of the intervertebral discs. Type III forms part of the wall of blood vessels, heart valves, dermis and the network of connective tissues in the walls of organs. Type IV is present in basement membranes. Type V is widely distributed in membranous sheaths of muscles, Schwann cells and in basement membranes.

2. Collagen was once thought to be relatively static but it can be rapidly laid down or degraded. Excessive collagen formation occurs in hypertrophic and keloid scars, and also in rheumatoid arthritis. In old age, collagen atrophy is progressive. It is defective in the syndrome described in 1896 by the French physician Bernard Marfan (1858–1942) and in the overstretched collagen syndrome descibed by two dermatologists, Edvard Ehlers (1901) in Germany and Henri Danlos (1908) in France.

Elastic fibre

1. This is composed of the protein elastin enclosed within elastic fibrils. It occurs in the aorta and its large branches, in the ligamentum nuchae, the lungs and the skin. It may be difficult to distinguish between elastic fibres and altered collagen fibres.

2. Elastin is generated by fibroblasts and elastic fibres appear to be produced by smooth muscle cells. Although stable in most circumstances, elastic fibres are rapidly destroyed by elastase, an enzyme produced by some microorganisms. Elastic fibres are reduced in old age, the most obvious feature being the loss of tautness of skin.

Ground substance

This consists of glycoproteins and proteoglycans (previously called mucoproteins), which include hyaluronic acid and chondroitin. They are synthesized in fibroblasts and osteoblasts.

Muscle

1. Skeletal muscle is often stated to be incapable of regeneration but this is not entirely so. A damaged muscle cell initially undergoes degeneration, followed by regeneration. Recovery depends heavily upon the adequacy of revascularization from surrounding tissues. Necrotic tissue is removed initially and replaced by satellite pluripotent undifferentiated cells in the near vicinity, as mature myofibroblasts lack ability to regenerate and divide. The cells of the original syncytium dedifferentiate, undergo cell division, then fuse, recreating the fibre. The satellite cells may account for one-third of all muscle nuclei of newborns, but this falls to less than 5% in adults, clearly affecting the relative ability of newborns and adults to recover from injury. Myoblasts appear and fuse to form myotubes, which coalescence into muscle fibres. This occurs within a newly laid down extracellular matrix and basal lamina surrounding the muscle fibres.

2. If part of a muscle is destroyed, function is restored, not by cell hyperplasia (Greek *hyper* = over + *plassein* = to form) but by hypertrophy (*trephein* = to nourish); the individual fibres thicken up, at best creating a muscle mass comparable with the original bulk. When a muscle is transected, the ends contract and separate, the intervening space being filled with haematoma. This is eventually replaced by collagenous scar tissue, so that a single bellied muscle is transformed into a double bellied one.

3. Muscle is frequently incised to facilitate exposure. Whenever possible, split muscle along the line of the fibres rather than dividing it across them. Incisions parallel to the fibres are expected to disrupt functional recovery less than transection of the muscle belly. However, it has been shown that fibroblasts lay down collagen fibrils at right angles to the axis of the surgical incision in the

muscle. Where scar tissue intervenes between muscle fibres and the motor endplate, the isolated fibres exhibit features of denervation. Excessive scar tissue formation affects the ability of a muscle to contract and lengthen normally. A muscle transected at mid-belly recovers only about half its ability to develop tension and exhibits about 20% reduction in shortening during contraction.

4. Apart from direct laceration by scalpel, scissors or diathermy, muscle is injured by excessive pressure from instruments causing contusion (Latin *tundere* = to bruise), resulting in postoperative oedema, bleeding and acute inflammation. Provided the muscle unit remains vascularized and the patient can mobilize, functional recovery is usually adequate, with minimal scarring.

5. Ischaemia results from devascularization, or from excessively long application of a tourniquet. Transient ischaemia usually recovers completely but, if it exceeds several hours, irreversible changes occur in the myofibrils, with dilatation of mitochondria and sarcoplasmic reticulum.

6. Postoperatively, ischaemia may develop secondary to compartment syndrome. Muscle that is starved of blood supply undergoes fibrosis, described in 1881 by the German surgeon Richard Volkmann (1830–1889). Too tight bandaging, or application of plaster, and limb swelling within them may cause ischaemia.

7. If a muscle is denervated or transected, functional recovery depends upon the degree of nerve regeneration across the surgical incision, and the completeness of reinnervation.

8. Within the healing environment, dense scar tissue forms and can interfere with muscle regeneration and functional recovery. Experiments in the small muscles of rodents suggests that, in a fully revascularized area, complete muscle regeneration is possible. This seems unlikely in humans and partial recovery is generally the norm. The gap usually fills with dense scar tissue. Myotubes may penetrate the fibrous tissue but complete regeneration is unusual.

9. Following division of the Achilles tendon, there is some evidence of a change in the proximal muscle fibre type from type I slow-twitch fibres to type II fast-twitch fibres.

10. Prolonged immobilization adversely affects the functional recovery of muscles following injury. Indeed, it has been reported that protein synthesis starts to decrease within 6 h of applying an immobilizing cast. On the other hand, repetitive loading increases the number and size of the muscle cell mitochondria, muscle glycogen concentration and oxidative capacity. Active mobilization favours a rapid and more complete regeneration. Low-tension high-repetition exercise promotes muscle endurance, while high-tension low-repetition exercise promotes muscle strength.

Key point

- **Disuse atrophy occurs in skeletal muscle following prolonged immobilization.**

11. These features can be minimized by immobilizing muscles under tension. Muscle mass and strength are lost quickly following immobilization, and fatiguability increases. For example, lying in bed with knee extended causes more rapid functional decline in the relatively relaxed quadriceps than in the hamstrings, which are relatively stretched. Therefore, when placing an external fixator fine wire through muscle and into bone, preferably hold the muscle in an eccentric position while passing the wire. For instance, as a wire passes through the gastrocnemius–soleus complex dorsiflex the ankle to ensure the muscle is transfixed in a lengthened position, minimizing the risk of the development of an equinus (plantar-flexed) deformity at the ankle.

12. Muscle sensitivity to insulin is decreased during immobilization so it is more difficult for glucose to enter it, depriving it of energy supplies and allowing lactate to accumulate. Aerobic metabolism of fat is reduced. During postoperative recovery the ability of muscle to synthesize protein is reduced because of increased levels of corticosteroids.

13. Heterotopic (Greek *heteros* = other + *topos* = place; displaced) ossification occurs in some patients within soft tissues, especially muscle, and following certain procedures. The pathogenesis is uncertain but may involve damage to muscle, tendon and periosteum, residual bone debris, and haematoma formation in the presence of pluripotent (Latin *pluris* = more + *potentia* = power; multiple potential), uncommitted fibroblasts. On careful inspection, up to 30% of postoperative hip replacement radiographs reveal evidence of ossification although re-exploration and bone excision is required in less than 1% of patients. The incidence is greatest in males, younger patients and following an anterolateral approach to the hip joint. The new bone is found within fascial connective tissue with extensions into the muscle mass. There is an acute rise in the levels of serum alkaline phosphatase during the early weeks following operation.

Tendons

1. Tendons (Greek *tenon* = sinew) are composed of fascicles (bundles) of collagen. Each fascicle contains fibrils of predominantly type I collagen, produced by fibroblasts, embedded in a proteoglycan matrix. Each bundle is surrounded by an endotenon of loose connective tissue and the whole tendon is surrounded by an epitenon.

2. Many tendons are enclosed in a tendon sheath, especially those that change direction abruptly, such as flexor tendons of the hand. The tendon sheath acts as a pulley and prevents 'bow-stringing' of tendons. The synovial membrane on its inner surface combined with the epitenon serve as sources of lubricating fluid for the tendon. The tendons themselves are relatively avascular; blood reaches them at isolated points through flimsy attachments termed vinculae (Latin *vincire* = to bind). These tendons possibly have a dual pathway for tendon nutrition – through blood vessels and also by synovial diffusion. Tendons not surrounded by a sheath have a paratenon surrounding them, such as the Achilles tendon; they are known as vascular tendons and receive vessels from many points.

Key points

- **Damage to the vinculae that bring blood vessels to the tendons seriously prejudices healing.**
- **Damage to tendon sheaths and paratenon roughens the surfaces and generates irregularities and adhesions.**

3. Repetitive loading is a stimulus for increase in strength, size, matrix organization and strength of the insertion into bone. Endurance training in optimal position, with minimal resistance, facilitates revascularization and can result in an increase in strength of up to 30–40%.

4. However, the overall blood supply of tendons is not bounteous and certain areas within them are recognized as being relatively avascular. They are prone to damage and disability because of their inability to repair; for example, the supraspinatus tendon in the shoulder, the Achilles tendon, and the tibialis posterior tendon at the ankle.

5. 'Vascular' tendons undergo repair by the normal inflammatory response. Macrophages and fibroblasts fill the tendon gap. Type I collagen predominates in the initial healing process, orientated at this early stage perpendicular to (across) the long axis of the tendon. Subsequent remodelling and reorientation follows but maximum strength is not achieved for 5–6 months.

6. The timing of mobilization is crucial following tendon repair. Too early mobilization weakens the repair and leads to gap formation between the tendon ends. Early controlled passive motion appears to stimulate intrinsic repair from the epitenon itself, and improves tendon strength.

7. Prolonged immobilization of flexor tendons of the hand leads to increased adhesions and stiffness resulting from ingrowth of scar tissue from the surrounding sheath.

Again, early controlled passive movement gives optimal restoration of flexibility and strength, especially of the finger flexors.

Fascia and compartment syndromes

1. The upper and lower limbs are divided into relatively inelastic compartments bounded by fascia and bone (Fig. 33.1). Each contains soft tissues, principally muscle, tendon and neurovascular structures. The development of a compartment syndrome after trauma is well recognized (see Ch. 2). Similar changes can occur after elective surgery to the limbs. The boundaries of each compartment allow only a finite amount of expansion before ischaemic changes develop. Fig. 33.2 outlines the pathogenesis of a compartment syndrome.

2. Postoperative swelling and bleeding increase the volume, and therefore the pressure, within compartments.

3. Monitor 'at risk' patients clinically after operation by testing sensation and movement; this is not possible if you have used nerve block anaesthesia. It is possible to measure objectively the pressure within, for example, the anterior tibial compartment, to detect an abnormal rise in pressure.

Key points

- **Avoid excessive tourniquet inflation times because this results in postoperative swelling within compartments.**
- **Drain compartments within which postoperative bleeding is likely.**

Ligaments

1. Ligaments (Latin *ligare* = to bind) span joints and provide stability. Additionally, they have important proprioceptive (Latin *proprius* = one's own + receptive; sense of one's position) and nocioceptive (Latin *nocere* = to hurt; pain perception) functions because of the specialized nerve endings embedded within them.

2. Fibroblasts within the ligaments lay down collagen (90% type I), and some elastin fibres in an extracellular matrix. The collagen fibres are generally laid down along the direction of the tensile forces but not as rigidly as in tendons. Ligaments are relatively avascular, the most important source of vessels being the surrounding soft tissue rather than the osseous attachments. The anterior cruciate ligament within the knee derives most of its blood supply from the synovial membrane, which surrounds it.

3. Repetitive loading promotes increased strength, size, matrix organizition and attachment to bone.

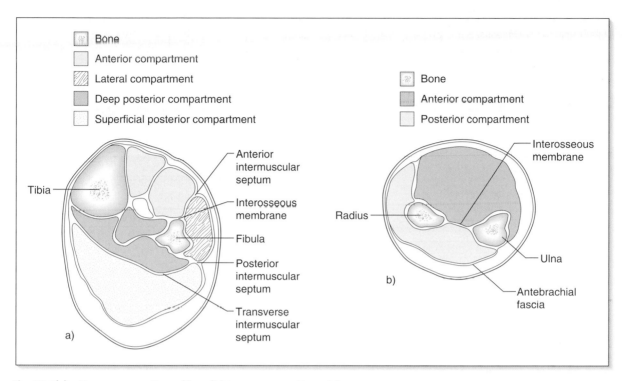

Fig. 33.1(a) Transverse section of leg, **(b)** transverse section of forearm.

4. Repair of a damaged extra-articular ligament, such as the medial collateral ligament of the knee, is induced by the normal inflammatory response. The resulting haematoma is rapidly invaded by inflammatory mediators. Vascular granulation tissue contains many fibroblasts, laying down predominantly type III collagen, which provides early stability. After several weeks, a period of remodelling and maturation commences, which may be completed only after a year. The collagen type is gradually converted back to type I.

5. Operative repair of intra-articular ligaments, such as the anterior cruciate ligament of the knee, is not associated with great success. The blood supply is sparse and synovial fluid dilutes the initial haematoma, inhibiting the normal repair mechanisms. Usually reconstruction is necessary, either with a hamstring tendon or with a part of the patella tendon that includes at one end a portion of bone from the tibial tubercle and at the other end a portion of patella.

Key point

- **Careful apposition of the divided ends, with minimal disturbance of the local soft tissues which carry the blood supply, are essential requirements for successful repair.**

6. Immobilization of a joint following operation compromises the biomechanical properties of a previously healthy ligament. Tensile strength, elasticity and toughness deteriorate, only slowly reversed as joint movement is resumed.

7. Joints immobilized after operation need to be splinted in a 'position of function' to avoid unnecessary contractures of the ligaments. Immobilization should be minimized to encourage recovery of the normal biomechanical properties of the stabilizing ligaments.

Synovial membrane

1. The function of synovium within articulations and around moving tendons is to provide synovial fluid for lubrication and nutrition and to remove unwanted elements from the area. Its superficial cells are served by a dense subsynovial plexus of vessels. Muscle bellies also slide over each other with minimal friction, although this is often ignored or overlooked. The apposed smooth external investing fascias must be separated by some form of synovial fluid. A.K. Henry, the poetic Irish surgeon-anatomist, eloquently describes the appearance of vastus intermedius muscle, when the overlying muscles are separated, as a 'silvery fish-like belly'; it is shiny and slippery like the scales of a freshly caught fish (Henry 1945).

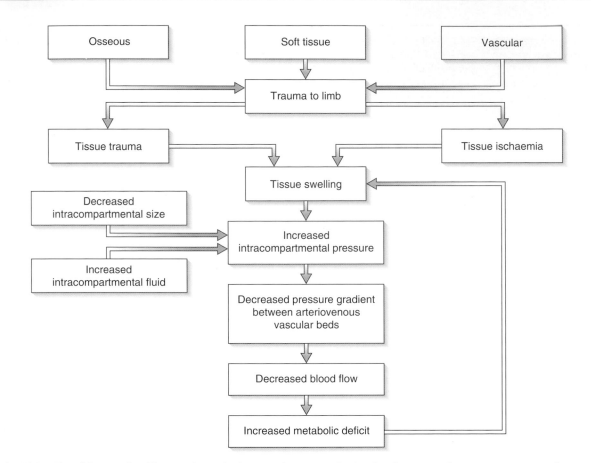

Fig. 33.2 The vicious cycle of haemodynamic changes that occurs in the development of a compartment syndrome.

2. Although the secreted fluid resembles white of egg (Greek *ovon* = egg), the origin of the name is obscure. The membrane invests many tendons and joints within the body. Membrane injury from trauma or operation increases its vascularity, cellular content and permeability, resulting in increased production of synovial fluid and white blood cells. Vacuum drainage of the joint may be valuable in removing excess synovial fluid.

3. Synovial fluid is viscous, lubricating and nourishing joint and tendon surfaces. Its viscosity and pH varies in diseases such as osteoarthritis and rheumatoid arthritis. Changes in the constituents can be detected by infrared spectroscopy, and as the viscosity falls the lubricating function is reduced.

4. Haemarthrosis (Greek *haima* = blood + *arthron* = joint + *-osis* = morbid process), following injury or operation, stimulates the synovial layer to phagocytose the erythrocytes and haemoglobin molecules. Type A synovial cells are probably the most active phagocytes. Ingested blood may form whorled bodies, known as siderosomes (Greek *sideros* = iron), within the cells. The haemarthrosis induces

a chronic inflammatory response within the subsynovial layer and there is evidence of angioneogenesis (Greek *neos* = new), cellular hyperplasia and some villous proliferation within the membrane. Large amounts of ingested blood may be toxic to the phagocytic cells, killing them. The dead cells release enzymes such as collagenase and neutral proteinase, which are potentially harmful to the joint and, in particular, to articular cartilage. Synovial iron deposits can still be found for up to 2 years following a major haemarthrosis.

5. Inflammatory disease processes, such as rheumatoid arthritis, mediate many of their pathological processes by direct action upon the synovium. The inflammatory stimulus causes cellular proliferation and increased vascularity. The inflammation, secondary to synovitis and effusion, causes joint swelling and distension of the joint capsule and ligaments. The latter may lose their stabilizing influence upon the joint, increasing deformity and joint destruction. The joint articular cartilage is gradually destroyed by the formation of a pannus of inflammatory vascular tissue, which spreads from the junction of the

cartilage and synovium until it envelops the whole articulation. The detrimental effect of the pannus is due to the direct proteolytic effect of its enzymes and the mechanical effect of its covering presence, depriving the articular cartilage of the benefits of the synovial fluid.

A combination of the osteoclastic cytokine action within the overlying pannus, relative inactivity and drug treatment causes the subchondral bone to become relatively demineralized and osteoporotic.

Joint instability can cause life-threatening changes to the cervical spine, affecting the safety of surgical procedures. Replacement will be undertaken in a joint more prone to instability and periarticular fracture. At times, different artificial joint designs will be required, e.g. increasingly stabilized prostheses. Wound healing may be compromised as a result of the patient's drug therapy and the generally more delicate nature of the adjacent soft tissues. Any inflamed synovial tissue, with its hypervascularity, is more at risk of infection from systemic causes.

The extra-articular sites of synovial tissue undergo changes causing similar damage to tendons, affecting strength and ultimately leading to rupture in many cases. Tendon repair following rupture may be impossible because of the poor quality of the tissue: a series of tendon transfers have been described for such eventualities.

Key point

- **Be aware of the changes that synovial tissue has undergone, and the consequent limitations placed upon you.**

JOINTS

Some joints may not permit movements, such as synarthroses (Greek *syn* = together) between the bones of the skull. Amphiarthroses (Greek *amphi* = both) joined by fibrocartilage, as in intervertebral discs, or synovial membranes, as in the pubic symphysis, permit very little movement. Diarthroses (Greek *dia* = through) are freely moveable, as in the hip and shoulder joints; the bone ends are covered in articular cartilage and they are enclosed in a synovial membrane (Table 33.1).

Joints can be damaged if weight is exerted through them in an abnormal fashion. This is very true of the complex knee joint. Weight should be transmitted equitably between the femoral condyles, through the menisci and the tables of the tibial platform.

Be aware of the importance of axes and alignments in determining the forces on joints and strains and stresses on musculotendinous units. In the lower limb, there are various lines along which bones rotate or are conceived to revolve, or about which the parts are symmetrically arranged (Greek *axon*, Latin *axis* = an axle) (Fig. 33.3):

- **Anatomical axis of bones**: a line running along the midpoint of the femur and tibia.
- **Vertical axis**: from the body's centre of gravity to the ground.
- **Mechanical axis**: a line that normally passes from the centre of the femoral head to the centre of the ankle joint through the centre of the knee. Any deviation of this axis, such as congenital deformities, operative or post-traumatic deformity, may cause uneven loading on joints, with consequent arthritis and instability.

Lubrication of synovial joints

Synovial joints are lubricated by synovial fluid. The science of friction, wear and lubrication is known as tribology (Greek *tribein* = to rub). Lubrication acts to

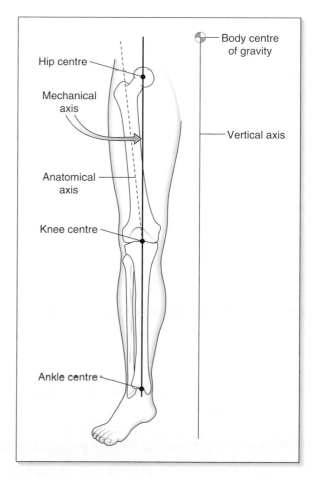

Fig. 33.3 Lower limb axes.

Table 33.1 Classification of joints

Joint type	Subtype	Examples	Characteristics	Movement
Fibrous		Skull sutures; syndesmosis of the inferior tibiofibular joint; interosseous membrane of the forearm	Bones joined by fibrous tissue continuous with periosteum or perichondrium	Variable from nil, e.g. skull sutures, to considerable, e.g. interosseous membrane
Cartilaginous	Primary	Physeal plate of the growing long bones	May be temporary, e.g. during bone growth and converts to bone at the end of growth	None
	Secondary	Pubic symphysis; manubriosternal joint; intervertebral discs	Joints are found in the midline. Each bone is covered with hyaline cartilage and joined by a central fibrous tissue which may cavitate, e.g. gel for discs	Slight movement
Synovial			Bone covered by hyaline cartilage. Enclosed by fibrous capsule, which is lined by synovial membrane. Joint cavity is filled with synovial fluid derived from membrane	
	Plane	Acromioclavicular joint	Flat surfaces	Permits gliding or sliding
	Hinge	Elbow joint	Hinge joint	Moves in one plane
	Saddle	First metacarpotrapezial joint	Biaxial joint	Permits circumduction
	Condyloid	Metacarpophalangeal joints	Biaxial	Permits movement in two planes
	Ball and socket	Hip; shoulder	Multiaxial	Circumduction. Amount of movement depends upon depth of socket and ligamentous arrangement
	Pivot	Forearm pronation/supination; atlantoaxial joint	Uniaxial	Rotation

reduce frictional resistance and wear. The coefficient of friction for a synovial joint is lower than that achieved in any synthetic (Greek *syn* = together + *thesis* = a placing; putting together) bearing surface yet designed.

There are several mechanisms of lubrication (Fig. 33.4):

1. Hydrodynamic
2. Elastohydrodynamic
3. Weeping
4. Mixed
5. Boundary
6. Squeeze film
7. Hydrostatic.

A normal synovial joint relies predominantly upon mechanisms 2, 3 and 5. Artificial joints rely on 2 and 5.

Menisci

1. The menisci (Greek *meniskos*, diminutive of *mene* = moon) increase the contact area in certain joints, participate in load distribution, act as shock absorbers and aid in distribution of lubricating synovial fluid.

2. The long-term absence of all, or a substantial part of, a meniscus is associated with increased risk for the development of osteoarthritis.

3. The meniscus is composed primarily of type I collagen, with lesser contributions from types II, III, V and VI. The cellular elements responsible for the synthesis of collagen and other constituents of the extracellular matrix are termed fibrochondrocytes. The collagen fibres are orientated predominantly circumferentially, with a few

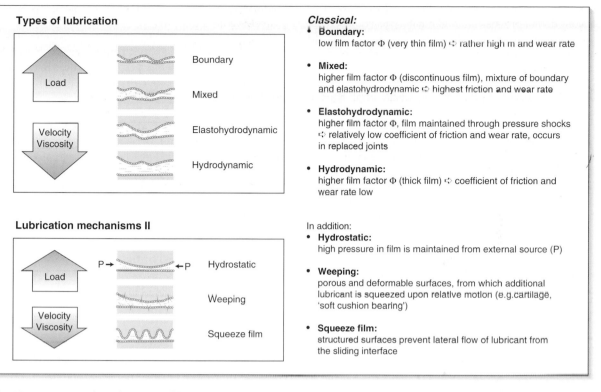

Fig. 33.4 Types and mechanisms of lubrication.

positioned radially, tying together the other fibres and limiting motion.

4. The vascular arrangement of knee menisci is important for nutrition and the ability to repair. A circumferentially arranged perimeniscal plexus sends radially orientated vessels into the meniscus. Unfortunately, they penetrate only 10–30% of the peripheral area. This has led to the concept of the outer 'red zone' and inner 'white zone'. The synovium extends for a couple of millimetres over the peripheral edges of the meniscus and contains blood vessels. Within the 'white zone', nutrition is dependent upon diffusion from the synovial fluid.

5. The ability of the meniscus to repair following a sporting injury or degenerative tear depends upon the site of damage. Within the 'red zone', repair can take place along similar lines to other connective tissue structures. Vessels from the synovium and circumferential plexus support this process. Success depends upon the size of the lesion, the delay between injury and repair, and the adequacy of the blood supply. Apposition of the torn edges can be aided by meniscal suturing.

6. Most meniscal tears occur in the avascular zone and are incapable of repair. Operation, usually through the arthroscope, involves excision of the torn fragment to prevent further propagation of the tear and to abolish pain, clicking and occasional joint locking experienced by the patient. If unstable segments are excised, later development of osteoarthritis is minimized. While not capable of repair, the meniscus may undergo remodelling following partial excision in the 'white zone'. The 'raw area' resulting from the surgical removal of the torn fragment fills with a fibrin clot and synovial-derived cells. Later, the tissue appears, on gross inspection, to be similar to fibrocartilage. It seems that this process is related to the ability of meniscal fibrochondrocytes to proliferate in the presence of haematoma-derived factors.

Articular cartilage

1. Articular cartilage is composed largely of an extra-cellular matrix populated with relatively few chondrocytes. It consists of predominantly water, collagen (mostly type II) and proteoglycans with link proteins. In contrast to the opaque fibrocartilage seen in menisci, articular cartilage is hyaline. Synthesis of the matrix is increased by moderate repetitive loading.

2. Mechanical loading of normal joints contributes to maintenance of the articular cartilage but high shear stress causes degeneration and loss of function.

3. Small defects may heal spontaneously. Superficial lesions do not provoke an inflammatory reaction because there is no bleeding and chondrocytes cannot repair the damage. They do not inevitably progress to full thickness damage and osteoarthritis, as a thin layer of matrix may form over the damaged surface. For deeper lesions, not only the cartilage but also the subchondral bone is breached. This allows bleeding from the deeper bone to fill the defect and induce an inflammatory response. Some mesenchymal cells assume the appearance of chondrocytes. However, even 6 months after the injury, the cartilage is not fully repaired. While areas of hyaline cartilage may appear, there is a substantial amount of fibrous tissue present. The ultimate composition of the repair tissue is usually a hybrid of hyaline and fibrocartilage.

4. Operative repair of damaged articular cartilage rarely reproduces the original structure. This failure results from the relative avascularity of articular cartilage and a paucity of cells available to provide the necessary materials. A lack of blood vessels disrupts the normal connective tissue response to injury: haemorrhage, fibrin clot formation, inflammatory reaction, phagocytosis and the synthesis of extracellular matrix components. Hyaline cartilage is uniquely composed of predominantly type II collagen and large cartilaginous macromolecules. The pluripotent (Latin *pluris* = several + *potentia* = power), undifferentiated cells available for repair do not consistently metamorphose into mature cells capable of replacing these elements.

5. When treating fractures involving an intra-articular element, aim to reduce the joint surfaces as anatomically as possible and stabilize the fragments to minimize steps and gaps that will cause later degeneration of the joint.

6. Osteoarthritis is a condition affecting predominantly the articular cartilage. The severity of the wear is classified accordingly:

Grade I: Softening of the articular cartilage
Grade II: Fibrillation and fissuring of articular cartilage
Grade III: Partial thickness cartilage loss, clefts and chondral flaps
Grade IV: Full thickness cartilage loss with exposed bone

Once the articular cartilage surface is breeched, the hyaline structure rapidly deteriorates. There is a loss of the proteoglycan and collagen in the matrix. The damaged cartilage breaks up and becomes free within the joint. It is regarded as irritant to the articulation and induces a synovitis as the lining attempts to phagocytose the fragments.

NERVOUS TISSUE

1. The organization of peripheral nerves is well described. An individual nerve fibre is separated from others by a loose connective tissue network, known as endoneurium. Some nerve fibres are enveloped by myelin (Greek *myelos* = marrow).

2. A group of nerve fibres form a fascicle, defined by a circumferential layer of perineurium. A group of fascicles forms an individual nerve. The fascicles are separated by epineurium, which is condensed to form a sheath around the whole nerve.

3. The blood supply to a nerve has both intrinsic and extrinsic components. Within the nerve are vascular plexuses at epineurium, perineurium and endoneurium levels. Externally, blood reaches the nerve at intervals from segmental regional vessels, which run in the connective tissue around the nerves. There are longitudinal anastomoses between the different supplying vessels, ensuring a rich microvascular network to support the metabolic activity of the nerve.

4. The environment of the individual nerve fibres is regulated and protected by the physical diffusion barrier of the perineurium and the structural and functional characteristics of the endoneurial capillaries, which function as a blood–nerve barrier similar to the blood–brain barrier in the central nervous system. Injury can affect these barriers and affect nerve function.

5. When mobilizing a nerve, as in ulnar nerve transposition, handle it and its surrounding tissue as little as possible to avoid damaging the nerve and its supplying vessels. Avoid tension and unnecessary dissection to minimize interruption of the longitudinal anastomoses. Avoid compressing the nerve (Fig. 33.5).

Nerve injuries are classified in a number of different ways. In 1951, injuries were classified into five degrees (Table 33.2).

6. Nerves can be damaged by undue traction during surgery. Depending upon the force of stretching and the duration of the insult, the nerve may suffer any injury between the first and fifth degrees.

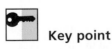

Key point

- **Ensure that you revise the anatomy of neurological structures before, not during, operation.**

7. Certain approaches are associated with particularly high rates of inadvertent nerve damage, such as the ulnar nerve at the elbow and radial nerve at mid-humeral level. At the beginning of the procedure, identify, appropriately mobilize and preserve the 'nerve(s) at risk'. Exercise particular care when undertaking procedures through previously explored areas, as the nerve position may have changed and identification is more difficult in dense scar tissue.

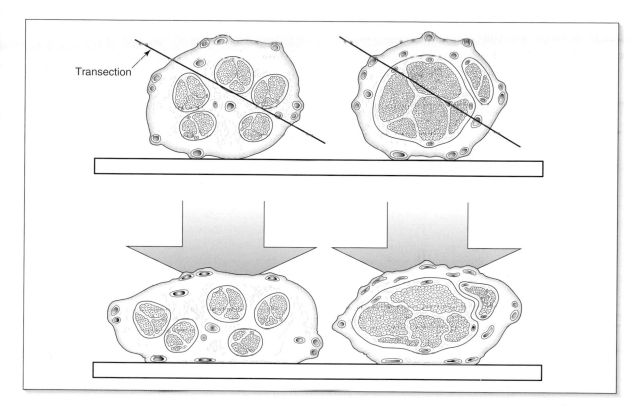

Fig. 33.5 Protective effects of the epineurium when a nerve is subjected to mechanical trauma. Several small fascicles embedded in a large amount of epineurium (left) are less vulnerable to transection injuries and compression than large fascicles in a small amount of epineurium (right).

8. Nerve damage at sites distant from the operative area may be caused during operation. Ensure that vulnerable nerves are suitably protected when positioning the patient before operation, particularly the radial nerve in the arm and the common peroneal nerve in the leg.

 Key point

- **Beware prolonged inflation, and overinflation, of tourniquets.**

Table 33.2	**Nerve injury classification**	
Degree	Description	Previous classification (1943)
I	Conduction block	Neurapraxia
II	Lesion confined to the axon. Wallerian degeneration occurs within an intact endoneurial sheath	Axontmesis
III	Both the axon and endoneurium lose continuity within an intact perineurium	Neurotmesis
IV	Loss of the perineurium around the fascicles. Only the epineurium remains to provide continuity	
V	Complete loss of division of the nerve	

9. If you inflate a tourniquet much beyond the patient's systolic pressure, the cuff may deform and damage peripheral nerves beneath it. The effects are mediated by mechanical pressure and ischaemic change. Mechanical compression causes obstruction of intraneural blood vessels and ischaemia causes damage to the same vessels, affecting permeability and leading to intraneural oedema. To minimize the effects of tourniquet ischaemia on nerve and muscle, make sure the pressure in upper limb tourniquets is no more than 50–100 mmHg above systolic pressure and no more than double systolic pressure in the leg. Do not exceed 2 h maximum tourniquet pressure.

10. When planning surgical incisions, take into account the concept of 'internervous planes'. Consider the skin areas and muscles supplied by individual peripheral nerves. When possible, incise between the 'territories' of major nerves. For instance, Henry's approach to the volar (palmar) aspect of the forearm is placed between brachioradialis muscle, supplied by the radial nerve, and flexor carpi radialis, innervated by the median nerve.

11. Neurological structures are clearly in danger of thermal injury from injudicious use of diathermy close to nerves. In such situations, use bipolar diathermy.

12. The outcome following nerve repair depends heavily upon surgical technique and operator experience. Prepare the nerve ends carefully, appose and realign individual fascicles, and leave a small gap between the ends, with minimal tension, to achieve the best results.

Key point

- **If there is a neuropathy, always consider diabetes.**

13. Diabetes is frequently affected by neuropathy. Musculoskeletal tissue, especially in the extremities, can be prone to trauma because of loss of normal protective mechanisms triggered by an intact sensory system. Frequently, the situation is exacerbated by a concomitant arteriopathy. As a result, diabetics are more prone to the development of ulcers, deep sepsis (including osteomyelitis), delayed wound healing postoperatively, and Charcot joints (after repetitive trauma).

GAIT

1. Normal gait (Old Norse *gat* = way, path; a way of walking, pattern of leg movements) is extremely complex. It requires equilibrium, the ability to stand upright in balance, and also to initiate locomotion (Latin *locus* = place + *movere* = to move). In order to achieve both of these requirements, the skeletal, muscular, sensory and motor nervous systems must work in concordance.

2. Different people walk in a wide variety of ways, depending upon the body shape and weight, urgency of moving, and other factors. The variation is so great that it is often possible to identify a close companion at a distance by recognizing the gait.

3. Carefully observe the gait of people and identify the stages of the cycle (Fig. 33.6).

4. You should be able to describe the main stages of the normal walking pattern.

5. Patients may limp (Old English *lemp-healt* = halting) for several reasons. The Latin word is *claudus*, and the Emperor Claudius was so named because he was lame. The main causes are listed in Table 33.3.

BONE

1. Bone forms the skeleton (Greek *skellein* = dry; originally + *soma* = body; dried body), a supporting structure. It is a highly vascular hard tissue with the capacity to grow in width (accretion, as a tree trunk expands) and length by endochondral ossification. The body is composed of flat bones and long bones. The long bones have

Table 33.3	Major causes of limp
Cause	Example
Pain: antalgic (Greek *anti* = against + *algos* = pain; pain relieving) gait	Arthritis of a joint, fracture, ligament injury
Weakness: paresis (Greek *parienai* = to relax; diminished function) or paralysis	Gluteal muscle weakness (= Trendelenburg gait); neurological injury
Leg length discrepancy	Congenital deformity; post-traumatic
Stiffness	Arthritis of a joint Post-traumatic soft tissue swelling

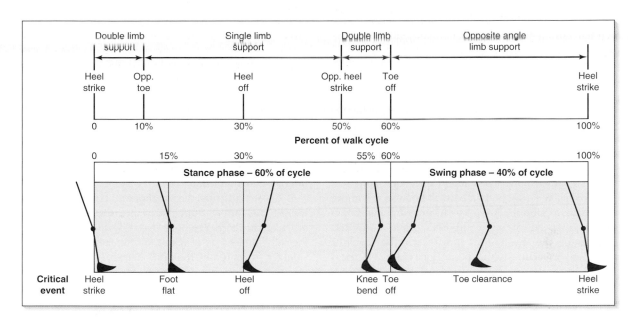

Fig. 33.6 Phases and events of walking cycle. Stance phase constitutes approximately 62% and swing phase 38% of cycle.

a central tubular structure, the diaphysis (Greek *dia* = through + *physis* = nature, growth), and an expanded end, the metaphysis (Greek *meta* = after), which incorporates the growth plate, the physis, and the subchondral bone plate covered by the articular cartilage of the adjacent joint. At skeletal maturity the architecture of the metaphysis becomes homogeneous, with loss of the cartilaginous growth plate. Bone is largely composed of type I collagen. It contains cells (osteocytes) embedded in an amorphous, fibrous collagen matrix interspersed with calcium phosphate, an inorganic bone salt. Osteoporosis is characterized by a reduction in bone mass. Loss of structural strength may lead to fracture and also affects implant fixation.

2. Bone exists in two forms, depending on the arrangement of the collagen fibre and the osteocytes. *Immature bone* has fibres and osteocytes irregularly arranged. The osteomucin is basophilic and there is a sparsity of calcium. It forms, during development of differentiating mesenchyme, into the bones of the skull vault, mandible and clavicle, and when bone is laid down in differentiating mesenchyme, as in fracture healing. It also occurs in various bone diseases, including osteogenic tumours.

Adult bone has the collagen arranged in parallel sheets or bundles, as flat plates or, in long bones, as tubular vascular canals surrounded by concentric systems of cortical bone, described in 1689 by the English physician Clopton Havers (1650–1702). The bone is less compact in the central canal of long bones and is termed cancellous

(Latin *cancellus* = lattice; *porous*). Most of the skeleton is formed on a cartilagenous model from ossification centres in the diaphysis and epiphyses (Greek *epi* = upon) which spread in all directions, replacing cartilage with bone. During growth, the cartilagenous physis grows as it is invaded from both sides, so the bone continues to lengthen. At the interface between expanding ossification and the cartilage, osteoblasts, resembling fibroblasts, lay down collagen and osseomucin, which becomes osteoid, which immediately becomes calcified with calcium phosphate deposition. This interferes with cartilagenous nutrition so the chondrocytes die, being replaced by osteocytes, the mature osteoblasts, which are locked in the newly created bone. At maturity the cartilagenous physis plate is invaded from both sides, which eventually fuse across it, so further growth in length ceases. A similar process occurs during the healing of bony fractures. Adult bone replaces membrane bone so that the whole skeleton of adults is composed of it.

3. There may be varied stimuli for changes in bone, including fatigue damage, stress-generated potentials, changes in the hydrostatic pressure of the extracellular fluid, and changes in the cell membrane diffusion resulting from direct loading. In 1892 the German-born orthopaedic surgeon Julius Wolff stated that if bone is mechanically stressed it is stimulated to build up bone in response to the force. It is considered likely that stretch receptors are associated with ion channels on osteocytes.

A minimum level of repetitive load is necessary to maintain normal bone. A number of biochemical changes can be detected during the process including raised prostacyclin, prostaglandin E2, intracellular enzyme glucose-6-phosphate dehydrogenase (G6PD), nitrous oxide (NO) and growth factors, including insulin-like growth factor 1 (IGF-1), which is a mediator of metabolic activity. Bone remodelling is accomplished by large multinucleate osteoclasts (Greek *clasis* = a breaking), which absorb bone, creating spaces or lacunae, described in 1841 by the London surgeon John Howship; osteoblasts lay down bone elsewhere. Cancellous bone has more extensive surfaces than cortical bone so it is more responsive to stimuli. Advances in imaging, combined with high-speed digital computers, have permitted analysis of the mechanical stresses to the level of individual trabeculae within bone. Bones carry electrical potentials at rest, resulting from metabolic processes. Active growth plates are electronegative. If bones are loaded to bend them, a negative charge develops on the compressed side and a positive charge is generated on the distracted side. Bone deposition occurs on the negative compressed side, and resorption on the positively charged distracted side. The electrical changes were thought to be the result of a piezo-electric (Greek *piezein* = to press) effect – compression of a crystalline structure generating an electrical charge. This mechanism has been challenged. Bone behaves as a composite viscoelastic material (Latin *viscosus* = sticky). It has multiple channels and lacunae within it, the lining of which may have a charge. Ions in the fluid within the channels tend to stay in the vicinity of the ions in the lining which carry an opposite charge. If the fluid flows, as a result of bone deformation, the ions are separated, resulting in an electrical field and a potential difference. This is called a streaming potential. The alternative explanation to a piezoelectrical effect is that when the bond is strained, movement of the non-mineralized matrix produces fluid movement, resulting in streaming potential which sensitizes the osteocytes and osteoclasts (Greek *klasis* – fracture; hence, absorption). The osteocytes respond by laying down bone and the osteoclasts by absorbing bone; the result is a remodelling to adapt the bone structure to any change in the forces exerted on it. In the hope of exploiting this mechanism, direct current, capacitative coupling, and pulsed electromagnetic fields have been used to stimulate osteogenesis in fractures and osteoporosis.

4. Bones and soft tissue respond to the loads placed upon them. Regular exercise has been shown to improve muscle strength and endurance and has important, although less obvious, ramifications for the structure and function of bone. This is particularly important for the elderly in an attempt to partially offset the development of osteoporosis. Bone conforms to Wolff's law. Julius Wolff was a German scientist, who in the late 1800s, stated that 'every change in the form and function of bones or of their function alone is followed by certain definite changes in their configuration in accordance with mathematical laws' – to borrow a modern sporting phrase 'use it or lose it!'. Increasing the load upon a bone increases the overall bone mass and causes remodelling of the bone to best withstand the types and directions of stress placed upon it. In normal long bones, the bone is strongest in resisting compressional forces, weakest in shear and intermediate in tension.

5. In osteoarthritis, the subchondral bone reacts to the loss of cushioning from the progressively diminishing articular cartilage. The bone becomes thicker and radiologically denser as a result of the loss of its 'stress shielder'. Eventually, the bone decreases in height as a result of successive trabecular fractures. Witness the increased work required to resect the medial femoral condyle compared to the lateral side during knee replacement surgery for a varus osteoarthritic joint.

6. The bone is continually repairing small defects developing within it. Usually, that process takes place before more major fractures occur. However, in impaired bone or bone subjected to higher than normal forces, fractures may occur. Patients who inhale nicotine, take catabolic steroids, or regular long-term non-steroidal anti-inflammatory medication, represent common groups with impaired ability to heal bone under various circumstances. The beneficial effect of postsurgery rehabilitation, with early weight-bearing and joint mobilization, is clear.

7. Certain conditions can lead to markedly increased density of bone. Sickle cell anaemia causes bone to undergo repeated infarcts as a result of vascular insults. The medullary cavity of long bones can be converted from a lattice-work pattern to an ivory-dense bone mass. Be aware of this or you can experience considerable problems in breaching such bone, as when placing an intramedullary implant.

8. Surgical operations to bone may be required for many reasons. The most common indication is to facilitate fracture healing. Bone may need to be divided to realign it, an osteotomy. Bone biopsy is carried out to obtain specimens to determine suspicious pathology. Bone may require resection because of infection or neoplasia. An increasingly common reason for operations is to replace worn articulations with prosthetic implants.

9. Healing of bone may be stimulated in a number of ways, including the use of demineralized bone matrix harvested from donor bones. Electrical stimulation has been in use since the 1880s. It is now known that when a bone breaks it generates a low-level electrical field, which stimulates repair.

Osteoporosis and osteomalacia

Distinguish between osteoporosis (Greek *poros* = a passage; permeable) and osteomalacia (Greek *malakos* = soft) in terms of the way the bone responds (Fig. 33.7). In both pathological conditions the bone is less able to withstand repetitive stresses or abnormal loads. As a result, such patients are more liable to develop pathological fractures and are at increased risk of developing perioperative injury.

Neoplastic bone lesions

1. Bone can be affected by primary and secondary tumours. In primary lesions, a number of different cells of origin can be implicated, such as osteoblasts in osteogenic sarcoma and chondrocytes in chondrosarcoma.

2. Some tumours are osteosclerotic, with increased bone formation, for example, prostatic secondaries, but the majority are osteolytic. Whatever the pattern, the bone involved with such lesions is abnormal and does not follow predictable biomechanical patterns when placed under stress. As a result, the patient experiences pain and potential fracture at the point of weakness.

3. Repeated imaging can monitor the progress of such lesions, and the healing response following such treatment as radiotherapy. However, there are certain parameters which gauge the potential for impending fracture and provide information about the desirability of prophylactic surgical intervention:

a. Long bone lesion greater than 2.5 cm increases the risk.

b. Lytic destruction of more than 50% of the bone's circumference has a greater than 50% risk of fracture.

c. Persistent pain on weight-bearing despite radiotherapy treatment is an ominous signal of impending fracture.

Periosteum

1. This is a thin lining tissue which surrounds the bone. It consists of two layers when examined histologically, an outer layer and an inner cambial layer (Latin *cambium*, is the exchange layer between the bark and wood of trees), although the layers cannot be separated macroscopically. It is easily peeled off the bone except at the juxta-articular region, where it is densely adherent at the point of attachment of the joint capsule, and at the insertion of muscles and tendons. For example, the insertion of the patellar tendon into the tibial tuberosity requires sharp dissection. In childhood, the periosteum is thick but it becomes thin with age.

2. Periosteum is relatively inelastic and is therefore difficult to suture and repair. It has a rich blood supply, often with prominent blood vessels on its surface, so that it bleeds readily when incised.

3. Periosteum is the most important structure involved in bone repair, so protect it. When performing an osteotomy it may be incised by cutting hard down onto the bone with a scalpel, elevating it to separate it from the bone, followed by formal bony division, or it can be perforated at intervals using a drill or fine osteotome (Greek *osteon* = bone + *temnein* = to cut) as part of a percutaneous osteotomy.

4. Occasionally it is released circumferentially in an attempt to accelerate growth in children. It is also elevated and separated from underlying bone in infection and in neurological conditions such as spina bifida – a congenital cleft of the vertebral column with meningeal protrusion.

Bone blood supply

1. The blood supply to long bones is well defined, coming from both endosteal (within the bone) and periosteal (around the bone) surfaces. Normal blood flow is centrifugal, vessels running distally away from the

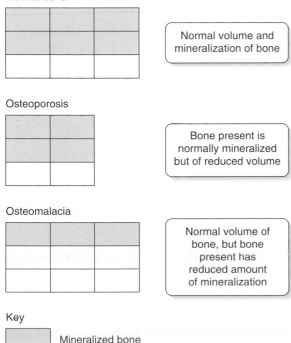

Normal bone

Normal volume and mineralization of bone

Osteoporosis

Bone present is normally mineralized but of reduced volume

Osteomalacia

Normal volume of bone, but bone present has reduced amount of mineralization

Key

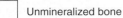

Mineralized bone

Unmineralized bone

Fig. 33.7 The volume of bone is represented by the total number of boxes. The amount of mineralized bone is represented by the dark shaded boxes.

heart. The bone receives most of its blood supply from medullary vessels.

2. Fracture disrupts the blood supply and revascularization occurs from the periosteum and surrounding soft tissues. In the early stages of repair, blood flow is predominantly centripetal (Latin *petere* = to seek; flowing proximally).

3. There are three primary components of the blood supply in long bones: the nutrient artery, metaphyseal arteries and periosteal arterioles. The diaphyseal supply is from the nutrient artery, which divides into ascending and descending medullary arteries supplying the majority of the diaphyseal cortex. The metaphysis is supplied by a rich network of metaphyseal arteries. It is much more vascular than the diaphysis and this is reflected in its ability to undergo repair following a fracture or osteotomy. The periosteal arterioles supply the outer third of the diaphyseal cortex in a patchy manner and anastomose with terminal branches of the medullary arteries.

4. The efferent vascular drainage is through large emissary veins and venae comitantes of the nutrient artery, which drain the medullary contents almost exclusively, whereas the cortex drains through cortical venous channels into periosteal venules.

5. In flat bones the blood supply is closely reflected in its periosteal attachments and is therefore tenuous in the navicular and scaphoid bones, which are at risk from avascular necrosis following fracture and dislocation. Also at risk is the head of the femur following femoral neck fracture, as it receives one-fifth of its blood supply through the ligamentum teres.

In children, haematogenous spread of osteomyelitis may occur to the joint if there is an intracapsular physis.

6. Under certain circumstances, the vascularity of bone may be increased, with an effect upon surgical procedures. In Paget's disease, described in 1877 by the London surgeon Sir James Paget (1814–1899), the increased metabolic activity induced by osteoclastic and osteoblastic activity necessitates an increased blood supply and may induce a high-output cardiac failure in the patient. The increased activity renders the bone more brittle and more liable to fracture following injury or during operation.

Certain tumours are associated with an increased blood supply. A common example that of metastatic lesions to bone from renal cell carcinoma. The leash of vessels around the deposit can cause profuse bleeding during surgical procedures.

In osteoarthritis, much of the pain is thought to be derived from the altered subchondral bone, with its hypervascularity and venous stasis.

Natural bone healing

1. Following fracture or osteotomy, bone enters a repair cycle of overlapping processes involving inflammation, haematoma formation, development of granulation tissue, callus formation and remodelling. Healing is influenced by the amount of damage, and therefore the local tissues available for repair. Callus (Latin = hard) is woven bone, cartilage, or a mixture of the two.

2. Primary callus response develops following a fracture and is initiated from the bone itself. It is short lived, lasting a few days to weeks, and sustained by bone contact. The second process is that of bridging external callus, which is a rapid process, tolerant of fracture movement and dependent on recruitment from the surrounding soft tissues. A third response, in which fibrous tissue is replaced by bone, is seen within the medulla. It is relatively independent of movement and is termed late medullary callus. The response depends on the amount of motion at the fracture site (interfragmentary strain).

3. If movement is obliterated, following, for example, rigid plate fixation, a different form of healing occurs, without intermediate callus formation. This is known as primary cortical healing. In most cases fixation reduces but does not entirely abolish strain, leading to the conversion of bridging fibrous tissue into cartilage, and, as the strain diminishes, bone is laid down. If tissue viability is poor, if there is excessive motion, a fracture gap, or if infection supervenes, healing is impaired.

Implants

Plates

1. Plate fixation involves extensive dissection of the soft tissues, with incision and elevation of the periosteum. The fracture site is exposed, the haematoma is evacuated and the periosteal circulation of the bone is interrupted. Preservation of the haematoma may be valuable, although whether the haematoma provides cellular elements contributing to fracture healing is controversial.

2. Following fracture or osteotomy, blood flow becomes centripetal and the periosteal circulation becomes dominant, primarily through dense connective tissue attachments. A plate reduces the local cortical blood supply. Blood perfusion is reduced by the close plate-to-bone contact because of periosteal damage and, by drilling through the bone for bicortical screw anchorage, both endosteal and intramedullary damage.

3. Rigid plate fixation eliminates micromotion at the fracture site, facilitating primary cortical healing. Terminal bone death is minimized and union occurs slowly, mainly by creeping cortical substitution. The plate

reduces stress on the bone and so may lead to bone atrophy, with the risk of refracture following plate removal. New low-contact compression plates inserted with minimal access may reduce the effects.

Intramedullary nails

1. A nail can be inserted without disturbing the fracture site or fracture haematoma. High intramedullary pressures may be induced while inserting the awl, guide rod and reamers and they may produce local damage and embolization. The nail is inserted down the length of the medullary canal, providing stability through areas of endosteal contact and also by the insertion of locking screws that pass through both cortices. Intramedullary nails permit more fracture motion than do compression plates, although nails vary significantly in their resistance to torsion (twisting) and to bending.

2. Reaming (Old English *ryman* = to open up) may be used to allow larger diameter nails to be inserted, increasing the contact area between the nail and the internal surface of the bone; however, although this benefits fracture stability, it can weaken the bone. Rigid nails providing stress protection may prejudice full recovery of strength.

3. Cortical reaming and nail insertion both injure the medullary vascular system, resulting in avascularity of significant portions of the diaphyseal cortex; nails inserted without preparatory reaming show more rapid revascularization.

4. Healing is more rapid than with plates, and refracture is rare. The limb reacts to medullary damage by exhibiting a significantly raised extraosseous blood supply. Primary callus response and bridging external callus both occur but medullary healing is inhibited. Reliability and speed of healing are both affected by fracture motion.

5. In animal studies the blood flow at the fracture site and within the whole bone was higher when using nails compared with plates, and it remained elevated for a long period.

External fixation

1. This can be applied without invading the fracture area. Unilateral fixators are applied with large, 5–6 mm diameter screws across the medullary canal, possibly temporarily disrupting the medullary blood flow. The bone is supported more effectively on the near cortex, referred to as 'cantilever loading'. Bridging external callus is seen more readily on the far cortex.

2. Dynamization (permitting movement within the body of the fixator within 3–6 weeks of injury) reduces the amount of fracture movement and allows slight fracture collapse, resulting in reduced pin site stresses and more rapid healing. Micromotion may speed up healing rates.

3. Fine-wire circular fixators are believed to produce less interference with the blood supply because the wires are only 1.5–2 mm in diameter. They provide an entirely different mechanical environment compared to unilateral fixators, with relatively even support for the whole bone ('beam loading'), permitting more fracture motion. Unusually, as the limb is loaded the fixator becomes stiffer, hence supporting high activity levels while controlling fracture motion. Rapid healing rates with little visible callus may be seen, perhaps reflecting a rapid medullary response unique to this device.

Osteotomy

1. There is complete transection of the bone; studies in dogs have shown a 50% decrease in blood flow at 10 min and 66% at 4 h. Following double osteotomy in the dog tibia, 80% of the intermediate fragment had vessels in the haversian canals that were derived from the endosteal circulation. Both the intermediate fragment and the bone ends showed bone resorption and new bone formation in the haversian systems.

2. In order to spare the tissues, corticotomy, a low-energy osteotomy of the cortex, preserving the local blood supply to both periosteum and medullary canal, may be used. In open corticotomy the periosteal structure is preserved. Preservation of the periosteum and intramedullary vessels are both important in the formation of new bone.

Distraction

1. Controlled mechanical bone distraction after osteotomy can produce unlimited quantities of living bone and direct the new bone formation in any plane following the vector of applied force. The new bone spontaneously bridges the gap and rapidly remodels to the normal macrostructure of the local bone.

2. Within the distraction regenerate three zones can be recognized, according to morphology and the calcium content. They are a fibrous interzone, a primary mineralization front and a new bone formation zone. Other connective tissues and skin respond to the distraction process; the pioneer Russian surgeon Gavril Ilizarov (1921–1992), working in Kurgan, Siberia, described the Law of Tension Stress: gradual traction on living tissues. As ossification occurs in the callus between the bone ends, if the bone ends are carefully and slowly distracted the callus is extended in a similar manner to growth of a physis during normal bone growth. In consequence the bone lengthens.

3. 'Law of tension stress' – gradual traction on certain living tissues creates stresses that can stimulate and maintain the regeneration of active growth. Slow, steady traction of tissues causes them to become metabolically activated, resulting in an increase in their proliferative and biosynthetic functions.

Bone cement

1. Polymethylmethacrylate (PMMA) has been used as a self-curing grout (filler) for implants since the Manchester orthopaedic surgeon Sir John Charnley (1911–1982) began replacing hips in the 1960s. Mixing the powder and liquid components induces polymerization. This is an exothermic (Greek *ex* = out + *therme* = heat) reaction, generating significant heating of local tissue and the potential for bone necrosis. This has been extensively researched as a possible cause of later implant loosening.

2. Orthopaedic surgeons are aware of the potential for cardiovascular collapse following the insertion of PMMA, especially into the femoral canal. It seems likely that the resulting elevated pressures (up to 900 mmHg) within the canal force fat and marrow contents from the bone into the circulation. These elements reach the pulmonary circulation within 2 min, initiating the aggregation of platelets and other clotting elements.

 Key point

- Cardiovascular collapse can be partially prevented by ensuring the patient is well hydrated before inserting bone cement.

> ## Summary
>
> - Have you appreciated how dynamic are the connective tissues, including bone?
> - Do you have a basic understanding of the responses of bone and connective tissues to trauma?

- Can you name some of the factors that modify the strength and growth of connective tissues, and how they act?
- Are you able to name some redundancies that function in spite of injury or disease?
- Do you appreciate the importance of preserving and restoring function resulting from injury and disease?

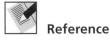 **Reference**

Henry AK 1945 Extensile exposure applied to limb surgery. Livingstone, Edinburgh, p 101

 Further reading

Aronson J, Good B, Stewart C, Harrison B, Harp JH 1990 Preliminary studies of mineralization during distraction osteogenesis. Clinical Orthopaedics 250: 43–49

Bolander ME 1994 Regulation of fracture repair and synthesis of matrix molecules. In: Brighton CT, Friedlander G, Love JM (eds) Bone formation and repair. American Academy of Orthopedic Surgeons, Rosemont, pp 186–187

McKibbin B 1978 The biology of fracture healing in long bones. Journal of Bone and Joint Surgery 60B: 150–162

O'Sullivan ME, Chao EYS, Kelly PJ 1989 The effects of fixation on fracture healing. Journal of Bone and Joint Surgery 71A: 306–310

Rhinelander FW 1968 The normal microcirculation of diaphyseal cortex and its response to fracture. Journal of Bone and Joint Surgery 50A: 784–800

Rhinelander FW 1974 The normal circulation of bone and its response to surgical intervention. Journal of Biomedical Materials Research 8: 87–90

Smith SR, Bronk JT, Kelly PJ 1990 Effect of fracture fixation on cortical bone blood flow. Journal of Orthopeadic Research 8: 471–478

Yang L, Nayagam S, Saleh M 2003 Stiffness characteristics and interfragmentary displacements with different hybrid external fixators. Clinical Biomechanics 18: 166–172

34 Postoperative care

J. J. T. Tate

Objectives

- **Understand the principles of patient management in the recovery phase immediately after surgery.**
- **Understand the general management of the surgical patient on the ward.**
- **Consider the initial management of common acute complications during the postoperative period.**

INTRODUCTION

Postoperative care of the surgical patient has three phases:

1. Immediate postoperative care (the recovery phase)
2. Care on the ward until discharge from hospital
3. Continuing care after discharge (e.g. stoma care, physiotherapy, surveillance).

The intensity of postoperative monitoring depends upon the type of surgery performed and the severity of the patient's condition.

THE RECOVERY PHASE

Basic management

Immediately after surgery patients require close monitoring, usually by one nurse per patient, in a dedicated recovery ward or area adjacent to the theatre. Monitoring of airway, breathing and circulation is the main priority, but a smooth recovery can only be achieved if pain and anxiety are relieved; monitoring the patient's overall comfort is essential. The nature of the surgery will determine the intensity of monitoring and any special precautions, but children, the elderly, patients with coexisting medical disease and patients who have had major surgery all require special care.

Management of the general comfort of the patient includes:

- Relief of pain and anxiety
- Administering mouthwashes (a dry mouth is common after general anaesthesia)
- The patient's position, including care of pressure points
- Prophylactic measures against:
  - atelectasis by encouraging deep breathing
  - venous stasis by passive leg exercises.

These steps, including the prophylactic measures, all start in the recovery area and will continue on the main ward.

Airway and breathing

Patients may have an oral airway, a nasopharyngeal airway or, occasionally, may still be intubated on arrival in recovery; all secretions must be cleared by suction and the artificial airway left until the patient can maintain his or her own airway. Breathing may be depressed and a patient hypoxic due to three factors:

- Airway obstruction
- Residual anaesthetic gases
- The depressant effects of opioids.

Oxygen is given, ideally by mask, and the oxygen saturation monitored by a pulse oximeter. Special care is needed for patients with a new tracheostomy. If there is concern about vomiting and the risk of aspiration, patients can be sat up or nursed head-up rather than supine.

Circulation

Blood pressure is recorded quarter-hourly or, after major surgery, continuously via a radial artery cannula. The pulse rate is recorded regularly and continuously monitored by a pulse oximeter. The wound and any drains are monitored for signs of reactionary bleeding.

Fluid balance

Before patients are returned to the ward their calculated fluid losses should be replaced with blood, blood products or crystalloids, and, ideally, fluid balance achieved. Monitoring of central venous pressure (CVP) can assist fluid balance management in severely ill patients or after major surgery. Urine output measurement may also provide useful information.

Core temperature

The patient's temperature is monitored, as there may be a significant drop during surgery, which should be corrected before the patient leaves the recovery room (e.g. with a space blanket). As the temperature rises, peripheral vasodilatation may occur; if not anticipated this can lead to hypotension after the patient has returned to the ward.

Special factors

Specific medical conditions and certain types of surgery will require additional monitoring. Some examples are:

- Diabetes mellitus – blood sugar monitoring
- Cardiac disease – electrocardiogram (ECG) monitor
- Orthopaedic surgery – monitoring of distal perfusion in a treated limb, position of limb, maintenance of fracture reduction, examination for peripheral nerve injury
- Neurosurgery – quarter-hourly neurological observations, intracranial pressure monitoring (intraventricular catheter or a transducer in the subarachnoid space)
- Urology – catheter output (after transurethral prostatectomy bladder irrigation is usually implemented and pulmonary oedema can develop if glycine has been absorbed into the circulation; fluid balance is particularly important)
- Vascular surgery – distal limb perfusion.

Pulse oximeter versus arterial blood gas

The pulse oximeter is an essential piece of equipment for the management of the postoperative patient. It monitors three parameters: pulse rate, pulse volume and oxygen saturation. The fingertip sensor contains two light-emitting diodes (LEDs): one red, measuring the amount of oxygenated haemoglobin, the other infrared, measuring the total amount of haemoglobin. The actual amount of oxygen carried in the blood relative to the maximum possible amount is computed – this is the oxygen saturation (SaO_2). The delivery of oxygen to the tissues depends on:

- Cardiac output
- Haemoglobin concentration
- Oxygen saturation (SaO_2).

The relationship between oxygen in the blood and SaO_2 is linear and thus easy to interpret. A fall in oxygen reaching the tissues can be detected far more rapidly with SaO_2 monitoring than by clinical observation of the lips, nailbeds or mucous membranes for cyanosis (which may only be apparent when the SaO_2 is 60–70%) or by measuring arterial blood gases. It should be noted that pulse oximetry does not indicate adequate ventilation; the SaO_2 can be normal due to a high inspired oxygen level.

Blood gases

Arterial blood gases measure pH, arterial oxygen and carbon dioxide tensions (PaO_2, $PaCO_2$), bicarbonate and base excess. These measurements are affected by many variables and can be difficult to interpret. The PaO_2 has a non-linear relationship to the oxygen content of the blood (the oxygen dissociation curve), and hence oxygen saturation is easier to use in practice.

$PaCO_2$ reflects the rate of excretion of carbon dioxide by the lungs and is inversely proportional to the ventilation (assuming constant production of carbon dioxide by the body). The base excess and bicarbonate reflect acid–base disturbances and may be used in conjunction with the $PaCO_2$ to distinguish respiratory from metabolic problems.

The recovery phase

- **Management of pain and anxiety is as important as care of airway, breathing and circulation.**
- **Restoring body temperature is important for prevention of circulation and clotting problems.**
- **SaO_2 (pulse oximeter) has a linear relationship to the amount of oxygen in the blood, giving a sensitive indication of tissue oxygenation.**

CARE ON THE WARD

Patients may be discharged from the recovery area when they are able to maintain their vital functions independently (i.e. full consciousness and stable respiratory and cardiovascular observations).

On the ward, the aim is to maintain a stable general condition and detect any complications early. Initially, closer and more frequent observation is necessary and the priorities are the same as in the recovery room. Nursing staff perform routine observations; medical staff must undertake additional, clinical monitoring dictated by the nature of the case, including daily review of drug prescriptions (Table 34.1).

General care

General care includes those measures described previously and control of pain. Early ambulation can reduce the risk of thrombotic complications. Patients who cannot mobilize require particular attention to skin care and pressure areas. Appropriate explanation of the results of the operation and the expected postoperative course should be given to the patient and relatives. The nature of the surgery or underlying disease will determine additional specific management (e.g. physiotherapy after orthopaedic surgery, stoma care for a new stoma).

Pain control

It is impossible for a patient to make a smooth recovery from surgery without adequate pain control (see Ch. 35). There has been a general shift from intermittent intramuscular analgesia to intravenous analgesia, either by continuous infusion or patient-controlled bolus, or epidural analgesia after major surgery. An epidural is particularly useful after major abdominal surgery, but insertion of an epidural catheter in patients who have received a preoperative dose of heparin for deep vein thrombosis prophylaxis is controversial and contraindicated if the patient has a coagulopathy.

For day surgery or minor operations oral analgesia is suitable and is most effective when prescribed regularly. Narcotics can still be used if required. Non-steroidal anti-inflammatory drugs (NSAIDs) are popular but must be avoided in some patients, including asthmatics and those with a history of peptic ulcer or indigestion. Rectal administration of NSAIDs to a sedated patient should only be given with preoperative consent.

Fluid balance

Fluid balance is important after major surgery and easier if a urinary catheter is in situ, allowing accurate charting of urine output. Visible fluid losses are recorded on a fluid balance chart at regular intervals (e.g. hourly for urine output, 4-hourly for nasogastric aspirations, and 12- or 24-hourly for output into drains) and totalled every 24 h. Unrecorded fluid losses (e.g. evaporation from skin and lungs, losses into hidden spaces such as the intestine, and diarrhoea) must be estimated and added to the recorded losses to calculate the patient's subsequent fluid requirements (see Ch. 9).

Table 34.1   The postoperative ward round: a daily checklist

A fresh assessment of each patient is required at each ward round, often daily but more frequently for seriously ill patients. Only a few factors may change on each occasion but all should be considered.

Look at the patient, look at the charts, look at the drug chart and communicate.

Enquire
- General comfort
- Pain control
- Thirst
- Specific symptoms

Examine
- General condition
- Respiration and chest (oxygen saturation if appropriate)
- Surgical wound
- Peripheral circulation/nerves (vascular/limb surgery)
- Drains and tubes (content, kinks or blockage, loss of vacuum)
- Pressure areas
- Drip sites

Check
- Pulse and blood pressure
- Temperature
- Urine output
- Fluid balance (assess insensible loss, e.g. sweating, diarrhoea)
- Special monitoring (e.g. diabetics – blood sugars)
- Results of blood tests/investigations

Review
- Nutrition/oral fluid and dietary intake
- Analgesia management
- Intravenous fluid prescription (volume, sodium and potassium need)
- Antibiotic prescription
- Other postoperative drugs
- Regular prescription medicines (when to start oral medication)

Inform
- What operation/treatment has been done and result
- Comment on progress over previous 24 h
- Expected course over next few days
- Results of investigations/histology
- Likely day of discharge (identify any special requirements early)

Communicate
- Receive reports from named nurse, physiotherapist, etc.
- Advise changes of management
- Advise frequency/nature of observations required
- Write in the notes

Fluid requirement

For the typical 70 kg patient, intravenous fluid requirement after operation is 2.5 litres per day, of which 0.5 litre is normal saline and the remainder 5% dextrose; potassium is added after the first 24 h once 1.5 litres of urine have been passed. Typically, the sodium requirement is 1 mmol kg^{-1} (normal saline contains 140 mmol l^{-1} of sodium) and potassium 1 mmol kg^{-1}.

If the dissection area at operation has been large, there will be a greater loss of plasma into the operation site and this may need to be replaced with colloid (e.g. Haemaccel) in the early postoperative period. In addition to these basic requirements, gastrointestinal losses are replaced volume-for-volume with normal saline with added potassium. Daily plasma urea and electrolyte measurement are advisable while the patient is dependent on intravenous fluids.

Monitoring

Clinical monitoring should include asking the patient about thirst, assessing central and peripheral perfusion, examination of dependent areas for oedema, and auscultation of the chest. Tachycardia is an important sign that can indicate fluid overload or dehydration, but is also caused by inadequate analgesia.

Patients in whom fluid balance is difficult to manage, or where there is a particular risk of cardiac failure, may require central venous pressure monitoring or even left atrial pressure recording.

Hypovolaemia

Oliguria (defined as a urine output of less than 20 ml h^{-1} in each of two consecutive hours) in postoperative patients is caused by hypovolaemia in the majority of cases, but always consider a blocked catheter or cardiac failure. Hypovolaemia may be due to:

- Unreplaced blood loss
- Loss of fluid into the gastrointestinal tract
- Loss of plasma into the wound or abdomen
- Sequestration of extracellular fluid into the 'third' space.

Blood transfusion

Haemoglobin measurement will be a guide to the need for blood transfusion unless plasma or extracellular fluid loss causes an artificially high measurement; this is most likely in the first 24 h after surgery and it is generally not necessary to monitor haemoglobin levels more than 72 h postoperatively. In a stable patient, a top-up transfusion is indicated if the haemoglobin level is less than 8 g% (determined by studies in Jehovah's Witnesses), while above this level patients should be given oral iron. An unstable patient, one who may rebleed, requires a higher threshold for transfusion of at least 10 g%. If blood transfusion is given, frequent, regular monitoring of pulse, blood pressure and temperature are routine to detect a transfusion reaction.

Complications

A major ABO incompatibility can result in an anaphylactic hypersensitivity reaction (flushing/urticaria, bronchospasm, hypotension). Incompatibility of minor factors is usually less severe and is indicated by tachycardia, pyrexia and possible rash and pruritus. The transfusion should be stopped, some blood sent for culture (both from patient and donor blood) and the remainder of the unit returned to the blood bank for further cross-matching against the patient's serum. However, if the reaction is mild it may be appropriate to give steroids or an antihistamine and to continue the transfusion (see Ch. 8).

Nutrition

Nutrition in postoperative patients is frequently poorly managed and treatment delayed. Dietary intake should be monitored in all patients, but usually only requires specific management in patents undergoing major abdominal surgery or in whom eating or swallowing is impossible. A basic indication for postoperative nutritional support is inability to eat (actual or expected) for more than 5 days. Serum protein is a crude but easily measured index of nutrition, and measurement of weight is useful over a period of time; more specific tests such as skin-fold thickness or estimation of nitrogen balance are used infrequently (see Ch. 10).

If nutritional support is required, enteral feeding is preferable, if possible, because it has a lower complication rate than parenteral nutrition. Fluid balance and electrolyte monitoring are required and treatment should be given to reduce diarrhoea, which may be precipitated by high calorie regimens. Parenteral feeding requires monitoring of the venous access point for sepsis, plasma and urinary electrolytes, blood sugar, plasma trace elements (e.g. magnesium) and liver function. The patient's fluid balance must be carefully managed.

Surgical drains
Nasogastric tubes

Nasogastric tubes drain fluid and swallowed air from the stomach and should be left on free drainage at all times with intermittent aspiration (4-hourly). There is rarely a need to leave a nasogastric tube spigoted; once drainage has fallen below 100–200 ml per day the tube can be removed.

Chest drains

Pleural drains are attached to an underwater seal because the pleural space is at subatmospheric pressure. If the lung does not expand fully, then low pressure, high volume suction may be added. When a drain is bubbling it should not be clamped because there is a danger of tension pneumothorax if the clamp is forgotten or left too long; however, it is essential that the bottle is never raised above the level of the patent's chest, as there is a risk that fluid will syphon back into the pleural cavity.

The drain is removed when:

• Bubbling has stopped for 24 h
• There is no bubbling when the patient coughs
• The daily chest X-ray shows that the lung is fully expanded.

Check X-rays should be taken at 24 and 48 h after removal of the drain.

Drains at the operative site

Drains at the operative site are used for the removal of anticipated fluid collections, not as an alternative to adequate haemostasis, and are usually simple tube drains or suction drains (check daily that the vacuum is maintained). Such drains should be removed early; if left in place they will not reduce the risk of a subsequent abscess and may introduce infection, if there is a chronic collection of fluid (such as an abscess or empyema) the drain may be left for several days to create a track. This type of drain is often removed a few centimetres at a time over several days (shortening) in an attempt to prevent the track closing too quickly; a sinogram may be used to confirm that the abscess cavity is shrinking.

Complications

All drains have similar potential complications:

• Trauma during insertion
• Failure to drain adequately due to
  – incorrect placement
  – too small size
  – blocked lumen
• Complications due to disconnection
• Introduction of infection from outside via the drain track

• Erosion by the drain of adjacent tissue
• Fracture of drain during removal (retained foreign body).

DAYCASE SURGERY

After daycase operations the postoperative period is inevitably short, but management should follow the same basic principles outlined above. Special considerations are:

• Is the patient being discharged to a suitable environment?
• Can adequate, non-parenteral pain control be achieved?
• Possible side-effects of sedation and anaesthesia.

Patients who have had a general anaesthetic or sedation must be accompanied home and should not drive for at least 24 h. Written advice and instructions should be given both to the patient and to the accompanying relative or friend.

Local anaesthetic

The main problems with local anaesthesia are systemic toxicity of the anaesthetic agent and reactionary haemorrhage if adrenaline (epinephrine) has been employed.

Toxicity

All the commonly used local anaesthetics (lidocaine (lignocaine), bupivicaine and prilocaine) are cardiotoxic. Initial symptoms are paraesthesiae around the lips, tinnitus and/or visual disturbance. These are followed by dizziness, which may progress to convulsions and cardiac arrhythmia and collapse. Such complications are prevented by strict adherence to maximum dosage schedules (Table 34.2).

Treatment of systemic toxicity is directed firstly towards maintaining ventilation (hypotension is uncommon in the absence of hypoxia):

Table 34.2	Maximum doses of anaesthetic agents	
	Plain solution (mg)	With adrenaline (epinephrine) (mg)
Lidocaine (lignocaine)	200 (20 ml of 1%)	500 (50 ml of 1%)
Bupivacaine	150 (30 ml of 0.5%)	200 (40 ml of 0.5%)
Prilocaine	400 (80 ml of 0.5%)	600 (120 ml of 0.5%)

- Give 100% oxygen and maintain the airway (by intubation if necessary)
- Control convulsions with intravenous diazepam
- Establish an ECG monitor; various arrhythmias can occur
- If cardiac arrest occurs, start with high energy (360–400 J) DC shock and continue resuscitation attempts for at least 1 h.

Sedation

For sedoanalgesia or sedation alone (e.g. endoscopy patients), particular attention is paid to monitoring respiration. During upper gastrointestinal endoscopy, delivery of oxygen by nasal spectacles is mandatory. All sedated patients should have a pulse oximeter attached during the procedure and until they are fully awake. The use of the antagonist flumazenil to reverse the sedative effects of benzodiazepines can be associated with delayed respiratory depression as the reversal agent may have a shorter half-life than the sedative itself. Midazolam, with a shorter half-life, is preferred to diazepam. All patients given sedation should be observed for at least 2 h before being sent home.

CARE AFTER HOSPITAL DISCHARGE

The key is good communication. The patient should understand what treatment he or she has had, its effect, the likely time period required to complete recovery and special restrictions on normal activity. Whenever appropriate, the relatives should also have this information. As many complications (e.g. wound infection) occur in the first week or two after hospital discharge, it is essential that the patient's general practitioner is aware of the diagnosis and treatment given and also what information the patient has received. Ensure arrangements are made to communicate histology results to the patient and plans for additional investigation or treatment have been made and explained to the patient.

Postoperative care

- **Adequate management of postoperative pain is essential.**
- **Poor management of fluid balance is probably the greatest cause of avoidable morbidity after major surgery.**

- **It is essential to know the maximum dosage for local anaesthetic agents and how to manage toxicity.**
- **Clear and concise communication with the patient and other health professionals involved in care will prevent problems and confusion.**

PROBLEMS IN THE POSTOPERATIVE PATIENT

The incidence and nature of postoperative complications depends upon the nature and extent of the operative intervention (see Ch. 36). Many are self-evident, but some specific problems are discussed below.

Cyanosis/respiratory inadequacy

The time between onset of respiratory problems and surgery may suggest the cause. In the recovery phase, it may be due to inadequate reversal of anaesthesia or excess opiates and the anaesthetist should be called.

Opiate overdosage usually presents in a drowsy patient with shallow, infrequent breaths, while airway obstruction is associated with obvious efforts to breathe, undrawn intercostal muscles and agitation.

Airway obstruction

If a patient is in respiratory distress, give verbal reassurance and 100% oxygen by mask. If cyanosed, check the pulse, as the most common cause is cardiac arrest. If breathing appears obstructed, call for anaesthetic help and:

- Inspect the mouth for foreign bodies (e.g. vomit, slipped denture and surgical swab after surgery in the mouth).
- Extend the neck and pull the jaw forward to clear the tongue from the back of the mouth and get an assistant to maintain the position.
- Insert an oral airway.
- If the patient has had a thyroidectomy, open the wound (skin and deep fascia) at the bedside.
- If the patient has had surgery in the mouth, throat or neck, or if there is no improvement with an airway in place perform a cricothyroidotomy without delay.
- Check that the patient can exhale.
- Monitor the oxygen saturation and obtain blood gases and chest X-ray as soon as possible.

Do not attempt to intubate a patient after surgery in the mouth or neck unless experienced: do a cricothyroidotomy and call an anaesthetist. In an emergency, a large-gauge intravenous cannula can be used for cricothyroidotomy but requires jet ventilation, whether the patient is breathing or not, because of the small lumen (attach a rigid oxygen line to the cannula via the barrel of a 5 ml syringe). During insertion, check that the needle is in the trachea, which may be displaced, by aspiration of air and be careful not to pass it straight through the back. The cannula can kink or displace and should be replaced as soon as possible with a purpose-made device.

Normal breathing

Cyanosis in a patient who appears to be breathing normally may be due to a problem in the lungs or circulation. Listen to the chest for bronchospasm (wheeze is absent in severe bronchospasm) and for uniform air entry. Is the patient asthmatic? Is this a hypersensitivity reaction? Loss of air entry in the upper chest suggests pneumothorax, and in the dependent part of the chest, haemothorax or pleural effusion. Has the patient had attempts at intravenous line insertion in the neck?

Acute circulatory problems that can cause cyanosis are loss of venous return (massive sudden blood loss), pump failure (myocardial infarct) and obstruction (massive pulmonary embolus). Check the blood pressure and get an ECG. Other possible causes include severe adverse drug reaction and severe sepsis (air hunger).

Hypotension

The commonest cause of hypotension in a postoperative patient is hypovolaemia, either due to inadequate fluid replacement or to bleeding. Myocardial infarction needs to be considered and excluded. Poor management of pain control, either too much or too little analgesia, may be a factor and hypotension is a side-effect of an epidural (local anaesthetic drugs may cause dilatation of the main capacitance vessels). It is difficult to confirm that an epidural is responsible without turning it off; however, treatment by volume replacement is the same whether hypotension is caused by hypovolaemia or the epidural.

An assessment of the overall clinical situation may suggest an obvious cause of hypotension in a given patient. If not:

- Increase the rate of intravenous fluids.
- Elevate the legs.
- Give oxygen up to 50% by mask.
- Obtain an ECG (dysrhythmia, acute ischaemia, signs of pulmonary embolus).

If the ECG is normal, place a central venous pressure line while giving additional intravenous fluid. Listen to the chest to exclude tension pneumothorax (chest trauma, chest surgery, surgery around the oesophageal hiatus, or failed neck line) and consider pulmonary embolus and septicaemia. If no cause is apparent, and the blood pressure responds to volume infusion, hidden blood loss is likely.

Hypertension

This may be dangerous in patients with ischaemic heart disease, cerebrovascular disease or following vascular surgery. Obtain anaesthetic assistance with the management of such patients if a cause cannot be found; the commonest causes of hypertension are inadequate control of pain and/or anxiety, urinary retention and shivering.

Postoperative infection

The patient's temperature is a basic, but crude, observation for infection. Clinical monitoring includes examination of the chest and inspection of the wound. The upper limit of normal temperature is 37°C, but there is considerable variation and occasionally a patient may be pyrexial despite a temperature below this 'magic' figure. The timing of postoperative pyrexia may suggest a cause (e.g. after a large bowel resection: pyrexia within the first 48 h – chest infection; fifth or sixth day – an anastomotic leakage or wound infection; tenth day – venous thrombosis).

If a patient develops a pyrexia, a routine 'infection screen' is carried out:

1. Examine the chest – chest X-ray; sputum for culture; ECG (if ?pulmonary embolus).
2. Examine the wound – wound swab for culture.
3. Enquire about urinary symptoms – urine culture.
4. Examine for signs of deep vein thrombosis.
5. Examine intravenous sites (phlebitis) and other catheter sites (epidural).
6. Examine pressure areas.
7. If a child – look in the ears and mouth.
8. If cause uncertain – send blood cultures; measure white cell count.

9. Consider the underlying disease (e.g. pyrexia of malignancy).
10. Consider hidden infection (e.g. subphrenic or pelvic abscess).

Delayed gastric emptying/aspiration

Abdominal surgery is frequently associated with delayed gastric emptying and impaired colonic motility, even though small bowel activity, and hence bowel sounds, may return relatively early. If there is intra-abdominal sepsis, metabolic disturbances or retroperitoneal haematoma or inflammation there may be prolonged inactivity of the small bowel also (paralytic ileus). Colonic pseudo-obstruction occurs most often in elderly patients confined to bed (e.g. after fracture or orthopaedic surgery) and postpartum. Reintroduction of diet too soon can lead to gastric dilatation with vomiting and the risk of aspiration. Monitoring nasogastric aspirates, abdominal distension and the passage of flatus determines the timing of reintroduction of normal diet. However, a restricted intake of oral fluids (30 ml h^{-1}) is permissible almost without exception, and increases patient comfort.

Gastric aspiration can be life-threatening:

- Place the patient head-down in the recovery position.
- Suction out the mouth.
- Give 100% oxygen by mask.
- Pass a nasogastric tube to empty the stomach.
- Examine for bronchospasm – if present, give nebulized salbutamol ± intravenous aminophylline and consider intubation and ventilation.
- Obtain chest X-ray.
- Arrange early chest physiotherapy.

Steroids are not thought to be helpful.

Summary

- Postoperative care is divided into three phases.
- The recovery phase is the immediate care of patients after surgery until they can maintain all vital functions independently.
- The second phase is care on the ward, during which the three most important general considerations are pain control, fluid balance management and nutrition.
- The third phase of care follows discharge from hospital and includes consideration of appropriate follow-up and/or surveillence.
- The intensity of monitoring in the postoperative phase depends on the severity of disease and/or the nature of surgery.
- Many specialized features of postoperative care are determined by the type of operation.
- Good communication is essential throughout postoperative care to ensure the best outcome.

 Further reading

In addition to the chapters in this book referred to in the text, several pocket-sized texts aimed at trainee anaesthetists are available and provide useful guidelines on the management of acute postoperative problems, for example:

Eaton JM, Fielden JM, Wilson ME Anaesthesia action plans. Abbott Laboratories Ltd, Abbott House, Norden Road, Maidenhead, Berks SL6 4XE

35 Management of postoperative pain

V. Sodhi, R. Fernando

Objectives

- Define the pathophysiology of pain.
- Define the effects of pain on the postoperative patient.
- Discuss pharmacological and non-pharmacological methods of analgesia.
- Discuss the assessment of postoperative pain.
- Discuss the causes and treatment of postoperative nausea and vomiting.

INTRODUCTION

Key points

- Up to 75% of postoperative patients experience moderate to severe pain.
- In many cases this pain is not relieved adequately.

A joint working party was set up by the Royal College of Surgeons and College of Anaesthetists in 1990 to address these findings. They concluded that the main failures were:

- That postoperative pain is given low priority in ward regimens
- Lack of education among medical and nursing staff
- Lack of provision of responsible personnel to manage postoperative pain.

Despite some advances in our understanding of the physiology of acute pain and the introduction of some new analgesics, improvements in the quality of acute pain management in the past 10 years have tended to focus on using existing drugs and techniques more effectively. Better postoperative pain control has been demonstrated following the sequential introduction of a staff education programme, pain scoring and a more proactive regimen for administering intramuscular morphine. Further, although less dramatic, improvements were seen when the more expensive 'high tech' interventions, such as patient-controlled analgesia (PCA) and epidural infusion analgesia were added.

WHAT IS PAIN?

The International Association for the Study of Pain (IASP) defined pain as 'an unpleasant sensory and emotional experience associated with actual or potential tissue damage'. This definition is important, as it states that pain is never only a physical sensation but always ultimately a psychological event, and responses to a given stimulus are variable between individuals. Pain perception threshold is defined as the least experience of pain that a subject can recognize. It is highly reproducible in different individuals and in the same individual at different times. Pain tolerance threshold, defined as the greatest level of pain that the subject is prepared to tolerate, is, in contrast, highly variable. That is, it can vary from person to person and within the same individual on different occasions. It is highly dependent on psychological variables, including cultural factors, past experience and the meaning of the pain for the individual

HOW DOES POSTOPERATIVE PAIN ARISE?

Pain involves four physiological processes: transduction, transmission, modulation and perception. Pain begins when local tissue damage, a noxious stimulus, occurs during surgery, causing the release of inflammatory substances (prostaglandins, histamine, serotonin, bradykinin and substance P). This leads to the generation of electrical impulses (transduction) at peripheral sensory nerve endings, or nociceptors. These electrical impulses are conducted by nerve fibres (A-delta and C fibres) to the spinal cord (transmission). Further relay to the higher brain centres can be modified within the spinal cord (modulation) before an individual perceives a painful stimulus (perception). Therefore pain can, in theory, be *blocked* at various levels in this complex chain. Non-steroidal anti-inflammatory drugs (NSAIDs) can reduce the peripheral inflammatory response by reducing prostaglandin production. Local anaesthetic drugs injected into the epi-dural or subarachnoid spaces can block impulses to the spinal cord by acting on spinal nerve roots. Opioids can produce analgesia through modulation by binding to opioid receptors in the spinal cord and other higher brain centres such as the periaqueductal grey, the nucleus raphe magnus and the thalamus, whereas binding to opioid receptors in the cerebral cortex can affect the perception of pain (Fig. 35.1).

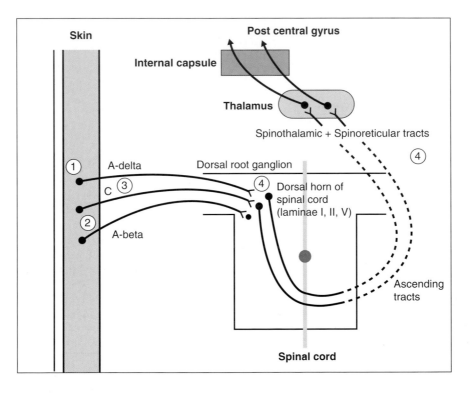

Site of action	Analgesic/effect
1. *Nocioceptors in skin and subcutaneous tissues* These receptors are stimulated by inflammatory substances, e.g. prostaglandins	NSAIDS, e.g. diclofenac, ibuprofen, ketorolac, block pathways involved in the formation of inflammatory agents
2. *A-beta fibres* Stimulation of these fibres inhibits transmission of pain to higher centres	Transcutaneous electrical nerve stimulation (TENS); stimulates A-beta fibres
3. *Primary afferent neurons (A-delta, C fibres)* Transmit impulses from nocioceptors to the spinal cord	Local anaesthetics, e.g. lidocaine, bupivacaine, ropivacaine. Block the transmission of impulses along neurons
4. *Dorsal horn of spinal cord and higher centres* Further relay/transmission of painful stimuli to the cerebral cortex	Opioids, e.g. morphine, pethidine, diamorphine, fentanyl, act as agonists at opioid receptors [also ketamine]

Fig. 35.1 Sites of action of common analgesics.

WHY SHOULD WE TREAT POSTOPERATIVE PAIN?

Apart from the humanitarian aspect, it is accepted that effective postoperative pain relief is fundamental to good quality patient care and is a legitimate therapeutic goal. There is increasing evidence relating good postoperative analgesia to reduced clinical morbidity. Some authorities suggest that there may be economic benefits associated with enhanced patient well-being and early rehabilitation. There are also several physiological reasons for treating postoperative pain.

Respiratory effects

Surgery involving the upper abdomen or chest reduces vital capacity, functional residual capacity and the ability to cough and deep breathe. This in turn can lead to retention of secretions, atelectasis and pneumonia. Inadequately treated pain aggravates these changes, while analgesia improves respiratory function.

Cardiovascular effects

Pain causes an increase in sympathetic output (tachycardia, hypertension and increasing blood catecholamines), which leads to increasing myocardial oxygen demand, which may in turn increase the risk of postoperative myocardial ischaemia, especially in those patients with pre-existing cardiac disease.

Neuroendocrine effects

The stress response to surgery and pain includes the secretion of catecholamines and catabolic hormones. This increases metabolism and oxygen consumption and promotes sodium and water retention.

Effects on mobilization

Mobilization of a patient in the postoperative period may be delayed if the patient is experiencing pain. This may in turn increase the risk of developing a deep vein thrombosis and also prolong hospital stay.

METHODS AVAILABLE TO TREAT POSTOPERATIVE PAIN

NON-PHARMACOLOGICAL

Preoperative counselling

The management of postoperative pain does not begin after the completion of surgery. Therefore inform your patient *preoperatively* as to the nature of the operation, likely postoperative pain and methods of analgesia available. Ideally, assess each patient jointly with the anaesthetist and a member of the nursing staff, to discuss the site and nature of the surgery (Table 35.1), the extent of the incision and the physiological and psychological make-up of the patient, which are all relevant in planning intraoperative and postoperative analgesia. Once these things have been ascertained, the various methods available for postoperative analgesia (including opioids, NSAIDs, isolated nerve blocks and epidural and spinal anaesthesia and analgesia) can be discussed between the patient and medical staff in order to reach a mutually agreeable postoperative treatment plan.

Transcutanenous electrical nerve stimulation (TENS)

A TENS machine consists of a pulse generator, an amplifier and a system of electrodes. It acts by stimulating afferent myelinated (A-beta) nerve fibres at a rate of 70 Hz. This activates inhibitory circuits within the spinal cord that reduce the transmission of painful nerve impulses to the higher cortical centres, thereby theoretically reducing the level of postoperative pain. However, in a systematic review of studies of TENS in postoperative pain relief, 15 out of 17 randomized control trials found no benefit compared with placebo. TENS has been shown to exert maximal relief in neurogenic pain, which is experienced in phantom limb pain and following nerve damage.

Acupuncture

Acupuncture has been clinically evaluated in postoperative patients. Although there is some variability in the way in which acupuncture is administered, there are a number of studies that suggest that it reduces pain and analgesic consumption after dental and abdominal surgery.

Other methods

Massage, hypnosis or application of superficial heat or cold are sometimes used.

Table 35.1 Pain associated with different surgical procedures (decreasing order of severity)

- Thoracic surgery
- Upper abdominal surgery
- Lower abdominal surgery
- Inguinal and femoral hernia repair
- Head/neck/limb surgery

Key point

- Although there is little evidence to support the effectiveness of unconventional methods, certain patients do derive some benefit from them, so do not dismiss them without consideration.

PHARMACOLOGICAL

In the majority of cases, acute pain is managed solely with drugs. There is good evidence that patients benefit from the use of multimodal, or balanced, analgesia after surgery. This involves the use of a variety of different classes of analgesics in combination, perhaps given by different routes, to achieve pain relief with a reduction in the incidence and severity of side-effects.

Paracetamol

Paracetamol is effective for mild to moderate pain, and as an adjunct to opioids in more severe pain. It has both analgesic and antipyretic effects but is not thought to be anti-inflammatory. Although there remains some controversy regarding its mechanism of action, it is generally thought to act by inhibiting the cyclo-oxygenase enzyme in the central nervous system, while sparing peripheral prostaglandin production. It is rapidly absorbed from the gut, and peak plasma levels are reached 30–60 min after oral administration. Paracetamol is metabolized in the liver and excreted by the kidneys, thus its dose should be decreased in renal and hepatic impairment. Contraindications include acute liver disease, alcohol-induced liver disease and glucose-6-phosphate dehydrogenase deficiency. Oral paracetamol is more effective when combined with other compounds such as codeine, dihydrocodeine or dextropropoxyphene. Numerous different compound preparations are available.

Key point

- Be careful to avoid inadvertent overdose of paracetamol when prescribing by mixing different compound preparations.

If the oral route is inappropriate, paracetamol may be given rectally. In some European countries the drug is given intravenously, as the precursor propacetamol, 2 g of which is converted to 1 g of paracetamol. Studies have shown propacetamol to be a more effective postoperative analgesic than paracetamol. A recent study demonstrated a 46% decrease in opioid requirement in orthopaedic patients given regular propacetamol.

NSAIDs

Sodium salicylate, a chemical manipulation of the glycoside salicin obtained from extracts of willow bark, was introduced in 1875 to treat rheumatic fever. Acetylsalicylic acid (aspirin) was introduced about 25 years later and since then numerous NSAIDs have been marketed, including diclofenac, ibuprofen and ketorolac.

NSAIDs do not relieve severe pain when used alone, but they are valuable in multimodal analgesia because they decrease opioid requirement and improve the quality of opioid analgesia. They have the benefit of improved analgesia without sedation or respiratory depression, and are more effective for the pain associated with movement than opioids. There is no evidence that NSAIDs given rectally or by injection perform any better or more rapidly than the same dose given orally. These routes become appropriate when the patient cannot swallow or absorb drugs from the gastrointestinal tract.

Key point

- The adverse effects of NSAIDs are potentially serious, and it is imperative that you respect any contraindications to their use.

The most important adverse effects for surgical patients are:

- Gastric ulceration – avoid NSAIDs in patients with symptoms of gastrointestinal intolerance and ulceration.
- Nephrotoxicity – risk factors include concomitant use of nephrotoxic antibiotics (e.g. gentamicin), increased intra-abdominal pressure (e.g. at laparoscopy), hypovolaemia and age greater than 65 years.
- Impaired haemostasis – NSAIDs inhibit the production of prostaglandin thromboxane A_2 within platelets, resulting in reduced platelet aggregation. They may also increase the risk of bleeding.
- Aspirin-induced asthma – NSAIDs may induce bronchospasm in susceptible patients.

NSAIDs block the synthesis of prostaglandins by inhibiting the enzyme cyclo-oxygenase, of which there are at least two isoenzymes, COX 1 and COX 2. Research has shown that COX 1 synthesizes prostaglandins responsible for physiological housekeeping functions, which include gastrointestinal and renal protection. COX 2, on the other hand, is responsible for the biosynthesis of inflammatory prostaglandins. Thus it would seem logical that by selectively inhibiting COX 2 it would be possible to develop an NSAID which retained the anti-inflammatory, analgesic and antipyretic actions required, without the undesirable side-effects of gastric irritation and renal injury. Two highly selective COX 2 inhibitors (celecoxib, rofecoxib) are now available, and have been shown to cause significantly less gastric mucosal injury than non-selective NSAIDs in patients without gastrointestinal pathology. However, some caution has been expressed over these findings. Chronic treatment with selective COX 2 inhibitors in patients with pre-existing gastrointestinal injury or inflammation may show a significant increase in damage. COX 2 appears to have an important role in promoting the healing of ulcers. The overall effectiveness of this group of drugs therefore awaits the outcome of long-term trials.

Opioids

The analgesic properties of opium were first described over 6000 years ago, and opioids are still the first-line treatment for severe postoperative pain in most patients. They act at opioid receptors in the spinal cord and higher brain centres to produce analgesia. The three main subtypes of receptor have most recently been classified as OP1, OP2 and OP3 (formerly δ, κ and μ, respectively). Opioids mimic endogenous opioid peptides at these receptors, causing their activation within the central nervous system. This decreases the activity of the dorsal horn relay neurons that transmit painful stimuli, thereby reducing the transmission of these stimuli to higher centres and producing analgesia. Activation of the receptors also causes the unwanted side-effects of opioids, namely, itching, sedation, respiratory depression, nausea and vomiting, euphoria or dysphoria and bladder dysfunction.

Opioids may be administered orally, intramuscularly, intravenously or centrally (into the epidural or subarachnoid space by an anaesthetist). Although novel techniques such as transdermal, inhalational and rectal administration of opioids have been used, and may offer certain advantages over conventional routes, their place in mainstream postoperative care is unproven.

The *oral route* for opioids is not recommended initially after major surgery for the following reasons:

- The use of opioids during general anaesthesia can lead to postoperative nausea and vomiting and delayed gastric emptying.
- Intra-abdominal surgery can result in postoperative ileus.

- Orally absorbed opioids from the gut reach the liver, via the splanchnic blood flow, where they are highly metabolized (first-pass metabolism), causing insufficient plasma concentrations of drug, e.g. 70% of orally administered morphine is eliminated through first-pass metabolism. Pethidine, morphine and codeine are all available as oral preparations.

The *intramuscular route* is the traditional method of administration. It is convenient and is associated with few side-effects, although the degree of analgesia varies between patients. Up to 40% of patients on a p.r.n. intramuscular opioid regimen may have inadequate pain relief. The dose prescribed should be based on the patient's age and medical condition. The onset of analgesia following intramuscular morphine begins after about 20 min, with a peak effect at about 60 min. With careful patient selection, and nursing staff trained to use this administration technique correctly, intramuscular opioids can thus be highly effective.

Key point

- **Take care when administering multiple doses of intramuscular opioids to shocked patients with poor peripheral perfusion. A large depot of opioid can accumulate intramuscularly, to be later released into the bloodstream when the peripheral circulation is restored, with unpredictable and often dangerous results.**

Morphine, diamorphine and pethidine are also commonly administered via the *intravenous route*. Intermittent intravenous bolus doses allow titration to effect, although care must be taken not to 'overshoot'. The peak effect of intravenously injected morphine is reached at about 15 min, and most of the effect by 5 min. Thus incremental titration with a 1–2 mg bolus every 5 min generally represents the best compromise between rapid pain relief and safety. Continuous infusion of opioid can abolish the wide swings in plasma drug concentration found with the intramuscular route and allow adjustment of the rate to the individual needs of a patient. Unfortunately, plasma drug concentrations may continue to increase with such regimens, leading to sedation and respiratory depression.

Key points

- **Side-effects of opioids are reversed by the drug naloxone, which should always be available on the ward.**

- **Optimum safe analgesia requires reliable infusion devices, frequent assessment and monitoring, with appropriate adjustment of the infusion rate. In UK practice, this level of care may not always be achievable in a general ward setting.**

Intravenous opioid patient-controlled analgesia (PCA) was developed to address the need for an improved mode of administering standard opioids. The first demonstration of a PCA machine was in 1976 at the Welsh National School of Medicine, and this became the first commercially available PCA machine, 'The Cardiff Palliator'. Modern PCA regimens have been shown to provide greater patient satisfaction and improved ventilation compared with other conventional routes of opioid administration.

PCA is superior to both intramuscular and continuous infusion routes because it allows the patient to self-administer small doses of opioid when pain occurs. PCA is administered using a special microprocessor-controlled pump which is triggered by depressing a button held in the patient's hand. When triggered, a preset amount (the *bolus* dose) is delivered to the patient, usually via a separate intravenous line. A timer prevents the administration of another bolus for a specified period (the *lock-out interval*). Before PCA is started, a loading dose of opioid must be given to achieve adequate analgesia. Background infusions of opioid are no longer used with PCA because of increasing side-effects. From a safety aspect, if patients become oversedated on PCA, they cannot give themselves another bolus. This will lead to a fall in plasma opioid concentration to safer levels. Regardless of this, regular monitoring of patients with PCA is essential. Naloxone should once again be available to treat respiratory depression and excessive sedation.

Patient selection is again an important factor in the effectiveness of PCA. The patient must have adequate preoperative instruction in its use, and be mentally able to understand the concept of self-administration of pain relief, as well as be physically able to press the button to activate the device.

PCA is suitable for many patients:

- After major surgery and who are fasting
- With marked 'incident pain' (e.g. pain associated with physiotherapy or dressing changes)
- During acute episodic pain (e.g. vaso-occlusive sickle cell crisis)
- When intramuscular injections are contraindicated (e.g. coagulopathy).

Relative contraindications for use of PCA are:

- History of illicit drug abuse
- Major metabolic disorders (e.g. sepsis) or severe fluid and electrolyte abnormalities

- End-stage renal or hepatic disease
- Severe chronic obstructive airways disease
- Sleep apnoea.

Miscellaneous routes of opioid administration

Transdermal. Fentanyl, a potent short-acting opioid, has been used in a drug-containing patch which adheres to the skin. The drug diffuses through the skin and into the bloodstream. Unfortunately the dose cannot be titrated to the patient's needs and it may take several hours to achieve adequate pain relief.

Sublingual. Since the drug is delivered directly into the bloodstream via the sublingual route, first-pass metabolism is avoided. Sublingual buprenorphine, a partial agonist, is available, but has a 20% incidence of nausea and vomiting and a 50% incidence of sedation or drowsiness.

Rectal. The rectal route is useful for providing a high systemic bioavailability of drugs that have a low oral bioavailability. Absorption, however, is slow, with peak concentrations being reached 3–4 h after administration. Pethidine and pentazocine are commonly administered by this route in Europe.

Subcutaneous. Morphine is commonly administered by the subcutaneous route in cancer patients and is occasionally used for postoperative pain. This route is better tolerated than the intramuscular route of administration but the entry site must be changed every 24–48 h to avoid infection, and rapid titration of the dose of drug against patient response is difficult to achieve.

Nebulizer. Morphine, diamorphine and fentanyl have all been administered as nebulized solutions, with the advantage that the lungs can provide a large surface area on to which the opioids can be rapidly absorbed; however, systemic absorption is variable, probably because an indeterminate amount of the agent is swallowed by the patient.

Intra-articular. In orthopaedic surgery, morphine may be of benefit by binding to opioid receptors that are present in inflamed tissue formed after injury within the joint spaces. Systematic review of the literature has so far failed to reveal evidence of efficacy for this route of administration.

Epidural and spinal (intrathecal). These routes are discussed below.

Tramadol – a new opioid

Tramadol is a synthetic analgesic, which has been used in Germany for over 20 years, but has only been available in the UK since 1994. It acts as a weak agonist at some opioid receptors, but also has important non-opioid and central nervous system effects via noradrenergic and serotoninergic pathways. It can therefore be classified as both an opioid and a non-opioid analgesic. When given parenterally, tramadol produces equivalent analgesia to morphine, except in severe postoperative pain, when it has been shown to be equipotent to pethidine. The advantage of tramadol is that it is analgesic with minimal respiratory depression, sedation, gastrointestinal stasis or abuse potential. Its disadvantages are its relative expense and side-effects, including dizziness, nausea, dry mouth and sweating. It may also lower seizure threshold.

Relative efficacy of commonly used oral drugs and intramuscular morphine

Relative analgesic efficacy can be expressed in terms of the number needed to treat (NNT); that is, the number of patients who need to receive the active drug for one to achieve at least 50% relief of pain compared with placebo over a treatment period of 6 h. For analgesics to be considered effective they require an NNT of 2–3 or less. Table 35.2 shows the relative efficacy of some common analgesics. The results have been gleaned from many meta-analyses of hundreds of clinical trials involving thousands of patients. The results should, however, be interpreted with some caution as they may hide effects such as non-standardization in the pain being treated.

Local anaesthetics and regional anaesthesia

The use of local anaesthetics for the treatment of acute pain can be traced back to the time of the Pharaohs. Hieroglyphics show that the ancient Egyptians used a topical substance to ease the pain of circumcision. Local anaesthetic (LA) drugs (e.g. bupivacaine, ropivacaine and lidocaine (lignocaine)) are sodium channel blockers and as such prevent the propagation of nerve impulses when applied to peripheral nerves or nerve roots. Sensory and sympathetic nerve fibres are blocked by smaller amounts of LA than are motor nerves. In the treatment of postoperative pain, LA drugs can be used in many ways:

- Local wound infiltration (e.g. after an inguinal hernia repair)
- Injection close to a peripheral nerve (e.g. digital nerves in a ring block)
- Injection close to a plexus of nerves (e.g. brachial plexus in an axillary block)
- May be used to provide central neural blockade (e.g. a spinal or epidural).

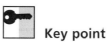

Key point

- **All local anaesthetic drugs can cause toxic effects if given in large doses or if accidental intravascular injection occurs. Central nervous system and cardiovascular toxicity can result in restlessness, hypotension, convulsions, cardiac arrhythmias and even cardiorespiratory arrest.**

Suggested safe maximum doses of LA are 2 mg kg^{-1} for plain bupivacaine and 3 mg kg^{-1} for plain lidocaine. LA solutions are also available with small amounts of adrenaline (epinephrine) (e.g. 1 in 200 000), which, acting as a vasoconstrictor due to its action on alpha-1 receptors, reduces the absorption of the LA, thereby allowing larger volumes of LA to be given. Adrenaline (epinephrine) has also been found to act on alpha-2 receptors in the spinal cord, which helps to potentiate the analgesic effect of local anaesthetics at spinal cord level.

Key point

- **Remember that injection of adrenaline (epinephrine)-containing solutions is *absolutely* contraindicated in areas supplied by end arteries, such as the fingers, toes and the penis, as prolonged ischaemia may lead to tissue necrosis.**

Bupivacaine is the most commonly used LA drug for both central and peripheral nerve blockade by virtue of its relatively long duration of action (2–3 h). It is prepared commercially as a racemic mixture of its R and S isomers.

Table 35.2	Relative efficacy of common analgesics
Analgesic	Number needed to treat
Paracetamol 1 g	4.6
Paracetamol 1 g + codeine 60 mg	3
Codeine 60 mg	18
Dihydrocodeine 30 mg	10
Tramadol 50 mg	8.9
Tramadol 100 mg	4.8
Tramadol 150 mg	2.9
Diclofenac 50 mg	2.3
Diclofenac 100 mg	2.1
Ibuprofen 200 mg	5.5
Ibuprofen 400 mg	2.9
Morphine 10 mg (single i.m. dose)	2.9

The R isomer is thought to be responsible for the main drawbacks of bupivacaine, that is its greater potential for cardiac and central nervous system toxicity, and the fact it can also cause profound motor block in high concentration. The drive within the pharmaceutical industry to produce single isomer drugs with improved safety has resulted in the manufacture of two new LA drugs, ropivacaine and levobupivacaine.

Ropivacaine is the S isomer of the propyl homologue of bupivacaine, and was claimed by its manufacturers to be less cardiotoxic than its parent drug, and also to have a more selective blockade on A-delta and C fibres, producing less motor blockade. However, further research has shown that it is about 40% less potent than racemic bupivacaine, so that in equipotent doses there may be no significant difference between them.

Levobupivacaine is the S isomer of bupivacaine itself, and has a more favourable safety profile in laboratory testing than the racemate. Clinical trials have shown it to have similar potency to racemic bupivacaine.

Epidural analgesia

The epidural space is a fat-filled space within the spinal canal. Anaesthetists inject local anaesthetics into this space, and, by doing so, block nerve root transmission of pain. Epidural opioids can also modulate pain pathways once within the epidural space by diffusion through the dura mater into the cerebrospinal fluid (CSF) and so to the opioid receptors of the spinal cord. A continuous epidural infusion using an indwelling epidural catheter, through which drugs are given for postoperative analgesia, is the most common catheter technique used for acute pain.

Most hospitals in the UK nowadays use epidural infusions consisting of combinations of low dose LA (e.g. bupivacaine 0.1%) and opioid (e.g. fentanyl 0.0002% or 2 μg ml⁻¹). Such low dose combinations are synergistic. Side-effects related to epidural opioids alone include nausea and vomiting, pruritus, sedation and delayed respiratory depression. Low dose mixtures, by reducing the amount of both LA and opioid, actually reduce the side-effects of both drugs. However, monitoring of the patient is still important. Naloxone should once again be available to reverse opioid side-effects such as excessive sedation and respiratory depression. Typically, patients receiving low dose LA plus opioid epidural infusions have superior analgesia, improved cardiovascular stability, and the ability to mobilize due to a reduction in motor block. A relatively novel method of epidural pain relief, which may become more common, is patient-controlled epidural analgesia (PCEA). Similar to the PCA, it allows the patient to titrate the analgesia required. The same low dose mixture of bupivacaine and fentanyl can be used for a PCEA regimen.

Indications for epidural analgesia include:

- Surgery (intraoperative and postoperative)
- Trauma (especially fractured ribs or pelvis)
- Labour pain
- Acute ischaemic pain
- Severe angina not controlled by conventional means (seldom used but some papers have shown a clear benefit).

Absolute contraindications are patient refusal, allergy to LA drugs, infection at the site of insertion, and lack of resuscitation equipment or skills. Relative contraindications require an assessment of the individual's risk and benefit, and include hypovolaemia, coexisting neurological disease, coagulopathy and compartment syndrome.

The benefits of epidural analgesia include:

- Effective analgesia (especially thoracic and major abdominal surgery)
- Reduced opioid requirement
- Reduction in the stress response after surgery
- Reduction in the incidence of deep vein thrombosis and pulmonary embolism
- An earlier return of gastrointestinal function after abdominal surgery
- Reduction in mortality and serious morbidity postoperatively.

There are, however, several complications that may arise following epidural analgesia:

1. *Cardiovascular.* The LA causes a sympathetic block, which can result in hypotension due to peripheral vasodilatation. If the cardiac sympathetic fibres (T1–T4) are involved, this can cause bradycardia and reduced contractility. This obviously causes reduced cardiac output and further contributes to hypotension.

2. *Respiratory.* Motor blockade of the intercostal muscles causes respiratory depression, and may cause respiratory arrest. Epidural morphine can cause late onset respiratory depression (up to 24 h after administration), as it is the least lipophilic of the epidural opioids and hence takes the longest time to diffuse through the dura mater.

3. *Dural puncture.* This may be caused by the epidural needle or catheter and, if not recognized, can result in extensive or total spinal block, which may require cardiorespiratory support. Leakage of CSF at the puncture site can lead to 'postdural puncture headache'.

4. *Infection.* This is uncommon but can result in meningitis; thus strict asepsis during epidural insertion by the anaesthetist is mandatory.

5. *Spinal haematoma.* This is a rare but potentially devastating complication. It may occur spontaneously or be triggered by antiplatelet or anticoagulation therapy.

Although it is difficult to determine the incidence rate accurately, a rate of 1/150 000 for epidurals and 1/220 000 for spinals has been quoted. This risk increases if there is a haemostatic abnormality or there has been difficulty with needle insertion (87% of reported cases of spinal haematoma had one of these problems). The signs and symptoms of spinal haematoma are:

a. Increasing motor block
b. Increasing sensory block
c. Back pain.

If spinal haematoma is suspected, an urgent CT or MRI scan and a neurosurgical opinion must be obtained. If a haematoma is present, a laminectomy is required to decompress the spinal cord and prevent or limit permanent neurological damage. (Note that epidural abscess presents in a similar fashion, with the additional signs of fever and a raised white cell count. Investigation and management are similar to those for spinal haematoma.)

Key point

- Successful acute pain management with epidural catheters requires regular assessment of the patient to detect signs of any complications early. Large audits of closely supervised epidural analgesia show the safety of the technique to be equivalent to traditional analgesic methods when coordinated by an acute pain service, with appropriate patient observations and monitoring.

Epidurals and thromboprophylaxis. Patients at risk of venous thrombosis postoperatively often require regular subcutaneous injections of heparin. Although unfractionated heparin is still used, there is a growing move towards the use of low molecular weight heparins (LMWH), e.g. dalteparin and enoxaparin. Guidelines have therefore been drawn up to deal with the obvious safety issues regarding the siting and removal of epidural catheters in these patients. It is imperative that the nursing and medical staff caring for the patient are aware of these recommendations:

- *Low dose (unfractionated) heparin.* Following administration of low dose heparin, there should be a minimum of 4 h before the epidural is sited. A minimum of 1 h is recommended following the siting, or removal, of an epidural catheter before low dose heparin is given.
- *LMWH.* An interval of **10–12 h** is required after LMWH before performing epidural blockade. The recommended interval between epidural blockade and giving LMWH is 4 h. This 4 h interval also applies to catheter removal.

It is accepted that aspirin and NSAID therapy per se do not increase risk, but in combination with low dose heparin or the increasingly used low molecular weight heparins, the risk of spinal haematoma may potentially increase.

A *caudal epidural* is a single shot epidural injection via the sacral hiatus (sacrococcygeal membrane), which can be used to provide perineal analgesia for a limited period. It is most commonly used in children for postoperative pain relief after circumcision, and for some gynaecological procedures.

Spinal analgesia

Local anaesthetic drugs with or without an opioid may be administered intrathecally as a 'single shot' spinal injection. An opioid such as morphine or diamorphine may provide useful postoperative analgesia for up to 12–24 h. Side-effects and complications are similar to epidural analgesia. Intrathecal (spinal) catheters are available, but owing to some case reports of cauda equina syndrome and arachnoiditis, they are not widely used in the UK.

Methods of treating postoperative pain

- Preoperative patient counselling and education.
- Administration of opioids by various routes.
- Wound infiltration and regional blockade with local anaesthetics.
- Non-steroidal anti-inflammatory agents.

Pre-emptive analgesia

A hypothesis exists that surgery, which produces a barrage of pain signals to the spinal cord, is a 'priming' mechanism which sensitizes the central nervous system. This is said to lead to enhanced postoperative pain. The rationale behind several studies is that, by providing presurgery, or pre-emptive, analgesia using parenteral opioids, regional blocks or NSAIDs, either individually or in combination, these sensitizing neuroplastic changes can be prevented within the spinal cord, leading to diminished postoperative analgesic requirements. Therefore the concept of pre-emptive analgesia may have implications in reducing not only acute postoperative pain, but also chronic pain states such as post-thoracotomy chest wall pain and postamputation lower limb stump pain. Taken to an extreme, a single dose of analgesic drug administered before surgery could theoretically abolish postoperative pain. Unfortunately, no current study proves the existence of pre-emptive analgesia in humans.

Specific patient groups

Day surgical patients

The ability to perform increasingly complex surgery on a daycase basis highlights the need for appropriate screening, selection, preoperative preparation, treatment and discharge of these patients. The brevity of the patient's hospitalization and contact with healthcare professionals make adequate pain management a particular challenge.

Pharmacological options for postoperative analgesia include opioids, NSAIDs and local anaesthetics. Try if possible to prescribe opioids with shorter half-lives, to avoid side-effects which may delay discharge from hospital. The use of NSAIDs may reduce postoperative opioid requirements and offer a better tolerability profile, and is highly recommended after ambulatory surgery. The use of LA drugs in laparoscopic surgery, e.g. in wound infiltration or intraperitoneally at the time of operation, is also effective in the treatment of postoperative pain, and can produce a prolonged analgesic effect. Once again, multimodal analgesia has been shown to be more effective in day surgical patients than any of these agents administered alone.

Elderly patients

When treating pain in the elderly, you must appreciate their generally reduced reserve and high incidence of concomitant disease and polypharmacy. Use NSAIDs with caution, as the elderly have an increased incidence of gastric and renal toxicity. Consider coadministration of a proton pump inhibitor (e.g. omeprazole) if gastric ulceration is of particular concern. Opioids are effective, with patients experiencing a higher peak and longer duration of pain relief, but remember that these patients are more sensitive to sedation and respiratory depression – probably as a result of altered drug distribution and excretion.

 Key point

• **Titrate opioid dosage carefully in the elderly to take into account analgesic effects and side-effects, including possible cognitive impairment.**

Children

Preparation of the patient starts at home, as psychological support may decrease anxiety and fear of surgical procedures. The presence of parents or carers in the anaesthetic room decreases postoperative pain and reduces the risk of adverse psychological sequelae. Make sure that drugs are given by the least painful route, and analgesic efficacy is assessed at regular intervals. It has been clearly demonstrated that children as young as 5 years old can understand the principles and workings of a PCA device.

Opioid tolerance and addiction

Tolerance describes the decrease in efficacy of a drug as a result of its previous administration. This is manifest as a high requirement for opioid analgesia and relative resistance to side-effects. Patients taking chronic opioid therapy require significantly increased doses of opiate in the acute situation. If the oral route is available, continue chronic oral opiates, with parenteral supplementation as required. Use non-opioid alternatives, if at all possible, as adjuncts or even as sole therapy.

 Key point

• **Surgical review is warranted if opioid requirements appear to increase rapidly, in order to rule out any surgical complication.**

Opioid addiction is unlikely to occur following the use of opioids for postoperative pain in opioid naïve patients. However, when treating patients with known opioid dependence or addiction it is important to realize that pain-scoring systems are unreliable. In patients still using opioids, PCA may be advantageous, as it allows the use of high doses of opioids and may reduce confrontation with staff members. Background infusions are a reasonable way of delivering the patient's daily requirement. Non-opioid therapies should always be considered, and epidural analgesia can be valuable after major surgery. In the reformed addict there is significant onus on clinical staff to avoid re-establishing dependency. Patients in this category presenting for major surgery are a particular challenge, but make every effort to avoid opioids without subjecting the patient to unrelieved pain.

MONITORING OF POSTOPERATIVE ANALGESIA

The effectiveness of any postoperative analgesic regimen, as well as any side-effects, needs to be assessed regularly. Ensure that the patient is monitored regularly to determine the level of pain, sedation and respiration.

Monitoring of pain

The simplest method of monitoring pain is through observation of the behaviour of the patient, for example the time taken for the patient to sit or stand or the ability of the patient to cough. You can also monitor the analgesic requirements of the patient (e.g. the total dose of analgesia administered over a 24 h period or the number of demands of a PCA pump). Physiological measures such as heart rate and blood pressure may also increase in the presence of pain, but these parameters at best simply improve the discriminatory power of other measures. However, patient self-report is the most reliable and valid measure of pain in the clinical situation, and this is usually done using unidimensional scales, as illustrated (Fig. 35.2).

Pain scores can be difficult to interpret because individual patients vary in their perception of pain. The verbal rating scale (VRS) and visual analogue scale (VAS) are the most commonly used methods when adjusting

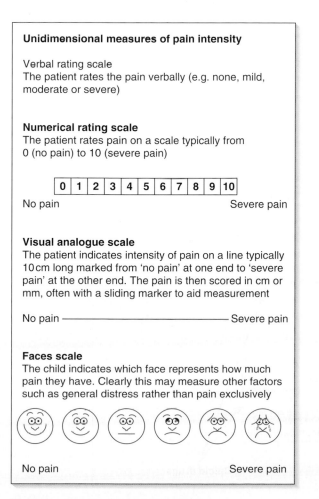

Unidimensional measures of pain intensity

Verbal rating scale
The patient rates the pain verbally (e.g. none, mild, moderate or severe)

Numerical rating scale
The patient rates pain on a scale typically from 0 (no pain) to 10 (severe pain)

0	1	2	3	4	5	6	7	8	9	10

No pain   Severe pain

Visual analogue scale
The patient indicates intensity of pain on a line typically 10 cm long marked from 'no pain' at one end to 'severe pain' at the other end. The pain is then scored in cm or mm, often with a sliding marker to aid measurement

No pain ——————————————— Severe pain

Faces scale
The child indicates which face represents how much pain they have. Clearly this may measure other factors such as general distress rather than pain exclusively

No pain   Severe pain

Fig. 35.2 Commonly used pain scales.

analgesic regimens such as opioid PCA or epidural infusions. Most pain scores only measure pain when the patient is resting. Obviously such a score will change when, for example, a patient after upper abdominal surgery attempts to cough to clear secretions or receives chest physiotherapy. Therefore pain scores on coughing or moving will be just as important as those at rest.

Monitoring of sedation and respiration

The major fear with opioids, administered by any route (intravenously, intramuscularly or epidurally) is that of respiratory depression. Epidural opioids have the added risk of delayed respiratory depression. This risk is extremely small. Highly lipid-soluble opioids such as fentanyl have a lower risk of this complication, administered epidurally, than does morphine, which is less lipid soluble. Of course you must also consider the general medical condition of the patient, as elderly patients with cardiorespiratory disease are at a higher risk of this potentially dangerous complication. Traditionally it has been assumed that intermittent observation of a patient's respiratory rate by a ward nurse is adequate to detect respiratory problems. It should be noted, however, that a decrease in respiratory rate has been found to be a late and unreliable indicator of respiratory depression. Sedation is a better indicator and all patients receiving opioids should be monitored using a sedation score, for example:

0 = None
1 = Mild, occasionally drowsy, easy to rouse
2 = Moderate, constantly or frequently drowsy, easy to rouse
3 = Severe, somnolent, difficult to rouse
S = Normal sleep

 Key point

- **A sedation score of 3 or respiratory rate less than 8 breaths per minute should be treated immediately with intravenous naloxone.**

The development of pulse oximetry, which allows a patient's blood oxygen saturation (SpO_2) to be measured non-invasively using a simple finger probe, is already a minimum monitoring standard during anaesthesia and the immediate recovery period. Several studies, which have extended the use of pulse oximetry to the postoperative period on the ward, have detected periods of hypoxaemia 3–4 days after major surgery. The relationship of these events to the risk of myocardial ischaemia is a subject of ongoing research.

Key point

- If using pulse oximetry, treat an Sp_{O_2} of less than 94% in a patient breathing air with supplemental oxygen through nasal prongs or a face mask.

POSTOPERATIVE NAUSEA AND VOMITING (PONV)

The vomiting centre is found in the reticular formation of the medulla. It receives afferent impulses from various pathways, including the chemoreceptor trigger zone (CTZ). This area is located within the floor of the fourth ventricle and is activated by various stimuli (Fig. 35.3). Risk factors associated with postoperative nausea and vomiting include:

- History and examination
  - Past history of PONV
  - History of motion sickness or migraine
  - Prolonged starvation
  - Recent oral intake
  - Obesity
  - Female sex
- Type of surgery
  - Gastrointestinal
  - ENT/ophthalmic
  - Gynaecological
  - Orthopaedic
  - Emergency
- Drugs, e.g. thiopentone, opioids.

A number of general measures may be employed in the treatment of PONV, including:

- Hydration and maintenance of adequate blood pressure
- Avoiding excessive movement in the immediate postoperative phase
- Reducing the patient's anxiety.

The following agents may be useful in treating PONV:

- Anticholinergic agents, e.g. cyclizine/hyoscine
- Antidopaminergic agents, e.g. domperidone and metoclopramide
- 5-HT3 antagonists, e.g. ondansetron.

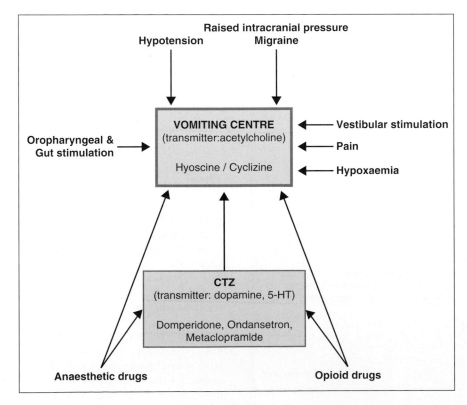

Fig. 35.3 Management of postoperative nausea and vomiting.

ACUTE PAIN SERVICE (APS)

An anaesthesia-based multidisciplinary team approach to acute pain relief was first described by Ready in Seattle, USA. In 1990 the Royal College of Surgeons of England and the Royal College of Anaesthetists recommended that each hospital should have an APS team. The establishment of an APS requires medical, nursing and pharmaceutical expertise. Anaesthetists have a major role to play, as they not only initiate postoperative analgesic regimens, such as PCA and epidural infusions, but are also familiar with the drugs and equipment used in such cases. Many hospitals have an acute pain team consisting of a dedicated pain nurse, consultant anaesthetist and sometimes junior anaesthetic staff.

The role of the acute pain team includes:

- Devising, implementing and auditing pain protocols
- Reviewing patients in whom postoperative analgesia is proving difficult
- Reviewing patients with epidural and intravenous infusions
- Managing patients with chronic pain.

CONCLUSION

Currently, in the treatment of postoperative pain, there is no single analgesic therapy that can treat all aspects of pain without causing side-effects. The emphasis should be on a 'balanced analgesic' technique, especially after major surgical procedures, using NSAIDs in combination with other drugs such as opioids or local anaesthetics. The future of acute pain management lies in better education of healthcare staff, universal introduction of pain scoring and improved use of existing facilities. The challenge lies in disseminating knowledge and expertise to ensure that best practice is adopted universally.

Summary

- Pain can be treated by various methods which affect the transmission of a painful stimulus at different levels along its pathway to the central nervous system.

- Treatment of pain may reduce the incidence of some postoperative complications and hence reduce hospital stay.
- Opioids, given i.v. or i.m. remain common analgesics for the treatment of postoperative pain. Regional blockade using a low dose combination of local anaesthetic and opioid is also now popular. The concurrent use of NSAIDs is useful in reducing opioid requirements.
- The degree of analgesia and sedation must be carefully monitored on the ward.
- In most hospitals an acute pain service is available to advise on the methods available for the treatment of postoperative pain and potential complications associated with such methods.

 Further reading

1998 Guidelines on the use of NSAIDs in the perioperative period. Royal College of Anaesthetists, London

Liu S, Carpenter RL, Neal JM 1995 Epidural anesthesia and analgesia, their role in postoperative outcome. Anesthesiology 82: 1474–1506

Lumley JSP, Craven JL (series eds) 2001 Pain. Anaesthesia and Intensive Care Medicine **2**(11).

McQuay HJ 1992 Pre-emptive analgesia. British Journal of Anaesthesia 69: 1–3

National Health and Medical Research Council 1999 Acute pain management: the scientific evidence. NHMRC, Canberra

Ogilvy AJ, Smith G 1994 Postoperative pain. In: Nimo WS, Rowbotham DJ, Smith G (eds) Anaesthesia. Blackwell, Oxford, pp 1570–1602

Rawal N 2002 Editorial: Acute pain services revisited – good from far, far from good? Regional Anaesthesia and Pain Medicine 27: 117–121

Ready LB 1990 Acute postoperative pain. In: Aitkenhead AR, Smith G (eds) Anesthesia, 3rd edn. Churchill Livingstone, Edinburgh, pp 2135–2145

Rowbotham DJ 1994 Gastric emptying, postoperative nausea and vomiting and antiemetics. In: Nimo WS, Rowbotham DJ, Smith G (eds) Anaesthesia. Blackwell, Oxford, pp 350–371

Sabanathan S 1995 Has postoperative pain been eradicated? Annals of the Royal College of Surgeons 77: 202–209

COMPLICATIONS

36 Complications: prevention and management

J. A. R. Smith

Objectives

- Accept that complications are best anticipated and avoided.
- Recognize the incidence of comorbidity.
- Understand the importance of matching the procedure to the associated risks.
- Appreciate the importance of recognizing complications early and treating them vigorously.

RISK FACTORS

- General – applicable to all procedures, *or*
- Specific to the operation and/or the complication concerned.

Old age

In older age, some conditions are encountered more commonly:

1. Neoplastic conditions.
2. Peripheral and cardiovascular disease. The incidence of cardiovascular disease rises with age (Table 36.1) and this is associated with an increased risk of postoperative myocardial infarction. Over age 50 years the risk is 6%, with a 70% mortality rate. There is also an increased incidence of atrial fibrillation and hypertension and therefore of serious dysrhythmia and death.
3. Respiratory disease. Several changes occur in the elderly. These include reduced arterial oxygen tension, especially over 80 years of age. There are also: increased physiological dead space; decreased lung capacity, vital capacity, maximal breathing capacity, forced expiratory volume and peak expiratory flow rate.
4. Renal function deteriorates with age because of peripheral vascular disease, loss of nephrons, and impaired cell function. Therefore fluid overload and disturbance of both acid–base and electrolyte balance are more common in the elderly.

Table 36.1	Risk of cardiovascular disease with age
Age (years)	Incidence of cardiovascular disease (%)
40–50	6
60–70	41
70–80	100

5. Medication. Elderly patients are more likely to be on regular medication for a number of disorders. The risk of drug interaction is therefore increased.

Neonatal period

At the other end of the age spectrum, neonatal surgery is also hazardous:

1. Tolerance of intravenous fluids is poor.
2. Gastrointestinal losses by vomiting and diarrhoea are common and can be life threatening. There is increased susceptibility to disturbance of acid–base balance, and accurate replacement of fluid and electrolytes and correction of disturbance of pH is much more difficult.
3. Thermal regulation is poor, resulting in an increased risk of hypothermia. Enzyme systems are immature, so that jaundice is more common, and both general and drug metabolism may be impaired.
4. Congenital abnormalities are often multiple and major, and surgery is more demanding because of the physical size of the patient and the delicacy of the tissues.

Obesity

Patients may be overweight (up to 10% above their ideal bodyweight), obese (10–40% above) or morbidly obese (more than 40% above their ideal).

Anaesthetic difficulties include difficulty in intubation and in the placement of intravenous lines. Chest wall compliance is reduced, with consequent difficulties with ventilation. Positioning the patient on the operating table while avoiding pressure injuries requires considerable skill. In morbidly obese patients, cardiomyopathy and respiratory dysfunction may be severe enough to be life threatening. In some series, mortalities of 10–25% because of anaesthetic risks alone have been reported.

Surgery is complicated by technical difficulties; these can include limited exposure, adipose tissue obscuring the view and making trauma to associated structures more likely, and problems in minimally invasive surgery because of difficulty in gaining access to the peritoneal cavity.

In addition, blood vessels are less well supported and tend to retract if divided. Control of haemorrhage is therefore more difficult and haematoma formation more common. As a consequence, wound infection and impaired wound healing are encountered more often. The risk of venous thromboembolism is increased because fat patients tend to be less mobile, their weight exerts greater pressure on the calf veins during surgery, and there is an increased likelihood of endothelial trauma. In some obese patients there is an association with atherosclerosis and therefore with peripheral vascular disease.

In orthopaedic practice, obesity increases the incidence of arthritis, makes joint replacement more difficult from a technical view point and places an extra strain on lower limb prostheses. Indeed, such patients may require bariatric surgery, such as vertical banded gastroplasty, to allow weight loss before joint replacement. A reduction of between 50 and 75% of the excess bodyweight over 12 months can be anticipated.

Key point

- **There is no scientific evidence that weight reduction is rewarded by a reduction in the incidence of postoperative complications.**

Cardiovascular disease

Myocardial infarction. A recent infarct is the most serious predisposing factor (Table 36.2). The more recent the infarct, the greater the risk of a further infarct. The risk remains higher than normal even after an interval of 3 years. The mortality from recurrent infarcts is also time related, being 75% in the first 6 months and falling to 25% after 1 year. Therefore, defer operations with a low risk of morbidity and mortality for at least 6 months post infarct.

Angina. The severity of angina dictates the risk of cardiovascular complications in general and myocardial infarction in particular.

Dysrhythmias. Dysrhythmias such as atrial fibrillation and heart block carry the worst prognosis. Correction

Table 36.2	Risk of myocardial infarction with time
Time since infarct	Incidence of further infarction after surgery (%)
0–6 months	55
1–2 years	22
2–3 years	6
>3 years	1
No infarct	0.66

of the dysrhythmia reduces but does not abolish the risk of cardiovascular complications.

Cardiac valve disease. The presence of an artificial valve causes a major risk of bacterial colonization following surgery. Administer prophylactic antibiotics for all procedures. Mitral valve disease increases the risk of atrial fibrillation and of atrial thrombosis. Significant valve disease impairs cardiac responses to surgery and to infused fluids.

Cardiac pacemakers. These are 'foreign bodies', therefore administer prophylactic antibiotics. If a pacemaker is at a fixed rate, an inability to increase heart rate renders the patient vulnerable to hypovolaemia. Take care when using diathermy, especially if it is unipolar.

Atherosclerosis. The incidence of atherosclerosis tends to increase with age, e.g. at age 50 the incidence is 23% with a 0.7% risk of myocardial infarction, while at age 70 the incidence of arteriosclerosis is 100%. The risk of cardiovascular complications shows a similar pattern to the incidence of atheroma.

Hypertension. This does not increase the risk of myocardial infarction in abdominal surgery, but there is an increased risk as a result of cardiac surgery. Remember that surgery for phaeochromocytoma, and sometimes for carcinoid disease, can be associated with wide fluctuations in blood pressure. This increases the risk of cerebral vascular accident.

Key points

- **The combination of respiratory and cardiovascular disease is more serious than one of them alone. A combination results in arterial hypoxaemia and is more common in older patients.**
- **If renal function is also impaired, the risk of fluid overload is greatly increased.**
- **A *normal* myocardium can compensate well down to a haemoglobin level of 10 g dl^{-1}. Below this level, or if there is myocardial**

disease, peripheral hypoxaemia is more likely. Even at this level, subendocardial ischaemia and fibrosis may occur.

Respiratory disease

There is an increased risk of respiratory complications in smokers, in patients with bronchiectasis and emphysema, and if surgery is undertaken in the presence of tonsillitis, bronchitis or even coryza (Greek *kara* = head + *zeein* = to boil; a head cold). In this group postpone elective surgery until the infection has cleared.

As indicated above, with advancing years there is a reduction in arterial oxygen tension and various changes in lung physiology. This results in a greater difference in alveolar–arterial oxygen tension and thus any respiratory complication produces more severe hypoxaemia.

 Key point

- **A combination of cor pulmonale and ischaemic heart disease produces a mortality of about 50%.**

Diabetes mellitus

Insulin-dependent diabetics are high risk patients for a number of different reasons.

Metabolic factors

The metabolic response to surgery results in hyperglycaemia. Maintenance of blood sugar can be difficult in the perioperative period and even non-insulin-dependent diabetics may require insulin for a short time. If complications such as infection arise, both hyperinsulinaemia and hyperglycaemia may coexist – so called insulin resistance. The major danger is the development of severe ketoacidosis. This is seen most commonly in poorly controlled diabetic patients, or indeed in those who are previously undiagnosed. Remember that one presentation of diabetic ketoacidosis is as an 'acute abdomen'. It is always sensible to measure blood and urinary glucose in all patients with abdominal pain.

Infection

In diabetes mellitus, polymorphonuclear phagocyte function is impaired. There is an increased incidence of peripheral vascular disease affecting both medium and small vessels. Diabetic neuropathy reduces sensation to touch and to pain. Skin ulceration commonly acts as a nidus for infection. Where diabetes is poorly controlled there may be a higher sugar level in blood and tissues; this also encourages bacterial growth.

Wound healing

The disease in medium and small vessels reduces blood supply to healing tissue. The impaired polymorph phagocyte function interferes with the acute inflammatory reaction. As described, there is an increased risk of infection. All of these factors contribute to impaired wound healing.

Peripheral vascular disease

The increased risk of atheroma affecting both medium and small arteries increases the risk of gangrene. Neuropathic ulcers are more common. If infection does occur in the presence of gangrene, wet gangrene is more likely to be encountered.

Renal disease

If diabetes mellitus has been present for 20 years there is a 15% incidence of glomerulosclerosis. This impairment of renal function makes fluid and electrolyte balance more complex. Diabetic patients are more sensitive to protein depletion, and are at increased risk of severe ketoacidosis during a surgical illness.

DRUG THERAPY

Antibiotics

Misuse of antibiotics is said to be a major cause of litigation in the USA. Anaphylactic reactions are rare but can be life threatening. Hypersensitivity reactions, however, are slightly more common and only marginally less serious. Ask about drug allergy during the systematic enquiry of every patient.

Misuse of antibiotics may result in the development of resistance. The most serious from the point of view of the patient and the surgical department is the methicillin-resistant *Staphylococcus aureus* (MRSA). It is important to have a hospital antibiotics policy, with clear indications for the use of antibiotics. Use them for a specific period only and take advice from the microbiologist for complex infections or immunocompromised patients.

The risk of MRSA infection in healthy individuals is very small but to ill patients in hospital can be life threatening. Isolate patients who have bacteriological evidence of MRSA infection and barrier nurse them. In patients who are unwell, administer appropriate antibiotic therapy according to advice from the microbiologist.

Pseudomembranous colitis

This may present as a surgical emergency. Exposure to antibiotics combined with a period of hypovolaemia or hypotension are joint factors in pathogenesis. Diagnosis is made on the basis of a frozen section biopsy taken at sigmoidoscopy and confirmed by the demonstration of the *Clostridium difficile* toxin in the faecal fluid. Intravenous vancomycin or metronidazole are usually effective in treatment. Occasionally total colectomy is required for resistant cases.

Aminoglycocides

Gentamicin causes ototoxicity in 3% of patients. The elderly and those with impaired renal function are at increased risk. It causes nephrotoxicity in 2% of patients. For that reason monitor peak and trough blood levels in all patients receiving this therapy.

Corticosteroids

The greatest risk of complications occurs in patients on high dosage or on long courses of therapy.

Corticoids act to interfere with the mobility and phagocytic activity of polymorphonuclear leucocytes. This means that acute inflammation and the handling of bacteria are impaired, including the inflammatory reaction which is an essential part in the repair of wounds. Therefore deficient wound healing and wound infection are more common.

The production of ground substance is reduced. Therefore capillary fragility is increased and wound haematoma is more common. This contributes to impaired wound healing and also provides a nidus for infection. Note, however, that in experimental circumstances the short term use of methylprednisolone has not been associated with impaired healing of colonic anastomoses.

Stress response

Steroid therapy within the 6 months before surgery depresses the endogenous production of glucocorticoids. The output of endogenous glucocorticoid is an essential part of the response to surgery and anaesthesia. In order to avoid this complication the patient should receive 100 mg of hydrocortisone intravenously at the induction of anaesthesia and at 6-hourly intervals for 48 h. Over the next 5–7 days reduce the intake of glucocorticoid either to zero or to the preoperative level.

Delay in diagnosis

Because of the depression of the acute inflammatory reaction, steroid therapy may delay the diagnosis of postoperative complications. It may also render some complications more likely to occur. For example, if a peptic ulcer perforates in someone on steroid therapy the diagnosis may be delayed, with resulting increase in morbidity and mortality.

There is some evidence that glucocorticoids in dosages used for immunosuppression may encourage the development of certain virally induced tumours. In transplant patients there is evidence that the incidence of head and neck tumours and the virally induced tumours may be increased. This has not been reported in more common tumours of lung, breast or gastrointestinal tract.

Orthopaedic practice

Patients who are on steroid therapy in general, and those on steroids for rheumatoid arthritis in particular, have an increased risk of osteoporosis, which makes them more prone to suffer pathological fractures. Joint replacement is more difficult in such patients because of bone thinning and because of the general complications mentioned above.

Cytotoxic agents

Patients on cytotoxic chemotherapy have well-recognized problems of gastrointestinal upset and hair loss. Depression of the white cell count and white cell function interfere with acute inflammation. This produces an increased incidence of wound infection and of impaired wound healing. Bone marrow depression is common. This also increases the risk of infection, especially with opportunistic organisms. It also risks purpuric eruption and frank bleeding. The expected reduction in cell-mediated immunity increases the risk of developing a second neoplasm; for example, in patients successfully treated for primary lymphoma there is a 3% risk of a second tumour developing.

Ciclosporin

Ciclosporin A carries all the risks of depressing immune responses. More specifically, it can result in depression of renal function. This is the usual reason for having to discontinue therapy with this agent.

BLOOD TRANSFUSION

Incompatibility

Major incompatibility reactions are now rare, even with emergency crossmatching. Minor group incompatibility is more common, especially in patients who have had repeated transfusions. This involves, in order of importance, the Kell, Duffy or Kidd systems. It is common to attribute febrile reactions to incompatibility. Remember that transfusion of pyrogens or antibodies to white cells are alternative explanations for a febrile reaction.

Consequences of storage

The lifespan of red cells is finite and therefore lysis is an inevitable consequence of storage. This may produce transient jaundice but is not of dire consequence. More importantly, there is a potential for hyperkalaemia after massive blood transfusion because of the release of the intracellular potassium ion. Careful monitoring of such patients by regular assessment of urea and electrolytes and of ECG changes, which begin to occur above a level of 6 mmol l^{-1}, are essential.

Acid citrate dextrose

This is the most commonly used anticoagulant. Transfused citrate may bind free calcium, resulting in hypocalcaemia. Careful monitoring of the ECG is essential. Both platelets and clotting factors are consumed within some hours of storage. As a consequence, transfused stored blood cannot be relied upon to correct haemorrhagic tendencies and transfusion of fresh platelets or fresh frozen plasma may be required.

Oxygen carriage

The level of 2,3-diphosphoglycerate falls in stored red cells. This produces a shift of the oxyhaemoglobin dissociation curve to the left, resulting in an increased affinity of haemoglobin for oxygen. Delivery of oxygen at tissue level is therefore reduced. Stored red cells become more rigid. This impairs capillary circulation and encourages sludging.

Transmission of disease

In the past, both syphilis and hepatitis B were transmitted by transfusion (see Ch. 21). These diseases have been virtually abolished by stringent screening methods. Hepatitis C remains a significant risk in some countries where screening is not well established. Earlier serological tests were unsatisfactory but more specific immunological tests, such as immunoblotting, are now available. In Britain most case of hepatitis C are associated with drug abuse. More recently, the human immunodeficiency virus (HIV) has been transfused, mainly to haemophilic patients, with disastrous consequences.

Alteration in immunity

In transplantation surgery it is clear that the risk of renal rejection is reduced after blood transfusion. In patients undergoing resection for colonic cancer, perioperative transfusion results in a poorer prognosis, even when groups are matched for stage of disease, degree of operative trauma, age, sex and other factors. This is attributed to a reduction in cell-mediated immunity. Other neoplastic processes and the relevance of blood transfusion to prognosis remain under investigation. In colorectal surgery, the use of blood transfusion is also associated with an increased risk of infective complications in the postoperative period. This risk has not been identified in patients undergoing joint replacement in orthopaedic practice.

TYPE OF PATHOLOGY

Obstructive jaundice

1. *Effect on coagulation*. Patients with obstructive jaundice have an increased risk of haemorrhage in the perioperative period. The absorption of the fat-soluble vitamin K is impaired in the absence of bile salts. This interferes with the production of the vitamin K-dependent factors II, VII, IX and X. The liver manufactures most clotting factors and therefore back pressure from obstruction may interfere with the synthesis of these factors and also factors V, XI, XII and XIII. The liver also clears activated coagulation factors such as fibrin degradation products (FDPs). When there is severe impairment of liver function there may also be disseminated intravascular coagulation.

All patients with obstructive jaundice should have a full clotting screen. Depending on the results of that screen, patients should be given systemic vitamin K_1 and/or fresh frozen plasma. The intravenous route for vitamin K_1 is recommended because it reduces the risk of intramuscular haematoma.

2. *Effect on wound healing*. Back pressure interferes with hepatocellular function and therefore disturbs protein metabolism. There is clear evidence that where obstructive jaundice is due to a malignancy there is impairment of healing of wounds and anastomoses. It is also taught that the same problem occurs in all patients with obstructive jaundice. The evidence for this is less clear. However, sufficient doubt remains for all patients with obstructive jaundice to be considered at high risk of wound failure.

As already indicated, an increased incidence of wound haematoma and infection will also interfere with wound healing.

3. *Effect on infective complications*. Stasis within the biliary system increases the risk of infection, particularly

with Gram-negative organisms. It is well established that opening the common bile duct produces a threefold increase in the incidence of wound infection relative to cholecystectomy alone. Where obstructive jaundice is secondary to stones or to postoperative stricture, the incidence of infected bile is at least 75%. With malignant obstruction, incidences of infection of 25% have been reported. The more often the bile duct is operated upon, the more likely there is to be infected bile with a consequent increase in postoperative infective complications.

The whole picture is complicated by the fact that there is reduced efficacy of the reticuloendothelial (Kupffer) cells in the liver. In the presence of infected bile there is an increased incidence of septicaemia, but also an increase in the production of endotoxins. Furthermore, there is a possibility of translocation of bacteria from the small bowel. This combination may overcome the capacity of the reticuloendothelial system. The result is increased mortality and morbidity, particularly from ascending cholangitis. This means that the incidence of septicaemia and endotoxinaemia is increased. Increased mortality and morbidity result, particularly from ascending cholangitis.

4. *Effect on renal function.* Following surgery for obstructive jaundice, patients are at risk from acute renal failure – the 'hepatorenal syndrome'. There are a number of theories as to aetiology.

Acute renal failure is also a complication of Gram-negative septic shock, believed to be caused by the effects of endotoxins. The effects include activation of complement by the alternative pathway, the release of a number of cell mediators, including tumour necrosis factor and interleukins, and inappropriate disseminated intravascular coagulation (DIC). DIC results in microthrombi being found in the renal parenchyma, thus interfering with renal function.

It is also said that at least some part of renal failure occurs because the tubules are blocked by excess bilirubin. Histological evidence of this is variable and, at most, it is likely to be no more than a contributing factor.

The hormones responsible for maintaining fluid and electrolyte balance, such as antidiuretic hormone (ADH), aldosterone and natriuretic factors, are metabolized in the liver. Disturbance of hepatic function may interfere with the activities of these hormones. Because of the increasing problems of haemorrhage, patients with obstructive jaundice are at greater risk of hypovolaemia. Protection against the effects of obstructive jaundice on renal function are to ensure adequate perioperative fluid infusion and a good diuresis, e.g. by the use of the osmotic diuretic mannitol. Give prophylactic antibiotics.

5. *Effects on drugs and metabolism.* It is assumed that general drug metabolism is altered in the presence of obstructive jaundice. The evidence in support of this is not strong. However, a particular problem does arise for drugs which are oxidized in the liver. In surgical practice great caution is required with analgesic and sedative therapy with, for example, morphine-like agents.

6. Take note of the specific problems relating to warfarin and the interference with the International Normalized Ratio (INR) produced by certain antibiotics.

Neoplastic disease

Venous thromboembolism

The association between superficial thrombophlebitis migrans and pancreatic carcinoma is well established. However, it seems likely that malignant tumours secrete factors, such as thromboplastins, which affect the thrombotic cascade. In general terms, oncological procedures tend to be prolonged, they are associated with greater operative trauma, and they often require blood transfusion; all of this increases the incidence of deep vein thrombosis. Both in urology and in gynaecology, major procedures in the pelvis are at particular risk of this complication. In addition to the factors mentioned above, pressure on the iliac veins is a significant problem.

Wound healing

It is generally accepted that patients with carcinoma are at increased risk both of primary wound failure and later incisional herniation. This relationship has been most clearly confirmed in malignant obstructive jaundice. In this condition malnutrition is combined with impaired protein metabolism in the liver.

The whole concept of cancer cachexia is complex, and in patients who have lost more than 10% of their premorbid bodyweight, or who present with a serum albumin of less than $30 \, g \, l^{-1}$, there is impaired healing both of wounds and anastomoses.

Patients with ovarian cancer have a high incidence of ascites with omental and peritoneal deposits. In contrast to gastrointestinal malignancy, radical surgery in these patients can be rewarding. However, this involves the rapid loss of protein-rich fluid. If the ascites reaccumulates rapidly in the postoperative period there will be associated abdominal distension and leaking through the wound. Both of these factors also impair wound healing.

TYPE OF SURGERY

Minimally invasive surgery

No field of surgical practice has escaped the introduction of minimally invasive procedures. The picture is most clearly established in laparoscopic cholecystectomy, where there is evidence of more rapid recovery from surgery, earlier discharge from hospital and earlier return to normal activities. The operation of minicholecystectomy has been compared with the laparoscopic route, with no clear benefit of the latter being proven.

The learning curve for this new form of operation can be long. This is because hand–eye coordination is different from conventional surgery and because the handling of tissues at a distance means that tactile sensitivity is reduced. Visual fields are limited, which is of particular importance when diathermy, laser or intracorporeal suturing are being applied. Take great care to visualize probes and needles and to keep them within your visual field at all times.

More recently, the concept of hand-assisted laparoscopic surgery has been developed. This is of particular relevance to gastrointestinal surgery. Only time will tell whether such a combined approach avoids some of the problems of laparoscopic surgery, for example, radical ablation of neoplastic disease and port-site recurrence.

A particular problem exists when diathermy is used when capacitance coupling may occur, resulting in burn injuries at the trocar sites. Initially there was a vogue for the use of laser-assisted dissection; this has largely been overtaken by diathermy. However, if you use laser, take all the normal precautions for the use of lasers, and gain a clear understanding of the characteristics of the different forms of laser in current use.

With specific reference to cholecystectomy, it is clear that there is at least a fivefold increase in the incidence of bile duct injury in comparison with conventional surgery. Take great care to identify the anatomy and be willing to convert to open cholecystectomy if you encounter difficulty or if your field of view is obscured.

Orthopaedic surgery

Thromboembolism

Operations on the hips and pelvis have an increased risk of deep venous thrombosis (DVT), so prophylactic warfarin is often administered. Recent reports have demonstrated the value of low molecular weight heparin. The risk is higher if surgery is performed after major trauma. Blood transfusion also increases the risk of DVT.

Wound infection

Most orthopaedic procedures are classified as clean. Therefore the incidence of wound infection is low. However, the consequence of infection, for example after joint replacement, is catastrophic. If a foreign body such as a joint prosthesis becomes infected, the chance of eradicating the infection by antibiotics is minimal. It is necessary to remove the prosthesis.

Use of tourniquets

In orthopaedic surgery tourniquets are widely used and it is recognized that tourniquet time must be kept to a minimum. However, it is vitally important that you assess the vascular supply, especially to the lower limbs. If you do not, the potential hazard of, for example, knee replacement is greatly increased. Remember also that skin ischaemia may complicate badly planned incisions.

Steroid therapy

The problem with steroid therapy has already been mentioned. Especially in patients on steroids for rheumatoid arthritis, surgery is more difficult and anaesthetic problems may be faced, for example if the cervical spine is involved.

Gynaecological surgery

In operations within the pelvis, and particularly those lasting over 45 min, there is increased risk of trauma to the pelvic veins. This increases the risk of iliofemoral thrombosis. Extensive oncological eradication carries, in addition, all the risks relevant to cancer surgery (see above).

Thoracic and upper abdominal procedures

Incisions used for this type of surgery usually cause exceptional postoperative pain. Respiratory movement may be restricted, increasing the risk of atelectasis and infective complications, especially in elderly patients.

Prolonged operations

Traditional teaching is that prolonged operations increase the risk of respiratory difficulties, fluid and electrolyte imbalance and deep vein thrombosis. Experience with prolonged keyhole operations by the laparoscopic route have proved them relatively free of complications. This seems likely to be related to reducing the influence of such factors as:

- Intraoperative trauma
- Need for blood transfusion
- Loss of fluid and heat from exposed cavities
- Minimal damage to tissues.

 Key point

- **Prolonged time spent on the operating table does not inevitably cause respiratory, thrombotic, fluid balance and electroyte disturbances.**

Remember that although the incidence of complications may be lower in minimally invasive surgery, they are not abolished. Deep vein thrombosis, wound infection and wound hernia at port sites do occur. Therefore take prophylactic measures and carefully monitor patients in the postoperative period.

COMPLICATIONS AND THEIR MANAGEMENT

Venous thromboembolism

Risk factors

These include obesity, old age and malignant disease. Long operations, pelvic and hip surgery, a past history of DVT or pulmonary embolism and varicose veins increase the risk. Other provoking factors are pregnancy and the oral contraceptive pill.

Incidence

The incidence varies with the type of operation and the risk factors mentioned.

Key point

- **It is estimated that for every 1000 operations there are 100 deep vein thromboses, ten pulmonary emboli and one death.**

Diagnosis

Early diagnosis is difficult and clinical diagnosis inaccurate. Experimentally, ^{125}I-fibrinogen scanning is sensitive in detecting developing thrombi but is of no value for established thrombosis. It is likely this test overestimates the incidence of clinically significant thrombi. The new D-dimer assay is a very sensitive screening test which can be performed at the bedside. Validation is still required but it seems likely that, if the test is negative, DVT is not present. Be cautious in interpreting the result as it may be positive, for example in the presence of an inflammatory process. Doppler ultrasound scans are valuable detecting peripheral sites. However, isolated calf vein thromboses are probably of no significance.

For suspected iliofemoral thrombosis a colour duplex scan is the investigation of choice. Where this is negative, repeating the scan in 1 week is probably preferable to venography. Venography has been the gold standard for diagnosis in the past but colour duplex appears to be more accurate and is clearly less invasive.

Prophylaxis

Because of the difficulties of diagnosis, prophylaxis is the cornerstone of management. Correct risk factors such as obesity, or stop the taking of the contraceptive pill if clinically possible. The time of maximum risk of a thrombosis developing in surgical practice is during the operation, when the three factors of stasis, endothelial trauma and increased coagulability are most prevalent.

Electrical methods of stimulating muscle function and thereby maintaining blood flow have been superseded. Mechanical methods, such as intermittent pumping of the calves by air insufflation of below knee stockings, are again popular.

Subcutaneous calcium heparin (5000 units), injected 2 h before surgery and continued postoperatively 12-hourly until the patient is fully mobile, is a well-established method of reducing the incidence of DVT. Calcium heparin causes less bleeding than sodium heparin. More recently, the low molecular fragment heparin has been shown to be at least as effective for general, gynaecological and orthopaedic surgery. It may reduce the risk of perioperative bleeding, although this is still debated. A once per day dosage regimen saves nursing time, decreases patient discomfort and is cost effective. Some orthopaedic surgeons favour full anticoagulation with warfarin as prophylaxis for major joint replacement, especially for revision surgery. Shorter operating times and earlier mobilization have contributed to the decreased risk.

Treatment

Do not anticoagulate the patient if the thrombus can be shown to be confined to the calf and is less than 5 cm long. Analgesics and support stockings may well be helpful. Take care when actively treating patients with a dyspeptic history or with a history of cerebrovascular accident.

Most patients require intravenous heparin; give a loading dose of 10 000 units, followed by continuous intravenous infusion to prolong the activated partial thromboplastin time (APTT) by twice the control level. Thereafter, continue anticoagulation with warfarin for at least 3 months. Especially in hip replacement, the risk of DVT persists for several weeks. Low molecular weight heparin by subcutaneous injection is being used increasingly for established DVTs.

Complications

Pulmonary embolism may be fatal. Multiple emboli produce pulmonary hypertension. Diagnosis is on the basis of a radioisotope ventilation/perfusion lung scan.

More recently spinal computerized tomography (CT) scans have proved of greater value. If surgery is contemplated, as for a major embolism in a specialist centre, perform pulmonary angiography if time allows. Alternatively, stimulate thrombolysis using streptokinase or urokinase, or fully anticoagulate the patient, as described for DVT.

Postphlebitic limb is more likely to follow an occlusive iliofemoral thrombosis. Treatment is symptomatic with support stockings and analgesics or aimed at treating the venous ulcers, which can complicate this condition, probably secondary to dermatoliposclerosis.

Respiratory complications

Postoperative respiratory complications are the most common, but because of the various risk factors involved a true incidence is difficult to establish.

Risk factors

Arterial oxygen tension falls gradually with age, more rapidly over the age of 80. Vital capacity, lung capacity, peak expiratory flow rate and postexpiratory volume are all reduced. Cardiovascular disease is more common with advanced years and a combination of cardiovascular and respiratory problems is particularly serious.

The risk of respiratory complications is increased with obesity, excessive sedation, immobility, pre-existing lung disease and myocardial disease, especially following cardiothoracic, upper abdominal and vertical wounds, all of which reduce expiratory movements.

Pathology

The commonest problem after surgery is atelectasis (Greek *a* = not + *telos* = complete + *ektasis* = stretching out, expansion). Small plugs of mucus block minor air passages and cause localized collapse. The plugs can usually be coughed clear with the aid of physiotherapy, but if they are not, superinfection may result. Pulmonary embolus (see above) may also predispose to infection. Pulmonary effusion often complicates pulmonary pathology such as infection, infarct or metastatic disease. An effusion may also result from a subdiaphragmatic abscess or pancreatitis, or complicate congestive cardiac failure and hypoalbuminaemia. Pneumothorax may complicate ventilation, or cannulation of central veins, either for monitoring central venous pressure or for parenteral nutrition.

Adult respiratory distress syndrome (ARDS) is the most serious pulmonary complication in surgical practice. It may complicate severe sepsis, fluid overload, chest trauma, fat emboli, burn injury and inhalation pneumonitis. The cause is unclear but contributing factors are:

- Changes in type I and II alveolar cells, resulting in loss of surfactant and alveolar collapse.
- Impaired capillary to alveolar diffusion.
- Arteriovenous shunts.
- The effects of endotoxin resulting in complement activation by the alternate pathway and disseminated intravascular coagulation (DIC).
- Consequent upon the effects of endotoxin, numerous mediatory cytokines such as tumour necrosis factor or interleukins are released; these contribute to pulmonary damage.
- The effects of hyperoxide radicals.

Management

Where possible, correct clinical risk factors such as obesity and smoking habit prior to surgery. Ensure that the patient receives adequate analgesia without excessive sedation. Encourage regular physiotherapy administered both by the therapist and by the nursing and medical staff. Time physiotherapy so that the patient is free of pain but not oversedated.

Carefully monitor the pulse, respiratory rate and temperature. Administer appropriate antibiotics to patients who are pyrexial despite conservative measures, clinically ill, at high risk, especially if there is combined myocardial and pulmonary disease, and all patients with features of ARDS.

 Key point

- **Give supplementary oxygen by mask; if despite that, the Pao$_2$ falls below 75 mmHg, consider ventilatory support.**

Figure 36.1 illustrates the procedure when a 'trigger' necessitates considering transferring a patient to the high dependency unit for more intensive monitoring and treatment.

Infective complications

Risk factors

Alimentary surgery generates a higher incidence of infection; this is often associated with endogenous organisms. In 'clean' surgery, infection is usually secondary to exogenous agents. Wounds may be classified as:

- Clean, such as thyroid or hernia surgery
- Potentially contaminated, as in elective gastrointestinal surgery

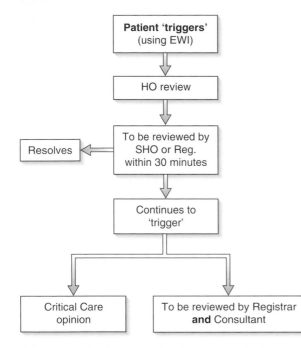

Fig. 36.1   Patient referral algorithm. EWI = Early Warning Indicator.

- Contaminated, as following bowel perforation
- Dirty, when there is faecal contamination.

The incidence of infection, morbidity and mortality increases from clean to dirty. The risk of infection is greater in all categories if surgery is performed as an emergency.

In 'clean' operations, infection is usually secondary to exogenous agents such as *Staphylococcus aureus*. Whenever there is a series of infections in one unit following clean procedures, seek a source of carriage of such organisms. In alimentary surgery the infecting organisms are usually endogenous. These are usually Gram-negative aerobes. Where surgery is performed in the lower ileum and in the large bowel, remember the importance of anaerobic infection.

Key point

- **Although the incidence of wound infection is low after clean procedures, its consequences may be catastrophic, as following joint replacement or valvular heart surgery.**

The risk of wound infection is increased in the presence of obesity, in haematomas and in patients with diabetes mellitus. Other factors are glucocorticoid therapy, immuno-suppression, malnutrition and obstructive jaundice.

Prophylaxis

Identify the patients at risk. This includes those in whom the incidence of infection is higher and those for whom infection is particularly hazardous. Reduce or control risk factors if possible. Ensure that your surgical technique is as perfect and as meticulous as possible, with particular reference to haemostasis, avoiding excessive use of diathermy, leaving dead space or traumatizing tissues by rough handling.

Select the appropriate antibiotic to give the greatest protection and tissue penetration at the time of surgery. Remember to take account of possible patient allergies and the cost involved. It is sufficient to give one dose intravenously at the time of induction. Alternatively, give one dose intramuscularly with the premedication. Give more than one dose only if the operation lasts longer than 4 h or if there has been contamination during gastro-intestinal surgery. In this case you are practising treatment rather than prophylaxis.

Remember the value of mechanical bowel preparation, which reduces loading at the time of large bowel anasto-mosis but does not remove pathogens from the gastro-intestinal tract.

There is continuing controversy about the need for, and timing of, shaving the operative area (see Chs 15, 22). There is some evidence that shaving increases the number of potential pathogens on the skin. There is also contro-versy about the agent used for skin preparation. Chlorhexidine in spirit (Hibiscrub) or aqueous povidone-iodine (Betadine) are both acceptable. Debate continues about the value of intracavity antibiotics or antiseptics and these have probably been superseded by prophylac-tic antibiotics.

In potentially contaminated surgery there is no value in using plastic drapes; these tend to increase the number of pathogens on the skin. The use of danger towels, separate knives for incising skin and deeper tissues and changing gloves after performing anastomoses are now of histori-cal interest only.

The principles of antibiotic prophylaxis are:

1. Identify patients at risk.
2. Select an appropriate antibiotic according to the type of operation.
3. Take account of the patient's allergies and the costs involved.
4. Administer the antibiotic, either intravenously at induction or intramuscularly with the premedication; ensure adequate serum and tissue levels at the time of surgery.

5. Repeat the administration of antibiotic in operations lasting longer than 4 h.

Key point

- **Antibiotics are no substitute for gentle handling of tissues, careful haemostasis, judicious use of diathermy and avoiding strangling tissues with ligatures and sutures.**

Treatment

Wound infection. Open the wound to allow adequate drainage. Obtain pus for culture to establish the infecting organism(s) and their antibiotic sensitivity. Irrigate the wound for adequate drainage and debridement. Formally reopen and surgically debride dirty wounds. If clean wounds become infected, consider cross-infections and investigate the likely sources.

Use antibiotics only if specifically indicated (for cellulitis or septicaemia) or if the consequences of infection would be disastrous (see above).

If the wound infection is chronic, consider the possibility of specific organisms such as *Actinomyces*, a foreign body, such as a suture in the wound, an associated fistula as may occur in Crohn's disease, or associated factors such as irradiation and perineal wounds. Remember the danger of synergistic infections and dermal gangrene.

Postoperative abscess. These are usually intraperitoneal but can occur deep in the wound. Localize the abscess and attempt drainage, if necessary under ultrasound or computed tomography (CT) control. Monitor resolution of the cavity radiologically if necessary. Exclude anastomotic leakage as a cause (see below).

If the patient remains toxic or the cavity fails to resolve, proceed to operative drainage and definitive treatment of any underlying sepsis. If you strongly suspect an abscess, this may involve an exploratory laparotomy, even when the scan is inconclusive.

Septicaemia and septic shock. The septic complications mentioned above may progress to septicaemia and septic shock in patients who are debilitated by disease or drug therapy such as steroids or cytotoxic chemotherapy. However, some organisms may be particularly virulent from the outset.

Remain alert after operation for all septic problems. The danger signs are:

- Persistent, often swinging pyrexia with tachycardia
- Signs of toxicity – flushed warm skin, glazed eyes, tachypnoea
- Falling urinary output – less than 40 ml h^{-1}
- Hypoxaemia.

Key point

- **Treat suspected septic shock effectively to avoid low output septic shock with its associated high mortality (>50%).**

The nature of death in such patients is multiple organ failure, and while a patient may survive failure of a single organ system such as the kidneys, the more organs which fail the higher the mortality (Table 36.3).

This problem is most likely to be encountered if you delay identifying and localizing a septic focus, and fail to institute adequate initial treatment.

The principles of treatment are:

1. Ensure adequate circulating blood volume using a mixture of crystalloid and colloid fluids, aiming for a central venous pressure of 10–15 cmH$_2$O in a ventilated patient.
2. Oxygen supplementation.
3. Broad-spectrum intravenous antibiotic(s).
4. Ventilatory support if the PaO$_2$ is less than 75 mmHg despite 40% oxygen by mask.
5. Cardiac support with such drugs as dopamine, dobutamine, digitalis and catecholamines, as indicated.
6. Attention to renal function with dialysis for established renal failure.
7. Early recognition and treatment of any evidence of multiple organ failure.
8. Collaborate closely with specialist colleagues in intensive care, and where required with cardiac, respiratory and renal physicians.

More controversial are the methods used in some centres to ensure gastrointestinal decontamination. This involves a combination of enteral antibiotic and antiseptic agents, combined with a parenteral antibiotic, and this is gaining popularity. The value of enteral glutamine and/or α-ketoglutarate is considered vital in several intensive care units. This is yet to be proven in a controlled trial. However, enteral nutritional support is preferable to the parenteral route.

Table 36.3 Multiple organ failure: rates of survival	
No. of organs	Survival (%)
1	90
2	40–50
3	5–10

Anastomotic leakage

Anastomotic leakage may complicate any anastomosis, but is seen most commonly following oesophageal and colorectal surgery. In the latter group, leakage results in a threefold increase in operative mortality.

Colonic anastomoses below the pelvic peritoneal reflection are associated with an increased risk of leakage, both clinically and radiologically detected (Table 36.4). The clinical rate always underestimates the true incidence of leakage, as detected by Gastrografin or barium enema.

Predisposing factors

The general factors are similar to those which apply to wound healing in general, such as nutritional deficiencies (particularly protein, vitamin C and zinc), old age and impaired local blood flow from general conditions such as arteriosclerosis and cardiac disease.

Local factors include tension at the anastomosis and poor surgical technique with regard to preparing the bowel ends, handling of tissues, excessive use of diathermy and the insertion and ligation of sutures. Contamination of the anastomosis with liquid faeces prejudices healing, as does an inadequate vascular supply to one or both sides of the anastomosis. Less important factors are the suture material, the number of layers employed, and whether a stapling or suturing technique is used. However, there is preliminary evidence that tumour recurrence is lower in experimental studies when stainless wire is used for the anastomosis and, in clinical work, if the anastomosis is stapled.

Presentation

Gastrointestinal contents may be identified in the wound or at a drain site. An intra-abdominal abscess or more serious septic complication may develop. There may be prolonged adynamic ileus, unexplained pyrexia or

tachycardia, sudden collapse postoperatively or development of an internal fistula.

Where there is any doubt, confirmation can often be obtained from a gently performed X-ray using a contrast medium. In this regard, Gastrografin, which is water soluble, is preferable to barium because leakage of barium has much more serious consequences if present free in the peritoneal cavity.

Management

If the patient is adversely affected by peritonitis, shock or infection, be prepared to intervene with:

1. Adequate resuscitation
2. Antibiotic cover
3. Operation.

The surgical procedure depends on the operative findings, but the principles are:

1. Thorough peritoneal lavage with cefuroxime and warmed saline (1.5 g l^{-1}).
2. Identification of the leak and any associated pathology, such as Crohn's disease.
3. Resection of the affected area. Never try to insert a few extra sutures, as the tissues are very friable and you may cause more damage rather than achieve repair.
4. Be prepared to establish a proximal stoma and a distal mucous fistula or carry out a Hartmann's type procedure of closing the distal rectal stump.
5. Very occasionally, if contamination is slight, conditions are satisfactory and you are expert, you may elect to excise the margins and reform the anastomosis.
6. As a rule, after restoring the patient's health and nutritional status over a minimum of 6–12 weeks, you may reanastomose the bowel ends.

In the presence of a fistula, management depends on the state of the patient and the volume draining. When the volume is small (i.e. less than 500 ml per 24 h) and the patient is well, initially treat the patient conservatively:

1. Restrict oral intake.
2. Give intravenous fluids.
3. Correct fluid, protein, electrolyte, acid–base and vitamin deficiencies (see Chs 9, 10).
4. Treat associated sepsis.
5. Institute nutritional support.
6. Consider the somatostatin analogue octreotide to reduce gastrointestinal secretion and motility. If such treatment fails or the output is high (>500 ml day^{-1}) or there is associated sepsis, you must intervene surgically.

Table 36.4 Rates of clinically evident and radiologically detected leaks following colonic anastomoses performed above and below the pelvic peritoneal reflection

Location of anastomoses	Detected leaks (%)	
	Clinical	Radiological
Above pelvic peritoneum	1.2	18.3
Below pelvic peritoneum	16	33

Problems with the wound

Failure of wound healing may result (in descending order of importance) in wound dehiscence, incisional hernia or superficial wound disruption. Wound dehiscence should now be less than 0.1%. Incisional hernia is more common but should occur in less than 10% of abdominal wounds.

Risk factors

General risk factors include respiratory disease, smoking, obesity, obstructive jaundice (especially secondary to malignant disease), nutritional deficiencies of protein, zinc and vitamin C, malignant disease, steroid therapy, and following emergency procedures.

Local risk factors include wound infections, impaired blood supply, foreign body in the wound and previous irradiation to the area. Clean incised wounds heal better than ragged traumatic wounds. The site of wound is important: the anterior tibial area is notorious for wound breakdown, as are flap wounds with inappropriate length-to-width ratio. Poor surgical technique is another important factor.

Prevention

As in all complications, the cornerstone of success is to recognize risk factors, correct those that can be corrected and use an appropriate surgical technique for all wounds. For closing the abdominal wall, the best results are obtained by suture with a non-absorbable material, such as nylon, or an absorbable suture with prolonged tensile strength, such as polydioxanone. The Jenkins technique of mass closure is now well-established: take 1 cm bites, 1 cm apart, avoiding too much tension in the closed wound.

Key point

- **To avoid wound complications, ensure that your surgical technique is perfect, and choose your materials appropriately.**

Management of superficial disruption

- Evacuate haematoma and/or pus.
- Excise and remove slough.
- Remove any foreign body.
- Irrigate with, for example, hydrogen peroxide and povidone–iodine.
- Pack gently to avoid too rapid healing over of the skin, but avoid trauma to granulation tissue.
- Carefully monitor healing by secondary intention.

- Use newer materials such as Kaltostat or Sorbsan, which are well tolerated, highly absorbent alginates for wounds containing slough.

Management of wound dehiscence

The mortality reported following abdominal wound rupture varies from 24% to 46%.

- Recognize the problem early.
- Do not overlook premonitory serous discharge from the wound, a prolonged ileus, or low grade pyrexia.
- Resuscitate the patient.
- Re-explore the abdomen and perform adequate peritoneal lavage.
- Proceed to resuture the abdomen under general anaesthetic, using an adequate length of non-absorbable suture without tension.
- Use 1 cm bites about 1 cm apart.
- Avoid pulling the suture tightly in the tissues.
- It may be helpful to decompress the small bowel in retrograde fashion to reduce intra-abdominal tension.

Recurrence is uncommon but incisional herniation complicates approximately 25% of cases.

Management of incisional hernia

The indications for surgical intervention are obstruction, pain, or increasing size that makes control difficult. First spend time reducing such risk factors as obesity, smoking, constipation and prostatism. Assess the overall prognosis. Not all patients require or want surgical repair. Repair is unrewarding in the presence of unresected neoplastic disease. An abdominal support will control symptoms in most elderly and high risk patients.

Historically, a number of options are available as regards surgical technique, including Mayo or Keel repairs. However, except where the hernia is very small, a mesh repair is now the treatment of choice. Operative mortality should be less than 1% and the recurrence rate 5–10%. If a patient is morbidly obese at the time of repair a satisfactory result is less likely. The main problem with mesh repair is if infection supervenes. Under those circumstances it is most unusual that the repair will heal because of the presence of a foreign body. You will need to remove the mesh, allow the sepsis to settle completely, then start afresh. Meshes impregnated with antibiotics for high risk recurrent cases are under trial.

Hypertrophic and keloid scarring

Hypertrophic scars are limited to the wound area and do not advance after 6 months. Keloid (Greek *kele* = claw + *eidos* = like) scars are more extensive and continue to expand beyond 6 months, but fortunately are much less common. Predisposing factors are pigmented skin, burn trauma, wounds on posterior aspects, younger age groups, and a past history of keloid scarring.

There is excessive production and contraction of fibrous tissue. The synthesis of collagen is increased but the scar contains embryonic or fetal collagen. Only in hypertrophic scars is there an increased lysis of collagen. The main complication is joint deformity, but the cosmetic problems can be considerable in exposed sites and with younger patients.

Successful treatment is difficult, and should not be contemplated until 6 months from injury. There is no treatment for hypertrophic scars; do not attempt to treat keloid scars until they are mature. Re-excision with and without pressure or plastic procedures are as disappointing as radiotherapy. Greater success has been claimed for injection of steroids into the wound. The mode of action appears to be increased collagen lysis, with depression of the proliferation of fibroblasts. Injection of triamcinolone can be repeated at intervals of 1 or 2 weeks, depending on the result achieved.

Haemorrhage

Incidence

The incidence and severity of haemorrhagic complications are not easy to quantify. It is uncommonly necessary to re-explore a wound, evacuate haematoma and secure haemostasis. Wound haematoma and local bruising are sufficiently common to make it difficult to differentiate a complication from a normal sequel of surgery.

Where bleeding complicates intra-abdominal surgery, warning signs are haemodynamic instability with rising pulse and falling blood pressure, reduction in hourly urine volume to less than 40 ml h^{-1}, and excessive volume draining from the abdominal drain.

Predisposing factors are obesity, long-term steroid therapy, and jaundice. Recent transfusions of stored blood, coagulation diseases, platelet deficiencies and anticoagulant therapy may result in haemorrhage, and in old age there is increased capillary fragility. Severe sepsis may result in disseminated intravascular coagulation.

Pathology

It is conventional to consider primary haemorrhage as that occurring within 24 h of surgery. This is usually a technical problem of haemostasis. The operative area appears dry but with restoration of normal blood pressure or continuous infusion of intravenous fluids a vessel may dilate and bleed. In secondary haemorrhage, bleeding usually occurs 5–10 days after operation. It is due to local infection, sloughing of a clot or erosion of a ligature.

Prevention

 Key points

- **Recognize patients at risk of bleeding and reverse the risk factors before operation.**
- **Control infection.**
- **Ensure your surgical technique is meticulous.**

In patients on long-term warfarin it is relatively straightforward to convert the anticoagulation to intravenous heparin, which can be reversed more rapidly than warfarin by the injection of protamine.

Cooperate with a haematologist (see Ch. 8) in managing patients with coagulation disorders. Infuse specific factors as required. Timing is vital; for example, if fresh platelets are required for patients undergoing splenectomy, they must be given after the spleen has been removed. Give vitamin K by the intravenous route to reverse the problems associated with the obstructive element of jaundice.

Management

The need for intervention is dictated by the patient's symptoms and vital signs. Where haemorrhage is overt it is usually easier to decide whether exploration of the wound and cavity is indicated or not. When bleeding is internal you cannot rely on the effectiveness of an intra-cavity drain.

- Check a clotting screen to assess any established problems and to identify any new ones.
- Correct any deficit appropriately with vitamin K by injection for problems with the clotting mechanism, expressed as the international normalized ratio (INR). Use specific factors for deficiencies, fresh frozen plasma, and fresh platelets as indicated by the results of the coagulation study.
- Do not undertake surgical exploration until you have corrected any deficit, at least in part.
- It is unusual to identify a specific bleeding point at exploration.

The principles of surgery are to evacuate the blood and clot, identify any bleeding point or points, and control them appropriately. If a troublesome ooze persists, try the effect of a haemostatic agent such as Spongistan, or a collagen derivative. If you still cannot control the bleeding, pack the raw surface for 24–48 h. Consider leaving the superficial wound open. When you suspect a deeper source, and fear recurrent bleeding, as following a pancreatic operation, consider creating a laparostomy; leave the main wound open, packed with sterile packs. This facilitates re-exploration.

Summary

- Do you realize that the combination of cor pulmonale and ischaemic heart disease, or low output septic shock, carry up to 50% mortality?
- Do you appreciate the importance of correcting comorbidity factors before operation whenever possible?
- Are you aware that there are many complications that are common to all types of operation?
- Will you study the special risks you will encounter in each form of surgery?

 Further reading

Cuschieri A, Giles GR, Moossa AR 1988 Essential surgical practice. Wright, Bristol

Pollock AV 1991 Postoperative complications in surgery. Blackwell Scientific, Oxford

Smith JAR (ed.) 1984 Complications of surgery in general. Baillière Tindall, London

Tayfor I, Karran SJ (eds) 1996 Surgical principles. Edward Arnold, London

37 Intensive care

J. Jones, R. C. Leonard

Objectives

- **To identify the signs of impending critical illness.**
- **To understand the early and ICU management of critical illness.**
- **To appreciate the limitations of intensive care.**

INTRODUCTION

Although it has never been proved, it is likely that very sick patients can be managed better and more efficiently in a separate area specially equipped for their needs. In the UK, the Department of Health has recommended that intensive care units (ICUs) should represent 1–2% of acute hospital beds. This proportion is lower than in almost all other Western countries, and is now manifestly inadequate.

Organization

1. Critical care is labour intensive, and properly trained staff represent by far its most valuable resource. There should be one nurse for each ventilated patient and a senior nurse whose sole responsibility is to manage the unit.

2. There should always be at least one doctor capable of managing the airway on duty within the ICU and free from other commitments. A consultant must be immediately available. Although in the past most intensive care consultants in the UK have been anaesthetists, care of the critically ill requires close cooperation across many disciplines. The recent emergence of intensive care as a specialty in the UK has resulted in the creation of a small number of specialists capable of directing this complex multidisciplinary process. There is now evidence that intensive care units controlled by intensivists have better outcomes and shorter patient stays than those that are not (Carson et al 1996, Ghorra et al 1999, Baldock et al 2001).

Decision making

1. Advice on critically ill patients must be provided at a senior level. Never take it upon yourself to manage the sickest patients in the hospital without asking your consultant for support. Events proceed much more quickly in ICU than elsewhere, and what would be an acceptable delay on the wards is often not tolerated by ICU patients or staff.

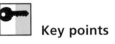

Key points

- **Offer intensive care only to those who need it and will benefit from it.**
- **Respond quickly to requests for advice or assistance from the ICU staff.**

2. It is often said that it is not reasonable to refuse admission to ICU simply on the grounds of advanced age, and that old people have been shown to respond to intensive care just as well as younger ones with similar disorders. While this is true, death cannot be postponed indefinitely, and the humane and reasonable use of intensive care over the age of 80 requires particular care in patient selection. Regardless of age, when the appropriateness of ICU admission is in question, an assessing intensivist needs the following information:

a. Current diagnosis and its prognosis

b. Comorbidities

c. Functional status; often a decisive factor – exercise tolerance, mobility, ability to do housework, shop, and venture outside the home.

3. Clearly judgements regarding the possible withholding of life-sustaining treatment can be difficult. They should be made at a senior level, whenever possible involving the patient (see Chs 14, 47). If the patient is not competent, the role of the next of kin is to represent the likely wishes of the patient regarding treatment. However, it is inhumane and morally irresponsible to leave such decisions to the relatives alone. The current fashion of seeking written agreement from the next of kin

before making an order not to attempt resuscitation often leaves families feeling that they must bear ultimate responsibility for their relative's death. Conduct discussions in terms of 'working together to decide what the patient would want us to do', not of 'asking consent to withdraw or withhold treatment'. Dealing explicitly with death can be painful and difficult, but should not be avoided until it is too late; patients and their families are sometimes surprisingly grateful for the chance to discuss these issues openly.

4. Intensivists often receive requests for manifestly inappropriate admission to ICU, justified by the words 'The family wants everything done'. Such requests represent failures of communication during the decision-making process outlined above. The intensivist should not be asked to take on the responsibility for communication, which lies with the referring specialist.

5. It has been shown that some patients are admitted to ICU too late in the course of their disease (McQuillan et al 1998). Earlier treatment might improve outcome and perhaps even avoid ICU admission altogether. For this to succeed, it is necessary to detect deterioration early and then provide staff capable of intervening effectively. The concept of a medical emergency team, called in response to defined physiological criteria, has been suggested as a solution. While this is theoretically attractive, outcome benefits have yet to be demonstrated (Bristow et al 2000). It may be impossible to detect deterioration soon enough to affect the course of the disease.

6. Successful management of the critically ill patient requires that two processes occur simultaneously:

a. Resuscitation from the pathophysiological derangement

b. Diagnosis and specific treatment of the underlying disease.

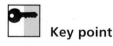

Key point

- **Critically ill patients need resuscitation, diagnosis and specific treatment.**

CORRECTING THE PHYSIOLOGY OF CRITICAL ILLNESS

We shall consider the vital systems serially (in succession); in reality they must be dealt with simultaneously – in parallel. Safe threshold limits for physiological values are given in order to provide practical guidance but there are some for whom these limits are too permissive or too stringent. If you ignore these limits without seeking senior advice you endanger the patient and will be called to account.

Cardiovascular pathophysiology

The function of the circulation is to transport oxygen and nutrients to the tissues and to remove metabolic waste products. There must be:

- Enough oxygen in the blood
- Enough blood flowing (cardiac output)
- Enough blood pressure to let tissues regulate their own perfusion.

1. The *oxygen content of blood* is determined by the concentration and oxygen saturation of haemoglobin.

2. *Blood pressure* is determined by the equation

$$BP = CO \times TPR$$

where BP = blood pressure, CO = cardiac output, and TPR = total peripheral resistance. Thus hypotension can be due either to low cardiac output or to inappropriate vasodilation. Treatment usually requires correction of the abnormal variable.

3. *Cardiac output* is determined by:

a. *Rate*. Too high a heart rate prevents adequate filling of the ventricle and reduces preload and cardiac output. Bradycardia reduces cardiac output as ejection simply does not happen often enough.

b. *Rhythm*. Loss of atrial contraction in junctional rhythms or atrial fibrillation also reduces preload and hence cardiac output by up to 30%.

c. *Preload*. The law of the heart, described by Henry Starling in 1915, states that the force of contraction of a cardiac muscle fibre is proportional to its initial length. The fibre length is determined by the ventricular volume. However, volumes are difficult to measure clinically, and the simplest substitute is the central venous pressure (CVP). The relationship between pressure and volume is not linear and is described by the ventricular compliance, which varies both between individuals and within each individual over time. For this reason, and because of the shape of the ventricular compliance curve (Fig. 37.1), it is usually not possible to determine the true preload or volume status from a single measurement of the CVP.

Key point

- **To check the volume status, observe the response of the CVP to a fluid challenge.**

Give 250 ml colloid over 10 min. The response indicates the volume status (Gomersall & Oh 1997):

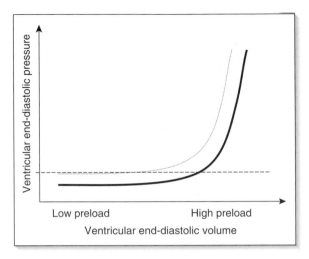

Fig. 37.1 The ventricular end-diastolic pressure–volume curve shows how, for a given pressure, the preload may be low or high because of the shape of the curve and the fact that compliance can vary between individuals and within individuals over time.

– if the CVP rises by more than 7 mmHg the patient is hypervolaemic
– if the CVP settles to within 3 mmHg of the original value, the patient is euvolaemic
– if the CVP rises by less than 3 mmHg the patient is hypovolaemic.

Serial fluid challenges may be given until the response suggests volume replacement is adequate.

d. *Contractility* is defined as the intrinsic ability of the myocardium to contract, independent of loading conditions. It is impossible to measure directly even under laboratory conditions, and must be inferred clinically from the CVP, blood pressure and assessments or measurements of the cardiac output. If preload is adequate, and blood pressure remains low, with evidence of a low cardiac output, contractility is usually impaired.

e. *Afterload.* Cardiac output is inversely related to the afterload, which may be defined either as the aortic input impedance or as the systolic ventricular wall tension. Afterload is reduced by:
– vasodilation (including rewarming of hypothermic patients)
– positive intrathoracic pressure
– intra-aortic balloon counterpulsation.

Manipulation of afterload in cardiogenic shock is complex and difficult, and is outside the scope of this introduction.

It is not often necessary to measure cardiac output in clinical situations. It is debated, but with very unreliable evidence, whether there is an association between the use of pulmonary artery catheters to measure cardiac output

and an apparent increase in mortality (Connors et al 1996). Less invasive methods of monitoring cardiac output are gaining in popularity.

4. *Shock* may be defined as inadequate tissue perfusion. It can be categorized into four types:

a. *Hypovolaemic shock* is due to a reduction in circulating volume following haemorrhage or dehydration. Venous return to the heart and hence ventricular preload are reduced, and the cardiac output and blood pressure fall. Reflex tachycardia and vasoconstriction partially compensate for the hypotension.

b. *Cardiogenic shock* results from primary myocardial dysfunction, reducing contractility and cardiac output. Causes include myocardial infarction and myocarditis. Once again, blood pressure is low, and reflex tachycardia and vasoconstriction occur in an attempt to compensate, but CVP is raised as the heart fails to eject the venous return adequately.

c. *Obstructive shock* occurs when an adequately filled heart is unable to eject its contents because of pericardial tamponade, tension pneumothorax or massive pulmonary embolism. CVP is again high because of the failure to eject, while cardiac output and blood pressure are low and the usual compensatory reflexes ensue.

d. *Distributive shock* refers to a condition of pathological vasodilation and capillary leak, which result in hypotension with a normal or high cardiac output. The condition is seen in sepsis, burns, pancreatitis and anaphylaxis. As the disease progresses, the capillary leak produces hypovolaemia. Multiple organ failure is characteristic of septic shock, and causes acute lung injury, renal failure and coagulopathy. Although there is a high cardiac output, it appears that there is a defect of tissue oxygen utilization. It is presently uncertain whether this is due to derangement of the microcirculation or of mitochondrial function.

Anaphylaxis (Greek *ana* = without + *phylaxis* = protection) usually follows immediately after the administration of drugs, colloids or contrast media. As in septic shock, there is profound vasodilation and increased capillary permeability. Urticarial rashes and bronchospasm are also common.

Inadequate tissue perfusion produces the signs of shock listed in Table 37.1. As can be seen, the disorder involves several systems.

5. *Hypotension.*

Table 37.1 Signs of inadequate tissue perfusion

Hypotension (BP < 90 mmHg)
Tachypnoea
Oliguria
Agitation, confusion or coma
Slow capillary refill (not in early sepsis)

Key points

- **Patients with the signs of shock are critically ill and are liable to rapid decompensation.**
- **They need urgent resuscitation.**

While there may be patients for whom a slightly lower BP is acceptable (for instance the rule does not necessarily apply under anaesthesia), if you are inexperienced, do not take such a decision alone. Conversely, if a patient has a systolic BP of 100 mmHg, but shows all the other signs of inadequate tissue perfusion, treat them with the same urgency as a shocked hypotensive patient.

The early management of hypotension follows from the physiological principles above, and is described in Table 37.2. ICU admission may become necessary at any stage in this process, but is usually inevitable if vaso-active drugs are required.

The most important point to realize is that, contrary to the myths instilled into all trainees at medical school, it *is generally far safer to give fluids than to withhold them.*

It is not clear what the appropriate goals of resuscitation are. The past fashion for targeting supranormal values of oxygen delivery (the product of oxygen content and cardiac output) is no longer sustainable. In the absence of convincing evidence, aim for these endpoints:

- Mean BP > 70 mmHg
- Resolving tachycardia
- Improved peripheral perfusion
- Urine output improved above at least 0.5 and prefer-ably 1 ml kg^{-1} h^{-1}
- Resolving acidosis and falling lactate.

Key points

- **A non-pregnant adult with systolic blood pressure below 90 mmHg has dangerous hypotension and requires immediate treatment.**
- **It is generally far safer to give fluids than to withhold them.**

Respiratory pathophysiology

The respiratory system transports oxygen to the blood and removes carbon dioxide from it. Success requires an adequate volume of gas to ventilate the alveoli and close matching of the degree of ventilation and perfusion of each lung unit. Failure results in hypoxaemia, hypercarbia (raised blood carbon dioxide) or both.

Table 37.2 Management of hypotension

- Check for **airway, breathing and circulation**
- **Check the BP yourself**
  Automatic BP machines measure the mean arterial pressure; the systolic and diastolic pressures they display are calculated and may therefore be inaccurate
- **Give high flow oxygen**
- Check for **signs of shock**
- Establish **large-bore venous access** (14 gauge or 16 gauge) and draw blood for…
- **Investigations**: FBP, coagulation studies, U&E, amylase, cardiac enzymes, arterial blood gases, chest X-ray, ECG
- Examine for **signs of pulmonary oedema**. If a hypotensive patient has pulmonary oedema, he or she is desperately ill and needs expert assistance from the ICU immediately. **If there is no pulmonary oedema it is safe to give fluid**
- **Give 500 ml of any fluid except 5% dextrose,** and repeat as necessary
- **Take a history, examine the patient, MAKE A DIAGNOSIS AND GIVE SPECIFIC TREATMENT**
- If there is no response after between 1000 and 2000 ml fluid, insert a central venous catheter and titrate filling using **serial fluid challenges** as described above
- If hypotension persists despite adequate filling, give **vasoactive drugs**: **inotropes** (adrenaline (epinephrine)) if cardiac output is low or uncertain; **vasoconstrictors** (noradrenaline (norepinephrine)) if cardiac output is high. It is sometimes necessary to measure cardiac output directly in order to make this distinction

---

Ventilation–perfusion (V/Q) matching

Consider the idealized alveolar–capillary unit represented in Fig. 37.2. If perfusion and ventilation are either perfectly matched or completely mismatched, then there are three possible situations:

1. Perfect matching of ventilation to perfusion (V/Q = 1).
2. Normal ventilation but no perfusion (V/Q = ∞), as shown in Fig. 37.3, analogous to that existing in the anatomical dead space, which refers to that part of the tidal volume which does not reach a surface where gas exchange can occur.
3. Normal perfusion but no ventilation (V/Q = 0), as shown in Fig. 37.4, resembles what happens to the venous blood which is shunted anatomically past the lungs without participating in gas exchange because it passes through the thebesian or bronchial veins (in normal subjects) or a right-to-left intracardiac shunt (in patients with cyanotic congenital heart disease). These

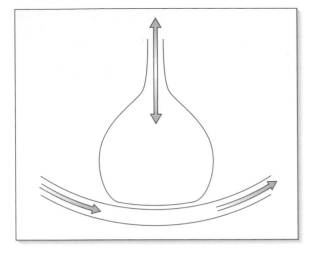

Fig. 37.2 Idealized alveolar–capillary unit showing ventilation of the alveolus and perfusion of the capillary.

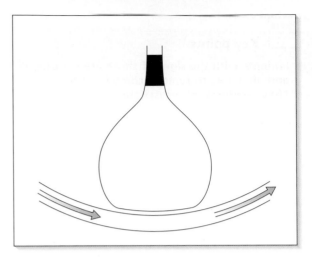

Fig. 37.4 Normal perfusion but no ventilation (V/Q = 0), referred to as shunt.

situations are therefore referred to as representing the physiological dead space and the physiological shunt.

Dead space ventilation decreases the proportion of each breath that participates in gas exchange, and hence alveolar ventilation falls. Unless the respiratory rate rises to compensate, hypercarbia will ensue.

The consequence of blood being shunted through the diseased, unventilated lung tissue without engaging in gas exchange is that unoxygenated venous blood is mixed into the blood that has been oxygenated; hence, arterial oxygen content falls.

In reality, there exists a spectrum of V/Q relationships from 0 to ∞. The vast majority of lung units of healthy subjects are tightly clustered around the ideal situation, with a few outliers, as shown in Fig. 37.5. However, when the lungs are diseased there is an increase in the scatter of the V/Q ratios, which causes an increase in physiological shunting and dead space ventilation.

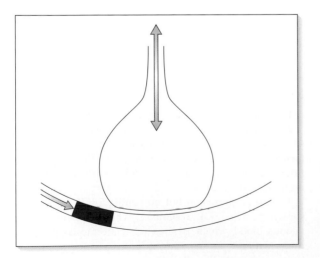

Fig. 37.3 Normal ventilation but no perfusion (V/Q = ∞), referred to as dead space ventilation.

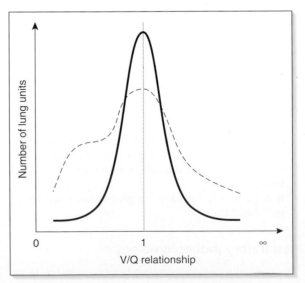

Fig. 37.5 Scatter of V/Q ratios in a healthy subject (solid line) and in a patient with respiratory disease (dotted line). Note the increase in physiological shunt and dead space.

Hypercarbia

Caused by reduced alveolar minute ventilation, hypercarbia results from:

1. Reduced respiratory rate (hypoventilation)
2. Increased physiological dead space ventilation.

Both of these can be corrected or compensated by increasing the respiratory rate.

Hypoxaemia

Hypoxaemia is caused by:

1. Hypoventilation. When the rate at which fresh inspiratory gas is presented to the alveoli falls, but oxygen consumption remains the same, the partial pressure of oxygen within the alveoli must also fall. As a result the oxygen tension within the pulmonary capillary and hence the systemic arteries (PaO_2) is reduced. Postoperative patients may hypoventilate because of pain from upper abdominal incisions, or because of opioid analgesia. Clearly, the hypoxaemia of hypoventilation can be corrected by increasing the respiratory rate, either pharmacologically or mechanically, but also more simply by increasing the inspired oxygen fraction (FiO_2).

2. Shunting. True anatomical shunting cannot be corrected by an increased FiO_2, because by definition no gas exchange occurs. Postoperative patients may develop a shunt because of basal atelectasis (Greek a = not + *telos* = end + *ectasis* = expansion; hence, collapse) or chest infection. However, relative physiological shunting caused by imperfect V/Q matching can be partially corrected by increasing the FiO_2. Techniques available to reduce shunt involve raising the mean airway pressure in order to recruit collapsed lung units.

 Key point

- **Hypoxaemia is a far more dangerous and rapidly lethal state than hypercarbia.**

Hypoxaemia may be treated by oxygen therapy.

Oxygen therapy. It is incorrect to withhold oxygen in the presence of chronic obstructive pulmonary disease (COPD) for fear of inducing hypercarbic narcosis. The false reasoning for withholding oxygen is that, although in healthy humans the normal source of ventilatory drive is the carbon dioxide response, patients with COPD have a blunted response to hypercarbia and are dependent on hypoxaemic ventilatory drive. Treatment with oxygen is then assumed to remove this stimulus to breathe and thus to cause hypoventilation, hypercarbia and coma. It is true

that some patients with COPD do experience an increase in arterial carbon dioxide tension when hypoxaemia is treated with oxygen, but it is irresponsible to treat this response with a return to hypoxaemia. The increase in arterial carbon dioxide tension ($PaCO_2$) rarely causes problems as long as oxygen therapy is controlled to ensure safe but not excessive oxygen saturations (say 90–92%). If hypercarbia does occur, and is causing problems, do not add hypoxaemia to the patient's difficulties, but instead refer urgently for ventilation.

Oxygen therapy is always prescribed in the early postoperative period to treat hypoxaemia from the causes mentioned earlier. It is known that patients continue to experience episodic nocturnal hypoxaemia for at least three days after surgery. This coincides with the period of highest risk for perioperative myocardial infarction, and anaesthetists commonly prescribe oxygen for 3 days following operation in patients who are at particular risk of this dangerous complication. Do not countermand these orders or you will be putting your patient at risk.

Oxygen can be given by the following devices:

1. Nasal cannulae deliver 2–4 l min^{-1} O_2; Hudson masks deliver up to 15 l min^{-1} O_2. Although they deliver a known flow, the FiO_2 is determined by the amount of air entrained by the patient during inspiration. This in turn is determined by the peak inspiratory flow rate, which of course varies.

2. Venturi masks (G. B. Venturi, 1746–1822, was an Italian physicist) deliver 24–60% O_2. They use Bernoulli's principle (as the velocity of a moving fluid increases, the pressure within the fluid decreases) to deliver a high enough flow of known FiO_2 to exceed the patient's peak inspiratory flow rate, thus avoiding entrainment of further air.

3. Continuous positive airway pressure (CPAP) represents the next level of respiratory support from oxygen supplementation. A tight-fitting mask connected to either a large reservoir or high gas flow permits an FiO_2 of up to 1.0, while at the same time a positive pressure is applied continuously to the patient's upper airway. This positive pressure recruits alveoli which are collapsed due to lung disease, and results in:

a. Reduced shunt and therefore increased PaO_2

b. Increased lung volume and therefore (usually) improved pulmonary compliance and reduced work of breathing. CPAP usually has little effect on $PaCO_2$, despite the reduced work of breathing.

4. Mechanical ventilation (Latin *ventus* = wind) may be applied invasively (via a tracheal or tracheostomy tube) or non-invasively via a tight-fitting face mask. The latter technique is only suitable for conscious patients with adequate ventilatory drive who require a modest reduction in their work of breathing and shunt. The indications for mechanical ventilation are:

a. Respiratory failure refractory to less invasive treatments

b. Elective postoperative ventilation

c. Physiological control (as for instance in raised intracranial pressure).

The decision to ventilate a patient with respiratory failure is complex, and takes into account the following factors:

- Respiratory distress
- Respiratory drive
- Level of consciousness
- Natural history of underlying disease
- Arterial blood gas results.

Elective postoperative ventilation is often used in anticipation of respiratory failure in the following situations:

- Major surgery (e.g. cardiac surgery, thoracoabdominal aneurysm repair)
- Hypothermia
- Massive transfusion
- Haemodynamic instability
- Staged procedure (e.g. following penetrating abdominal trauma or faecal peritonitis).

Mechanical ventilation carries a number of complications. Do not seek to embark upon it without proper indications. The complications include:

- Cardiovascular compromise
- Fluid retention
- Pneumothorax
- Ventilator-associated lung injury
- Ventilator-associated pneumonia
- Accidental disconnection
- Complications relating to the artificial airway (e.g. tracheal stenosis).

The various modes of ventilation are confusing, and classifications of them are unhelpful. Essentially, other than the basic goal of delivering tidal volumes of respiratory gas to the lungs a certain number of times a minute, the different modes are aimed at one of the following:

- Facilitating the patient's spontaneous respiratory efforts
- Improving oxygenation in refractorily hypoxaemic patients
- Limiting dangerously high airway pressures

Respiratory distress

This is one of the earliest indicators of impending critical illness, as well as the major determining factor of the need for mechanical ventilation. The signs of respiratory distress are:

1. Tachypnoea (Greek *tachys* = swift + *pnoia* = breathing)
2. Use of accessory muscles of respiration – the most obvious being the sternocleidomastoid muscles, which contract during inspiration
3. Difficulty speaking
4. Pulse oximeter (SpO_2 = oxygen saturation from pulse oximeter) reading < 90%
5. Agitation, confusion or coma.

 Key points

- **Respiratory rate > 30 or < 8, inability to speak half a sentence, agitation, coma, SpO_2 < 90%, indicate potentially serious illness.**
- **Provide immediate treatment.**

Unless a patient with these signs improves rapidly, he or she may require early intubation and ventilation. In the setting of respiratory distress, agitation or coma are particularly worrying, as they make it very difficult to manage the patient without securing the airway.

1. SpO_2 < 90% requires immediate correction, as further desaturation is likely to be rapid.

2. A satisfactory SpO_2 reading does not rule out severe respiratory problems. Oxygen therapy can maintain a normal saturation until shortly before respiratory arrest occurs.

 Key point

- **Monitor the respiratory rate: it is a crucial indicator in a potentially unstable patient.**

Renal dysfunction

Renal failure is a frequent problem in surgical wards and in ICU. By far the commonest cause is acute tubular necrosis. The cells lining the renal tubules are metabolically very active and have a high oxygen requirement; if they are deprived of it, they swell, die and are shed into the lumen. The same effects result when toxic substances are excreted by the kidneys, such as gentamicin, amphotericin B and cisplatin. Fortunately, the cells can regenerate. Inadequate renal perfusion is usually due to a combination of hypovolaemia, hypotension, sepsis, nephrotoxic drugs and pre-existing renal disease.

In the case of sepsis, renal failure may occur as part of the syndrome of multiple organ dysfunction, when it carries a grim prognosis. However, if the patient survives the acute illness, renal function usually recovers.

Key point

- **Monitor urine output hourly; if it falls below 0.5 ml kg^{-1} h^{-1}, correct it without delay.**

Early correction of underlying renal hypoperfusion may prevent the development of acute tubular necrosis. Therefore:

1. Correct hypovolaemia, if necessary using CVP guidance as described above.
2. Correct hypotension and low cardiac output, using vasopressors or inotropes.

In previously hypertensive patients it may be necessary to raise the blood pressure to levels close to their normal pressure (which may be higher than the usual target mean arterial pressure in ICU of around 70 mmHg). Only then can the kidneys autoregulate their blood flow, allowing renal perfusion to occur.

There is no evidence of benefit from other strategies, including low dose 'renal' dopamine (Bellomo et al 2000). Furosemide (frusemide) given to promote a diuresis is common; at least it has the theoretical benefit of reducing renal oxygen consumption and protecting the struggling kidney against ischaemia. However, it is essential to correct hypovolaemia first.

Key point

- **Do not treat oliguria with excessive early doses of furosemide (frusemide); hypovolaemia *must* be corrected first.**

Other causes of oliguria in a surgical patient are urinary obstruction, of which the commonest cause by far is a blocked catheter, and sodium and water retention due to the neuroendocrine stress response to surgical trauma.

If oliguria persists despite correct treatment, it is likely that established renal failure will develop. A high urinary sodium (> 20 mmol l^{-1}) or a low urinary osmolality (280–320 mOsm l^{-1}) in the absence of recent diuretic treatment suggest renal failure. Seek the advice of an intensivist or nephrologist. Meanwhile:

1. Maintain euvolaemia, which usually involves fluid restriction to 20 ml h^{-1} plus the previous hour's output. Be particularly careful to avoid fluid overload in patients who are not ventilated.
2. Monitor closely for hyperkalaemia and metabolic acidosis.
3. Measure serum creatinine and urea twice daily.

Renal replacement therapy in the form of haemofiltration or haemodialysis is indicated for hyperkalaemia, acidosis, fluid overload or an inexorably rising creatinine. Once dialysis is inevitable there is nothing to be gained from procrastination; arrange for it without delay.

Acute neurological problems

You will encounter many patients with an acutely depressed conscious level resulting from trauma, drugs, acute intracranial event (such as infarction or haemorrhage) and encephalopathy of critical illness.

Key points

- **Never forget to check the blood sugar level.**
- **Glasgow coma score (GCS) < 8 or failure to localize to pain are indications for intubation, ventilation, investigation and specific treatment.**

You should only ignore this recommendation for intubation if it has been decided that the patient should not have active management under any circumstances, following an intracranial disaster. If a CT scan shows an unrecoverable situation, then treatment can be withdrawn at that point.

Nutrition

1. Nutritional support is needed when the patient is unlikely to resume normal oral intake within 7–10 days of it ceasing (Klein et al 1997). If nutritional support is inevitable, start it as soon as the patient is stabilized (see Ch. 10). Discuss the timing of commencing feeding with the intensivists.

2. Enteral feeding is cheaper, easier and therefore preferable. Evidence for a protective effect on the intestinal mucosa is weak, and complications of enteral feeding are underreported (Lipman 1998). It has been definitely indicted as an independent risk factor for ventilator-associated pneumonia (Drakulovic et al 1999). Thus it is reasonable to consider parenteral feeding in patients with doubtful ability to tolerate enteral feeding within

7 days (Woodcock et al 2001). Meanwhile, make strenuous efforts to establish enteral feeding.

3. When nasogastric feeding is not tolerated despite giving prokinetic agents, try passing a nasojejunal tube. This route is now commonly used in patients with pancreatitis. Traditionally, such patients were fed parenterally, but jejunal feeding is now known to be safe and perhaps associated with better outcomes (Pupelis et al 2001).

4. The optimal content of feeding solutions is uncertain. Carbohydrates, essential lipids, protein, vitamins and trace elements are needed, and it is clear that there is an upper limit to the amount of both energy and protein that the body can use. Excessive feeding is at least as dangerous as underfeeding. There is a vogue for using regimens containing immunologically active nutrients such as arginine, glutamine, RNA and omega-3 fatty acids; they are expensive and not well evaluated.

General considerations

Intensive care medicine consists mainly of the vital process of nursing patients back to health, and requires meticulous attention to detail. Four areas deserve mention:

1. Nosocomial infection with resistant organisms is an enormous problem. You must adhere strictly to infection control measures:

a. Wash hands before and after touching every patient.

b. Wear gloves and a plastic apron when examining a patient.

c. Use full sterile technique, as for a surgical procedure, when inserting a central venous catheter, both in ICU and on the wards. This reduces catheter-related bacteraemia rates sixfold.

2. Thromboembolism prophylaxis is needed for most patients, usually with subcutaneous heparin. Compressive stockings may be useful.

3. Stress ulcer prophylaxis is necessary, at least until enteral feeding is established. On current evidence give H_2 antagonists (Cook et al 1998). If the patient has no history of, or special risk factors for peptic ulceration, enteral feeding alone is adequate.

4. Patients' families are under enormous stress; try to alleviate this with frequent, early communication and support (see Ch. 47). It can be one of the most rewarding aspects of working in the ICU.

Summary

- Do you understand that intensive care depends on the availability of highly skilled, dedicated staff, so that selection of patients for admission must be justified by expectation of survival with acceptable quality of life?
- Do you recognize that intensive care is not different from standard patient care, but performed in an exemplary fashion?
- Are you aware of the need to adhere strictly and unremittingly to infection control measures?
- Will you try to alleviate the stressful situation of the patients' families by maintaining good communication and support (see Ch. 47)?

References

Baldock G, Foley P, Brett S 2001 The impact of organisational change on outcome in an intensive care unit in the United Kingdom. Intensive Care Medicine 27(5): 865–872

Bellomo R, Chapman M, Finfer S, Hickling K, Myburgh J 2000 Low-dose dopamine in patients with early renal dysfunction: a placebo-controlled randomised trial. Australian and New Zealand Intensive Care Society (ANZICS) Clinical Trials Group. Lancet 356(9248): 2139–2143

Bristow PJ, Hillman KM, Chey T et al 2000 Rates of in-hospital arrests, deaths and intensive care admissions: the effect of a medical emergency team. Medical Journal of Australia 173(5): 236–240

Carson SS, Stocking C, Podsadecki T et al 1996 Effects of organizational change in the medical intensive care unit of a teaching hospital: a comparison of 'open' and 'closed' formats. JAMA 276(4): 322–328

Connors AF Jr, Speroff T, Dawson NV et al 1996 The effectiveness of right heart catheterization in the initial care of critically ill patients. SUPPORT investigators. JAMA 276(11): 889–897

Cook D, Guyatt G, Marshall J et al 1998 A comparison of sucralfate and ranitidine for the prevention of upper gastrointestinal bleeding in patients requiring mechanical ventilation. Canadian Critical Care Trials Group. New England Journal of Medicine 338(12): 791–797

Drakulovic MB, Torres A, Bauer TT, Nicolas JM, Nogue S, Ferrer M 1999 Supine body position as a risk factor for nosocomial pneumonia in mechanically ventilated patients: a randomised trial. Lancet 354(9193): 1851–1858

Ghorra S, Reinert SE, Cioffi W, Buczko G, Simms HH 1999 Analysis of the effect of conversion from open to closed surgical intensive care unit. Annals of Surgery 229(2): 163–171

Gomersall CD, Oh TE 1997 Haemodynamic monitoring. In: Oh TE (ed.) Intensive care manual. Butterworth Heinemann, Oxford, 831–838

Klein S, Kinney J, Jeejeebhoy K et al 1997 Nutrition support in clinical practice: review of published data and recommendations for future research directions. Summary of a conference sponsored by the National Institutes of Health, American Society for Parenteral and Enteral Nutrition, and American Society for Clinical Nutrition. American Journal of Clinical Nutrition 66(3): 683–706

Lipman TO 1998 Grains or veins: is enteral nutrition really better than parenteral nutrition? A look at the evidence.

JPEN. Journal of Parenteral and Enteral Nutrition 22(3): 167–182

McQuillan P, Pilkington S, Allan et al 1998. Confidential inquiry into quality of care before admission to intensive care. BMJ 316: 1853–1858

Pupelis G, Selga G, Austrums E, Kaminski A 2001 Jejunal feeding, even when instituted late, improves outcomes in patients with severe pancreatitis and peritonitis. Nutrition 17(2): 91–94

Woodcock NP, Zeigler D, Palmer MD, Buckley P, Mitchell CJ, MacFie J 2001 Enteral versus parenteral nutrition: a pragmatic study. Nutrition 17(1): 1–12

38 Dialysis

A. Davenport

Objectives

- **Be aware of the indications for dialysis.**
- **Understand the principles of haemodialysis and peritoneal dialysis.**
- **Recognize the limitations to artificial replacement of renal function.**

INTRODUCTION

Dialysis (Greek *dia* = asunder + *lyein* = to lose; hence separation of substances through a septum or partition) offers a method of treating patients with loss or severe impairment of renal function. The membrane is synthetic in haemodialysis but the peritoneum forms the membrane in peritoneal dialysis.

Loss of the renal function threatens intracellular homeostasis (Greek *homos* = like, similar + *stasis* = a standing; hence, a state of equilibrium) resulting from failure to maintain salt and water balance. There is an additional hormone disturbance. Erythropoietin (Greek *erythros* = red + *poiesis* = a making) is produced by peritubular cells in response to hypoxia. The final step in the synthesis of active vitamin D takes place in the kidney; vitamin D increases uptake of calcium in the gut and the resorption of bone.

Surgical patients may present with impaired renal function. It may develop as a complication of treatment following the stress of an operation there is increased arginine vasopressin (also known as antidiuretic hormone, ADH) release, resulting in water retention. Acute renal failure may develop secondary to hypovolaemia and/or septic shock.

The increased availability of, and survival on, dialysis makes it likely that you will encounter patients on dialysis requiring surgical treatment.

PRINCIPLES

Fluid and chemical exchanges take place across a semipermeable membrane (Latin *semi* = half or partly + *per* = through + *meare* + to pass). On one side is natural fluid such as blood, on the other is dialysate, a specially formulated liquid. In peritoneal dialysis the peritoneal mesothelium is the natural membrane; in haemodialysis it is synthetic and the size of the pores determines what can cross the partial barrier. Across the membrane, interchange takes place of water, electrolytes and other solutes under the influence of hydrostatic and osmotic forces. Dialysis exploits two physical principles: diffusion and convection.

Diffusion

1. Molecules within a medium are constantly moving, the speed determined by the temperature. As they collide, they bounce off each other and separate. The Scottish botanist, Robert Brown, observed the result of these collisions in 1827 and this movement is named after him: brownian movement. In an area of high concentration there are more collisions and an increased tendency to separate. This is diffusion (Latin *dif*, *dis* = asunder + *fundere* to pour out; thus, to pour out in all directions). It results in an even distribution of the molecules throughout the medium (Fig. 38.1).

2. If blood is separated from prepared fluid – dialysate – by a semipermeable membrane that permits the passage of molecules of a substance in high concentration in the blood, the molecules will pass through into the dialysate provided the substance is absent or in lower concentration in the dialysate.

3. In peritoneal dialysis the membrane is the peritoneum; in haemodialysis the membrane is artificial and has pores of predetermined size in order to control the size of the molecules that can or cannot pass through.

4. In renal failure, urea, creatinine, potassium and other waste products accumulate in the blood. Since the dialysate used in peritoneal dialysis or haemodialysis

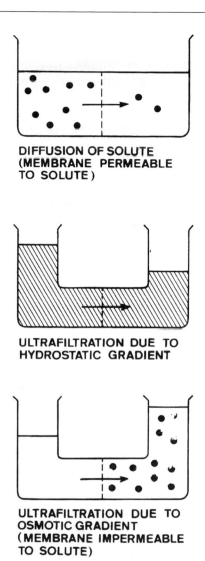

**DIFFUSION OF SOLUTE
(MEMBRANE PERMEABLE
TO SOLUTE)**

**ULTRAFILTRATION DUE TO
HYDROSTATIC GRADIENT**

**ULTRAFILTRATION DUE TO
OSMOTIC GRADIENT
(MEMBRANE IMPERMEABLE
TO SOLUTE)**

Fig. 38.1 Diffusion of a solute from a region of high concentration to one of low concentration.

contains none of these substances, the accumulated substances diffuse into it from the plasma.

5. Conversely, by adding bicarbonate to the dialysate at a higher than plasma concentration, so that bicarbonate diffuses into the plasma, metabolic acidosis can be corrected.

6. By similar adjustments of dialysate concentration, calcium can be introduced into or extracted from, the plasma.

7. Because the water content of both peritoneal dialysis and haemodialysis fluid is greater than that of plasma, water should diffuse from the dialysate into the plasma. This is prevented by the relatively higher hydrostatic plasma pressure during haemodialysis; it is prevented in

peritoneal dialysis by increasing the osmotic pressure of the dialysate with glucose, raising the concentration above plasma levels.

Convection

1. Convection (Latin *con* = together, with + *tehere* = to carry) is the transfer of substances or effects by means of currents. In haemodialysis, as blood is pumped through the haemodialyser, its hydrostatic pressure is higher than that of the dialysate, so that plasma water passes through the membrane into the dialysing fluid. Depending on the size of the pores in the membrane, any plasma solute that is small enough to pass through will be carried across with the plasma water. The rate of permeable solute removal corresponds to the solute concentration in the plasma water (Fig. 38.2).

2. Convection also occurs across the peritoneal membrane but there is no significant hydrostatic pressure difference. Therefore, the dialysate glucose concentration is raised to increase its osmotic pressure, creating a plasma water flow current into the dialysate (Fig. 38.3).

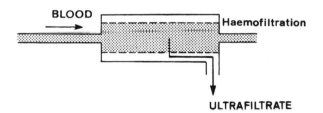

Fig. 38.2 During haemofiltration solute moves by convection, according to concentration in plasma water.

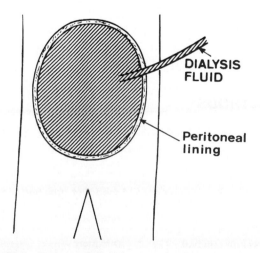

Fig. 38.3 Peritoneal dialysis.

Ultrafiltration

The separation of particles by filtration under pressure or suction is ultrafiltration (Latin *ultra* = beyond + *filtrum* = felt – from the use of fabric formed from fibres that can be matted together without weaving, through which to strain liquids). Because there is very little convection during standard haemodialysis, the transfer effect can be increased by reducing the pressure in the dialysate compartment. Normal kidneys ultrafiltrate 180 litres each day, depending on the pressure difference between the renal glomerular arteriole and the renal tubule (Fig. 38.4).

Key point

- **The majority of solute (dissolved substance) transfer during dialysis is by diffusion.**

Table 38.1 illustrates what can be accomplished by the different methods.

INDICATIONS

1. Acute dialysis may be required for:
   a. Hyperkalaemia refractory to medical treatment. A level above 6 mmol l^{-1} is dangerous; above 7 mmol l^{-1} it demands urgent correction.
   b. Severe metabolic acidosis unresponsive to supportive treatment.
   c. Pulmonary oedema not responding to medical management.
   d. Uraemia with serum urea above 30 mmol l^{-1} and/or creatinine above 500 μmol l^{-1}, or a rise in creatinine of more than 100 μmol l^{-1} in 24 h.
2. Chronic renal dialysis replaces long-term loss of excretory functions. It does not, of course, replace endocrine functions of the kidneys.

METHODS

1. Kolff in Holland devised the first practical haemodialysis machine during the Second World War.

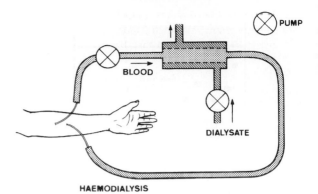

Fig. 38.4 Ultrafiltration can occur by applying hydrostatic pressure during haemodialysis, or osmotic pressure during peritoneal dialysis.

Scribner, in 1960, described a practical method of vascular access by uniting the cephalic vein and radial artery using an external shunt but this has been almost completely superseded by the side-to-side arteriovenous fistula between the vein and artery described by Simeno and Brescia. An alternative is a venous end-to-side anastomosis into the artery. Alternative sites may be needed, such as basilic vein to brachial artery. Care of these fistulae demands skilled management by trained attendants.

2. Chronic haemodialysis is increasingly performed using higher flux membranes than formerly, to reduce dialysis times. In the USA, blood flow rates have been increased up to 450 ml min^{-1}. To decrease dialysis times still further, ultrapure dialysate may first be administered to maximize subsequent haemofiltration.

3. The anaemia resulting from loss of renal production of erythropoietin can be corrected by administering recombinant human erythropoietin.

4. Acute dialysis may be required, often on critically ill patients.

5. Peritoneal dialysis became practical after the development of a semipermanent peritoneal catheter by Tenkhoff, followed by a variety of catheters and methods of inserting them. Peritonitis may develop, presenting with generalized abdominal pain, peritonism, absent bowel sounds, vomiting, dehydration and pyrexia. There is neutrophilia and cloudy peritoneal dialysate effluent.

Table 38.1 Comparison of modes of filtration.			
	Haemodialysis	Haemofiltration	Peritoneal dialysis
Solute removal	Diffusion	Convection	Diffusion
Water removal	Ultrafiltration	Convection	Convection
Dialyser type	Low permeability	High permeability	Peritoneal membrane

The diagnosis is confirmed by detecting in the dialysate, after a 4 h dwell, more than 100 leucocytes per millilitre, of which 90% are polymorphs. Because of changing trends in peritoneal dialysis, it may not be possible to differentiate between peritoneal dialysis peritonitis and an intra-abdominal catastrophe. For this reason always test a 4 h dwell specimen with a Gram stain. Peritoneal dialysis peritonitis, often resulting from coagulase-negative staphylococci, usually responds to intra-peritoneal antibiotics; an intra-abdominal catastrophe may demand operative intervention.

6. Peritoneal dialysis can be employed in the management of acute renal failure. To minimize the changes in intraperitoneal pressure, which can cause cardiovascular instability, prefer to use small volume changes, known as tidal peritoneal dialysis. Reduced mesenteric blood flow in septic, hypotensive patients may prejudice solute transfer. Because of technical problems, such as leaks, peritoneal dialysis may not be possible following abdominal operation.

Key point

- The management of patients on dialysis treatment demands skilled care from trained attendants – to maintain the system and avoid, anticipate, detect and treat complications.

OUTLOOK

1. The effectiveness of dialysis is not more than 7% of that of normally functioning kidneys.

2. Increasing the amount of dialysis increases survival.

3. Because of decreased $1,25(OH)_2$ vitamin D_3, patients tend to develop secondary hyperparathyroidism. Treat this with vitamin D analogues or patients will develop tertiary hyperparathyroidism with bone resorption, requiring operative treatment. It may be possible to prevent this by injecting vitamin D analogues into the parathyroid gland.

4. Chronic dialysis patients may develop a form of amyloid disease owing to the deposition of E_2 microglobulin. Deposits in the wrist may provoke carpal tunnel syndrome, in tendon sheaths causing trigger finger, in the palm causing Dupuytren's contracture, and elsewhere in the body.

5. The native kidney shrinks and develops cysts, which have an increasing malignant potential.

6. The effect of uraemia in reducing platelet function increases the risk of bleeding at operation. This may be made worse if the patient is taking prophylactic aspirin to counter the increased risks of cardiovascular disease in renal failure.

Key points

- **Carefully prepare patients with renal failure before operations by ensuring the haematocrit is above 30%.**
- **Ensure that the patients are well dialysed preoperatively.**
- **Avoid giving low molecular weight dextrans prior to operation because they will have a prolonged half-life.**

Summary

- Do you understand the physical principles on which dialysis is based?
- Do you know the aims of dialysis therapy: the maintenance of patient well-being until acute renal failure recovers, and the extension of life in chronic renal failure?
- Do you know what are the major methods used in a patient with renal failure?
- Do you appreciate the deficiencies of dialysis compared with normal renal function?

Comprehensive reference

Davison AM, Cameron JS, Grunfeld JP, Kerr DNS, Ritz E, Winearls CG (eds) 2002 Oxford textbook of clinical nephrology, 3rd edn. Oxford University Press, Oxford

Future reading

Davenport A, Will EJ, Davison AM 1993 Improved cardiovascular stability during continuous modes of renal replacement therapy in critically ill patients with acute hepatic and renal failure. Critical Care Medicine 21: 328–338
Ronco C, Bellomo R, Kellum J A 2002 Continuous renal replacement therapy: opinions and evidence. Advances in Renal Replacement Therapy 9(4): 229–244
Wester JP, de Koning EJ, Geers AB et al 2002 Analysis of renal replacement therapy in seriously ill (ARTIS) investigators. Catheter replacement in continuous arteriovenous hemodiafiltration: the balnce between infectious and mechanical complications. Critical Care Medicine 30(6): 1261–1266

39 Chronic illness, rehabilitation and terminal care

A. C. Kurowska, A. Tookman

Objectives

- **Recognize the importance of effective communication.**
- **Understand the principles of pain and symptom control.**
- **Prescribe analgesics appropriately (especially opioids).**
- **Be able to manage the process of dying.**

INTRODUCTION

In patients with chronic illness and advanced disease, effective symptom control forms the basis of management (Table 39.1). For such patients the primary aim of treatment is not necessarily to prolong life but to make it as comfortable and meaningful as possible. Effective palliative care enables this to happen. A significant number of patients experience functional limitations because of their disease or its treatment. Many of these can be treated by rehabilitation techniques that enable them to develop to their maximum potential.

Patients with malignancy form a large proportion of the patients you see with chronic and terminal illness. Since such patients present with complex problems, focus your approach on the whole patient, rather than simply on the disease. An interdisciplinary team approach, including the patient and 'family', is essential to achieve these aims.

The proportion of all deaths occurring in hospital has increased over the last 15 years. Patients can choose the most suitable place to spend their terminal illness if specialist palliative care support teams are used effectively. Such teams provide support and expert advice to the professionals and other carers involved in the patient's management. Make sure you are familiar with your local teams both within the hospital and in the community.

Table 39.1 Important definitions

- A *terminally ill* patient is one with a confident diagnosis that cure is impossible. Prognosis is usually months or less. Treatment is aimed at relief of symptoms. Most such patients have advanced cancer, but non-malignant disease also falls within this definition, such as the end stage of renal failure, chronic obstructive airways disease, multiple sclerosis, acquired immune deficiency syndrome (AIDS) and motor neuron disease.
- A *chronically ill* patient (Greek *chronos* = time; hence lasting a long time) has a longer and less predictable prognosis. Many of these patients have non-malignant disease, such as inflammatory bowel disease, peripheral vascular disease and post-trauma. Some malignant conditions have a protracted course, such as breast and prostatic cancer.
- The *palliative care approach* (Latin *palliare* = to cloak; disguise, extenuate) aims to promote both physical and psychosocial well-being. It is a vital and integral part of all clinical practice, whatever the illness or its stage, informed by palliative care principles.*
- *Specialist palliative care* is provided by those with palliative care as their core speciality. It is needed by a significant minority whose deaths are anticipated; it may be provided directly through specialist services, or indirectly through advice to the patient's normal professional advisers/carers.*

*National Council of Hospices and Palliative Care Services 1995 Specialist palliative care: a statement of definitions. Occasional Paper 8.

Key points

- Address the psychological, social, sexual, spiritual and financial needs of the patient as well as the physical symptoms.
- Provide effective symptom control.
- Offer control, independence and choice. This enables the patient to participate in decisions about management problems.
- In terminal illness this includes negotiating the most appropriate place for the patient to die – home, hospice or hospital.
- Support 'the family' (i.e. all those who are important to the patient) as well as the patient.
- Provide bereavement counselling for the terminally ill patient's 'family'.

COMMUNICATION

Communication is difficult with patients who have advanced incurable illness. Chronic and terminal illness can be seen as a failure by you and so generate feelings of inadequacy, fear and despair. These fears lead to the use of certain tactics in order to keep patients at a safe emotional distance (see Ch. 47):

- *Premature reassurance*. You reassure the patient that you can control physical symptoms when the real issue is the patient's underlying emotional fears.
- *Selective attention*. You avoid addressing the emotional issue by selecting the physical problem for attention.
- *Changing the topic when emotional issues are raised.*
- *Closed questions.*
- *Physical avoidance by walking past the end of the patient's bed.*

1. Give clear explanations of the physical and functional outcome of surgery. Patients handle side-effects better and gain trust in you if they understand the rationale for treatment. If they are given accurate facts about their diagnosis and treatment they adapt better to radical surgery. It gives them the opportunity to prepare psychologically for the major physical changes associated with procedures such as radical mastectomy, colostomy and head and neck surgery, thereby facilitating postoperative adaptation. Explore issues surrounding 'loss', such as altered body image (especially when associated with cosmetic deformity), sexuality, social role and anxieties related to death and dying. Be sensitive to patients' psychological needs and educate them in order to ease their acceptance of their new image and readjust their goals. Often these issues are not discussed at all. Start rehabili-

tation as soon as the diagnosis is made. Clinical nurse specialists such as breast, stoma and incontinence advisors play a key role.

2. Principles of good communication are to:

a. Deal with the patient's concern before yours

b. Fully cover each topic before proceeding to the next.

c. Elicit all the problems before offering advice or attempting solutions

d. Be sensitive to non-verbal clues

e. Clarify and summarize what the patient reports and what is the proposed plan of action.

Key point

- It is not always a question of 'What should the patient know?' but rather 'What does the patient want to know?'

COMMON EMOTIONAL REACTIONS

1. *Anxiety* is a normal reaction to a serious illness. One of the commonest emotional reactions to a life-threatening illness is fear. Patients with life-threatening illness commonly fear:

a. Unrelieved symptoms, especially pain

b. Death and the process of dying

c. Dying alone

d. Incompleted tasks (e.g. will has not been made)

e. Loss and separation (family, job, income, etc.)

f. Loss of dignity (confusion, incontinence, loss of control)

g. Altered body image

h. Retribution in the afterlife.

Find out precisely what the patient fears, as many of the fears on which the anxieties are based can be resolved. Acknowledge and accept normal levels of anxiety, but assess the patient for signs of clinical anxiety. Signs of clinical anxiety include:

a. Persistently anxious mood, which is subjectively different from normal worrying

b. Difficulty in distracting the patient from his or her worries

c. Feelings of tension and restlessness

d. Insomnia

e. Autonomic hyperactivity (e.g. palpitations, sensation of choking)

f. Panic attacks.

Offer treatment with anxiolytics (Latin *angere* = to press tightly + *lyein* = to loosen; release tension and anxiety) to these patients.

2. *Despair* or *depression* are normal reactions to a life-threatening illness. Recognize and acknowledge them. However, look for signs of clinical depression. The classical somatic symptoms of depression, e.g. weight loss, anorexia and lethargy, carry less importance in the assessment of patients with terminal illness as they are often a manifestation of cancer. Important clues are:

a. Persistently depressed mood, which is subjectively different from normal sadness

b. Difficulty in distracting the patient

c. Lowering of interest in and enjoyment of social activities

d. Crying, irritability, etc.

e. Insomnia

f. Feelings of guilt

g. Suicidal ideas may be present.

Offer treatment with antidepressants to these patients.

3. *Denial.* Assess whether this is causing harm, such as refusal of necessary medication or psychological turmoil. In many patients it represents a successful coping strategy, in which case breaking down the denial may cause unnecessary distress.

4. *Anger* can be displaced on to staff and/or on to the relatives. It is important not to react with anger but to try to accept and understand. Explain to the relatives that the patient is not really angry with them, but is displacing the anger he or she feels towards the disease, on to them.

SYMPTOM CONTROL

Take a positive but realistic attitude. Offer assurance that a considerable amount can be achieved. A problem-oriented individualized approach is the key to effective symptom control. For each symptom, undertake the following.

1. *Diagnose the cause and treat appropriately.* An accurate diagnosis is important for good symptom control. A careful history and examination can be more revealing than extensive investigations, which are often impractical and distressing. Investigations may be important but carry them out only if they alter subsequent management. The treatment of a symptom varies considerably, depending on the underlying pathology. For example, in a patient with cancer, vomiting may be due to:

a. Raised intracranial pressure

b. Drugs

c. Hepatomegaly

d. Intestinal obstruction, etc.

Each of these requires specific management. Since many symptoms are multifactorial in origin, recognize the contributory factors and tackle each as far as possible.

Other intercurrent illnesses are common in debilitated patients, hence it is vital to consider non-malignant as well as malignant causes. Do not assume that the symptom is related to the primary diagnosis, as this can lead to inappropriate management.

If the diagnosis is tentative but it is inappropriate to investigate further, give symptomatic relief. A therapeutic trial of drugs may be an option. For example, in a confused patient with suspected brain metastases consider a trial of steroids. If the patient improves, this is a therapeutic test.

2. *Explain symptoms to the patient.* Fear is an important contributory factor in the patient's interpretation of any symptom. The fact that you acknowledge the problem, understand the symptom, can explain its cause and offer treatment is therapeutic in itself.

3. *Discuss the treatment options.* Give the patient accurate and balanced information that is appropriate to the stage of the illness. This allows the patient to make informed choices about treatment and possible options, thereby enhancing his or her sense of control. Treatment with a palliative intent need not be limited to drugs. Other measures, such as surgery, radiotherapy, nerve blocks, physiotherapy, psychological therapy such as counselling and hypnotherapy, may be indicated.

4. *Set objectives that are realistic.* It is frustrating for both patient and staff alike if expectations are set that will never be achieved.

5. *Anticipate.* With advancing illness, symptoms (Table 39.2) may change rapidly. If such changes are anticipated, much distress may be avoided. For example, deterioration in a patient's condition with a progressive, advanced cancer may make it impossible for the patient to continue with oral medication. Such deterioration

Table 39.2 Common symptoms in patients with advanced cancer	
Symptom	Approximate incidence (%)
Physical	
Weakness	80
Pain	70
Anorexia	70
Dyspnoea	50
Cough	50
Constipation	50
Nausea and vomiting	40
Psychological	
Depression	30
Anxiety	30

should be anticipated and injectable preparations should be available. This particularly applies in the home care setting and can avert an unnecessary crisis.

6. *Ensure relatives remain informed and supported.* It is important to treat the 'whole family'.

PAIN

Pain is a common symptom in chronic and terminal illness and one that is particularly feared by cancer patients. Pain can be alleviated or modified in all patients. Proper pain assessment leads to effective management. The principles outlined here have been developed in the context of management of patients with advanced cancer, but are applicable to patients who have non-malignant pain secondary to chronic disease (see Ch. 35).

Diagnose the cause

The majority of patients with far advanced disease have pain at more than one site. Evaluate each pain individually.

In order to establish the cause of any pain, take a careful history, particularly noting:

- The site of pain and any radiation
- The type and severity of pain
- When the pain started and any subsequent changes
- Exacerbating and alleviating factors
- Analgesic agents already used.

Physical examination often confirms the diagnosis. If appropriate, investigate the patient with X-rays, isotope bone scans, CT scans, etc.

Key point

- **Pain may be due to a malignant cause but in up to a third of patients with advanced cancer the underlying cause is non-malignant.**

Always assess how significant the pain is for the individual patient – how does it affect and alter his or her life-style?

Common causes of pain in cancer patients

Pain in patients with advanced disease is often complex because it can be due to multiple pathologies. An accurate assessment of the cause of the pain leads to more effective management.

- *Bone pain* from metastatic disease or local infiltration by adjacent tumour is characteristically a deep gnawing pain made worse by movement. The bone is often tender on percussion.
- *Visceral pain* from a tumour mass in the lung or internal organs of the abdomen or pelvis causes pain by a variety of mechanisms:
  - *Soft tissue infiltration* causes deep-seated pain due to complex pathology. The tumour invades and/or stretches pain-sensitive structures such as parietal and visceral pleura, peritoneum, nerve plexuses, and local bony structures.
  - *Stretching of a capsule* of an organ is painful. The most common example is right hypochondrial pain due to stretching of the liver capsule. It can be very severe, and a sudden exacerbation of pain may stem from a bleed into a local deposit.
  - *Stretching of a hollow organ,* such as small and large intestines, bladder or ureters, can cause severe spasmodic colicky pain.
- *Nerve pain* from irritation, infiltration and/or compression is often a deep ache. Nerve destruction pain may be burning, lancinating and associated with abnormal sensations such as hyperaesthesia. When there is destruction of nerve plexuses, nerve roots or peripheral nerves, deafferentation pain may result. This type of pain is not uncommon and often coexists with visceral and somatic pain. Deafferentation pain is characterized by unpleasant pain that is difficult to describe. It is often associated with sensory changes in the painful area and patients complain of allodynia (pain that is evoked by a non-painful stimulus, such as stroking skin lightly).
- *Myofascial pain.* Musculoskeletal pains are common in chronically ill patients. They radiate in a non-dermatomal pattern. Typically there are localized hypersensitive areas of muscle known as trigger points, which are tender to pressure.
- *Superficial pain* may develop in weak, debilitated patients; bedsores may be unavoidable and give rise to distressing pain.

Realistic objectives

Pain can be significantly modified in nearly all patients and fully relieved in many. In a few of them it can be intractable and unresponsive to most treatments. These patients provide the greatest challenge so explore all avenues of achieving pain relief. Invariably involve your local specialist palliative care team in the management of these patients. Pursue realistic objectives. You should always be able to achieve freedom from pain at night, usually freedom at rest. Sometimes you may not succeed in relieving pain on mobility.

Treat pain appropriately.

Not all pain requires analgesia; for example, the pain of constipation is best treated with laxatives, not analgesics. However, when analgesics are indicated, prescribe them correctly.

Analgesic treatment of pain

The variety of analgesics available for use in the treatment of pain can be daunting. It is better to use a few drugs really well than many badly. The following 'three-step' regimen is effective in the majority of situations:

STEP 1 Non opioid +/– adjuvant, such as paracetamol. If the pain is not relieved with 2 paracetamol 6-hourly move on to:
STEP 2 Weak opioid +/– adjuvant, such as paracetamol/dextropropoxyphene, paracetamol/codeine, tramadol. If the pain is not relieved with 2 co-proxamol (or equivalent) 6-hourly move on to:
STEP 3 Strong opioid +/– adjuvant, such as morphine sulphate immediate release, morphine sulphate slow release, diamorphine subcutaneously.

Principles of prescribing opioids

- Give morphine orally unless the patient cannot tolerate oral medication.
- Prescribe it regularly to pre-empt pain. An 'as-required' basis results in poor pain control, increased incidence of side-effects and the use of higher doses overall.
- Give it an adequate trial at an adequate dose.
- Coprescribe extra doses for breakthrough and incident pain to be used as necessary – pro re nata (Latin = according to the condition arising, born).
- Side-effects should be anticipated so that they can be prevented.

Prescibe p.r.n. doses of analgesic for:

- **'Breakthrough' pain – that breaks through the background analgesia. Daily use of breakthrough analgesics implies the regular dose of analgesic is not adequately controlling the pain so increase it accordingly.**
- **'Incident' pain – that is precipitated by painful incidents such as dressing changes. The need for p.r.n. analgesics for incident pain does not imply that background pain is inadequately controlled. Therefore do not increase regular analgesics; this might increase side-effects.**

Strong oral opioids of choice

1. Morphine sulphate as tablets or solution are quick-acting preparations. Prescribe 4-hourly day and night. The short duration of action means there is rapid response to alterations of dose. Use them when the patient first starts on opioids in order to estimate the overall opioid requirement for that individual.

2. Morphine sulphate controlled release is a long-acting preparation. Prescribe it 12-hourly. When the patient's pain is stable on 4-hourly morphine convert to the equivalent dose of morphine sulphate controlled release to simplify the regimen.

3. If the pain is only moderate and urgent control is not necessary, you may start the patient on morphine sulphate controlled release initially.

4. The above two morphine preparations are suitable for most patients. Other strong opioids have a role in pain management (Table 39.3). These drugs are generally used when morphine is contraindicated or when opioid-sensitive pain has become resistant to morphine, when

---

Table 39.3 Alternative opioids

- *Fentanyl.* This is available in a transdermal preparation, Change the patch every third day. It takes several days to reach steady state (biological half-life of 17 h). It is therefore not indicated in patients who need quick titration nor in the opioid naïve. It is particularly useful in patients who cannot swallow, who have absorption problems or who are poorly compliant with oral medication. It is metabolized in the liver to inactive metabolites and is therefore useful in patients with renal dysfunction. It is said to cause less constipation than morphine. Switching between transdermal fentanyl and other opioids can be difficult; conversion tables are only a guide.
- *Hydromorphone.* This is similar to morphine but 7.5 times more potent. Its metabolites are less active than morphine metabolites.
- *Methadone.* Long acting opioid which may have a useful role in neuropathic pain. (Although opioids are said to be ineffective in neuropathic pain, clinical experience challenges this.) Its long half-life makes it a difficult drug to use because accumulation can occur.
- *Oxycodone.* A step II/III analgesic with inactive metabolites.

Table 39.4   Relative potency of opioids

Opioid	Relative oral potency (for repeated dosing)	Typical starting dose	Equipotent morphine dose (approx. – great individual variation)
Morphine	1	**10 mg 4-hourly**	**10 mg**
Codeine	0.1	30 mg 6-hourly	3 mg
Dihydrocodeine	0.1	30 mg 6-hourly	3 mg
Pethidine	0.125	50 mg 4-hourly	6.25 mg
Tramadol	0.2	50 mg 8-hourly	10 mg
Methadone	4–5	5 mg 8-hourly	20–25 mg
Hydromorphone	7.5	1.3 mg 4-hourly	10 mg
Fentanyl	250	25 mg h^{-1} 72-hourly	10–20 mg 4-hourly

morphine has been unexpectedly ineffective or when morphine is causing too many side-effects. They are generally second-line agents.

5. The dose depends on previous analgesic requirements:

a. If not on any previous analgesic, start with 2.5 mg morphine 4-hourly or 10 mg morphine sulphate slow release 12-hourly.

b. If on weak opioid (e.g. co-proxamol) start with 5–10 mg morphine 4-hourly or 30 mg morphine sulphate slow release 12-hourly.

c. If on other strong opioid, use Table 39.4 to convert to equivalent dose of morphine 4-hourly. Titrate the dose as indicated by the level of pain control achieved.

Key points

- **Treat significant pain with early, adequate, effective analgesics.**
- **Don't waste a terminally ill patient's time using ineffective moderate analgesics.**
- **Opioids are the most effective strong analgesics.**

Routes of administration

1. If the patient is able to swallow, use the oral route. However, at times it may be necessary to give opioids transdermally or parenterally; opioids can be given rectally, but this route is rarely necessary.

2. Indications for transdermal/parenteral opioids:

a. In the last few hours/days of life when the patient is unable to swallow

b. Dysphagia

c. Nausea and vomiting

d. Gut obstruction

e. Unable to tolerate taste/number of tablets.

3. Parenteral opioids. Diamorphine hydrochloride is highly soluble (1 g in 1.6 ml). It is the drug of choice for parenteral use because of the small volume needed. *Subcutaneous* injections are effective and this is the route of choice. Diamorphine undergoes first-pass metabolism in the liver, hence the subcutaneous dose should be half to one-third the oral dose.

4. If the patient is going to require more than two or three injections, consider a subcutaneous infusion pump. This is a small battery-driven device that injects the contents of a syringe over a 24 h period. It can be used in the home as well as in the hospital (Table 39.5).

5. Transdermal opioids. Fentanyl patches may occasionally be used in preference to subcutaneous infusion (see above under alternative opioids).

Fears of prescribing opioids

Fears about prescribing opioids are common and may lead to patients having effective analgesia withheld. Both professionals and patients have unfounded anxieties

Table 39.5   Equivalent dose of opioids

Equivalent doses of opioids
(Dose of oral morphine:dose of injected diamorphine = 2:1 or 3:1)
10 mg morphine sulphate orally 4-hourly
(60 mg oral morphine in 24 h)
is equivalent to
30 mg slow release morphine twice a day
(60 mg oral morphine in 24 h)
is equivalent to
5 mg of diamorphine s.c. 4-hourly
(30 mg s.c. diamorphine in 24 h)
is equivalent to
30 mg diamorphine in a 24 h s.c. infusion (syringe driver)

about opioids. An understanding of these myths will lead to improved communication, more appropriate analgesic prescribing and better compliance.

1. *Fear of addiction.* It has been shown in many studies that psychological addiction does not occur. Patients reduce and/or stop their opioid if their pain is controlled by another method (e.g. nerve block, surgical fixation). Since chemical dependence occurs (as is the case with many drugs), morphine should be gradually reduced. It must never be stopped abruptly.

2. *Fear of tolerance,* which occurs only to a minor degree and for practical purposes is not relevant. If the dose of opioid needs to be increased, it is as a result of an increase in pain secondary to disease progression.

3. *Fear of respiratory depression* but with careful attention to dosage this does not occur. In fact opioids are used in palliative care to alleviate dyspnoea by reducing ventilatory demand and hence the sensation of breathlessness.

4. *Fear of hastening death.* Opioids do not hasten death when correctly prescribed. The exhaustion caused by unrelieved pain may do so.

5. *Fear that a morphine prescription signals that death is imminent.* This is a common anxiety for patients, who may believe that a morphine prescription is given only when the doctor feels that death is imminent and has kept this information from them.

Predictable side-effects of morphine/diamorphine

- *Constipation* occurs in >95% of patients. Prescribe a regular prophylactic laxative.
- *Nausea and vomiting* occur in approximately 20% of patients. An antiemetic should be prescribed if nausea or vomiting occurs but it is not necessary to prescribe antiemetics prophylactically. The antiemetic of choice for opioid-induced nausea is haloperidol. Nausea due to opioids is usually self-limiting so the antiemetic can be withdrawn after 10–14 days.
- *Drowsiness* occurs in about 30% of patients. This side-effect wears off after approximately 5 days on a stable dose.
- *Other side-effects.* These include dry mouth, which is very common and should be treated with simple local measures; confusion and hallucinations are rare (<1% of patients) and other causes should be excluded; twitching can occur on high doses.

Key points

- **Morphine and its metabolites are dependent on the kidney for excretion.**

- **Toxicity will result unless you adjust the dose for a patient with renal dysfunction.**

Opioid-resistant pain

Some pains are either partially sensitive or insensitive to opioids. These pains will need to be managed with an additional or alternative drug or some other technique.

Bone pain. Although partially sensitive to opioids, bone pain frequently requires the addition of a non-steroidal anti-inflammatory drug. Localized bone pain can often be treated with radiotherapy. Surgical fixation may be indicated if there is a pathological fracture. Consider prophylactic fixation if more than 75% of the cortex is eroded, because a spontaneous fracture is highly likely. Generalized bone pain in malignancy may need systemic therapy with bisphosphonates. Chemotherapy, hormone therapy and strontium-89 all have a role in the management of bone pain.

Nerve pain. This is very often opioid insensitive; however, a trial of opioid is usually indicated. Methadone seems to be particularly effective. Steroids are useful in nerve compression. Nerve infiltration/irritation/destruction pain may respond to drugs that alter neurotransmission (e.g. low dose tricyclic antidepressants, anticonvulsants, membrane stabilizers). Radiotherapy and nerve blocks may also be indicated.

Liver capsule. This pain is partially opioid sensitive. Steroids are very useful in this context as they may reduce liver swelling and relieve capsular stretching.

Colic. If caused by constipation, this demands treatment with laxatives. Stop drugs causing hyperperistalsis. Colic from tumour obstruction may respond to antispasmodics.

Meningeal pain/raised intracranial pressure. Steroids are the drug of choice. Consider using radiotherapy.

Lymphoedema. Non-steroidal anti-inflammatory drugs and steroids can be helpful. Physical treatment plays an important role (massage, compression hosiery and manual lymphatic drainage).

Muscle spasm. Benzodiazepines or baclofen can be used.

Infection. It may be appropriate to treat infections in order to relieve pain.

Joint/myofascial pain. Use non-steroidal anti-inflammatory drugs in conjunction with opioids. Local injections of steroid into joints and trigger points may be of value. Physiotherapy can also be helpful.

Superficial pain. Patients with bedsores need to be kept off the pressure areas with regular turning. An effective mattress to support the patient is essential.

Psychological pain. If management is solely directed at physical factors, you may fail to control pain adequately in some patients. It is important to treat co-existent depression or anxiety, and if appropriate offer counselling and diversionary activities.

Complementary therapies

Although scientifically unproven, these seem to benefit some groups of patients. If the patient perceives these therapies as adding to their overall well-being then support the patient, provided the treatment does no harm and does not interfere with their conventional management.

Injection techniques in cancer pain

Nerve blocks have a place in palliative care. They are highly effective when used in a selected group of patients (approximately 4% of patients with pain will benefit).

Consider using nerve blocks for:
- Unilateral pain
- Localized pain
- Pain due to involvement of one or two nerve roots
- Abdominal pain arising from 'upper' gut
- Rib pain.

1. Carefully assess the cause of the pain before carrying out a block and determine the exact site at which the pain pathways should be interrupted.

2. Many procedures can be performed using local anaesthetics and steroids. These blocks can give good pain relief, outlasting the effect of the anaesthetic, and they are safe procedures. The pain relief from a nerve block may be transient and repeated blocks may be necessary.

3. Select the patient carefully and offer a nerve block only if there is a reasonable chance of success.

4. In addition to neural blockade, spinal analgesics have an important role in selected cases. Epidural and intrathecal administration of opioids (and local anaesthetics) by a catheter system are particularly useful in patients with opioid-sensitive pain who are experiencing unacceptable side-effects with systemic therapy.

5. Major neurolytic procedures may carry the risk of serious side-effects, so first assess the patient carefully. For example, intraspinal neurolysis for nerve root pain can produce urinary and faecal incontinence. Coeliac plexus block for upper abdominal pain can cause postural hypotension.

SPECIFIC PROBLEMS

Weakness and immobility

1. Weakness is a common and distressing symptom in patients with advanced illness. When due to general debility it is very difficult to treat. Exclude reversible causes such as cord compression and cerebral metastases. Acknowledge the problem and explain to the patient that it is a result of the illness. This allows realistic goals to be set, which in itself can reduce the patient's distress. Even very sick patients need to feel a sense of control. Simple measures such as a wheelchair can help them achieve this.

2. Steroids improve weakness in a proportion of patients. The response, however, is often short lived so take into account side-effects such as proximal myopathy and poor wound healing. Select patients carefully and assess the time at which steroids are introduced.

3. A patient who is immobile and confined to bed loses muscle strength. A normal person loses 10–15% of muscle strength when completely rested for 1 week and it takes 60 days to restore that strength. It is therefore not surprising that muscle weakness quickly develops in the immobile cancer patient, especially in the common situation where protein catabolism is increased. If immobility continues, contractures can develop, leading to impaired ability to self-care. Contractures are more likely when soft tissue damage is present and with improper positioning in bed. Good nursing care and regular physiotherapy are essential for these patients.

4. When patients are debilitated and immobile, pressure sores can rapidly develop. This is aggravated by increased protein catabolism and negative nitrogen balance as well as other factors (e.g. diabetes, steroids). Damage can be minimized if pressure on the skin is intermittent. Limit the damage and prevent the consequent pain by early prophylaxis with scrupulous nursing attention and the use of effective patient support systems (e.g. special mattresses, low-loss airbeds).

5. Autonomic dysfunction and impaired peripheral circulation are the cardiovascular consequences of immobility. There is an increased likelihood of deep venous thrombosis and pulmonary embolism.

6. Atelectasis results from reduced aeration of the posterior lungs and predisposes patients to chest infection.

7. Urinary retention and urinary infection are more common in immobile patients.

8. Immobility, anorexia and weakness lead to reduced peristalsis and constipation.

9. Loss of proprioceptors in the skin of the feet will lead to an inability to balance, which can take many weeks to recover.

Anorexia

1. This occurs in approximately 70% of patients with advanced cancer. It is important to decide whose problem it is – the patient's or the carers'. The family need to understand that as death approaches it is normal to lose

interest in food. At this stage the goal of eating is enjoyment, not optimal nutrition.

2. Causes of anorexia are:

a. Tumour bulk and associated biochemical abnormalities (hypercalcaemia, uraemia, etc.)

b. Oral problems (e.g. thrush, oral tumour)

c. Constipation

d. Drugs, radiotherapy

e. Depression or anxiety.

3. Remember that fear of vomiting may lead to avoidance of food, as opposed to true anorexia. Psychological factors such as anxiety and depression can manifest as lack of appetite. Presentation of food is important – it should be in small portions and well presented.

If the above factors have been attended to and it is still felt to be a problem for the patient, consider progestogens or steroids as appetite stimulants.

Dysphagia

1. The site of dysphagia can be predicted from the symptom complex. Drooling, leaking of food and retention of food in the mouth indicate a buccal cause; nasal regurgitation, gagging, choking and coughing suggest pharyngeal pathology; a sensation of food sticking behind the sternum and pain between the shoulder blades imply oesophageal obstruction.

2. It is important to explain the cause (Table 39.6) to the patient so that any dietary adjustments are understood. If necessary, restrict intake to liquids or soft foods.

3. Treat any associated pain. Mucaine is useful for the local pain of *Candida* or radiotherapy, but many patients require opioids for satisfactory pain relief. Actively treat *Candida* with topical or systemic antifungals. If patients are unable to swallow even liquids, give drugs by another route. A subcutaneous infusion of drugs (analgesics, etc.) is both effective and well tolerated.

4. If it is appropriate to attempt to relieve the obstruction, then possibilities include radiotherapy, endo-oesophageal tubes, stents, dilatation and laser therapy. Steroids, by reducing oedema, may palliate dysphagia for a significant period. They can be particularly useful in the management of dysphagia syndrome associated with head and neck tumour. Consider endo-oesophageal tubes and stents in patients who are relatively independent and active; they are not for the moribund. Percutaneous gastrostomy may be an option in patients with incurable malignant obstruction but it does not solve the problem of saliva aspiration. There is a significant morbidity associated with percutaneous gastrostomy insertion, so select patients carefully.

5. In irreversible total obstruction or terminal neuromuscular dysfunction reduce secretions to a minimum using hyoscine.

6. Regard dehydration as a natural process in the last few days of life. It can help relieve a number of symptoms. Intravenous fluids may exacerbate discomfort by increasing bronchial secretions, gastrointestinal fluid (increased likelihood of vomiting), urine flow (leading to need for catheter), etc. However, hydration may be indicated in selected patients, for example if a patient is complaining of thirst/dryness. Usually these patients can be managed with subcutaneous fluids, preventing the repeated trauma of cannulation.

Nausea and vomiting

1. These occur in approximately 40% of patients with far-advanced cancer. Find the cause in order that rational treatment can be offered (Table 39.7).

2. If an antiemetic is needed, most nausea and vomiting in patients with advanced illness can be controlled using the antiemetic drugs in Table 39.8. Most antiemetics act at one of the sites shown in the table. Sometimes more than one antiemetic is necessary. If this is the case it is common sense to combine drugs that act at different sites, i.e. a neuroleptic with an antihistamine.

Table 39.6 Common causes of dysphagia in patients with advanced disease		
Problem	Implication	Example of cause
Solids then liquids	Obstruction	Tumour mass External compression
Solids and liquids simultaneously	Neuromuscular cause	Terminal neuromuscular dysfunction in very weak patients Perineural tumour infiltration with head and neck tumours which damage cranial nerves (V, IX, X) Bulbar palsy
Painful	Mucosal causes	*Candida* (Note: only 50% of patients with oesophageal *Candida* have clinically apparent oral *Candida*) Post-radiotherapy

Table 39.7   Common causes of nausea and vomiting in advanced cancer

Cause	Symptomatic treatment
Drugs	If possible withdraw the drug
Metabolic (hypercalcaemia, uraemia. etc.)	Treat with centrally acting antiemetic
Bowel obstruction	Centrally acting antiemetic (see below)
Squashed stomach syndrome*	Prokinetic antiemetic, proton pump inhibitor/H_2 antagonist
Gastric irritation (e.g. NSAIDs, gastric ulceration)	Prokinetic antiemetic, proton pump inhibitor/H_2 antagonist/misoprostol
Constipation	Laxatives
Liver metastases	Centrally acting antiemetic/steroids
High bulk disease	Steroids, centrally acting antiemetic/ondansetron
Raised intracranial pressure	Steroids

NSAIDs, non-steroidal anti-inflammatory drugs.
*Squashed/small stomach syndrome is a constellation of alimentary symptoms seen in patients with a large epigastric mass/gross hepatomegaly. It is manifested as early satiation, epigastric fullness, flatulence, hiccoughs, nausea, vomiting and heartburn.

Table 39.8   Sites of action of antiemetic drugs

Main site of action	Class of drug	Example
Central		
Chemoreceptor trigger zone	Neuroleptic	Haloperidol
Vomiting centre	Antihistamine	Cyclizine
5HT3 receptors	5HT3 receptor antagonists	Ondansetron
All central sites	Phenothiazine	Levomepromazine
Peripheral	Prokinetic	Domperidone

3. The antiemetic must be delivered by a suitable route. There is little point in giving a drug orally if the patient is vomiting! Choose rectal or parenteral routes in these situations. A 24 h subcutaneous infusion by means of a syringe driver is a simple and effective method of drug delivery. (Syringe drivers are discussed in more detail later.)

Bowel obstruction

1. Gastrointestinal obstruction occurs in approximately 4% of patients with advanced cancer, more commonly in those with colonic primary (10%) and ovarian primary (25%). Manage these patients surgically if they are in good general condition, if they have low-bulk disease and if an easily reversible cause seems likely. Take into account previous laparotomy findings. Surgery remains the primary treatment because in selected patients 10% of obstructions prove to be non-malignant, 10% represent a new primary and approximately 60% will not reobstruct.

2. With conservative treatment, 30% of obstructions resolve spontaneously. Therefore consider this management prior to proceeding to surgery. The medical management of bowel obstruction is given in Table 39.9.

3. Do not resort to either of these strategies as part of the primary management of irreversible obstruction in patients with far-advanced cancer. The majority of such patients have obstruction at multiple sites. Aim for symptom control with drugs. Intravenous fluids and nasogastric tubes are rarely needed.

4. Obstruction may be proximal, in which case the predominant symptom is vomiting, or distal, when the predominant symptom is colicky pain. Nausea is often more

Table 39.9   Medical management of bowel obstruction

Diet	No restrictions but small meals appropriate.
Nausea and vomiting	Cyclizine 150 mg per 24 h via syringe pump. If partial/no success combine with haloperidol 5–10 mg per 24 h in syringe pump. Octreotide via the subcutaneous route has an important role in bowel obstruction, particularly in high volume vomiting.
Reverse obstruction	If constipated, attempt to clear with softeners. Docusate 100–200 mg t.d.s. Consider dexamethasone 16 mg per 24 h by subcutaneous infusion to reduce oedema. In certain cases, e.g. cancer of the ovary, chemotherapy may be effective.
Pain	Diamorphine in appropriate dose in syringe pump according to previous analgesic requirement and level of pain.
Colic	If colic persists despite the above, add hyoscine butylbromide 60–120 mg per 24 h to pump. Octreotide is helpful by decompressing the bowel and reducing the distension.

Gastrokinetic antiemetics such as metoclopramide or domperidone are contraindicated – they will exacerbate vomiting.

distressing than vomiting. The aim is to eliminate nausea, reduce vomiting to a maximum of once or twice a day and treat associated pain. Baines et al (1985) reported on this form of management in 38 patients with advanced malignant disease. They found that nausea and vomiting was well controlled in 90% of patients, colic in 100% and pain relief was total in 90%, with only mild residual pain in 10%. The median survival was 3 months and 24% survived >6 months.

Constipation

The need to treat constipation is usually a consequence of failing to use prophylactic laxatives (virtually all patients on opioids should have a regular laxative). A rectal examination is essential on any patient complaining of constipation or diarrhoea to assess for impaction.

Syringe drivers in symptom control

Syringe drivers delivering subcutaneous infusions of analgesics, antiemetics, anticholinergics or tranquillizers are commonly used in patients who require regular parenteral medication (Table 39.10). The subcutaneous route is simple, safe, effective and acceptable to most patients. Indications for the use of such syringe drivers have already been discussed above in the context of pain control.

TERMINAL PHASE MANAGEMENT

1. When a patient who has advanced illness enters into the terminal phase, normally a day or so prior to death, review *all* medication. Stop all drugs apart from those aimed at symptom control.

Table 39.10   Drugs commonly used in a continuous 24 h subcutaneous infusion pump

Reason for drug	Drug	Dose in 24 h
Analgesia	Diamorphine	According to need
Colic	Hyoscine butylbromide	30–60 mg
Antiemetic	Haloperidol	5–10 mg
	Cyclizine	150 mg
	Levomepromazine	12.5–25 mg
Bronchial secretions	Hyoscine hydrobromide	1.2–1.8 mg
	Hyoscine butylbromide	30–120 mg
	Glycopyrrolate	0.6–1.2 mg per 24 h
Anxiolysis	Midazolam	5–10 mg
Terminal agitation	Midazolam	15–60 mg
	Levomepromazine	100–200 mg
Other drugs	Dexamethasone	0.5–16 mg
	Octreotide	300–1200 µg

2. Communication is vital. Explain to the patient and the carers about anticipated changes in the patient's condition. Offer reassurance that symptoms will remain controlled and the patient kept comfortable. Often it is appropriate to use a syringe driver to administer medications.

3. Continue analgesia even if the patient becomes unconscious. The patient may still perceive pain and, in addition, abrupt withdrawal of opioids can result in an unpleasant physical withdrawal reaction. If a patient is on regular opioids, these will need to be continued at an equivalent dose subcutaneously. If the patient will require more than a few injections, start a syringe driver.

4. Agitation. Search for the causes and treat them if indicated; for example, retention of urine requires catheterization. However, it is not uncommon for patients to become agitated and confused shortly before death. If a tranquillizer is indicated, use subcutaneous midazolam (5–10 mg, 4–6-hourly). Midazolam (20–60 mg per 24 h) can be combined with diamorphine in a syringe driver.

5. Bronchial secretions can be controlled using subcutaneous hyoscine or glycopyrronium, as required. Either can also be added into the syringe driver together with diamorphine and midazolam.

6. Crises. In some circumstances it may be appropriate to prescribe drugs for an anticipated crisis such as a massive haemoptysis or rupture of a major vessel. Such crises cause great distress to the patient and the family, so handle them speedily and sensitively. Prescribe midazolam with or without diamorphine as required, and give the nurses instructions to give it *immediately* should such an 'end of life' crisis occur.

Key points

- **Always follow the rules of symptom control throughout.**
- **Evaluate symptoms and treat them appropriately.**
- **Anticipate crises.**
- **Communicate.**
- **A peaceful death alleviates the severity of bereavement in the family**

Bereavement

1. Provide support for the family both during the patient's illness and at the time of death. It helps them to cope better and also reduces the likelihood of future complications. Evidence suggests there is higher physical and psychiatric morbidity and possibly increased mortality in those recently bereaved.

2. People avoid grieving individuals because they feel helpless, awkward, embarrassed, they do not wish to feel sad themselves and they fear releasing strong emotions.

Bereavement counselling

1. Identify those who are likely to have a difficult bereavement, as they are at risk of developing psychiatric illness in the bereavement period, such as psychosis, clinical depression or extreme anxiety states. Some individuals may resort to alcohol, drugs, denial, idealization, etc. as a way of coping with loss. Refer them early to the appropriate agency, such as a psychiatrist or bereavement counsellor.

2. Individuals at increased risk of difficult bereavement include those:

a. With a close, dependent or ambivalent relationship

b. Undergoing concurrent stress at the time of bereavement

c. With memories of a 'bad' death (e.g. uncontrolled symptoms)

d. Who have a perceived low level of support (the carer's perception is more important than the actual support in determining outcome)

e. Experiencing strong feelings of guilt/reproach

f. Unable to say goodbye, who feel there are things left unsaid (e.g. sudden or traumatic deaths or absence at the time of death).

Summary

- Do you recognize the essential importance of clear, effective communication?
- Will you determine to treat the whole patient, not just the disease?
- Do you intend to assess fully each symptom before prescribing treatment and revise it as the disease progresses?
- Do you feel confident that you can control or modify pain?
- Do you recognize the value of using morphine sulphate as the first choice when a strong opioid is indicated?
- Will you continue to control symptoms with analgesia, sedation and antisecretory drugs for excessive respiratory secretions during the terminal phase?
- Will you remember to call upon the expertise of your local palliative care team/hospice?

References

Baines M, Oliver DJ, Carter RL 1985 Medical management of intestinal obstruction in patients with advanced malignant disease: a clinical and pathological study. Lancet ii: 990–993

Further reading

1998 Directory of hospice and palliative care services in the United Kingdom and Republic of Ireland. Hospice Information Service, St Christopher's Hospice, London

Buckman R 1992 How to break bad news: a guide for health care professionals. Papermac, London

Doyle D, Hanks WC, Macdonald N 1998 Oxford textbook of palliative medicine. Oxford University Press, Oxford

Faulkner A, Maguire P 1994 Talking to cancer patients. Oxford Medical Publications, Oxford

Kaye P 1996 Breaking bad news. (Pocket Book) EPL Publications, Northampton

Parkes CM 1972 Bereavement: studies of grief in adult life. Tavistock and Pelican, London; International Universities Press, New York

Regnard C, Davies A 1986 A guide to symptom relief in advanced cancer. Haigh and Hochland, Manchester

Stedeford A 1985 Facing death. Heinemann, London

Twycross RG 1997 Symptom management in advanced cancer. Radcliffe Medical Press, Abingdon, Oxfordshire

Twycross RG, Lack SA 1986 Control of alimentary symptoms in far advanced cancer. Churchill Livingstone, Edinburgh

Twycross RG, Wilcock A, Thorp C 1998 PCF1 Palliative care formulary. Radcliffe Medical Press, Abingdon, Oxfordshire

GENERAL CONSIDERATIONS

40 Genetic aspects of surgery

M. C. Winslet

Objectives

- **Recognize genetic disorders which may produce life-threatening complications during surgery and anaesthesia:**
  - **defects of haemoglobin and haemostasis**
  - **defects of muscle**
  - **defects of connective tissue**
  - **skeletal dysplasias.**
- **Become familiar with the disorders leading to a genetic susceptibility to cancer.**

RELEVANCE TO SURGERY

In certain genetic disorders life-threatening complications may occur during surgery and anaesthesia. Recognize family history and clinical signs suggestive of these genetic disorders in order to plan appropriate perioperative management. It is now possible to study the molecular basis of genetic disorders, human development, carcinogenesis and many other biological events. This stems from exciting advances in laboratory techniques for the analysis of the human genome.

Genes involved in the control of cell proliferation and transcription of genetic information have been shown to cause increased susceptibility to cancer if their function is defective. Thus, genetic analysis and the development of new methods for clinical diagnosis, monitoring of cancer progression and treatment are being reported in medical literature and incorporated in clinical medicine. These advances clearly illustrate the link between basic sciences and clinical practice. They emphasize your need to understand basic genetic concepts in order to keep abreast of new developments.

BASIC CONCEPTS AND TERMINOLOGY

1. *Genes* are units of genetic information which are passed on from generation to generation. Biochemically, genes are stretches of *DNA* (deoxyribonucleic acid) which direct the synthesis of a specific protein.

2. DNA is tightly coiled and packaged in *chromosomes*, which are visible under the light microscope in the nucleus of dividing cells. *Somatic cells* (non-germline tissue) have 23 pairs of chromosomes (*diploid* number 46): one chromosome from each pair is inherited from each parent. Chromosome pairs 1–22 are called *autosomes*, while the 23rd pair are the *sex chromosomes*, XX in females and XY in males. In the ovum or sperm (*germ cells* or gonadal tissue cells) one set of autosomes and a sex chromosome are present (*haploid* set), so that, on fertilization, a diploid set of chromosomes is restored. Thus, males determine the sex of the offspring.

3. When viewed under the microscope, each chromosome has a visible constriction (*centromere*). The part of the chromosome above the centromere is usually shorter, called the short arm or *p* (from petite); the long arm is termed *q*. Each arm of the chromosome is further divided into bands for easy reference. Thus, 5q21 is the position of the adenomatous polyposis coli gene on the long arm of chromosome 5.

4. *Mutation* is a change in the gene function which results either in activation (more protein is produced) or, more often, inactivation of the gene with reduction or loss of function. Some diseases with a gene component are sporadic (Greek *sporadikos* = scattered, from *sperein* = to sow); others, on which I shall concentrate, are familial, that is, characteristic of a family, because the mutation is passed on to subsequent generations.

5. *Single gene disorders* account for many defects. A single base substitution results in sickle cell disease. A single point mutation results in some forms of β-thalassaemia.

6. *Chromosomal disorders.* An extra, free-lying chromosome 21 accounts for most cases of Down syndrome.

7. *Multifactorial diseases* are the result of combined genetic and environmental factors, including some cases of cleft lip and palate, club foot, long segment Hirschsprung's disease and hypertrophic pyloric stenosis. Combined genetic and environmental factors are implicated in insulin-dependent diabetes, ankylosing spondylitis, peptic ulceration and atherosclerosis.

8. *Mendelian inheritance* (Gregor Mendel, 1822–1884, the Augustinian monk who studied the inheritance characteristics of peas) refers to the mode of transmission of genetic information from generation to generation. *Dominant inheritance* (autosomal or X-linked) is clinically expressed when a copy of the mutated gene is inherited from one parent but not from the other. In *recessive inheritance* the clinical signs of the disease are evident only when both copies of the gene have the mutation.

9. *Proto-oncogenes* (Greek *protos* = first + *onkos* = bulk, mass + *-gene* = born) are normal cellular genes which participate in normal proliferation. They may undergo mutation to form *oncogenes*, which initiate or stimulate neoplasia.

10. *Tumour suppressor genes* (or antioncogenes) have the opposite function.

11. *Family history* is essential for establishing the diagnosis of genetic disorders. The drawing of a family tree (pedigree – French *pied-de-grue* = crane's foot, possibly from the arrowhead on the scroll) is straightforward and shows in graphic form the mode of genetic transmission

(Fig. 40.1). When a complex of symptoms and signs occur together in a particular disorder, this is referred to as a *syndrome*, usually named after the authors of the first report, for example, in 1969, the Li–Fraumeni syndrome – the criteria for inclusion being an autosomal dominant cancer predisposition, a wide variety of cancer types, young onset and a potential for multiple primary sites. An important surgical familial condition is hereditary non-polyposis colon cancer, often referred to by the acronym HNPCC.

PREOPERATIVE ASSESSMENT AND PERIOPERATIVE MANAGEMENT

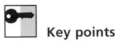

Key points

- Concentrate on the genetic disorders with which you, as a trainee surgeon, should be

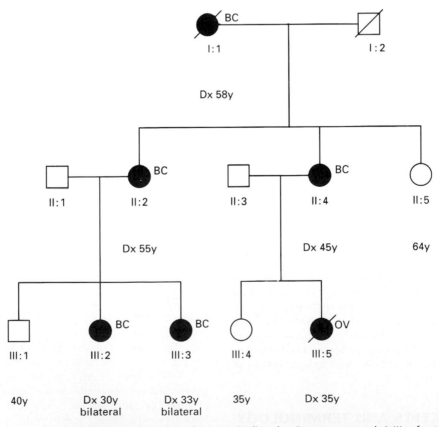

Fig. 40.1 A family tree for establishing a diagnosis of a genetic disorder. Roman numerals I–III refer to generations; arabic numerals refer to the individual (e.g. III:5, fifth individual from the third generation shown on the pedigree). (○) female; (□) male; shaded symbols = affected; crossed symbols = dead; BC, breast cancer; OV, ovarian cancer; Dx, diagnosed; y, years (present age or age at diagnosis).

familiar, because they may result in serious complications during surgery and anaesthesia.
- These genetic disorders can be divided into four groups: defects of haemoglobin and haemostasis; defects of muscle; connective tissue defects; and skeletal dysplasias.

Haemoglobin and haemostasis

1. Enquire about history of anaemia, bleeding tendency or recurrent venous thrombosis in the patient or relatives. The development of sickle cell crisis due to hypoxia during surgery and the need for factor VIII infusion in haemophilia A are well known. If you obtain a suggestive history, most rare defects of other clotting factors can be diagnosed on routine screening. For example, in Noonan syndrome, with a birth frequency of 1:2000, factor XI and XII deficiency and thrombocytopenia occur in 60% of patients. The clinical signs include short stature, neck webbing, congenital heart defects and usually subnormal intelligence. There is no chromosomal abnormality and both sexes are affected.

2. Patients with thromboembolic disease due to inherited protein C or S deficiency may give a history of superficial and deep vein thrombosis, thrombosis of the mesenteric, cerebral, renal and axillary veins and portal veins, and pulmonary embolism.

Muscle defects

1. Malignant hyperthermia is the most serious genetic disorder of muscle presenting in the operating theatre. It is estimated to affect approximately 1:15 000 paediatric patients and 1:40 000 adult patients. It is triggered by halogenated anaesthetic agents, with or without depolarizing muscle relaxants. The inheritance is autosomal dominant or recessive and approximately 50% of families have a mutation in the calcium ion channel gene on chromosome 19. The patient develops an acute onset of skeletal muscle rigidity, metabolic acidosis and malignant hyperpyrexia. Immediately reverse it, or it can lead to tissue damage and death. The mainstay of treatment is dantrolene, which acts directly to relax skeletal muscle. Administer 1 mg kg^{-1} by rapid intravenous injection, repeated up to a cumulative maximum of 10 mg kg^{-1}, either prophylactically or immediately you suspect a hyperthermic episode.

2. Hand-grip weakness and difficulty in walking are symptoms of myotonic dystrophy. There is usually a positive family history. Myotonic dystrophy affects approximately 1:10 000 individuals and the clinical expression is very variable. Myotonic dystrophy and the other less common myotonias are due to defects in the chloride and sodium channels of the muscle membrane. Patients show undue sensitivity to various anaesthetics and sedative agents, including opioids, barbiturates and benzodiazepines. Tonic spasms during operation, prolonged recovery from anaesthetic and depression of the respiratory centre necessitating prolonged ventilation have been reported. Cold and shivering also induces myotonia. Myotonic dystrophy usually presents between the ages of 15 and 35 years. The most noticeable clinical signs are facial and neck weakness with ptosis. Patients usually notice weakness of hand grip, inability to open the clenched fist and difficulty in walking due to weakness of foot dorsiflexion. This is a multisystem disorder: heart block frequently develops in adults. Fully evaluate these patients prior to operation. Because anaesthetic management may be difficult, prefer regional anaesthesia whenever possible.

Connective tissue defects

1. Is there evidence of poor wound healing, paper thin scar tissue, joint dislocations and possible aortic aneurysm in relatives? Connective tissue abnormalities may cause difficulty during suturing, resulting in a high incidence of anastomotic and wound dehiscence. In Marfan's syndrome, named for the Parisian paediatrician (1858–1942), the clinical signs are usually obvious: the patient is tall, thin, with long slim fingers, chest deformity, scoliosis and dislocated optic lens. Preoperative cardiac assessment is mandatory, as there is a high incidence of dissecting aortic aneurysm with aortic valve insufficiency at a young age.

2. Ehlers–Danlos syndrome was described in 1901 by the Danish physician Ehlers, and by Danlos a Parisian dermatologist in 1908. The arterial type IV, in particular, is characterized by friable arteries and veins, and spontaneous arterial rupture has been reported. Paper thin scars, joint dislocation and spontaneous colonic perforation may also occur. Arteriography and vascular surgery is particularly hazardous; if varicose vein surgery is absolutely necessary, perform it with the utmost care.

Skeletal dysplasias

1. Patients with such disorders may have odontoid dysplasia or C1–C2 subluxation due to ligamentous laxity. The patient is of short stature, with some body disproportion. The most commonly encountered conditions are achondroplasia and Down syndrome, described in 1866 by John Langdon-Down of the London Hospital, which are easily recognized.

2. Skeletal dysplasia due to mucopolysaccharidosis, an inborn metabolic storage disorder (such as Hurler syndrome), is characterized by a 'coarse' looking face and mental retardation. Take care to limit head and neck manipulation during surgical operations for fear of causing cervical medullary compression. In certain cases, elective cervical vertebral fusion may be required.

3. Congenital malformations and genetic disorders may indicate the presence of unsuspected anatomical abnormalities of obvious importance to the surgeon. Patients with Sturge–Weber syndrome have a port wine stain on the skin, which, if present over the face or cranium, is associated with epilepsy or mental retardation. Multiple arteriovenous malformations may be encountered during surgical manipulation of tissues beneath the port wine stain.

GENETIC MECHANISM OF CANCER DEVELOPMENT

Cancer development is the result of the accumulation of mutations in a number of genes (4–5 in colorectal cancer) over time in somatic tissues. Each mutation results in stepwise clonal proliferation of cells, with the next mutation giving rise to further expansion. The mutations are present in two types of genes which regulate cell growth. There is a mutational activation of oncogenes and mutational inactivation of tumour suppressor genes (see Ch. 26). A genetic model for colorectal tumorigenesis has been particularly well studied, for example by Fearon & Vogelstein (1990). Early mutations in the bowel epithelium in the oncogene *ras* and the tumour suppressor genes on 5q and 18q give rise to a colon adenoma. Additional mutation of the tumour suppressor gene p53 (localized at 17p) result in progression to carcinoma. Further tumour growth results from the accumulated loss of suppressor genes on additional chromosomes. This correlates with the ability of the carcinomas to metastasize and cause death.

GENETIC SUSCEPTIBILITY TO CANCER

Key points

- **Most malignant tumours are sporadic (in one individual in the family) and develop in older age.**
- **Cancer occurring in successive generations in a family is rare.**

1. Features which suggest the probability of the presence of a genetic predisposition to cancer are shown in Table 40.1. As molecular genetic analysis methods have become available, attention has focused over the last 10 years on unusual families where a particular type of cancer (breast/ovary, colorectal) has developed in many relatives, over several generations and at a young age.

2. Significantly, the tumours are often bilateral or multifocal. This clinical presentation could be explained by an inherited mutation of a tumour suppressor gene (which is present in all tissues). Subsequent mutations of further genes frequently result in multiple tumours at a young age of onset. This mechanism of genetic susceptibility to cancer was initially proposed by Knudson in 1986 (Knudson hypothesis) and has recently been confirmed. Among the first genes to be localized were those causing clinically well-characterized disorders such as familial retinoblastoma, Wilms' tumour and adenomatous polyposis coli (APC). Table 40.2 shows the gene localization and clinical presentation of some of the more common cancer susceptibility genetic disorders. Adenomatous polyposis coli is an important surgical example of an autosomal dominant disorder presenting in late childhood/early teens, with abdominal pain or bleeding per rectum due to multiple large bowel polyps. At colonoscopy numerous polyps are visible, almost replacing the bowel mucosa. Polyps may be present in the rest of the gastrointestinal tract. There is a high frequency of progression of such polyps to the adenoma–carcinoma sequence. Another serious complication in approximately 10% of patients with APC is the development of desmoid (Greek *desmos* = chain, bundle + *eidos* = like) tumours arising mainly from the peritoneum or abdominal wall; these are highly vascular and difficult to resect in their entirety. When you make the clinical diagnosis of APC, you must inform the patient's close relatives and counsel them about their increased cancer risk. They need to decide whether to have regular colonoscopy, as some gene carriers develop the polyps later, or opt for a predictive genetic test or CHIRPE (congenital hypertrophy of retinal pigment assessment).

Table 40.1 Features which increase the probability of the presence of genetic predisposition to cancer

- The development of specific (e.g. breast/ovary) or uncommon (e.g. adrenal/rhabdomyosarcoma) tumours
- Unusually early onset of cancer (<45 years)
- Multiple primary cancers in one individual
- Relatives with cancer (maternal or paternal side)
- Associated phenotypic or developmental abnormalities (rare)

Table 40.2　Gene localization and clinical presentation of disorders with a genetic susceptibility to cancer

Disorder	Mode of inheritance	Gene localization	Tumour susceptibility
Retinoblastoma	Autosomal dominant	13q14	Retinoblastoma, osteogenic sarcoma
Wilms' tumour	Autosomal dominant	11p13	Nephroblastoma
Adenomatous polyposis coli	Autosomal dominant	5q21	Colorectal, gastrointestinal tract
Li–Fraumeni syndrome	Autosomal dominant	17p12	Rhabdomyosarcoma, leukaemia, glioma, breast cancer
Breast and ovarian cancer	Autosomal dominant	BRCA1–17q21 BRCA2–13q12	Breast and ovarian Breast? Pancreas
Hereditary non-polyposis colon cancer	Autosomal dominant	hMSH2–2p12 hMLH1–3p21 hPMS1–2q31 hPMS–7p22	Colorectal and gastrointestinal, ureteric, endometrial, ovarian cancer
Neurofibromatosis 1	Autosomal dominant	17q11	Benign schwannoma, brain tumours (rare)
Neurofibromatosis 2	Autosomal dominant	22q13	Optic neuroma, acoustic neuroma, meningioma, glioma
von Hippel–Lindau syndrome	Autosomal dominant	3p25	Meningioma, renal
Peutz–Jeghers syndrome	Autosomal dominant	19p	Hamartoma, gastrointestinal tract

Key point

- **Predictive tests for adenomatous polyposis coli may carry a social stigma or be potentially misused by insurance and employment agencies.**

At the same time, for the patients and their families, the knowledge of cancer risk and subsequent need for major surgery is stressful. Mutation analysis in the APC gene must be performed on a sample from the affected family member, as many different mutations from different families may be found spanning the whole length of the gene. When the mutation is identified in a family, prenatal diagnosis is of course also possible, with all its associated problems regarding the decision to terminate pregnancy for late-onset disorder.

3. The cloning of breast/ovarian cancer susceptibility genes (BRCA1 and BRCA2) has been accomplished (Miki et al 1994, Wooster et al 1995). This constitutes a major advance in the study of these common cancers. Mutations have been identified in all areas of these large genes. For practical clinical application, less expensive and less laborious methods of gene analysis need to be developed.

4. Genetic susceptibility to breast and ovarian cancer is impossible to diagnose clinically in the absence of a convincing pedigree suggestive of autosomal dominant inheritance. Several mutations occur more frequently in the Ashkenazi Jewish population; the knowledge of the patient's background may facilitate mutation detection. The population risk for breast cancer in a woman aged 30–39 is 4 in 1000. While the numbers of cases analysed to date are relatively small, and with only preliminary data available, the percentage of breast cancer due to BRCA1 within that age range has been estimated at 5%.

5. A number of cancer syndromes have been described, showing a characteristic combination of cancers (Table 40.2). As relatively small numbers of families have been analysed to date; it is likely that a more accurate clinical spectrum will be available in the future.

6. The study of families with a high frequency of site-specific colorectal cancer and colorectal cancer associated with malignant tumours of the genitourinary tract, uterus, breast cancer and other malignancies has facilitated the recent discovery of several new genes. These syndromes

were initially described by Lynch et al (1988), but have subsequently been termed 'hereditary non-polyposis colon cancer' and 'cancer family syndrome'. The colorectal cancer is of early onset with a proclivity to the proximal colon and an excess of synchronous (Greek *syn* = together + *chronos* = time, hence simultaneous)/metachronous (Greek *meta* = after; hence occurring in sequence but separated by intervals) lesions. It is often, but not always, preceded by the development of colonic polyps. Colonoscopy is advocated every 3–5 years, with an increasing frequency in the presence of polyps. The surveillance for the associated cancers is problematic because, again, clinical diagnosis is difficult. Genetic diagnosis is now possible, but methodological problems will need to be overcome for potential clinical application, as is the case with BRCA1/2 genes.

7. It has been noted that tumours from these affected individuals contain a large number of DNA replication errors. The normal function of these newly discovered genes is to survey the fidelity of DNA replication and repair. Mistakes are frequently introduced during normal DNA replication and DNA repair has to take place, especially when the cell is exposed to carcinogens, ionizing radiation or alkylating agents. The clinical expression of mutations in these genes is compatible with their function as tumour suppressor genes. The frequency of these gene mutations in the population is unknown, but in patients with colorectal cancer, genetic susceptibility has been estimated to account for 5–10% of cases.

8. Advances in molecular genetics continue at an intense pace. With the current study of oncogene amplification to tumour stage and ultimately to prognosis, and the further development of tumour drug targeting and gene therapy, major practical advances in cancer prediction, detection and therapy should be forthcoming in the foreseeable future. Exciting recent developments include predictive genetic testing for relatives at high risk for developing cancer by mutation analysis. Clinical trials directed towards early cancer detection and chemoprevention in this group will provide statistically significant outcome data in a shorter time than other general population trials.

Summary

- Can you identify the genetic disorders that may predispose to life-threatening complications during surgery or anaesthesia?
- Which congenital defects in haemoglobin, haemostasis, muscle, connective tissue and the skeleton should you note?
- Do you understand the accumulation of mutations in oncogenes and in tumour suppressor genes that may increase susceptibility to cancer?
- Do you realize that genetic mutations in specific tumour suppressor genes were identified in approximately 20% of individuals with early onset and family history of cancer?
- While the great majority of cancers are sporadic, what salient features in the history and examination suggest a genetic increased susceptibility to cancer?

References

Fearon ER, Vogelstein B 1990 A genetic model for colorectal tumorigenesis. Cell 61: 759–767

Lynch HT, Lanspa SJ, Bonan BM, Smyth T, Walson P, Lynch JF 1988 Hereditary non-polyposis colorectal cancer, Lynch syndromes I and II. Gastroenterology Clinics of North America 174: 679–715

Miki Y, Swensen J, Shattuck-Eidens D et al 1994 A strong candidate for the breast and ovarian susceptibility gene BRCA1. Science 266: 66–71

Wooster R, Bignell G, Lancaster J et al 1995 Identification of the breast cancer susceptibility gene BRCA2. Nature 378(6559): 789–792

41 Screening for surgical disease

T. Bates

Objectives

- Identify essentials for justifying a screening programme.
- Appreciate the practical requirements.
- Recognize the cost-benefits, including mortality and quality of life.

INTRODUCTION

At first sight, screening the population for the common forms of surgical disease seems a good idea, as it should then be possible to cure the condition before it becomes symptomatic. Cancer of the lung, which is still the commonest malignancy, with 22 700 male and 11 000 female deaths in England and Wales per year (Office of Population Censuses and Surveys 1994), has such a poor prognosis that screening the population by mass miniature chest X-ray failed. In contrast, prevention, by a public health programme to stop smoking, has reduced death rates by almost a third in men. Screening programmes have been set up for carcinoma of the colon, stomach, breast and cervix, and more recently the prostate and ovary. It is possible that screening for non-malignant conditions such as abdominal aortic aneurysm may reduce the number of deaths in older men from leaking aneurysm. To be effective, early detection and treatment must lead to fewer deaths from the disease, or have a major impact on the quality of life in the screened population, but in some of these conditions there are still doubts that this can be achieved.

BIAS

Lead time bias

The term 'lead time' originated as the interval between a decision to begin a process and the completion of the project. An increased survival time from diagnosis to death could well be due to earlier, and therefore more prolonged, observation of the natural history of the disease, which might be unaffected by the treatment. This situation is known as *lead time bias* and in breast screening is usually reckoned to be about 2 years.

Length bias

1. If the interval between screening episodes is relatively long, the test detects those cases with slowly growing tumours, whereas rapidly growing cancers with a worse prognosis tend to present in between screens. Both lead time and length bias increase the apparent benefit of screening, without necessarily improving the natural history of the cancer in question.

2. The acid test for a screening programme is to compare a screened population with an identical non-screened population; this is ideally set up as a randomized controlled trial (see Ch. 45), to avoid unrecognized systematic biases (Shapiro 1981, Hardcastle et al 1996). If the disease carries a relatively good prognosis when adequately treated at an early stage, it may take many years of observation to show a difference in the number of deaths between the screened and non-screened groups; this requires considerable resources.

3. There are many questions which must be answered before considerable amounts of time, money and effort are committed to a screening programme. These questions must be addressed by several disciplines: clinical scientists in the relevant specialty, epidemiologists with expertise in screening, social scientists and economists.

4. Is the burden of the disease in the population sufficient to warrant an intervention? Is the screening test accurate in detecting cases in the population to be screened, and is the subsequent treatment effective in curing the disease? In trying to answer these three critical questions the following specific issues must be considered.

Key points

If longer survival from progressive disease is claimed to result from improved screening:

- **Was the diagnosis being made at an earlier stage of the disorder than previously?**
- **Were the patients suffering from a less rapidly aggressive form of the disease than is usual?**
- **Will early detection alter the natural history of the disease?**

REQUIREMENTS FOR A SCREENING TEST

1. Is the screening test sensitive: does it detect most of the cases, with few false negatives?

2. Is the test specific: does it detect only cancer cases, with few false positives?

3. Is the negative predictive value of the test high: does a negative test provide reassurance that the risk of the condition is very low?

4. Is the test safe, relatively inexpensive and capable of achieving adequate compliance in the population to be screened?

There are many examples of screening where these criteria have not been met. *O*-tolidine-based dyes for detecting occult blood increased the risk of bladder cancer in laboratory staff. The dose of irradiation initially used for breast screening mammograms is no longer regarded as safe. Investigation and treatment of false-positive cases may lead to psychological or physical morbidity. A few cases, only, of suicide precipitated by the anxiety of a positive or doubtful test negate or at least undermine any real survival advantage from early diagnosis and treatment.

False-negative screening tests, or clerical failure to notify people of positive results, cause a public outcry when a delay in diagnosis has led to the need for more radical treatment or even a premature or preventable death. Such failures have tended to undermine public confidence in the cervical and breast screening programmes in the UK. Sensitivity and specificity tend to be inversely related. The individual performance of screening radiologists is monitored; a radiologist in the breast screening programme with a high sensitivity has a high recall rate with more false-positive cases, and therefore a low specificity; and vice versa (Grimes & Schulz 2002).

To be effective a screening test must be:

- Sensitive – low false-negative rate
- Specific – low false-positive rate
- Of high negative predictive value – should effectively rule out the condition
- Safe and acceptable – with a high compliance rate
- Effective – treatment should reduce the number of deaths, the severity of treatment and improve the quality of life.

POPULATION TO BE SCREENED

The at-risk population must be defined. To screen young people for cancer does not make sense but cancer of the cervix has become more common in younger women; this has led to a lowering in the age at which screening is offered. It is essential to have an accurate register of the population to be screened, and in city areas this must be frequently updated if the clients are to receive invitations for screening. Screening the elderly is likely to show poor uptake (compliance) with age, and an increasing proportion of patients will die of intercurrent disease. The cost:benefit ratio is therefore less favourable but there may be political resistance to the omission of this age group.

Screening of high risk groups, such as those with a strong family history of cancer, poses special problems and different criteria must be used.

COLORECTAL CANCER

Colonoscopy is the 'gold standard' test (against which other tests are measured) for detecting colonic cancer or polyps. It has both specificity and sensitivity nearing 100%, but high cost and low compliance rule this out as a screening test except for those at very high risk from, for example, familial adenomatous polyposis, or longstanding ulcerative colitis. Those at risk from colorectal cancer should be ideal candidates for screening, as many cancers are preceded by benign adenomatous polyps. Furthermore, early cancer (Dukes' stage A) has a 5 year survival of 90% with conventional operative treatment. However, the best available test is poor. The guaiac-based Haemoccult test of three samples is probably the best available test for faecal occult blood but it has a relatively low sensitivity, especially for right-sided and rectal tumours. Immunologically based tests are more sensitive but less specific and give rise to false-positive cases which require expensive and unnecessary investigation.

Randomized controlled trials of faecal occult blood screening have shown a reduced number of deaths from colorectal cancer by 15–33% in the screened group (Hardcastle et al 1996, Kronborg et al 1996). It is intended to introduce systematic screening in the UK. The issues are well reviewed by Ransohoff & Sandler (2002).

CANCER OF THE BREAST

There have been four randomly allocated trials of population screening for breast cancer by mammography; of these, only the Swedish two-counties study has shown a significant reduction in mortality (Tabar et al 1989). However, an overview of these trials and other non-randomized studies shows that all report fewer deaths in the screened versus the non-screened population (Wald et al 1991). There has been a recent reduction in the number of deaths from breast cancer in many countries (Peto et al 2000) but the trend preceded screening and may be principally related to the increased use of adjuvant therapy (Latin *adjuvere* = to aid; something that enhances the effectiveness of medical treatment).

Key point

- **The incidence of cancer varies over time for many reasons. Do not automatically assume that screening programmes have generated observed improvements.**

There has been an unexpectedly high number of cancers presenting between 3-yearly screens (interval cancers) in the UK National Breast Screening Programme, which has led to the adoption of two-view instead of single-view mammography for the first screen (Blanks et al 1997), but a randomized trial of 2 versus 3 years showed no benefit from an increased frequency of screening (UKCCCR 2002). The upper age limit will be increased from 64 to 69 years in the UK, as compliance in this age group seems better than was expected and there is evidence of benefit. Screening women under the age of 50 achieves a relatively small reduction in the number of deaths and remains controversial. Recent criticism of the methodology used in the randomized trials of breast screening (Olson & Gotzsche 2001) has been countered by an updated overview of the Swedish randomized trials (Gelmon & Olivotto 2002, Nystrom et al 2002). This shows a 21% reduction in breast cancer deaths but the age-adjusted relative risk for total mortality was 0.98 (0.96–1.00).

CARCINOMA OF THE CERVIX

Unfortunately no randomized trial of cytological screening for carcinoma of the cervix has been carried out. Although death rates for this disease have fallen in many countries, this fall has often preceded the introduction of screening (Williams 1992).

Up to 60% of women who have developed cervical cancer in the UK had never been screened, and the false-negative rate for examination of the smears is about 10%. Not all smears are adequate, and cytoscreening is very labour intensive and susceptible to problems with quality control (Miller 2002). This is unsatisfactory because adequate treatment of cervical intraepithelial neoplasia (CIN) is highly successful. An efficient mechanism has been developed for recalling and treating patients with positive smears based on general practice, and compliance has reached 83% (Austoker 1994a).

CARCINOMA OF THE STOMACH

The incidence of cancer of the stomach seems to be falling as colon cancer rises but these changes may be confounded (an alternative explanation for the observed facts) by the vagaries of death certification.

Cancer of the stomach is much more common in Japan, where screening for early gastric cancer seems to be effective (Hisamichi & Sugawara 1984) with the use of barium studies, gastroscopy and, more recently, serum pepsinogen. In the UK the search has been less successful. It is suggested that screening by gastroscopy should be confined to symptomatic patients over the age of 55 (Hallissey et al 1990).

CARCINOMA OF THE PROSTATE

Screening for carcinoma of the prostate is controversial, as the disease mainly affects an elderly population and 30% of men over the age of 50 have histological evidence of prostatic cancer at necropsy but in only 1% of these is there clinically active disease (Austoker 1994b). The available screening tests, apart from rectal examination, are prostatic-specific antigen and transrectal ultrasound. Neither the sensitivity nor the specificity of these tests is high, either alone or in combination, and the treatment of localized prostatic cancer is also controversial. Radical prostatectomy, radiotherapy, hormonal manipulation and a watch policy are all used but there is as yet no randomized trial that is sufficiently mature to indicate survival benefit. It is important not to cause unnecessary morbidity in elderly men with asymptomatic disease (Donovan et al 2001).

CANCER OF THE OVARY

Evidence for survival benefit from screening for carcinoma of the ovary is lacking but a large randomized controlled trial has been organized. The main screening tests are antigen marker CA 125 and transvaginal ultrasound, but other tumour markers and colour Doppler are being evaluated. The sensitivity of CA 125 for early ovarian cancer may be as low as 50%. There is, however, a strong case for screening a high risk group with familial ovarian cancer syndrome (Austoker 1994c).

SCREENING FOR NON-MALIGNANT SURGICAL DISEASE

Neonatal screening

Congenital disease is increasingly diagnosed as a result of routine antenatal ultrasound screening but postnatal clinical examination must be carried out to exclude congenital cardiac and renal abnormalities as well as orthopaedic, sexual and anorectal malformations. Most congenital abnormalities usually present as a clinical problem in the first few days of life. Recognize also silent conditions, such as congenital dislocation of the hip, in which delayed diagnosis may worsen the outcome.

Abdominal aortic aneurysm

This accounts for 2900 male and 1040 female deaths per year in England and Wales.

There are several population screening studies from the UK and the USA, and in men over the age of 65 ultrasound screening of the aorta shows a prevalence (the percentage of population affected, as opposed to incidence, which is the rate of occurrence) of aneurysm of about 5%, depending on size criteria. This rate may be twice as high in men with hypertension or vascular disease, and the lifetime prevalence in first-degree male relatives may be as high as 50% (Collin 1994). Deaths from leaking abdominal aortic aneurysm can be reduced by screening men at age 65 years, combined with a policy of electively operating on fit patients with an aortic diameter of about 5.5 cm or more. (Multicentre Aneurysm Screening Study 2002).

WHAT COMPLIANCE IS TO BE EXPECTED?

Compliance, conforming to the advice of the screeners, varies with the social acceptability and public awareness of the disease, the inconvenience or discomfort of the screening test, and the perceived effectiveness of the treatment. Screening for breast cancer by mammography achieves 80% in areas with a stable population but may be less than 50% in inner city areas. Compliance is also sensitive to media exposure in the short term.

In screening for colorectal cancer, the acceptability of the faecal occult blood test is very low, leading to poor compliance; unless public awareness is increased at the time that screening is offered. There are many reasons why people decline screening invitations but failure to receive the letter is a common cause. The true refusers are an unusual group of people who have a poor outlook from both a health and a social standpoint. They neglect or abuse their health in many respects and cannot therefore be used as a control group for comparison with those who accept screening; whatever comparison is made, the refusers will be disadvantaged. Compliance for cervical screening is worst in the low socioeconomic group most at risk from the disease (Segnan 1997).

THE INTERVENTION TO BE USED

It has already been noted that an operation for early bowel cancer has a high cure rate but we cannot be sure that this is the case for breast cancer. Screen-detected breast cancer has many features known to indicate a good prognosis (Klemi et al 1992) but ductal carcinoma in situ is diagnosed in up to 20% of screened cases and the best treatment for this condition is still in doubt. It is possible that fear of overtreatment by mastectomy may lead to a sacrifice of survival advantage by inadequate surgery. Severe dysplasia of the cervix (CIN III) has an extremely good outlook with local treatment and close surveillance. Node-positive carcinoma of the stomach has a 5 year survival rate of less than 10% but in situ tumours carry a good prognosis with adequate surgical treatment. The Japanese have pioneered surgery for gastric cancer that is more radical than has been the norm in the West; clinical trials are currently in hand to try and repeat their excellent results in the UK. The place of radical prostatectomy in the treatment of screening-detected prostatic cancer remains uncertain.

Abuse of screening

Opportunistic screening may be offered or even advertised to give 'peace of mind' where there is no evidence of benefit. High technology tests, such as electron-beam computed tomography (CT) for detecting obstructive coronary artery disease and low dose spiral CT for detecting early lung cancer, have been criticized in this respect, and it seems likely whole body CT scans will be the next high technology test (Lee & Brennan 2002).

Key points

Controversies in screening

- **False negative tests cause public concern and fear of litigation, especially in carcinoma of the cervix and carcinoma of the breast.**
- **There is doubt as to the actual reduction in the number of deaths.**
- **False-positive tests lead to unnecessary investigations/operations.**
- **The high cost of screening might be better spent elsewhere.**

WHAT IS THE COST?

Economists wish to know the cost per case detected, per case treated and per life saved. Sociologists wish to know the psychosocial cost in those false-positive cases investigated unnecessarily and the quality of life in those patients who have cancer detected sooner than it otherwise would have been.

Summary

- How do you decide whether or not a screening test for cancer is capable of detecting disease at a stage when earlier treatment will lead to fewer deaths?
- What are the sensitivity and specificity of a test, and how can your assess them?
- What is meant by 'high negative predictive value'?
- Why does the treatment of a screened disease need to be effective?
- How do cost and quality of life enter into consideration?

References

Ashton HA, Buxton MJ, Day NE et al 2002 The Multicentre Aneurysm Screening Study (MASS) into the effect of abdominal aortic aneurysm screening on mortality in men: a randomised control trial. Lancet 360: 1531–1539

Austoker J 1994a Screening and self-examination for breast cancer. BMJ 309: 168–174

Austoker J 1994b Screening for cervical cancer. BMJ 309: 241–248

Austoker J 1994c Screening for ovarian, prostatic and testicular cancers. BMJ 309: 315–320

Blanks RG, Moss SM, Wallis MG 1997 Use of two view mammography compared with one view in the detection of small invasive cancers: further results from the NHS breast screening programme. Journal of Medical Screening 4: 98–101

Collin R 1994 Abdominal aorta: epidemiology. In: Morris PJ, Malt RA (eds) Oxford textbook for surgery. Oxford University Press, New York, pp 377–378

Donovan JL, Frankel SJ, Neal DE, Hamdy FC 2001 Screening for prostate cancer in the UK. BMJ 323: 763–764

Gelmon KA, Olivotto I 2002 The mammographic screening debate: time to move on. Lancet 359: 904—905

Grimes DA, Schulz KF 2002 Uses and abuses of screening tests. Lancet 359: 881–884

Hallissey MT, Allum WH, Jewkes AJ, Ellis DJ, Fielding JWL 1990 Early detection of gastric cancer. BMJ 301: 513–515

Hardcastle JD, Chamberlain O, Robinson MH et al 1996 Randomised controlled trial of faecal occult blood screening for colorectal cancer. Lancet 348: 1472–1477

Hisamichi S, Sugawara N 1984 Mass screening for gastric cancer by X-ray examination. Japanese Journal of Clinical Oncology 14: 211–223

Klemi PJ, Joensuu H, Toikkanen S et al 1992 Aggressiveness of breast cancers found with and without screening. BMJ 304: 467–469

Kronborg O, Fenger C, Olsen J et al 1996 Randomised controlled study of screening for colorectal cancer with faecal occult blood test. Lancet 3348: 1467–1471

Lee TH, Brennan TA 2002 Direct to consumer marketing of high-technology screening tests. New England Journal of Medicine 346: 529–531

Miller AB 2002 The (in)efficiency of cervical screening in Europe. European Journal of Cancer 38: 321–326

Nystrom L, Anderson I, Bjurstam N, Frisell J, Nordenskjold B, Rutgvist LA 2002 Longterm effect of mammographic screening: updated overview of the Swedish randomised trials. Lancet 359: 909–919

Office of Population Censuses and Surveys 1994 Series DH2, No. 19. Mortality statistics for 1992. Cause. HMSO, London

Olson O, Gotzsche PC 2001 Cochrane review on screening for breast cancer with mammography. Lancet 358: 1340–1342

Peto R, Boreham J, Clarke M, Davies C, Beral V 2000 UK and USA breast cancer deaths down by 25% in year 2000 at ages 20–69 years. Lancet 355: 1822

Ransohoff DF, Sandler RS 2002 Screening for colorectal cancer. New England Journal of Medicine 346: 40–44

Segnan N 1997 Socioeconomic status and cancer screening. IARC Scientific Publications 138: 369–376

Shapiro S 1981 Evidence on screening for breast cancer from a randomised trial. Cancer 39: 618–627

Tabar L, Fagerberg F, Duffy SW, Day NE 1989 The Swedish two counties trial of mammographic screening for breast cancer: recent results and calculation of benefit. Journal of Epidemiology and Community Health 43: 107–114

United Kingdom Co-ordinating Committee on Cancer Research 2002 The frequency of breast screening: results from the UKCCCR randomised trial. European Journal of Cancer 38: 1458–1464

Wald N, Frost C, Cuckle H 1991 Breast cancer screening: the current position. BMJ 302: 845–846

Williams C 1992 Ovarian and cervical cancer. BMJ 304: 1501–1504

42 Audit

B. Davidson, H. J. Schneider

Objectives

- Appreciate what audit is and its vital link with clinical effectiveness.
- Recognize that audit is but the first step, not an end in itself.
- Recognize the need to change clinical practice in the light of audit findings.
- Use audit as a valuable educational tool.

INTRODUCTION

Audit (Latin *auditus* = a hearing) is a critical appraisal of the care dispensed by clinicians. There have been many examples of audit activity in a number of guises over the last few centuries. One of the most notable surgeons to declare his failures as well as successes for the benefit of colleagues was the great 19th century German surgeon of Swedish origin, Theodor Billroth (1881).

The improvement in standards of care in surgery as a whole and in the practices of individual surgeons has, until recently, relied on the apprenticeship of the training years, and the dissemination of new learning and good practice through the medium of the book, the journal and the lecture by the 'expert'. Those who were prepared to listen and read were able to change practice where appropriate. Even now, many surgeons rely on the annual meetings of the various 'craft' associations for education in current surgical practice.

The roots of modern audit lie in the regular morbidity and mortality meetings held in many hospitals in the USA. The value of these meetings as a means of learning was recognized and formed the basis of broader audit activities. When transferred to the British Isles in the 1950s, the American drive for change based on the findings, and the educational importance, were missing.

In the early 1980s, microcomputers became available and made it possible to collect and analyse large amounts of information very swiftly. Most of us now have, or should have, access to reliable, peer-reviewed data on all aspects of medicine and surgery (see Ch. 12). This provides us with a powerful tool to assist in the interpretation of types of work done, throughput, complications, cost and mortality. We have the opportunity to see what are the best results, compare ours with them, determine the reason for differences and react to them.

Possession of an audit system is not synonymous with the successful practice of audit. Systems are merely tools with which we can get a grasp and some understanding of the activity for which we are responsible. Moreover, there is great variation in acquisition, recording, analysing and using information. For this reason some people deprecate attempts to collect and compare it – but imperfect information is better than none at all. A danger of having easy access to information is that it is collected but never utilized. Unless it is applied in an effort to produce improvements, it is merely bureaucratic detritus.

Every hospital in the UK is now responsible for ensuring the development of clinical audit in which all doctors participate. The requirement for audit is now written into the job descriptions for all new medical staff. However, effectiveness in securing worthwhile and lasting improvements in the quality of care for patients is still very variable (Walshe & Spurgeon 1997). These authors have developed a clinical audit assessment and improvement framework designed to improve the effectiveness of audit programmes and individual audit projects.

Until 1990 there was no funding or allocation of time for audit activity. Health authorities must now agree plans for audit, addressing local service and clinical priorities with trust managers and audit groups. As part of the audit contract with hospitals, health authorities can request audit of specific clinical areas.

DEFINITIONS

Clinical audit is defined by the Department of Health as: 'The systematic, critical analysis of the quality of medical care, including the procedures used for diagnosis and treatment, the use of resources, and the resulting outcome and quality of life for the patient', and states that 'an effective programme of medical audit will also help to provide reassurance to doctors, their patients, and managers that the best quality of service is being achieved, having regard to the resources available' (Department of Health 1989). The efficient and effective use of resources is important (Ellis et al 1990), but it is not the first priority of clinical audit.

Key points

- **Omitted from the Department of Health's definition is the vital educational component for you as a trainee surgeon.**
- **Clinical audit is not only a critical assessment of what has and has not been done but a potentially powerful and practical teaching aid.**

Clinical audit is the responsibility of clinicians and must be led by us. The terms 'clinical audit' and 'medical audit' are sometimes used interchangeably, but a consensus has developed whereby *medical audit* refers to the assessment by peer review of the medical care provided by the medical profession to the patient, and *clinical audit* refers to an assessment of the total care of the patient by nurses, professions allied to medicine (such as physiotherapists) as well as doctors. The multiprofessional team has an essential role in patient care and the quality of health care cannot be determined by doctors alone. Most hospitals have now focused their audit activity around clinical rather than medical audit.

A revised position statement on clinical audit identifies future goals:

- Clear patient focus
- Multiprofessional working
- Patient care managed across primary, secondary and continuing care
- Closer links with education
- Integration of effectiveness information
- Improvement of clinical effectiveness.

ATTITUDES TO AUDIT

1. You may argue that audit is practised already; that ward rounds, clinical presentations, research and morbidity and mortality meetings fulfil this function. However, there are differences between these and clinical audit. Audit must be seen as a systematic approach to the review of clinical care to highlight opportunities for

improvement and to provide a mechanism for bringing them about. As such, it endeavours to get away from the 'single interesting case' and look for patterns of care that should ideally be evaluated against research-based evidence or accepted best practice. Audit should initiate investigation into those areas of clinical care that are considered as high risk, high cost or very common. Audit investigation is also suitable for resolving issues of contention or local interest.

Key point

- **Discussing the rare and clinically interesting case is not audit. Leave it for the clinical conference.**

2. You may feel that the time spent on audit could be much better spent on other activities, such as treating more patients. This is not a wholly spurious argument; audit was introduced without any prior evaluation and, although there have been several subsequent evaluations, the results have, to date, failed to demonstrate clear value for money or effort expended (Walshe 1995).

3. There is, none the less, general agreement that a regular review of your own practice against agreed standards of best practice can lead to improved care of patients, who must be the principal beneficiaries of the process.

4. Clinical audit improves patient care not only through direct changes in clinical practice but also through indirect effects such as professional education and team development.

5. An effective clinical audit programme can give the necessary reassurance to patients, clinicians and managers that an agreed quality of service is being given within available resources.

6. Clinicians and managers share audit information within agreed rules of confidentiality. Many deficiencies revealed by audit relate to the organization of care and, although audit must remain clinically led, support from National Health Service (NHS) board directors and management is vital if it is to achieve the necessary changes in practice.

7. There is a growing need to base clinical practice on the knowledge obtained from rigorous research into the effectiveness of healthcare interventions.

8. However, your freedom to determine the treatment you offer individual patients must be preserved – but remember that you may need to justify it as accepted or evidence-based practice if there is an adverse outcome.

9. An important part of the national research and development strategy is to make information on research

findings easily available to clinical and managerial staff, both in printed form, such as Effective Health Care bulletins, and electronic media, such as the Cochrane Library.

AUDIT COMMITTEE

UK hospital clinical audit committees draw members from a range of clinical backgrounds, such as nurses, general practitioners, educational tutors, trainee doctors, pharmacists and physiotherapists, together with audit staff. The committee reports to the unit management. The chairman needs to be well motivated and prepared to devote time on a regular basis.

Audit committee functions are to:

1. Coordinate and foster clinical audit for everyone involved in patient care
2. Offer reassurance that audit is valuable for patients and clinicians, not threatening
3. Determine existing practice of audit
4. Assist clinicians to implement audit methods
5. Monitor the data, results, conclusions and reporting of the audit process
6. When changes are indicated, ensure they are implemented and the effects monitored
7. Promote the educational value of audit
8. Maintain confidentiality
9. Ensure effective liaison with general practitioners
10. Staff requirements include an audit officer and/or coordinator to enable the implementation of audit, and to assist clinicians in the execution of the audit process. They help plan and prepare audit programmes, plans and literature searches, and screen case records against determined criteria. They give computer assistance with databases, graphics, forms and help with the preparation of reports.

The Royal College of Surgeons of England has published guidance on audit, *Clinical Audit in Surgical Practice* (1995), as well as a number of clinical guidelines.

A National Centre for Clinical Audit (NCCA) was established in 1995. Publications include the *NCCA Clinical Audit Action Pack* (1996), a regular newsletter and a series of fact sheets. The centre runs an information service and has its own web site on the internet.

METHODS

Donabedian (1966) identified three main elements in the delivery of health care: structure, process and outcome.

1. *Structure* includes the quantity and type of resources available and is generally easy to measure. It is not a good indicator of the quality of care but should be taken into account in the assessment of process and outcome.

2. *Process* defines what is done to the patient. It includes consideration of the way an operation was performed, what medications were prescribed, the adequacy of notes, and compliance with consensus policies. There is an underlying assumption that the activities under review have been previously shown to produce an optimal medical outcome. This is the area of patient care that is most open to change by clinicians.

3. *Outcome* is the result of clinical intervention and may represent the success or failure of process. For example, outcome could be measured by studies of surgical fatality rates, incidence of complications, or patient satisfaction. It can be considered to be the most relevant indicator of patient care, but it is the most difficult to define and quantify. Mortality and length of stay in hospital are very easily measured outcome indicators, but variations in these outcomes are rarely related directly to the quality of the service being delivered. It may be more important to consider whether patients perceive that their problems have been solved, their quality of life improved and, where appropriate, the duration of their survival.

A number of audit techniques have evolved and found a place in the regular assessment of clinical practice.

Basic clinical audit entails analysing throughput and case type, and assessing complications, morbidity and mortality. A review of such data is undertaken by each clinical firm at intervals of approximately 3 months. The essential ingredient is to distil out of the data any notable deviations from an accepted 'norm' and then to investigate the reason for this observation.

Incident review involves discussing strategies to be adopted under certain clinical situations. An 'incident' may be a leaking aortic aneurysm or using a department for an investigation such as emergency intravenous urography. The discussions should lead to clear policies for future actions and use, with the construction of local guidelines. This audit method is particularly suitable for multidisciplinary or interdisciplinary audit.

Clinical record review. A member of another firm of the same or similar speciality reviews a random selection of case notes, preferably having been given criteria (Greek *krites* = judge; hence, standards) against which to assess them. Clinical record audit has the advantage of simplicity and requires relatively little additional time or other resources. However, there is a potential disadvantage in that discussion might concentrate too much on the quality of record keeping and not enough on patient care – these two are distinct facets of the clinical process, although related.

Criterion audit is a more advanced and structured form of incident audit. Retrospective analysis of clinical records is made and judged against a number of carefully chosen criteria. These criteria should encapsulate the key elements in management of a particular topic which are capable of unambiguous interpretation from the medical record, by a non-medical audit assistant. All cases falling within the scope of the topic in question are screened and those that fail to meet any of the criteria are brought forward for further clinical review. The criteria may relate to administrative elements such as waiting time, investigations ordered, treatments given, outcome and follow-up strategies. Criteria for adequate management of a particular condition can be derived easily from clinical guidelines. Clinicians need to participate actively in the preliminary discussion, but thereafter most of the work can be performed by audit assistants. The method is applicable to a variety of circumstances and allows data to be compared between different hospitals (Shaw 1989). The criteria can be used for setting standards, with targets identifying the proportion of patients in whom each criterion should be met. After review, new targets can be set to stimulate improvement. For example, a suitable target is the reduction of infection rates in colorectal surgery to those obtained in other published studies (Hancock 1990).

Adverse occurrence screening is intended to identify events that need to be avoided, such as wound infections, unplanned readmissions, delayed or erroneous diagnoses. Occurrences are recorded and those that are complex or serious are reviewed by clinicians. A database is accumulated which can then be interrogated to identify trends and, for example, perform comparative analyses. Cases can be considered in total or as samples. This technique can also be used for risk management (Bennett & Walshe 1990).

Comparative audit implies the collection of data and its comparison across units, health authorities and even through a whole region (Gruer et al 1986, Black 1991). Within a single hospital, comparisons may be difficult because the number of departments undertaking similar work is often very small, and the case mix even between two general surgical firms may be disparate. The Royal College of Surgeons (1991) set up a comparative audit service in which all surgeons supply information under a confidential number for comparison with their peers at regular meetings. Techniques in data presentation allow such sensitive information to be widely disseminated and discussed, while maintaining an individual clinician's confidentiality (Emberton et al 1991). In Scotland, a regional computerized audit system maintained by general surgeons over 15 years, recording clinical data which is regularly reviewed in a peer group setting, has provided clear evidence that regional audit

can significantly influence and improve surgical practice (Aitken et al 1997).

National studies were first used to study perinatal mortality in obstetric units. The report of the first confidential enquiry into perioperative deaths (CEPOD: Buck et al 1987) considered the factors involved in the deaths of patients who died within 30 days of operation within three regional health authorities. Much was learned, especially the need for doctors in the training grades to be given adequate support and supervision. Disaster was clearly associated with surgeons attempting procedures for which they possessed insufficient skill or training. Subsequently a national review (NCEPOD) was launched; data is submitted on a voluntary, confidential basis by surgeons and anaesthetists. Reports are published annually (Gallimore et al 1997). The findings can identify remedial actions and indicate appropriate topics for local audit, such as out-of-hours surgery (Campling et al 1997).

Outcome audit is a review of the whole process of healthcare delivery during a patient's hospital contact. It thus measures all the skills of the medical and nursing staff, the hospital administration and, indeed, all those with whom the patient comes into contact. Inevitably there are different perspectives of outcome by the patient, general practitioner and hospital clinician. Satisfactory measures have not yet been evolved. Outcome studies, especially in the surgical specialities, are likely to be important measures of the quality of care.

American surgical audit practice

Audit is used in American surgical practice for the early detection of poor surgical results (Kirk 2001, Singer 2001). There is a customer-oriented approach for cultural and economic reasons. It is a litigious society where the performance and outcomes of surgeons and surgical establishments are closely scrutinized. Recent changes in the UK in the wake of the Bristol affair, such as the publication of league and performance tables, suggest that some or all of the following audit practices, which are standard in the USA, will eventually become commonplace in the UK.

Morbidity and mortality meetings are closed, confidential, and attended weekly by the full surgical faculty, residents and surgical medical students. The departmental chairman supervises and guides the debate and, most importantly, reaches a conclusion regarding each complication or death. It is a basic premise that complications inevitably occur in surgical practice. The chief resident from each surgical team presents surgical throughput, complications and deaths for the previous 1 week period. The methods and outcomes of every surgeon are scrutinized in the light of current evidence and research, with the acceptance that complications are an inevitable part of surgical practice, and from which no surgeon is immune. These are discussed fully, openly, with reference to contemporary evidence-based literature, to define complications or deaths that were preventable, and identify corrective steps. This process is termed 'closing the audit loop'. Passive documentation is unacceptable. The corrective action is recorded, to be effected through letters, guidelines and alterations in departmental policy intended to reduce the risk of future similar errors. Trainees are educated to learn vicariously (Latin *vicarius* = substitute) from the errors of others, rather than from their own failures.

Tissue committee meets monthly to compare every preoperative diagnosis with the histological specimen report, to identify discrepancies and remedy them.

Quality assurance committee meets monthly to audit outcome. For a specific condition they select a sample of approximately 20 patients' case notes to compare outcomes with national standards. Any significant lapse in performance by individuals, teams, departments or equipment is rectified.

Insurance companies have access, by consent of the insured patients, to inspect the case notes on a periodic basis to identify discrepancies in practice, such as prolonged stay, complications and significant increase in the financial cost of patients' care.

ANALYSING AND CORRECTING FAILURES

1. For many years mortality and morbidity conferences and audit meetings considered isolated failures – now often termed 'adverse incidents'. A 'cause' was identified by the senior participants and the meeting passed on to the next incident. The atmosphere gradually changed with demands by the public, and therefore by the politicians, for accountability by doctors for errors, increasingly involving litigation. This was counterproductive because admission that a failure had occurred inevitably generated a demand for exposure of the 'culprit', so that doctors became reluctant to report failures.

2. Contrast this with the situation in the airline industry:

a. It is accepted that we all make mistakes and the investigation is pursued on a 'blame-free' basis.

b. It is mandatory (Latin *manus* = hand + *dare* = to give; a command given by hand, allowing no option) to report any failure. It is not assumed that there is a single 'cause'.

c. The failure can be compared with other potentially similar failures, from the accessible, international database.

d. The best and most cost-effective method of preventing subsequent failures is determined.

e. The correction is implemented – and monitored thereafter. The national and international aviation safety boards have the power to order changes in procedures, design, servicing and manning.

f. Whenever a disaster occurs, teams of skilled investigators search for the causes, aided by flight and speech recorders. The findings, and corrective actions required, are promulgated internationally.

Key point

- **We need to learn and apply the studies available within the medical profession and industry to avoid errors and improve safety, and particularly the US Federal Aviation Administration's methods of improving civil aviation safety.**

3. Some of the approaches used:

a. System analysis failures demand a clear understanding of the failure or failures. This often demands step by step examination of each piece of evidence, with immediate recording of the findings.

b. Fault tree analysis was originally developed for the US Air Force. After identifying the top 'undesired' event causing failure, the analysis continues sequentially to detect the subsidiary contributing causes.

c. 'What's different?' may be a valuable question when an unexpected failure occurs. Changes in assessment, decision making, technique, equipment, monitoring and aftercare may have been overlooked.

4. Corrective action may involve system changes – but some methods are preferable to others on grounds of safety, reliability or convenience:

a. *Improvement in methodology or equipment* may eliminate failure. The most effective measure may be physically to prevent an error being committed. For example, redesign of equipment may make it 'idiot proof'. If accidents have occurred because the wrong components were connected, the connections may be altered so the correct ones alone can be matched.

b. *Monitoring* systems may be introduced to identify potential failures, such as regular, routine checking for premonitory signs. In some cases automatic warning systems can be built in to identify impending failures. In medical practice, intensive care unit monitors relieve nurses of constantly checking basal measurements, allowing them to concentrate on other problems.

c. *Replacement*: components of equipment that fail may be exchanged for new ones after intervals that are shorter than the earliest recorded failure time.

d. *Duplication* and back up is an alternative to anticipating failure by early replacement of essential components.

e. *Training* methods may need to be adapted to make sure that the risk of error is avoided.

f. *Routines, protocols, algorithms* can be changed but the resulting benefit depends upon the conscientiousness with which they are followed.

g. *Checks* are often employed. A junior may need to ask approval from a senior to carry out a procedure. A junior nurse may require to have a drug chart countersigned by a senior before administering treatment. Routine checks suffer from overreliance on them; they may become routine and casually performed and are best reserved for exceptional circumstances.

h. *Warnings* are an unreliable method because they are overused. Visual warnings may not be seen, audible warnings may not be heard.

Key point

- There are two vital steps after identifying a solution, or it is useless. Implement it. Evaluate it.

Human factors

1. The human factor analysis and classification system (HFACS) was developed by the US military to investigate human causes of flying accidents, and was applied to civil aviation accident investigations. Errors are classified as skill based, decision errors, violations of safety rules, or perceptual errors. Other factors were adverse mental or physical states and supervisory or organizational defects.

2. Acceptance that the hierarchical system of command has defects (pilot > copilot > cabin crew) is defective and has led to vital information being ignored. The emphasis is on the aircraft crew working as a team, with each member having input.

Changes needed to reduce or prevent medical errors:

1. We cannot totally eliminate errors. They are inevitable in every human activity.

2. We need an easily accessible, national and international database of errors, adverse incidents and near misses – not just the ones that have been harmful, but also those that were averted or were potentially harmful. This information can be gathered only in an atmosphere of trust, without the threat of blame.

3. Errors, harmful or harmless, offer opportunities to study potential improvements for the future in equipment, systems, decisions and techniques.

Key points

- Although comparison between professions is valuable, remember that many airline problems are mechanical 'black and white'; many biological and clinical problems are immensely complex and are 'shades of grey'.
- Retrospective judgements and actions are less secure when analysing biological failures compared with mechanical and structural failures.

4. In the past, out of a misplaced reluctance to 'tell tales', we failed to challenge or report failures, mistakes, lazy corner-cutting, incompetence and lack of commitment by others. As with most failures, no harm usually follows. Unfortunately, on occasion, other failures develop simultaneously and disaster occurs. To avoid disasters, everyone must perform to a high standard all the time.

Ethics and confidentiality

You must protect the confidentiality of individual patients; the same principles apply as in clinical conferences, which form part of any academic programme. Avoid identifying details of a patient in verbal or written presentations; exclude them.

Protect the confidentiality of the professionals involved, although this is difficult when, for example, one consultant reviews the clinical records of another consultant's patient. Nevertheless, this can be successful if you foster an atmosphere of trust and collaboration. Obtain permission from all consultants involved beforehand.

Anticipate and provide for what should happen if audit reveals deficiencies in an individual's practice (Ellis & Sensky 1991). The Joint Consultants Committee recommends that you develop a plan of action, which they suggest. If necessary, check if the Ethical Committee requires to give permission before interviewing patients.

Computers

Acquire a working knowledge of the basic uses of a computer. You can utilize word processing and graphics and obtain access to databases such as MEDLINE from the postgraduate medical centre. This is faster and more versatile than searching *Index Medicus*. You may download abstracts and papers to a personal computer. The internet offers extensive and rapidly expanding reference sources, including the Cochrane Collaboration. There are now many programs available as clinical information systems, with outputs configured to aid audit, and also some pioneering ventures into clinical decision making and artificial intelligence.

Hospital information systems

Only a few hospitals have completely integrated hospital information systems covering every function, such as clinical records, the scheduling of clinics, to the provision of financial and manpower reports. Other hospitals have a patient administration system (PAS), including the 'master index' (patients' demographic details) and records of admissions and diagnostic codes. This represents the minimum upon which a hospital manager can rely for information. PAS systems regularly pass aggregated patient-level data according to a national minimum data set to the local health authority. This, together with contract activity information, enables local planning of services.

In hospitals with this minimum configuration some clinical departments have implemented their own information systems, and these may provide sufficient information on which to draw patient samples for audit projects and some limited clinical data.

Current trends favour the integration of all these disparate systems so that key patient-specific information, once entered, is available throughout the organization. The surgical trainee will almost certainly be involved in the gathering of information for the production of a discharge summary to the general practitioner and for clinical audit.

EDUCATIONAL COMPONENT

1. Because of the manner in which audit was introduced, with the intention of improving patient treatment and cost-effectiveness, the educational value was a secondary consideration. It is now seen as vital that doctors in training are taught the basic principles of audit. Equally, conclusions drawn from the audit process should be seen as an important feeder into education. The educational benefits of clinical audit have been considered in depth by Batstone (1990).

2. Acquire and update your knowledge by critically reviewing current practice and comparing it with predefined standards. The audit process also enables you to identify important features of clinical practice that help to make teaching explicit. Audit is an active process of review. If you are passive, and unclear whether your current practice is inappropriate, you are unlikely to respond to information through traditional channels such as journals or continuing medical education (Lomas 1993).

3. Audit helps you to identify areas for improving and increasing knowledge, or suggests the need for research. Remember that audit itself does not lead to new clinical knowledge.

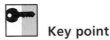

Key point

- **Research aims to identify 'the right thing to do'. Audit assesses whether 'the right thing has been done'.**

4. Self-evaluation and peer review, common activities in audit, are important components of postgraduate education. To realize the full educational potential of audit, you must learn the lessons arising from previous audit meetings and review the conclusions acted upon.

IMPLEMENTING CHANGE

1. Consider audit as a cycle, the first component of which is the observation of existing practice to establish what is actually happening (Fig. 42.1).

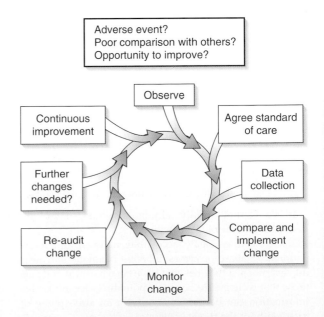

Fig. 42.1 The audit cycle. There should be no 'closure' in the terminal meaning of the word, but there should be 'closure' in the sense that no gap can be left in the circle of reacting to circumstances that demand action to improve them.

2. Now set standards of practice to define what ought to happen and make a comparison between observed practice with the standard.

3. Now implement change.

4. Observe again to see whether what has been planned has been achieved.

5. You may need to decide whether practice needs to change further, or whether the standards were unrealistic or unobtainable.

6. This process has become known as the 'cycle of audit' (Royal College of Physicians 1989) and the achievement of change has been termed 'closing the audit loop'.

7. However, 'closure' implies completion. Always continue to observe results.

Key points

- **Never cease to monitor results.**
- **Once you achieve improvement, If you relax attention your improvement may relapse.**

8. The provision of information on clinical activity without any evaluation or suggestions for improvement has almost no effect on clinical practice (Mitchell et al 1990). It needs to be targeted at decision-makers who had already agreed to review their practice (Mugford et al 1991). A systematic review of 160 interventions directed at changing clinical behaviour or health outcomes showed that effects were small to moderate (Davis et al 1995). Effective strategies were outreach visits, opinion leaders, patient-mediated interventions and physician reminders. Audit with feedback gives variable results.

9. The most commonly used approach involves the publication of guidelines, which have been shown to change practice and affect outcomes. Guidelines are more likely to be effective if they have local involvement and take into account local circumstances, are supported by active educational interventions and use patient-specific reminders, for example, in the medical notes (Effective Health Care 1994). Guidelines need to be reviewed regularly to establish 'ownership' and to incorporate the latest research findings.

THE NEW NHS

The government white paper *The New NHS: Modern, Dependable* (Department of Health 1997) outlines a new '10 year' structuring and modernization programme. The internal market is replaced by a system of integrated care based on a partnership between health and social care. The split between planning and providing care is maintained, with cooperation replacing competition. The quality of care is a priority for everyone.

Chief executives of trusts will be held accountable for the quality of services they provide. This responsibility for 'clinical governance' covers quality improvement (see Ch. 43). The importance of clinical audit, led by clinicians, in improving the quality of care for patients was recognized in the previous NHS reorganization in 1989. The new framework signals a more directed but integrated role for audit within the organization. This can be seen as an opportunity for audit to deliver the necessary changes in practice which have been identified, and fulfil its potential in improving patient care.

Summary

- Do you recognize the two aims of audit – improved health care and clinical education – must both be addressed?
- Do you accept that audit without application of the findings is a wasted 'paper exercise'?

References

Aitken RJ, Nixon SJ, Ruckley CV 1997 Lothian surgical audit: a 15-year experience of improvement in surgical practice through regional computerised audit. Lancet 350: 800–804

Batstone GF 1990 Educational aspects of medical audit. BMJ 301: 326–328

Bennett J, Walshe K 1990 Occurrence screening as a method of audit. BMJ 300: 1248–1251

Billroth TH 1881 Clinical surgery: reports of surgical practice, 1860–1876. New Sydenham Society, London

Black N 1991 A regional computerised surgical audit project. Quality Assurance in Health Care 2: 263–270

Buck N, Devlin HB, Lunn JN 1987 Report of a confidential enquiry into perioperative deaths. King's Fund, London

Campling EA, Devlin HB, Hoile RW, Ingram GS, Lunn JN 1997 Who operates when? A report of the national confidential enquiry into perioperative deaths. King's Fund, London

Davis DA, Thomson MA, Oxman AD, Haynes RB 1995 Changing physician performance: a systematic review of the effect of continuing medical education strategies. JAMA 274: 700–705

Department of Health 1989 Working for patients (paper no. 6). HMSO, London

Department of Health 1997 The new NHS: modern, dependable (Cmnd 3807). Stationery Office, London

Donabedian A 1966 Evaluating the quality of medical care. Millbank Memorial Federation of Quality 3(2): 166–203

Effective Health Care 1994 Implementing clinical practice guidelines. University of Leeds, Leeds, vol. 1: 8

Ellis BW, Sensky T 1991 A clinician's guide to setting up audit. BMJ 302: 704–707

Ellis BW, Rivett RC, Dudley HAF 1990 Extending the use of clinical audit data. BMJ 301: 159–162

Emberton M, Rivett RC, Ellis BW 1991 Comparative audit: a new method of delivering audit. Bulletin of the Annals of the Royal College of Surgeons 73: 117–120

Gallimore SC, Hoile RW, Ingram GS, Sherry KM 1997 The report of the national confidential enquiry into perioperative deaths, 1994–5. NCEPOD, London

Gruer R, Gordon DS, Gunn AA, Ruckley CV 1986 Audit of surgical audit. Lancet i: 23–26

Hancock BD 1990 Audit of major colorectal and biliary surgery to reduce rates of wound infection. BMJ 301: 911–912

Kirk J 2001 American mechanisms in place for the early detection of poor surgical results. Bulletin of the Annals of the Royal College of Surgeons 83: 307

Lomas J 1993 Diffusion dissemination, and implementation: who should do what? Annals of the New York Academy of Sciences 703: 226–235

Mitchell MW, Fowkes FGR 1990 Audit reviewed: does feedback on performance change clinical behaviour? Journal of the Royal College of Physicians 19: 251–254

Mugford M, Banfield P, O'Hanlon M 1991 Effects of feedback of information on clinical practice: a review. BMJ 303: 398–402

National Centre for Clinical Audit 1996 NCCA clinical audit action pack: a practical approach. National Centre for Clinical Audit, London

Royal College of Physicians 1989 Medical audit. A first report – what, why and how? RCP, London

Royal College of Surgeons 1991 Royal College of Surgeons confidential comparative audit service. Bulletin of the Annals of the Royal College of Surgeons 73: 96

Royal College of Surgeons 1995 Clinical audit in surgical practice. RCS, London

Shaw CD 1989 Medical audit: a hospital handbook. King's Fund, London

Singer A 2001 The Bristol affair – a view from New York. Bulletin of the Annals of the Royal College of Surgeons 83: 306

Walshe K 1995 Evaluating clinical audit: past lessons, future directions. Royal Society of Medicine Press, London

Walshe K, Spurgeon P 1997 Clinical audit assessment framework. Handbook Series 24. HMSU, University of Birmingham, Birmingham

 Further reading

National Centre for Clinical Audit 1996 NCCA criteria for clinical audit. NCCA, London

Royal College of Surgeons of England 1994 Guidelines for clinicians on medical records and notes. RCS, London

Royal Society of Medicine 1990 Computers in medical audit: a guide for hospital consultants to personal computer based medical audit systems. RSM Services, London

Trent Regional Health Authority 1993 Guidelines on confidentiality and medical audit. Trent RHA, Sheffield

Systems failure analysis

Berk J, Berk S 1993 Total quality management. Sterling, New York

Wiegman DA, Shappell SA, Christina E 2000 A human factors analysis of aviation accident data: an empirical evaluation of the HFACS framework. Aviation Space and Environmental Medicine 71: 328

These and many more are available on the internet by searching under the title 'Systems failure analysis'

Also consult:
Reason J 1990 Human error. Cambridge University Press, Cambridge

Useful links

http://www.ahrq.gov/qual/errback.htm Medical errors: the scope of the problem: fact sheet.

43 Clinical governance

B. Higgs

Objectives

- **Understand the concept of and need for clinical governance.**
- **Outline the framework/system of clinical governance.**
- **Understand the role of clinical governance in delivering quality health care.**

INTRODUCTION

Public, political and professional pressure has been growing to maintain and improve standards of patient care throughout the National Health Service (NHS). Clinical governance is one aspect of a system designed to set, monitor and maintain standards of patient care. The driving force for the introduction of clinical governance was the perceived lowering of public confidence in the NHS, a desire within the medical profession for systems to be established that set, maintain and improve standards, and a demand for the government to fulfil public expectations.

We should all aspire to improving the quality of health care. Although most health professionals already provide excellent quality care and many keep records or data supporting their practice, there are inequalities within the country, instances of substandard care and isolated cases of abuse of the public's trust.

Clinical governance should identify areas where patient care is suboptimal. However, not all of the issues relate directly to the quality of clinical care provided, but to other aspects that contribute to patient care which may be economic and managerial, such as underfunding, understaffing and lack of facilities, beds, equipment and support services.

Hospital trusts, like other business activities, need to be well organized to address these and other issues. Any organization that functions as a single unit can be called a corporate body. The system of corporate governance (Greek *kybernaein*, Latin *gubernare* = control) is well established in NHS Trusts, just as it is in the business world. Within the Trust the responsibilities of those working within a corporate structure are defined, and the rules and procedures for pursuing the aims of the business are decided and defined. The chief executives of NHS Trusts are the designated accountable officers for corporate governance.

Clinical governance is the clinical parallel of corporate governance and defines the responsibilities of all those who provide service for the patients, provide support for their activities, monitor the results and ensure that the quality of care provided meets the requirements of the patients. The chief executives of NHS Trusts are also the designated, accountable officers for clinical governance.

CLINICAL QUALITY

The World Health Organization defines clinical quality under four headings:

1. Professional management – quality of the technical aspects of care
2. Resource use – the efficiency of the management
3. Risk management – the risk of injury, illness or poor outcome resulting from the care provided
4. Patient satisfaction.

 To achieve optimal care we need to:

- **Set clear standards in each aspect of quality assessment**
- **Ensure that in each aspect the delivery of service is the highest attainable**
- **Monitor the outcome in each aspect and if necessary correct deficiencies.**

Audit is used to monitor clinical quality (see Ch. 42). Medical audit provides a means of determining the quality of the care by physicians and surgeons. This does not encompass all that is included in clinical quality, and clinical audit incorporates the total care by nurses and allied health professionals in addition to doctors.

SCOPE OF CLINICAL GOVERNANCE

1. For many years the majority of clinicians have checked results/outcomes and compared them with published results from highly respected centres. However, these have usually been restricted to survival and resulting major morbidity. Clinical governance incorporates these results, and more, with the overall service and quality of patient care.

2. A patient visiting the outpatient clinic or general practitioner, or one who is admitted to hospital, does not judge the experience on the outcome alone. Patient satisfaction does not depend only on your clinical skills, abilities and judgements, but on the whole episode, which involves medical, nursing, ancillary, technical, allied health professionals, managers and secretaries, as well as the availability of equipment and facilities. Good clinical care may not compensate for poor facilities or equipment. The process must, therefore, be a multi- and interdisciplinary event. Traditional boundaries and restrictive practices must be addressed and patient care needs to be more integrated, involving all staff at all levels.

Key points

- **Professional and clinical culture needs to place the patient at the centre of the health care organization.**
- **The effects must extend outside any institution into all aspects of patient care.**

REPORTING OUTCOMES

Following American experience, there is pressure for publicly available outcome results for comparison between units in the health service. Access to clinical information in order to allow monitoring of clinical and organizational practice appears to be a challenge for many organizations. The quality of recording and classification is not uniform and is often unreliable because of differences in facilities, equipment, trained staff and commitment to accurate recording. Moreover, the publication in 'ranked order' of crude survival rates is valueless and could be harmful. However, comparisons between different units with comparable data and informed interpretation may be useful to both staff and patients. As information and data collection improves, there can be no doubt that useful information will be gained, helpful to clinicians and patients alike.

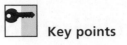

Key points

- **Clinical governance challenges us to identify and address clinical issues to improve them.**
- **Imperfect information is better than no information.**

COMPONENTS OF CLINICAL GOVERNANCE

1. *Clinical effectiveness* is concerned with ensuring that the best care is provided by delivering treatments that work. Clinical practice should be based on objective evidence. There are several components of clinical effectiveness that result in the delivery of evidence-based care (see Ch. 12). Health workers should know what is clinically effective practice, and how to apply that knowledge in day to day practice. We should make sure that changes in practice work to benefit patients.

2. *Clinical audit* (see Ch. 42) is a systematic and critical analysis of the quality of clinical care, including the procedures for the diagnosis, treatment and care, the associated use of resources and the resulting outcome and quality of life for the patient. It is used to examine current practice in relation to a standard. If there is a gap between current practice and the standard, then practice must be changed to close the gap. The process is then reaudited to make sure that the loop is closed and the audit cycle is completed.

3. *Risk management* is clinical and non-clinical, and is proactive – instigating changes in anticipation of future developments:

a. Clinical risk management is achieved by establishing a process of reporting by all members of the clinical team whenever unexpected, adverse or 'near miss' clinical incidents occur, whether or not actual harm results. The reports are reviewed to identify any immediate action that should be taken to avoid future potentially dangerous incidents. The aggregated data, together with recommendations, are fed back to all members of the care team. This process allows immediate action on incidents when required and the aggregate data draw attention to risks that may occur seemingly in isolation. When analysed over time, patterns may emerge, in isolation or across the whole establishment, so that steps can be taken to reduce or eliminate the risk.

b. Non-clinical risk management is applied to considerations such as fire and electrical safety.

4. *Research and development* supports clinical governance by providing the evidence base for good and effective health care. It is a popular misconception that to be of any value the research has to be funded by the Medical Research Council, be international, multicentred and published in a highly rated journal. While national and international research collaborations help to identify modern and effective treatments, many improvements to the provision of quality health care are made at local level. There is an obligation on all trusts to support, train and develop their staff to enhance the staff's research skills and hence improve the quality of care delivered.

5. *Quality indicators and monitoring of quality*: Trust boards identify quality indicators, monitor them and act accordingly. This is achieved by tracking all national indicators that apply to trusts (Department of Health and Dr Foster), the most important of which are the clinical indicators including mortality, other incidents and complaints. There are always problems with standardization and this makes comparisons difficult. It is vital that data relating to clinical quality are accurate. All clinicians have a responsibility to ensure that data about their patients are correct.

6. *User perspective is important*: services must be centred on patients' needs. Strangely, this is an area that previously was rarely addressed in a systematic, cohesive corporate manner. Clinical governance will not succeed unless the patients are involved in the initiation of trust strategy. There are many different mechanisms for seeking feedback from patients and involving patients in planning health care. In addition to clinical needs, it is necessary to address information, privacy, dignity and religious and cultural aspects. Feedback can be obtained by questionnaires, surveys, audit and interviews. However, direct involvement of patients in 'users' groups' is essential to enable new ideas, concerns and help with planning new and existing services to be dealt with.

7. *Education, training and continuing professional development* are essential for the provision of high quality care (General Medical Council 2001). There must be a balance between teaching and training. Support must be provided both for trainers and teachers. Lifelong learning should involve a systematic approach whereby doctors and other health professionals are helped to identify development needs that will enable them to do their jobs better and move toward their career goals. Postgraduate medical organizations are well placed to help carry this forward. All staff should have a personal development plan which balances service needs and career aspirations.

 Key points

- **All elements of clinical governance must be active in your trust.**
- **Are you involved in all these aspects?**

8. *Other systems and relationships* that support or complement clinical governance: in addition to long established organizations within the National Health Service, new ones have been created (see Fig. 43.1). 'Outside' bodies and national principles involved in clinical governance in your Trust are:

a. *National Institute for Clinical Excellence (NICE)*. This is a Special Health Authority. It was set up to provide a strong lead on clinical and cost-effectiveness by drawing up guidelines based on scientific evidence and to advise on best practice.

b. *National Service Frameworks (NSFs)*. These are designed to set national standards and define service models for a specific or defined service care group. They are, or put in place, strategies to support implementation/establish performance milestones.

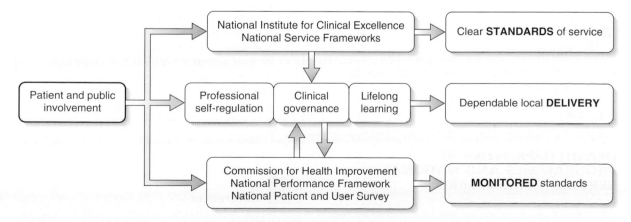

Fig. 43.1 It is important to note the central position of clinical governance.

c. *Commission for Health Improvement (CHI)*. Established to assure, monitor and improve the quality of care in the NHS in England and Wales. It will provide national leadership to develop and disseminate clinical governance principles. The Commission will visit every NHS Trust every 4 years and independently scrutinize local clinical governance arrangements to support, promote and deliver high quality services. By 2003 it is proposed that NHS performance indicators will be transferred to CHI and will be published.

d. *NHS Performance Framework*. This will be used to move toward assessing performance of the NHS in the round, covering quality and efficiency. A set of national indicators will measure progress against main targets. It will encourage benchmarking between similar NHS organizations and underpin national and local performance and accountability arrangements. High level performance indicators (e.g. deaths, surgery rates, cancer detection, hospital stay, etc.) will be used to ensure a more rounded assessment of NHS performance. Depending on their performance against the Performance Assessment Framework, all NHS organizations will annually and publicly be classified as 'green', 'yellow' or 'red'. Red organizations will be those who are failing to meet a number of the core national targets.

e. *Professional organizations and Royal Colleges*. The professional bodies as well as the newly established Medical Education Standards Board (replacing the Specialist Training Authority) will work together to maintain quality and improve training.

The Commission for Health Improvement will join with the Audit Commission to form the Commission for Healthcare Audit and Inspection (CHAI). This body will lead inspections in the NHS and the private health care sector and be responsible for all financial and performance audit as well for the quality of the assessment work which CHI has been doing.

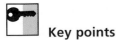

Key points

- **Do you understand the interrelationships of clinical governance?**
- **Do you understand the role of the outside bodies?**

HEALTH IMPROVEMENT PROGRAMMES AND NATIONAL SERVICE FRAMEWORKS

1. Clinical governance is an integral part of developing and implementing Health Improvement Programmes (HimPs). However, hospital trusts do not work in isolation! Health authorities, hospital trusts, primary care trusts and social services work together to develop a 3 year HimP. This plan should consider national and local priorities. The national priorities for 1999–2000 were coronary heart disease, mental health, cancer and antibiotic prescribing. Since then, National Service Frameworks (NSFs) for diabetes and care of older people have been introduced, and NSFs for renal services, children's services and long-term conditions focusing on neurological disorders are in preparation.

2. Local priorities take into account the needs and special circumstances of the local population. If these priorities are to be addressed there needs to be a mechanism for making certain that the standards required are monitored and delivered. Similarly there needs to be evidence that the priorities are being met and/or pointers toward where resources are being used effectively.

3. This combination of agreeing and setting priorities in planning, purchasing and delivering health care, introducing clinical governance and measuring the outcomes by means of the National Performance Assessment Programmes should result in more modern and effective healthcare delivery by including all the key partners in planning and tackling the root causes of ill health.

Summary

- Do you know who is ultimately responsible for maintaining overall clinical standards in your hospital?
- Do you know the range of people who come into contact with patients or provide a service to them?
- Do you appreciate the range of experiences on which patients base their assessment of outcome?
- Do you accept individual and collective responsibility for the reputation and quality of care delivered by your firm, unit, hospital, health service?

References

General Medical Council 2001 Good medical practice, 3rd edn. GMC, London (www.gmc-uk.org/standards/good.htm)

Further reading

Clinical governance: quality in the new NHS (HSC 1999/065). HMSO, London

Bloor K, Maynard A 1998 Clinical governance: clinician heal thyself. Institute of Health Service Management, London

NHS Executive 1999 Quality and performance in the NHS: high level performance indicators. HMSO, London

NHS Executive 1999 Quality and performance in the NHS: clinical indicators. HMSO, London

Secretary of State for Health 1997 The new NHS, modern dependable. HMSO, London

Swage T 2001 Clinical governance in health care practice. Butterworth-Heinemann, Oxford

44 Economic aspects of surgery

R. W. Hoile, G. Douglas

Objectives

- **Understand some basic principles behind economic considerations in surgical practice.**
- **Recognize the potential conflict between clinical freedom, medical ethics and the logic of health economics.**
- **Examine areas of clinical practice where surgeons can influence the costs of surgery.**

INTRODUCTION

This is probably a subject which, up to now in your surgical career, you have not needed to think about or understand. Before you progress much further you will undoubtedly be exposed to economic considerations and the consequences of your actions, so it is worthwhile discussing some of the principles used when addressing this topic.

The National Health Service was developed on the principle of fairness and that health care was free to the patient at the point of delivery. With rising costs of health care, limited resources and the heightened expectations of our patients, it is inevitable that questions are asked about cost. There is also a debate about the quality versus quantity of care and the total benefit to the community. Will the economic arguments take over and conflict with good patient care, or can good economic strategies mean better patient care? At all times in this debate keep central the outcome for your patients.

MEASUREMENT OF COST EFFECTIVENESS

The measurement of cost effectiveness can be considered, in simple terms, as synonymous with economic evaluation. The cost of surgery is not just monetary but also personal and social. For the patient, there is pain, suffering, time spent in hospital and the economic consequences

of the disease, hospitalization and time off work. While we should be striving to deliver a cost-effective healthcare system, we should not lose sight of these personal costs. Measuring cost effectiveness is an unfamiliar process to clinicians, but it is important in evaluating and practising modern surgery. Before the cost effectiveness of any surgical management is understood, it is necessary to understand some of the principles, definitions and accounting practices that are applied to problems of health care and the way in which they may affect clinical decision making.

COST EFFECTIVENESS: WHAT DOES IT MEAN?

There are four ways of interpreting cost effectiveness in clinical practice.

1. Cost savings: this can also be considered as avoided costs, or the estimated costs caused by the disease process that can be avoided by surgical intervention; for example, appropriate treatment of venous insufficiency in the leg can prevent the development of subsequent, costly (in all senses of the word) chronic venous ulceration.
2. Effective improvement of health care.
3. Cost savings with equal or better health outcome: this requires no compromise by accountants, financial directors or clinicians – it is a 'win–win' situation.
4. Additional benefits worth the additional cost: judgement is needed to decide whether additional cost is worth the anticipated benefit and to select the course of action with the least cost at the most probable benefit. Both a high dependency unit (HDU) and an intensive care unit (ICU) give high benefit for cost. Similarly, critical care outreach teams effectively identify critically ill patients and advise on management; they are expensive but cost effective.

Key points

- **Surgeons should consider both clinical benefit and cost effectiveness together.**

- **Clinical freedom allows you to choose the best treatment for a patient (based on the evidence, clinical knowledge and understanding) but remember that resources are limited.**
- **Unwise use of resources is poor cost effectiveness.**
- **An unnecessarily expensive remedy for one patient may deprive other needy patients of valuable treatment.**

HOW ARE BENEFITS MEASURED?

1. Cure.
2. Increased life expectancy.
3. Improved quality of life. One method of evaluating the value of a year of healthy life is the calculation of quality-adjusted life years (QALYs). One year of life in full health is 1 QALY.

HOW ARE COSTS MEASURED?

- *Direct costs* are those borne by the healthcare system, community and family.
- *Indirect costs* are those borne by the individual, family, society and employer, such as time spent in hospital, loss of earnings and loss of productivity.
- *Intangible costs* are those borne by the patient, such as pain, anxiety, grief, suffering and loss of leisure. Death following an operation is also often considered as an intangible loss.

Hospital attendances, medical and surgical risks, mortality, resulting disability, management of complications and failures, contribute to all three cost evaluations.

HOW CAN YOU INFLUENCE HOSPITAL COSTS?

1. Use resources efficiently and appropriately. The introduction of day surgery as a low cost/high throughput service reduces the cost of procedures without increased morbidity. Short-stay, 5 day wards, low dependency units and hotel use also reduce costs, are not detrimental and may be advantageous. Preadmission clinics, which may avoid last minute cancellations, are also proven to be cost effective.

2. Avoid investigative and operative techniques that are outdated or of unproven use (see Ch. 12). 'Routine' investigations for all admissions are valueless unless they influence subsequent management (see Chs 6, 15). Order the fewest tests that will provide the speediest, most specific

and reliable results. Tests requested out of hours cost more to provide so avoid them if they can be deferred. However, remember that sometimes a quicker diagnosis and prompt action may ultimately shorten hospital stay and speed recovery. Can you justify your requests?

3. Critically assess the value of procedures that demand expensive technological back-up or instrumentation. The gains must be balanced against the costs; laparoscopic colonic surgery reduces hospital stay, recovery and back-to-work time. On the other side of the balance sheet there may be the costs produced by a longer operating time, increased risks of thromboembolism, ureteric injury and concerns about the adequacy of resection. Patient preference must also be considered; for example, in hernia repair the cost effectiveness of the 'open' and endoscopic techniques are roughly comparable but many patients will express a preference for minimal access procedures. You could probably make considerable cost reductions and feel more at ease with resource implications if you and your clinical colleagues could agree 'best practices' for selected procedures, develop local protocols and adhere to them; for example, you might agree to perform laparoscopic procedures but carefully define the circumstances when it would be acceptable to use the more expensive disposable pieces of equipment.

4. Place the patient's interests above those of academia or research. Patient screening (see Ch. 41) must be shown to be cost effective. Society must participate in the decision to introduce screening or compliance will be poor.

5. Keep complication rates low. Postoperative complications are expensive and can spoil any attempt to improve the cost effectiveness of surgery. The management of complications may triple the costs of an uncomplicated procedure. Avoid complications at all stages of assessment, decision making, preparation, active treatment, recovery, discharge and review. Audit your results.

6. Do not be afraid to develop new ideas and think laterally if you can show a benefit. It is appropriate to seek funding if there is a proven or predicted benefit for the service or the patients. For example, an emergency admissions unit (such as that established at Eastbourne General and other hospitals) allows intensive preadmission assessment and may prevent 20% of admissions. This saving in bed occupancy more than justifies the cost of such a unit.

 Key points

- **Avoid unnecessary costs.**
- **Recognize that the benefit and outcome for the patient are the most important factors.**

- Choose relevant investigations.
- Assess the evidence concerning the efficacy and outcomes of operative interventions.
- Do not assume that you have to operate: think carefully about the benefits fIrst.
- Take precautions to minimize complications.
- Only adopt new techniques after proper evaluation.
- Develop guidelines for 'best practice' for selected common procedures.
- Liaise with departmental managers in order to determine the service requirements for your local population.

CONCLUSIONS

Thinking about the economics of health care raises issues that are sometimes uncomfortable. There are questions about waste, the inappropriateness of investigations and operations, rationing, cost containment, ethics, etc. The response to these questions needs to be well thought out and workable. It is possible to set professional standards and deliver appropriate care while eliminating the unwarranted use of medical resources. It is easy to 'do something', particularly when faced with an individual patient, but perhaps we should stand back, take a broader view and consider whether an action for the individual patient is appropriate and/or cost effective. A multitude of tests and complex procedures do not necessarily produce an accurate or speedy diagnosis, a lower morbidity or mortality, or 'better' health care. Professional guidelines and clinical audit may sometimes help us when it is necessary to say 'no'. A partnership between clinician and manager may help rationalize the provision of a surgical service, with maximum benefits to all concerned.

We have not found all the answers yet but you must begin to address these difficult issues.

Summary

- You should recognize that the costs of surgery (and health care in general) are rising but resources are limited.
- Health economics provides a logical framework for the allocation of resources.
- You can reduce costs without compromising clinical freedom and patient care by investigating wisely, operating sensibly and keeping complications low. 'Choose well, cut well, get well.'
- You may perceive a conflict between your medical ethics and the economic logic applied by your hospital accountants and trust financial director. However, having read this chapter, you will appreciate that the aim of both disciplines is to promote health and alleviate suffering. The surgical economic argument is just one more tool for you to use when making decisions about the care of your patients.
- Consider the wider implications of your decIsions and actions.

 Further reading

Gray AJ, Hoile RW, Ingram GS, Sherry KM 1998 The report of the national confidential enquiry into perioperative deaths 1996/97. NCEPOD, London

Hicks NR 1994 Some observations on attempts to measure appropriateness of care. BMJ 309: 730–733

Hodgson K, Hoile RW 1996 Managing health service contracts. WB Saunders, London

Jefferson T, Demicheli V, Mugford M 1996 Elementary economic evaluation in health care. BMJ Publishing Group, London

O'Brien B 1986 'What are my chances doctor?' A review of clinical risks. Health Economics Research Group, Brunel University

Williams A, Anderson R 1985 Efficiency in the social services. Blackwell, London

45 Statistical concepts: a tool for evidence-based practice

R. W. Morris

Objectives

- If you wish to apply up-to-date published research to your clinical practice, you need to grasp basic statistical concepts and common techniques that quantify the benefits of new interventions and diagnostic tests. You must be able to appraise critically the design of research studies, apart from understanding the handling of quantitative data in published research. You can then practise evidence-based medicine (see Ch. 12).
- If you wish to carry out your own quantitative research, you must have a firm grasp of statistical principles. In this chapter I shall aim to provide a comprehensible outline of various statistical techniques employed in surgical research, rather than attempt a detailed coverage. For this reason I have recommended useful books for further reading.

CLINICAL SCENARIO

Mr Dennis Gray is a 49-year-old gardener. He was diagnosed as having carcinoma of the rectum after presenting to his general practitioner with bleeding on defecation. A CT scan of the abdomen suggests that the tumour is about 3 cm in diameter and has not yet become locally invasive. There is no sign of metastatic spread. Mr Gray is scheduled for curative resection with preservation of anal function. You feel that adjuvant chemotherapy is not necessary in this case in view of the many favourable prognostic features. The consultant, however, wishes to maxi-mize Mr Gray's chances of complete cure by administering an intraportal regimen of fluorouracil, 500 mg m^{-2}, on the first day after surgery and a continuous heparin infusion for 7 days. The patient, who has three young children, is keen to follow any regimen that improves his chances of long-term survival.

Many clinical questions might arise during Mr Gray's encounters with both the general practitioner and the surgeon. These may include, in particular:

- *Diagnosis.* How important is bleeding on defecation in establishing the presence of a rectal carcinoma?
- *Prognosis.* What probability of long-term survival (e.g. for 10 years) does Mr Gray have?
- *Therapy.* Will adjuvant therapy increase Mr Gray's chances of a complete cure? If so, by how much?

All three of these questions may potentially be answered by appropriate studies.

DIAGNOSIS

1. It is unlikely that any routine test carried out to establish the presence or absence of disease will be entirely accurate. When applying such a test, however, knowledge of its accuracy will be helpful in interpreting the result gained. Traditionally this will be expressed in terms of two quantities, namely the sensitivity and specificity. These can be assessed by a study in which the routine test has been applied to a number of subjects where the true presence or absence of disease has been established, usually by a diagnostic test seen as the 'gold standard' (Table 45.1).

2. A study was carried out by Fischer et al (1991) on patients with new knee conditions. All subjects underwent arthroscopy, which was taken as the gold standard, as well as magnetic resonance imaging (MRI). A comparison was made for 911 patients on whether arthroscopy

Table 45.1 Test for presence/absence of disease

	Disease present	Disease absent	Totals
Test positive	True positive	False positive	*All test positive*
Test negative	False negative	True negative	*All test negative*
Totals	*All with disease present*	*All with disease absent*	*All in study*

and MRI showed the presence or absence of a medial meniscal tear. The results were as shown in Table 45.2.

Of 473 subjects who actually had a medial meniscal tear (according to the arthroscopy), 440 were correctly picked up by the MRI. Thus the *sensitivity* of the test was 440/473 = 0.93, or 93%. The MRI missed 7% of the meniscal tears.

Of 438 subjects who did not have a medial meniscal tear, 367 were correctly excluded by the MRI. Thus the *specificity* of the test was 367/438 = 0.84, or 84%.

Thus we know that if someone has a medial meniscal tear, there is a 93% probability that they will be picked up by an MRI. If they do not have a meniscal tear, there is an 84% chance that this diagnosis will be correctly excluded by an MRI.

3. As a clinician faced with an individual case, however, the sensitivity and specificity are of little direct value to you. The idea of performing an MRI is that its result will become available before an arthroscopy is performed. The question therefore is not 'If this patient had a meniscal tear, how likely is it that a positive MRI result would be shown?' but rather 'When given a positive MRI result, how likely is it that a medial meniscal tear is actually present?' The latter question leads to consideration of the *positive predictive value* (PPV).

From the data above, the PPV is 440/511 = 0.86, or 86%. In other words, 86% of all positive MRI scans indicate a true tear of the medial meniscus.

By analogy, another useful statistic is the *negative predictive value* (NPV). 'When given a negative test result, how likely is it that a medial meniscal tear is actually absent?'

The NPV is 367/400 = 0.92, or 92%. In other words, 92% of all negative MRI scans indicate absence of tear in the medial meniscus.

4. The PPV and NPV are of more intuitive use to you than the sensitivity and specificity. Unfortunately, their appeal may be illusory. They depend very heavily on the actual prevalence of the condition in the population under study. In the study generating the data shown in Table 45.2, the prevalence of a meniscal tear was just over 50% (473/911). If a similar study was carried out on a population where the true prevalence was lower, then the PPV would be less than calculated above. The NPV would be even higher. For example, if the prevalence were 33%, the PPV would fall from 86% to 74%. The NPV would increase from 92% to 96%.

5. Fagan's nomogram. A more directly useful approach comes through use of Bayes theorem. When applied to diagnostic testing, it runs as follows:

$$\text{pretest odds} \times \text{likelihood ratio} = \text{post-test odds}$$

The pretest odds will be based on a hunch from the clinician prior to application of a diagnostic test such as MRI. The clinician, having taken a clinical history, may have a rough subjective idea of how probable it is that the patient has a medial meniscal tear. The probability may then be converted into an 'odds', but this step can be omitted by using Fagan's nomogram (shown and explained in detail below).

The likelihood ratio (LR) will incorporate information given by the diagnostic test. When the test gives a positive or negative result, the LR can take one of two possible values. If the MRI result is positive:

$$LR+ = \frac{\text{sensitivity}}{100 - \text{specificity}}$$

$$= \frac{93}{100 - 84}$$

$$= 5.8$$

If the MRI result is negative:

$$LR- = \frac{100 - \text{sensitivity}}{\text{specificity}}$$

$$= \frac{100 - 93}{84}$$

$$= 0.08$$

Table 45.2 Presence/absence of a medial meniscal tear

	Tear present	Tear absent	Totals
MRI scan positive	440	71	*511*
MRI scan negative	33	367	*400*
Totals	*473*	*438*	*911*

If you think there is a 50% probability that a meniscal tear is present, then the pretest odds are 50/50 = 1.

A positive result means that post-test odds = 1 × 5.8 = 5.8. The post-test probability is then around 85%. This would probably be high enough to indicate a need for arthroscopy.

A negative result means that post-test odds = 1 × 0.08 = 0.08. The post-test probability is then around 7.5%. This is probably low enough to render arthroscopy unnecessary.

Fagan's nomogram (Fig. 45.1) allows direct mapping from pretest probability to post-test probability once we know values for the likelihood ratio for a positive and for a negative result. Use of a ruler will show that a pretest probability of 50%, combined with a likelihood ratio of 5.8, will translate into a post-test probability in excess of 80%. Similarly, a pretest probability of 50%, combined with a likelihood ratio of 0.08, will translate into a post-

test probability between 5 and 10%. Usually, approximate answers will be sufficient for decisions on clinical management.

Key points

- **Studies that generate the sort of data shown in Table 45.2 are more useful if their methodology is sound.**
- **Many studies are carried out on two independently selected groups of subjects: one group with confirmed disease, one healthy control group.**
- **This ignores the spectrum of pathologies seen in clinical practice. It is likely to produce an unduly optimistic picture of the test's ability to discriminate between differential diagnoses.**
- **A study will avoid *spectrum bias* if it has included a cohort of consecutive cases seen in a realistic clinical setting.**

6. It would be ideal (although perhaps difficult in practice) if the result from the test under consideration (e.g. MRI) and the gold standard diagnosis (arthroscopy) are independently ascertained. If you already know the result of the MRI before undertaking the arthroscopy, your judgement will inevitably be influenced in marginal cases.

THERAPY

Returning to the scenario of Mr Dennis Gray, the 49-year-old gardener, it might be asked whether there are studies that address the question of adjuvant therapy. The study by the Swiss Group for Clinical Cancer Research (1995) may help to resolve the question.

Answer the following questions before deciding whether the Swiss study will help the decision:

- Can the methods of the study be trusted?
- What do the results of the study actually show?
- Are the patients in the study like Mr Dennis Gray?

Methods

1. A study that evaluates the effects of a new intervention should be a *randomized controlled trial* (RCT). By this we mean that the patients entering the study should be allocated at random to one or other treatment (e.g. adjuvant therapy, or not). The purpose of this is that the two treatment groups should, on average, be like each other in every respect other than the treatment given. The two groups of

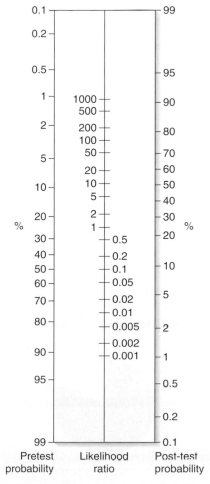

Fig. 45.1 Fagan's nomogram.

subjects should have the same average age, and the same ratio of males to females, and so on. Not only should there be a balance of *known* prognostic variables, there will also be a balance of *unknown* prognostic variables.

2. Random numbers are generated to produce an assignment to one of the treatment groups for each patient entering the study. This should to be done so that the investigators cannot predict the assignment before entering the subject into the study. Thus, assignment by whether the patient's date of birth is odd or even, or alternating assignments between the treatment groups, is unsatisfactory. Multicentre trials typically involve telephoning a central office to receive a random assignment.

3. Once patients are assigned to a particular treatment group, they should stay in that group for analysis purposes. This principle, known as 'intention-to-treat', should be adhered to even if the patients or doctors are unable to follow the treatment protocol.

Of course this depends on whether it has been possible to obtain outcome data on every patient. Sometimes patients drop out of a study altogether and it is not possible to analyse all patients according to their original treatment group, simply because the required data have not been collected. Sometimes it may be possible to impute plausible values, but often some subjects simply have to be omitted from analysis. The proportion of subjects 'lost' in this way, out of all those randomized, should not be too high.

4. 'Blinding' is desirable to prevent subjective bias. For placebo-controlled drug trials, neither the patient nor the doctor should know what treatment the patient has received. Such an ideal is difficult to achieve when surgical interventions are being assessed. In trials of coronary artery bypass grafting versus percutaneous angioplasty, neither the patient nor the surgeon may be blinded. Yet there may be scope for blinding study personnel who need to read X-rays or code death certificates to assess outcome in all the patients.

Results

1. The first table of results in papers reporting an RCT should compare the baseline characteristics of the two groups of subjects. The process of random allocation should demonstrate broad similarities. However this balance may not occur if the study is small. If so, any differences in outcome later reported should be weighed alongside possible differences in baseline characteristics of the groups.

2. You must be clear about the choice of the primary outcome variable, or endpoint. In the Swiss trial, there were two endpoints. One endpoint simply concerned death of the patient. The other concerned 'disease-free survival', which was defined when a patient did not die

and had no evidence of relapse or a second primary tumour. We shall consider the simpler 'death' endpoint.

3. It was estimated that of those who received adjuvant therapy, 43% died within 5 years. For those who did not receive adjuvant therapy, 52% died. A comparison can be made between these two rates, both in absolute terms and in relative terms.

Absolute differences

The *absolute risk reduction* (ARR) is the event rate in the control group minus the event rate in the intervention group = 52 − 43% = 9%. Thus, for every 100 patients who received adjuvant therapy, nine (9%) fewer subjects died than would have otherwise been the case.

A popular statistic to express this idea in another way is the *number needed to treat* (NNT). This is the reciprocal of the ARR: NNT = 100/ARR = 100/ 9 = 11. Thus for every 11 patients treated with adjuvant therapy, one fewer patient will die within 5 years.

Relative differences

When considering the ARR, we concentrated on subtracting one death rate from the other. Another approach is to divide one death rate by the other: Relative risk (RR) = 43/52 = 0.83. In other words, use of adjuvant therapy reduces the probability of death within 5 years to 0.83 (83%) of what it would have otherwise been; that is, 17% of the risk is removed (*relative risk reduction*, or RRR).

The pie chart (Fig. 45.2) shows the effect. Suppose the entire circle represents the risk of death in the next 5 years for Mr Dennis Gray if he is not offered adjuvant therapy. The white slice represents the proportion by which his risk is reduced if adjuvant therapy is administered (17% of the total). The black region represents the proportion of his risk still remaining.

Odds ratio

This is another relative measure and in many circumstances may be interpreted in a similar way to the relative

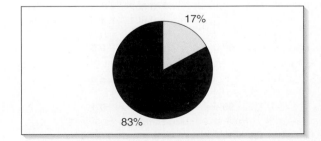

Fig. 45.2 Pie chart showing relative risk reduction.

risk; however, it uses the idea of an 'odds' rather than a 'risk'. In everyday life, the term 'odds' is most mentioned in the context of placing bets! When a horse is given odds of 4:1, it means that there is supposed to be one chance of it winning to four chances of it not winning. So its probability of winning is 1 in 5, or 20%.

The probability of death for Mr Gray if he is not treated with chemotherapy is 0.52 (or 52%). Therefore his odds is $52/(100 - 52) = 1.08$. Similarly, if he is treated with adjuvant therapy, his odds will be $43/(100 - 43) = 0.75$. The odds ratio is the odds if treated with adjuvant therapy/odds if not treated with adjuvant therapy = $0.75/1.08 = 0.69$.

When an event is uncommon (e.g. occurs less than 10% of the time), the odds ratio and the relative risk tend to converge to similar values. They are rather different in the present example, and the odds ratio is probably a more robust relative measure. However, if fewer subjects died when given the intervention (as here), then both the relative risk and the odds ratio will be less than one.

Confidence intervals

1. A group of subjects recruited to a study is a *sample*. Our true interest is not in the subjects studied but the underlying *population* from which the subjects were drawn. Any summary statistic (for example, a relative risk) calculated from a sample is an *estimate*. We want to know the true value of the relative risk, say, for the population. It is inevitable that if we repeated the whole study with a similar number of subjects included, we would get a slightly different estimate. We therefore wish to establish a *confidence interval* for the relative risk, based on the estimate from the study we have carried out.

2. The mathematical theory behind the construction of a confidence interval cannot be covered in this chapter, but the idea is to provide a range within which the true relative risk is likely to lie. Typically a 95% confidence interval is quoted.

3. In the Swiss study, the authors quote a hazard ratio (yet another relative measure!), which is a useful statistic when the data consist of differing follow-up times. The hazard ratio of death in those treated with adjuvant therapy was 0.74. This means that at any time point after surgery, those treated with adjuvant therapy are 0.74 times as likely to die at that point as those not given adjuvant therapy (26% reduction in the 'hazard'). The authors also quote the 95% confidence interval as 0.57 to 0.97. What does this mean?

4. Formally, there is a 95% probability that the confidence interval calculated and quoted above will contain the true hazard ratio for the entire population. In practice, we may assume that the true hazard ratio is unlikely

to be larger than 0.97, and it is unlikely to be below 0.57. At the optimistic end, the true hazard ratio may be as small as 0.57, suggesting that the hazard of death could be reduced by almost one half. At the pessimistic end, the true hazard ratio may be 0.97, suggesting the hazard would be reduced by only 3%. So the results of the study, which estimate a 26% reduction in the hazard, are also compatible with a substantial reduction on the one hand, or a miniscule reduction on the other. It could be argued that the results of the study are therefore not very precise.

Application

There is always some way in which your particular patient (e.g. Mr Dennis Gray) may seem unique. However the question 'Is my patient so different from those in the study that its results cannot apply?' should supply the right perspective.

Sample size calculation

If you wish to carry out an RCT you need to answer the question of how many subjects to study. This depends on answering several questions, including a specific guess of how much difference the new intervention might make.

First, there is the need to define a primary outcome measure. In the Swiss trial, this was either death, or disease-free survival. Secondly, we should estimate how much difference the intervention of interest (adjuvant therapy) would make to this primary outcome. The Swiss researchers do not tell us what they expected before commencing the study. But let us suppose that we wish to replicate their study. We might expect 50% of subjects to die within 5 years, and that adjuvant therapy will cause the risk of death to be reduced by one quarter, to 37.5%.

In any comparative study, there is a risk of making a type I error (claiming the new intervention makes a difference, when it fact it does not) or a type II error (concluding the new intervention makes no difference, when in fact it does benefit to the degree initially thought). We would like to avoid making such errors, but the probability of making such errors can only be diminished by increasing the sample size. In fact it is standard to set the probability of a type I error (called α) at 5%, and the probability of a type II error (called β) at either 10% or 20%. If β is 10%, the *power* of the study is 90%. The power is the probability of demonstrating a true difference of the specified magnitude.

Using tables provided by Machin et al (1997), we would need 329 subjects in each group (658 in all) to have 90%

power to demonstrate this sort of effect as statistically significant at the 5% level.

PROGNOSIS

1. Studies that outline the natural history of a disease are useful to gauge how worthwhile the application of treatment is. A relative risk reduction of 30% may be useful for someone at high risk, but less so for someone who is already at low risk.

2. Surgical studies frequently follow patients from the date of operation until some event such as death, or recurrence of a tumour. The resulting data can then be used to produce a Kaplan–Meier survival curve.

3. Not all patients will reach the endpoint within the time of the study. These are known as censored observations. They contribute to construction of the survival curve until the time of censoring.

4. The Swiss study shows a survival curve for each treatment group. However, the survival curve for the control group in a clinical trial may not always give a realistic estimate of prognosis. Those selected for a trial may be selectively fitter than average members of this population of patients. It is sometimes asserted that many aspects of medical care given to patients in a trial is superior to that given to other patients. A realistic survival curve will be obtained using an observational rather than an experimental study.

Points to consider when reading the literature

1. Inclusion criteria and selection of patients should be carefully documented. They should be assembled at a common, well-defined point in the course of their disease. The outcome should also be well defined and established by a standard methodology.

2. Assembling a cohort retrospectively is fraught with difficulty. Applying a clear selection criterion may be impossible. In addition, data may be unavailable for some or all of those who have died, thus producing a biased sample. In a prospective study, these questions may be tackled from the start. Prospective studies are likely to be expensive and take a long time to carry out if a long follow-up is required.

3. Subgroups within a cohort may have different prognoses (e.g. males versus females, older versus younger patients, stage I disease versus stage II versus stage III versus stage IV, etc.). Kaplan–Meier survival curves may be drawn for the whole group, or for a series of subgroups. Comparisons of survival curves between subgroups are carried out using the 'log-rank test'. Cox models are used to assess simultaneously the effect of several variables on survival (e.g. age, gender, stage of disease).

SYSTEMATIC REVIEWS/ META-ANALYSIS

1. The last decade has seen an explosion of interest in formal syntheses of research studies. It was recognized that single studies did not in themselves provide definitive answers to clinically important questions, and that bringing together several results was potentially powerful. Systematic reviews, however, differed crucially from the old-fashioned medical review, in that relevant studies were searched in a comprehensive and explicit manner, thus reducing potential charges of bias. Published systematic reviews will outline exactly which databases were searched, and which key words were used, so that the methods could be reproduced by the interested reader. Inclusion and exclusion criteria will be specified.

2. Once relevant studies have been located, they may be appraised by the reviewers. Those studies whose methodology is particularly poor may be omitted from further consideration. Again, explicit criteria for decisions made will be described.

3. Provided the data are provided in a compatible way in the studies concerned, it will then be possible to pool their results using a technique known as 'meta-analysis'. The confidence intervals from a pooled analysis will be narrower (i.e. more precise) than from any single study included.

4. The major drawback concerns the possibility of publication bias. Using electronic databases such as MEDLINE, one might reliably identify all *published* studies, but what of those studies which are never published? Many researchers embark on studies but never have them published, either because they are rejected by journal editors, or, more commonly, because they are never even submitted. It has been demonstrated empirically that published studies are more likely than unpublished studies to contain statistically significant results. Thus the published studies are biased towards showing a new treatment in a more exciting light than is strictly true. A famous example concerned the use of magnesium after myocardial infarction; many small trials had indicated a possible benefit, but a large trial demonstrated that this treatment was in fact useless, or even slightly harmful!

5. *Publication bias*, as defined above, tends to be particularly strong for small studies. Large studies, even if statistically non-significant, have a reasonable chance of being published, but this does not happen for small studies.

For this reason, systematic reviewers often attempt to locate unpublished studies and include them in their meta-analysis. Writing to experts in the field, and scanning abstract lists of conferences, are methods that have been used to some effect.

Example: Graduated compression stockings in the prevention of postoperative venous thromboembolism

Wells et al (1994) searched for articles on graduated compression stockings (GCS). They used MEDLINE, and also the bibliography of all retrieved articles. They searched Current Contents to find new reports that might not have yet appeared on MEDLINE. They found 122 articles, but only 35 referred to randomized trials. These articles were assessed by at least two authors. Some were deemed inadequate in their method of randomization, others did not contain an untreated control group, while others used inadequate diagnostic methods. In all, 12 studies were judged eligible for inclusion in a meta-analysis. Eleven of the studies were carried out in moderate risk, non-orthopaedic surgical procedures, including a total of 1752 patients. It was estimated that the use of GCS led to a relative risk reduction of about two-thirds.

This systematic review was itself later appraised by the Centre for Reviews and Dissemination, University of York. It was felt that the authors' insistence on use of studies with adequate forms of random allocation meant that the conclusions of the review were robust. However, it was pointed out that the authors had made no attempt to identify unpublished studies, thus leaving open the possibility of publication bias (see above).

The Cochrane Library now contains a more up-to-date and thorough systematic review on this subject, last updated in 1999 by Amaragiri and Lees. They found 16 randomized controlled trials, including some not identified by Wells and coworkers. This was partly because some trials were published after the Wells group carried out their review, but these authors searched EMBASE (an electronic database with good access to articles not published in English) and the Cochrane Controlled Trials Register, in addition to an ever more comprehensive MEDLINE. They also hand-searched relevant medical journals. Finally, in order to address the possibility of publication bias, they contacted companies that manufactured stockings.

In fact, Amaragiri and Lees do not mention finding unpublished trials. But at least they made efforts, and the results of their meta-analysis revealed essentially similar conclusions to those of Wells and coworkers. They divided their 16 trials into nine where patients were not undergoing any other form of venous thromboprophylaxis, and seven where all patients underwent another prophylactic intervention. The results for the former category are shown in a 'forest plot' (Fig. 45.3).

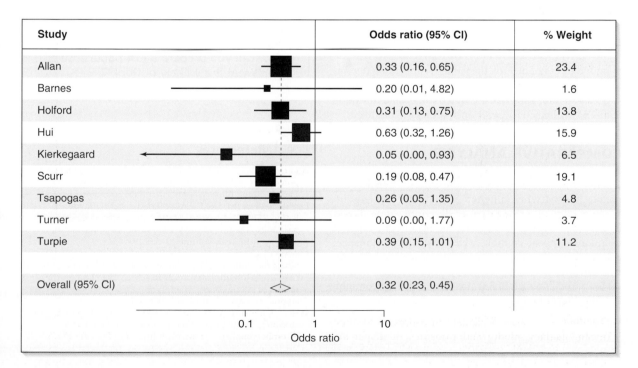

Study	Odds ratio (95% CI)	% Weight
Allan	0.33 (0.16, 0.65)	23.4
Barnes	0.20 (0.01, 4.82)	1.6
Holford	0.31 (0.13, 0.75)	13.8
Hui	0.63 (0.32, 1.26)	15.9
Kierkegaard	0.05 (0.00, 0.93)	6.5
Scurr	0.19 (0.08, 0.47)	19.1
Tsapogas	0.26 (0.05, 1.35)	4.8
Turner	0.09 (0.00, 1.77)	3.7
Turpie	0.39 (0.15, 1.01)	11.2
Overall (95% CI)	0.32 (0.23, 0.45)	

Odds ratio

Fig. 45.3 Forest plot.

A square is shown to denote the results of each individual trial. In most forest plots, we are hoping to see squares (representing the estimated treatment effect) to the left-hand side of vertical line representing the value 1. This is because stockings are supposed to *reduce* the risk of DVT. If the evidence was that stockings increased the risk of DVT, the squares would appear to the right of the value 1.

The nine squares seen in the diagram are of different sizes. The larger the square, the more weight that study carries. Thus the study of Allan carries most weight. This is mainly because it was based on more patients than any of the other trials (200). By contrast, the study of Barnes included only 18 patients, and thus has an appropriately small square.

Each square carries a horizontal line, and this represents the 95% confidence interval for the odds ratio. These tend to be wider for small studies such as that of Barnes. Those studies whose confidence intervals include the value 1 are not statistically significant (Barnes, Hui, Tsapogas, Turner, Turpie). Each of these studies (when taken in isolation) fails to demonstrate a statistically significant benefit of GCS. The other four studies (Allan, Holford, Kierkegaard, Scurr) all demonstrate the benefit of GCS in their own right.

The diamond shape at the bottom represents the result of meta-analysis. The centre of the diamond demonstrates the overall odds ratio of 0.32. This is a weighted average of the nine odds ratios for the individual studies. The width of the diamond represents the width of the overall confidence interval, which is narrower than any individual study's confidence interval. Because it is based on 1205 patients (compared with 200 patients for the biggest of the individual trials), it is a good deal more precise. The diamond does not include the value 1, confirming the statistical significance. Even the most conservative estimate suggests an odds ratio of 0.45, which still implies the odds of a DVT will be cut by over one-half if GCS are used.

COMPARATIVE ANALYSIS

You may become bewildered by the array of statistical terminology used when different analyses are carried out. When reading or writing a paper, descriptive data should be provided in such a way that the results of statistical techniques appear credible. The worst sort of statistical practice is to provide *p* values in the absence of descriptive data.

Here are a few guidelines as to the use of common statistical techniques.

- *Quantitative variables*. Calculate measures of location (mean, median, mode) and measures of dispersion (standard deviation, interquartile range), and compare between two (or more) groups.
- *Categorical variables*. Calculate proportions, or odds. Summary statistics to compare rates: relative risk reduction, absolute risk reduction, number needed to treat (to quantify effect of intervention).
- Comparative statistics need *confidence intervals*. A confidence interval (e.g. for the difference between two means, or the difference between proportions) puts limits on the likely size of the effect of intervention.
- *Hypothesis tests*. These test whether the comparative statistic calculated in a particular study is compatible with the 'null hypothesis'. Two sample *t* tests for comparing means, chi-squared tests for comparing proportions. Quantitative variables not following a Normal distribution (e.g. pain scores) may be compared with a non-parametric test such as a Mann–Whitney *U* test. All tests lead to a *p* value; a measure of strength of evidence against the null hypothesis.

Summary

- How can knowledge of the accuracy of a diagnostic test help you to arrive at a firm diagnosis in an equivocal case?
- What elements of a published randomized controlled trial are important in advising choice of treatment?
- What are the potential strengths and weaknesses of systematic reviews?
- How can you prepare a justifiable answer to: 'What is my likely outlook'?

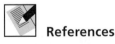 **References**

Amaragiri SV, Lees TA 2002 Elastic compression stockings for prevention of deep vein thrombosis (Cochrane Review). In: The Cochrane Library, Issue 2. Update Software, Oxford

Fischer SP, Fox JM, Del Pizzo W, Friedman MJ, Snyder SJ, Ferkel RD 1991 Accuracy of diagnoses from magnetic resonance imaging of the knee. Journal of Bone and Joint Surgery. American Volume 73-A: 2–9

Machin D, Campbell M, Fayers P, Pinol M 1997 Sample size tables for clinical studies, 2nd edn. Blackwell Science, Oxford

Swiss Group for Clinical Cancer Research 1995 Long-term results of single course of adjuvant portal chemotherapy for colorectal cancer. Lancet 345: 349–352

Wells PS, Lensing AWA, Hirsh J 1994 Graduated compression stockings in the prevention of postoperative venous thromboembolism. Archives of Internal Medicine 154: 67–72

Further reading

Bland M 1995 An introduction to medical statistics, 2nd edn. Oxford Medical Publications, Oxford

Campbell MJ, Machin D 1999 Medical statistics. A commonsense approach, 3rd edn. Wiley, Chichester

Egger M, Smith GD, Altman DG (eds) 2001 Systematic reviews in health care: meta-analysis in context, 2nd edn. BMJ Publishing Group, London

ACKNOWLEDGEMENTS

The clinical scenario was written by the NHS Research and Development Centre for Evidence-Based Medicine, Oxford (accessed at http://cebm.jr2.ox.ac.uk/docs/scenarios/sgu.html on 9 April 2002)

46 Critical reading of the literature

R. M. Kirk

Objectives

- Apply objective measures whenever possible – but do not rely only on measurable evidence to the exclusion of that which is not measurable.
- Have self-confidence. Do not accept received opinions – make up your own mind.
- Recognize that surgery does not stand still. Keep abreast of advances – do not become an expert in outdated practices.

Absence of evidence is not evidence of absence.

Not everything that can be counted counts, and not everything that counts can be counted.

Sign on the wall of Albert Einstein's office at Princeton University

INTRODUCTION

The two quotations should remind you that nothing is settled. However hard we try to think logically, we work in a complex and incompletely understood subject. We may know the full extent of the human genome but we do not understand what happens to change the chemical formula into something that is living. Although we wish to apply evidence-based disease prevention and treatment, we cannot ignore factors that are not yet amenable to scientific understanding.

Lord Kelvin, the distinguished physicist and mathematician, implied that only if we can describe a concept in numbers do we understand it. This may apply in mathematics but it is not totally applicable to biological phenomena. The study of living organisms is not yet sufficiently advanced for it to be described in numbers. In an attempt to be – or appear to be – scientific, we often ascribe numbers to phenomena and then treat them as objective measurements. But they are not. The numbers have been allocated subjectively, in an analogue fashion. Different observers may allocate different numbers.

An essential but indefinable characteristic of a good doctor is common sense. Beware of specious science. It is remarkable that if something is expressed in a formal, especially numerical, manner it takes on an appearance of authority and reliability. You need only read some of the commercial advertisements to appreciate the way in which statistics are misused.

You must keep up to date with the literature because the rate of change is rapid. However, try to obtain good evidence, especially of newly introduced methods. Remember the statement by Voltaire, 'Use the new treatment while it still works.' He had identified the powerful placebo effect of new treatments (Latin *placebo* = I shall please).

Favour evidence-based practice when it is available. Reports in prestigious journals are usually more reliable than those in which the papers are not refereed; however, no journals are totally reliable and you must make up your own mind. Remember, though, that investigation of practice must be narrowed, with exclusion of many of the possible variables. Your patients rarely present with exactly the same strictly limited features as those used in the trials.

Key point

- Literature (Latin *litera* = a letter) is not confined to books and journals but also to other media. Exploit the many sources of information that are now available. Remember, though, to maintain the highest critical standards because much of the information available on, for example, the internet has not been subjected to strict peer review before being promulgated.

LOGIC OF SCIENCE

1. Advances in science occur in a multiplicity of ways. We should all feel capable of making them, or recognizing

them if we encounter them. Do not dismiss the unexpected. Louis Pasteur stated, 'Dans le champs de l'observation, le hasard ne favorise que les esprits préparés' (In the field of observation, chance favours only the prepared mind).

2. Advances are often made as a result of encountered problems. Do not put aside problems that have so far resisted solution. There may be unique features that throw light on an individual unsolved problem. Consider discussing it with colleagues; we all view information differently, and someone may have a sudden idea that triggers a solution or a possible method of tackling it.

3. You may develop a possible reason or explanation for a phenomenon. This is a hypothesis (Greek *hypo* = under + *thesis* = placing; a supposition) or theory (Greek *theoreein* = to view; an idea that has not yet been proven). Your natural instinct is to attempt to prove it. The recommendation of the great scientific philosopher Sir Karl Popper (1902–1994) is that you should, on the contrary, try to disprove your supposition. If you fail, you may determine to use it for the time being. If you disprove your initial belief, this may lead you to develop an alternative that may be more robust. Popper declared that you can never prove a theory but you can disprove it. He used as an example the colour of swans: if every swan that you see is white, you can never prove that all swans are white, because you can never see every swan that exists, has ever existed, or will in the future exist. However, you need to see but a single black swan to disprove it – and of course you can see many black swans on the Freemantle River in Western Australia.

Key point

- We all pay lip service to Popper's logic. How many times have you seen a scientific paper that conforms to his teaching?

ORGANIZING YOUR READING

1. There is insufficient time to read every paper on your subjects of interest. You must be selective.

2. A valuable first step is to identify the journals that will form your core list. You should choose one or more general scientific journals that may have items of great promise in your field – *Nature, Science, New Scientist*. Each week, quickly scan the contents list.

3. Identify the authoritative journals dealing with your speciality and be prepared to scan through them.

4. You may read the titles of some articles, the summary of a few, the summary and selected parts of one or two, and occasionally the whole article. Rarely, read the article with obsessive critical attention.

CRITICAL READING

1. Some papers state a monumentally important advance in a short report. A classic example was the letter in *Nature* written by James Watson and Francis Crick announcing the construction of the DNA molecule.

2. More frequently, the idea has a less immediate impact and must be presented within a conventional format. Take advantage of the standard presentation.

3. The *Title* should clearly convey to you what the content is. It should convey the key words that allow it to be traced. Is it relevant to your interest?

4. The *Summary* must encapsulate the whole article. When you read it, you should know in outline a simple answer to each of the main questions posed by and answered in a paper reporting, for example, an investigation stimulated by a question or a hypothesis.

5. The *Introduction* answers the first question, 'Why did we do it?' You should be able to understand clearly what was the starting point, what has generated the need for an investigation and what is the question that was asked. Do you think the authors started with the correct premise?

6. The *Method* section must state clearly, 'What we did.' It must explicitly reveal every detail of how the investigation was organized, carried out and measured. Has the method been fully and openly described?

7. The *Results* answer, 'What we found.' All the results must be clearly displayed. Any inconsistencies should be identified and explained. Do you understand them, are they justifiable?

8. The *Discussion* states 'What it means.' This is often the shoddiest part of scientific papers. Until now the authors should have provided clear, simple facts. They should now limit themselves to stating how their results fit into or alter the position from the starting point. They may briefly suggest possible supplementary investigations that they or others could pursue to test the evidence. Are they overinterpreting their findings beyond the justifiable results of the investigation?

9. The *Conclusions* should not be a mere repeat of the summary but clearly and briefly summarize what has been added to our knowledge by the investigation.

Key point

- Apply your most important asset to the conclusions – your common sense. Are you convinced?

WHAT DID YOU LEARN?

1. Most importantly, you practice making up your own mind about the 'facts' that are presented to you on the basis of the evidence placed before you. You are not just a passive acceptor of the opinion of others. This gives you confidence to reject evidence you consider unreliable, and faith in your own good sense, rather than relying unthinkingly on 'experts.'

2. You may not know the fine points of statistics (see Ch. 45) but you can decide whether they have been applied correctly and with integrity. When two groups are compared, we may be assured that they differ in one respect only, but this is never so. Biological variation is so great and capricious that too much cannot be read into small differences.

Key points

- **If you are studying a prospective trial of, for example, two treatments, are you convinced that the authors had open minds beforehand – or were they hoping to prove one method superior?**
- **Make sure, when comparisons are made between groups of patients, that 'apples' are not compared with 'pears'. The groups must be closely comparable.**

3. You may detect imperfections in the manner in which two populations are to be compared, that are not clearly stated. Sometimes aspects such as the method of clinical follow-up is not clear; for example, was it by independent assessors, by personal interview or examination, prospective, performed blindly – when the assessor does not know the treatment or procedure to which the patients were subjected? Follow-up times may be given in a general way that does not make it clear that most of them were made too short, with very few long term follow-up times. Graphs and histograms may be used to avoid giving individual figures, in the same manner that advertisers use them to promote their goods.

4. Are the claimed benefits of one treatment over another genuine? There are so many variables: among diseases, such as site, extent, involvement of vital structures, virulence; among patients, such as age, sex, comorbidity; as a result of diagnosis, early, late, confidently or uncertainly; institution of treatment, promptly, effectively, long enough; and any ancillary treatment.

5. In cancer treatment, an improved method of detection may appear to produce improved results in two ways. Survival times may lengthen because the new method allows earlier detection, lengthening the recurrence-free time. The apparent improvement is the result of the 'lead time', the interval that transpired between the time of pick-up with the improved method, compared with later detection. In addition, the improved method may show that the disease is more extensive than would be shown by previous methods so that the earlier likelihood of recurrence is recognized. As a result the 'stage' is raised, whereas less effective methods may result in the tumour being classified as a lower grade. For example, when staging of breast cancer is limited to clinical assessment, a tumour may be diagnosed as stage I; imaging scans may demonstrate local, impalpable glands so that the tumour is classified in a higher stage, with a poorer prognosis. Chest X-ray may demonstrate, however, that rib metastases are present and the tumour must therefore be placed in stage IV – evidence of metastases. A series diagnosed by clinical examination alone and placed in stage I thus contains more advanced tumours and the results of treatment appears poor. If the tumours have been investigated with modern tests, these advanced tumours would be classified as stage II, III or IV, leaving only 'true' stage I tumours. Treatment of this smaller number produces better results than a mixture of early and undetected later tumours. This is often called the Will Roger's effect. (Will Rogers, an American homely sage, despised Californians. He described the often-despised (as mentally low grade) Oklahoma farmers who were forced to migrate to California during the 1920s drought – 'thus raising the IQ in both States.')

6. It is often accepted that authors provide only evidence that supports their hypothesis and those contradictory points that can be demolished. Seek out unstated weaknesses.

7. Papers sometimes appear too perfect. Were there no patients lost to follow up, people who did not fully comply with an arduous treatment regimen, tests in some that were equivocal?

8. Read other investigations in the same field of interest. You will be surprised that very often the results are not comparable. You may wonder how this can be: the populations may differ; among many other reasons, the expertise, case selection, and familiarity with the condition and the treatment methods may differ.

9. Why not just read authoritative reviews? Reviews are written by experts who already have a point of view. However honest and good intentioned they are, they inevitably argue for their own views – they would not adhere to them if they did not believe in them. If you read a review, seek out one that gives an opposing view.

10. During your career you are likely to see patients with unusual, perhaps unique, conditions. If you retain your inquisitive and critical enthusiasm you may recognize

what may be an important advance. Your familiarity with the literature will have nourished your thinking and writing abilities, allowing you to report your findings to your colleagues.

AVAILABILITY OF INFORMATION

1. We now have available a wealth of publications. In the past the *Index Medicus* – often called the greatest American contribution to medical science – was the 'browser' we consulted to find articles not in the journals to which we had normal access. We would then write for reprints of important articles.

2. Through the internet we now have available MEDLINE; many titles are accompanied by summaries. Other sources may provide access to the full text. Using the well-known search engines you can find an immense amount of information; remember, though, that you do not know the provenance of many reports that have not been subjected to independent review. However, you can find easily understood explanations of difficult subjects that give you a grasp of them, when the scientific papers assume you must be familiar with the terms used.

3. A list of available sources soon becomes outdated. Keep abreast of the advances and of the flow of new discoveries.

Summary

- Do you acknowledge how important it is that you do not fall behind and practise outdated medicine and surgery?
- Will you retain your critical faculties? However eminent the authors, or prestigious the journal, your common sense is your best protection against being misled by what you read.
- Since few of us try to falsify our hypotheses, will you determine always to read opposing articles after reading a seemingly convincing report?

47 Communication skills

R. M. Kirk, V. M. Macaulay

Objectives

- Good communication is essential in all areas of activity, not just in relation to patients.
- Recognize non-verbal as well as verbal communication.
- Empathize with the listener, especially when giving bad news.

'Communication skills' sounds like yet another facility to be learned, like operating; however, most of us already have inbred and acquired competence, as it pervades our contact with all other people.

VERBAL COMMUNICATION

The words we use, the tone of voice, the speed with which we speak, the pauses that we interject, all have an effect on the listener. If we are giving similar information to two different people, we usually do not attempt to employ the same words to each of them. Some people adopt the word patterns of those to whom they are speaking; others, wishing to impress, may use abstruse or jargon words or acronyms (words formed from the initial letters of other words).

The tone of voice and rhythm add a layer of meaning. Terse, staccato speech is sometimes commanding or threatening or signifies tension in the speaker. Quietly spoken words may be soothing or, if given in a sibilant (hissing) manner, may suggest potential threats.

Face to face communication is much richer than writing. Words have defined meanings and the writer is limited to choosing the ones nearest to the intended meaning plus a few symbols such as exclamation and question marks or underlining. The writer has to guess at the response to the message and cannot modify it if the receiver reacts unexpectedly. The words do not have to be cast on tablets of stone to be irrevocable in their effect. In contrast, the tone of voice, the emphasis placed on certain words and the reaction to the listener's responses help to guide the speaker to know how to proceed and estimate the effect of the words.

Telephone conversations are midway, containing vocal overtones but lacking the non-verbal expression and gestures that add a layer of meaning to the words.

It is self-evident that if you wish to communicate with someone over an important or delicate matter, you should always choose to do so face to face.

NON-VERBAL COMMUNICATION

This is a very deeply ingrained way of informing others of our mood and intentions. Our dress may indicate that we are relaxed and informal, or we may wish it to register professionalism and formality. Posture indicates depression and humility or confidence and command. Most revealing are our facial expressions. The giving out of signals and the reading of them is often unconscious.

Most of us acquire a social awareness of non-verbal communication. When one person is speaking and the listener wishes to interject a remark, he or she signals the wish or intention, perhaps by a movement to attract the speaker's attention, a raising of the hand, a seeking of eye contact with the speaker. The speaker responds, sometimes by returning the eye contact, by smiling and bringing the statement to a close, or resists by raising a hand with palm towards the person wishing to speak or raising the voice, to indicate resistance to stopping. The giving and receiving of signals can be confused and confusing. A smile and a sneer are not dissimilar – indeed one may change into the other. A gentle touch is a subtle method of conveying sympathy, a firm grip can convey authority and trust, but a push or a blow are threatening.

Actors, salesmen and confidence tricksters have always recognized, sometimes instinctively, the fundamentals of what is often called 'body language'. In recent years, non-verbal communication has been studied and brought to notice by those claiming to advise salespeople, job applicants, interviewers and 'interviewees.'

Key point

- Strenuously avoid giving potentially upsetting news, complaining or arguing, by letter or telephone. You need to watch the reaction of your listener to what you have just said, so that you can, if necessary, modify what you will next say.

COMMUNICATING WITH PATIENTS

1. Remember that you are familiar with clinical surroundings but patients associate them with anxiety and sometimes with dread. They may be apprehensive, confused or yearning for reassurance that all is well.

2. Because most patients are in later adult life, and often, therefore, more conventional, they may expect that doctors who dress and behave reasonably formally, take their responsibilities seriously. Immediate and casual use of first names is not welcomed by many older patients. Similarly, casual exposure of their bodies and clinical features is resented. We owe it to them to respect their wishes if we are to obtain their cooperation and trust.

3. Note that some colleagues adopt a serious and grave manner, others try to appear cheerful and light-hearted. There is no standard pattern. Sometimes we are serious with one patient and jovial with another. Avoid attitudes and speech that denote overbearing and curt superiority, or the overcasual 'jokeyness' that may suggest we take the patient's problems light-heartedly.

4. When you wish to discuss important information with a patient, ensure that the surroundings are quiet and that you will not be disturbed or distracted. Hand your 'bleep' to someone who can answer it for you. In appropriate circumstances suggest that a relative or friend of the patient is present.

5. The information you give the patient should be known to your medical and nursing colleagues, and to other paramedical carers. In many circumstances it is valuable for them to be present so they can participate in the discussion and know what has been decided. Patients' confidence is eroded if different people give them conflicting information.

Key point

- Patients you see are already apprehensive. Do not increase their insecurity by placing them in undignified circumstances.

Questioning

1. When taking a medical history (see Ch. 3), allow patients time to speak. Do not make them feel that what they have to say is of little account. If they are stuck for words, allow them time to choose a suitable one; do not immediately feed one that fits your prejudice. However, you must control the interview, so your timing when interjecting a question for clarification, or asking a new question, must be sensitively judged. A too rapid interruption cuts off the patient's train of thought, but if too long delayed it may allow the patient to take a new, diverting, train of thought.

2. Choose words suited to the patient before you. A simple person needs simple language spoken slowly, and repeated or rephrased without signs of impatience. For example, ask one person where is the pain in the belly if that was the term he or she employed to you. A professional person may resent the avoidance of the more formal 'abdomen'.

3. The ability to communicate is severely tested if the patient is a young child, deaf, has a speech defect, a behavioural anomaly, or has difficulty with the language. When talking to a person who is hard of hearing, always sit face to face. It can be impossible to communicate rationally with those under the influence of alcohol or other drugs, with people who are hysterical or violent, or with those suffering from diminished consciousness, whether it is the result of injury or disease.

Key point

- If you have difficulty in communicating, consider whether you need help from a senior colleague or an interpreter, or should you defer action if the patient's cooperation is likely to return later?

Telling and discussing

1. First find out what is already known, what that information signifies to the patient, and decide how the additional information should be presented. As a rule it is best to start by asking questions such as, 'Would you like to talk about the [problem]? I am not sure how much you know.' Later, you may ask questions in order to evaluate the patient's appreciation of the additional information you have given.

2. In most circumstances do not try to say too much all at once. Give the patient time to absorb what has already been said and wait for an indication of readiness to continue. From time to time ask questions to check that the patient really understands what has passed between you, for example, 'Can you tell me then, how you see the situation?'

3. Especially when discussing important problems, be extremely sensitive to the listener's reactions and signals. In some cases it may be better to defer the interview to a later date to allow the patient to absorb and react to what has already been said.

4. Patients anticipating bad news frequently demonstrate by their body language, or by suddenly ceasing to ask questions, that they do not wish to be told anything more at present. Do not ignore it. Allow the patient time to absorb what has passed between you and come back later. Before you restart further discussion, reassess the patient's comprehension of the situation; you may be surprised at the 'adjustments' made to the information so the patient can cope with it.

5. Remember that distress, anxiety or despair may be dealt with by total rejection, blame directed at others or at you, threatening behaviour or aggression. Do not react antagonistically.

Advising

1. Discuss with patients what options are available, what are the advantages and disadvantages of each. This is not always easy to do, as not many treatment choices can be scientifically justified. In biology there are few areas that are either black or white; most are shades of grey. This explains the differing advice that patients receive when they ask for a second opinion.

2. Surgeons have a reputation for being decisive, and in practice most of us are in no doubt about the advice we wish to give. Our advice is based on our professional experience – what we have encountered, read about and talked about. The patient needs to be encouraged to ask questions and, when there is no urgency, to go away, think about the advice, come back and discuss it again. However, we believe it is a rejection of professional responsibility merely to lay before our patients the pros and cons of each course of management and leave it to them to decide which one to follow. Patients are often not in a suitable state of mind to make the best decision, especially if they have just been told that they are suffering from a serious condition. Therefore, we should end with, 'So in my opinion ...' Of course, patients are free to reject the suggested course of action.

 Key points

- Anticipate aggression from an angry or threatening patient – but do not behave like a 'victim'.

- **Do not contradict or respond to aggressive behaviour. Stay calm, do not interrupt, be willing to listen.**

Relatives

1. Relatives deserve the same consideration that we give to patients. We hope that they will give encouragement, support and help to the patient throughout the management of the condition requiring treatment.

2. Occasionally there is conflict between the demands of the patient and those of the relatives. What do you say if a patient demands that you do not disclose what is happening, while the relatives press you for information? Your contract is with the patient and you must honour that relationship. The relatives may ask you not to give certain information to the patient. Again, judge for yourself the best course, on the patient's behalf.

COLLEAGUES

1. A vital professional duty is to inform colleagues about matters of patient care. Always write up notes, avoiding abbreviations, jargon and opinionated remarks that might be misinterpreted. Sign and date them. When you hand over before you go off duty, inform the on-call doctor personally of any outstanding problems.

2. If you have had a discussion with a patient about the future, or about treatment, ensure that you tell the nurses and your seniors. There is nothing that undermines the confidence of patients more than being given different information by different people.

3. Your colleagues include all those with whom you come into professional contact: doctors of all grades, students, nurses, physiotherapists, technicians, managers, clerical staff, porters, cleaners and tradesmen. Do not draw a line of 'importance', below which you do not acknowledge people, or bolster your dignity by trying to diminish others. Each of us counts as just one.

4. One of the most important qualities we have is our self-esteem. When we fail to carry out a task conscientiously we expect to be reprimanded. When we perform well, we rightly hope to be congratulated. If you expect to be acknowledged, remember there are others that hope you will acknowledge and encourage them.

IMPARTING BAD NEWS

1. Communicating with ill or distressed people requires great sensitivity. Your behaviour should

be influenced by your feelings of sympathy and compassion. Our reactions may be modified if we are able to enter our patient's personality in our imagination and think how we would feel if we were in a similar situation; this is termed empathy (Greek *em* = in + *pathos* = feeling, suffering). Obviously we cannot always achieve this, but in making the effort we can identify the likely reactions and apprehension of the patient and respond sensitively.

2. We have the duty to keep our patients and any close relatives informed of what is happening, and what it means. Of course, we must be guided by the patient's wishes about what we tell the relatives. This often entails telling them that recovery is failing, the patient has developed a complication, or our investigations reveal severe and perhaps terminal disease. At times of crisis you may be the only doctor present and are therefore responsible for dealing with the problem.

3. Prepare yourself before disclosing that the patient has a potential or actual terminal illness such as advanced cancer. Review the options by recalling or looking up the published results of the various choices before you go in to talk to the patient (see Ch. 39).

4. Ensure that this consultation takes place in a calm and private area. Ask someone to take over your 'bleep', so you cannot be interrupted. It is usually valuable to have a nurse with you so that she or he can tell colleagues what has been said.

5. As you approach, look at the faces of the patient and family, and try to judge how they are feeling. You are also being carefully studied in return, for hints of what you are about to say.

6. You should be prepared to structure the conversation. A suggested plan is as follows:

a. Ask the patient and the family what they understand of the situation.

b. Describe the situation as you see it, using terms with which they are familiar.

c. Outline what can be done.

At each stage you should allow the patient to ask questions so that you can explain the implications in a manner and speed that does not distress or confuse the patient. Be as optimistic as realistically feasible given the situation; if the outlook is poor, do not unthinkingly deliver the full extent in one encounter. Explain the reasons for recommending each aspect of the treatment, but if the results of trials are poor, you do not need to volunteer them unless the patient wishes to know them. Remember that the patient will be trying to come to terms with the diagnosis and may not be in the best frame of mind to absorb the consequences and make decisions about the practical implications. It may be necessary to defer making an important management decision until the patient has had time to assimilate information given during the first consultation.

7. It is sometimes stated that information belongs to the patient and the doctor has no right to withhold it. Indeed many patients are very knowledgeable, ask direct questions, and may wish to be told everything that is known about the situation and the consequences. Be aware that this will not apply to every patient, and you should not dismiss the minority who do not wish to be told the whole truth, by forcing information on them immediately. Occasionally a very anxious patient blurts out the words, 'I want to know everything', but their eyes are begging for reassurance that all is well. Be sensitive to verbal and non-verbal cues from the patient and relatives, and be ready to defer answering questions that are not asked.

8. In human relations we must retain a sense of balance and sensitivity. Rigid blanket rules are inappropriate. Just as in our personal life we try to avoid pouring out sensitive bad news, so we need to be as considerate to our patients and allow them to dictate the way in which we inform them. Our duty is to interpret the patient's often unspoken signals and be governed by them.

 Key point

- **The founder of the hospice movement in Britain, Dame Cecily Saunders, stated: 'The patient, not the doctor, or the nurse, or the relative, must retain control of information to suit his needs.'**

9. Provided you are sympathetic and sensitive, you are unlikely to make gross mistakes. Those who are told very serious news, and are later asked what was said, often give a different and more optimistic version if they are unable to cope with the full truth. There are some patients who indicate that they fully understand the circumstances but do not wish to have them spelled out in concrete terms. Respect their wishes.

10. Never leave a patient without hope or support. If treatment such as operation cannot be employed, it is possible to say, 'Operation is not appropriate but I shall continue to care for you.'

11. Remember that the news may be more distressing for the relatives and friends than for the patient, because they are not only sad for the patient but they are desolate at the prospect of being left alone. However, the information belongs to the patient, not the relatives. Ensure that you do not disclose anything to them against the patient's wishes.

Key point

- **Now write in the notes exactly what has passed between you and inform your colleagues including the family doctor and the nurses.**

COMPLICATIONS AND ERRORS

1. The outcome of any form of medical care does not always reach expectations. You cannot anticipate and warn the patient and relatives about every possible complication.

2. Every person makes mistakes from time to time by failing to notice a complicating factor, by misjudging a complex situation, by making the wrong decision or by technical error.

3. Do not attempt to hide the fact from a patient if something has gone wrong. Explain it and say what measures you will take to put it right. Just as we detect evasiveness when we watch a politician being asked an awkward question on the television screen, so our patients instinctively recognize any reluctance on our part to explain a misadventure.

4. One of the commonest complaints of patients is that when things go wrong, sympathy and openness are withheld. They naturally become suspicious.

Key point

- **Telling a patient that you are sorry if an unexpected complication occurs, is not an admission of guilt.**

Summary

- Do you appreciate that there are no rigid or absolute rules except to be sensitive to the patient's signals?
- Do you recognize that communication is more than mere words?
- Will you remember to give patients time to absorb your remarks, and time to respond in their own way?
- As you prepare to give patients information, will you first enquire how much they already know?
- Do you accept the need to recognize and honour the (often non-verbal) signs that patients do not wish to have more information forced on them at this time?
- Will you remember to keep your colleagues informed about the information passed between you and the patients?
- Do you recongize the danger of trying to conceal complications and errors from the patients?

 Further reading

Buckman R 1992 How to break bad news. Papermac, London
Lloyd M, Bor R 1996 Communication skills for medicine. Churchill Livingstone, Edinburgh
Myerscough PR 1992 Talking with patients. Oxford University Press, Oxford

48 The surgical logbook

D. M. Baker

Objectives

- **Understand the importance of maintaining a logbook.**
- **Understand how and what information to collect in your logbook.**
- **Know how to analyse the collected data.**
- **Recognize the difficulties in keeping a logbook.**

INTRODUCTION

A surgical logbook is a record of the activity you have undertaken. Although important during training, it remains a central part of the routine throughout your career. Of the different parts of a surgeon's job, the easiest to record are:

- Operations performed
- Patients seen in clinic
- Patients admitted and seen while in hospital.

I shall concentrate on logging actual operations undertaken. Although this is the most commonly kept record, the other two records are important, as you will see and treat many more patients than those operated upon. The outcome of surgical patients treated conservatively is as important as the outcome of those operated on.

WHY KEEP A LOGBOOK?

1. Just as airline pilots keep a log of every flight they make, so it is your duty and self-discipline to keep a record of the procedures you have performed. Although not yet legally demanded, you are required by the Surgical Colleges to keep a logbook during training. This is to demonstrate that you have been adequately trained in an operation or procedure before being considered fit to undertake it independently. It will soon be necessary to

demonstrate that, as consultant surgeon, you continue to demonstrate your competency.

2. The logbook provides a source of self-auditing surgical practice. If, for example, it demonstrates a series of wound infections following a particular procedure, you must identify and rectify this.

3. For you, the trainee, a logbook identifies strengths and weaknesses in your training. It may demonstrate significant experience of one procedure but show deficiencies in another. At the regular formal appraisal you should be guided to rectify the deficiency.

4. The logbook helps your trainers assess the standards within the specific posts of a surgical training rotation. If your log shows that you have undertaken unsupervised major procedures at night, this can be investigated to establish if you are very able, or the trainer should be informed on the training of surgeons!

COLLECTING THE INFORMATION

1. *Spreadsheets* are ideal for recording information, or a grid of data divided into rows and columns. Each operative procedure occupies a row, with each item of information occupying a separate column. There are a number of choices; the most simple is a lined school exercise book with vertical lines dividing the pages into rows and columns. The Royal Surgical Colleges have logbooks, and computer packages are available, at a range of prices, that are compatible with personal (PC) and palm-top computers. The data in computerized logbooks can be analysed quickly, presenting it clearly and neatly. More complex spreadsheets provide a full database.

Key point

It is not the logbook's complexity, type or cost that count but the accuracy and completeness with which you collect and record the data within it.

The operative information collected varies with your expertise and interest. This will change and develop throughout your career. However, some core information is always necessary. This includes:

2. *Patient details* – record name, age or date of birth, sex and hospital number as a minimum, otherwise your log cannot be externally audited (see quality assurance later), and you may fail to trace the notes, or follow up the patient.

3. *Demographic details* – complete the columns for hospital, operation, date and time, whether planned, emergency or 'next routine list'.

4. *Staff involvement* – what was your involvement, who performed the operation, who assisted, who was the most senior surgeon present? You may record the anaesthetist and even the scrub nurse – although this is entered in the hospital records.

5. *Operation* – devote at least three columns, each more specialized and specific than the last. Within your training programme you rotate, so enter the name of the speciality in the first column, such as orthopaedics or neurosurgery. In the second column name the subspeciality, for example within general surgery it may be colorectal or vascular. Record the name of the procedure in the third column. The Office of Population Censuses and Survey (OPCS) have developed specific codes for each operation to ensure uniformity for accurate subsequent analysis.

6. *Anaesthesia* – record the type, such as local or general, as a minimum.

7. *Selection of procedures* – you may decide what extra procedures you wish to record, for example, rigid sigmoidoscopies or central lines you insert.

8. *Complications* – record details of all adverse events following operation. Anastomostic leaks, wound infections and haemorrhage are obvious, but even though urinary tract infection and deep vein thrombosis may not be technical complications, record them.

9. *Mortality* – a perioperative death is one occurring within 30 days of operation. Record all deaths even though they may not be related to the procedure

Key point

The only way to avoid complications is not to operate. Be honest with yourself and record all complications.

PROBLEMS WITH KEEPING A LOGBOOK

1. Inaccurate and incompletely kept logbooks are a waste of time. Acquire an enthusiasm for keeping an accurate record of operative activities.

2. Develop a routine. Discipline yourself to complete the entries in your logbook every time – when you leave the operating theatre, or every night before going to bed. If you lag behind it is tempting to give up.

3. Record the data soon after the event while it is still fresh in your mind. Collect it little by little as you accumulate experience. If you defer it for intervals of once a month, you will miss patients and fail to remember the data accurately.

4. Collect your data from original sources, from what you know to have happened in the operating theatre, not from the operating room logbook or the hospital computer record of admissions and discharges, as this information is not reliably accurate.

5. Include all operations. Do not exclude minor procedures such as excision of sebaceous cysts because you have undertaken the procedure several times before. Avoid this temptation or your logbook will become inaccurate and incomplete.

6. Record all complications, even though it may demand courage to admit them.

Key point

Keep your logbook up-to-date, comprehensive and accurate

7. Analyse the data regularly. It is a stimulus to assessing your progress and identifying your strengths and weaknesses. It is both important and gratifying, demonstrating the value of keeping an accurate, complete logbook.

8. Quality assurance checks ensure that your data collection is accurate. At intervals of approximately 3 months, check your list of operations against an independent source such as the operating room logbook. Your record should be more accurate and complete than any other list, and if it is not, then your data collection is inadequate.

9. Keeping it legal: *register your log book with the data protection agency*. Your logbook must not infringe the patient's personal rights. You must avoid allowing this information to become publicly available. Ethical and legal restrictions on ensuring patient confidentiality apply here, as elsewhere in medicine. To ensure this, keep minimal patient information, such as the initials and not the names or hospital number. This creates difficulty for future audits and follow-up studies. If you keep your logbook always within the hospital where you work, it can be registered with the hospital's list of patient databases. This limits your access, as you must register it each time you move hospitals and you cannot take it to your home. If you are creating a surgical log for the whole of your working career, which you should be, then consider registering it under the Data

Protection Act, 1988. You need to fill in a form, obtainable over the internet (http://www.dpr.gov.uk), and pay an annual nominal fee.

ANALYSING THE DATA

The logbook contains a vast wealth of information from which many facts about training and, subsequently, surgical practice can be drawn. Analysing what you have done can be an exceptionally informative and often enjoyable reflection on your progress. Before starting to analyse your data, clearly determine what information is needed. For example, while in training it is important to know the number of operations you have done, their size, the degree of urgency and the level of supervision received. Using the above layout, this information can be extracted either manually or with the aid of a personal computer.

Problems with data analysis

Analysis takes too long

If the logbook data is stored in a paper book, analysis is done manually by counting through each case. This will take time once there are several years of cases. If the log is stored on a computerized spreadsheet, analysis time is considerably shortened. However, a limited basic knowledge of computers and computer spreadsheet analysis is necessary first. This should never be considered a hurdle and all surgeons in training should be prepared to sacrifice the single afternoon required to obtain these skills. The Colleges offer basic computer skill courses.

Analysis appears incomplete

Assuming complete data collection, a lack of uniformity between cases in recording similar data may result in a failure to detect all cases. For example, if abdominal aortic aneurysm repairs are sometimes recorded as 'aneurysm', at other times as 'AAA' and yet other times under the OPCS code L1940, computer analysis looking only for 'aneurysm' will miss cases coded with either 'AAA' or L1940.

The logbook is lost

Always keep at least one recently updated copy of your logbook separate from the original.

WHAT DATA DOES YOUR HOSPITAL KEEP?

Data collection is very important in reviewing progress and planning future changes. On an individual level, you as a surgeon need to undertake this. However, it is important at all levels of medicine. NHS trusts collect data about inpatients, outpatients and others on their patient administration systems. The data include demographic details of the patients, dates of admitted care and clinic appointments, the consultants in charge of their care, diagnostic and operative procedure codes, and a variety of other such information.

Trusts routinely send nationally specified subsets of these data to the NHS-wide clearing service (NWCS), which then electronically redistributes the information about patients to the appropriate commissioners of health care. This enables the local commissioners to monitor the workload of all the trusts serving large or small numbers of their patients.

Each quarter, a summary of the inpatient data held by the NWCS is sent to the Department of Health's own database, the hospital episode statistics (HES) system. It is HES that is used for the calculation of published clinical indicators – dubbed 'league tables' by the media – and for high level planning of the NHS, monitoring its performance and other government purposes.

The Department of Health is intending to add more detail to the data sets held at NWCS and HES, including the codes of surgeons and anaesthetists present in theatre during operations.

CONCLUSIONS

Keeping a record of your surgical activities is a central part of the discipline of being a surgeon. It requires dedication to ensure its accuracy and completeness, but if well done you have a valuable record of your activities as a surgeon.

Summary

- Keeping a record of all surgical activity is an integral part of a surgeon's job, both while in training and later in professional life.
- On every procedure, keep information relating to the patient's details, the site and time of the operation, the procedure undertaken and by whom and, importantly, record all complications.
- Ensure that the data are collected quickly, accurately and completely.
- Analyse and review your progress regularly.

49 The MRCS examination

D. Wilkins

Objectives

- **To explain the new format of the examination.**
- **To provide insights into the philosophy that underpins the examination.**
- **To provide advice on how to approach the examination.**

INTRODUCTION

The MRCS (Membership of the Royal Colleges of Surgeons) examination was devised and introduced in 1997 and has since been conducted by all four of the Royal Colleges of Surgeons of the United Kingdom and Ireland. Successful completion of the examination, which comprises a series of assessments, is designed to mark the end of basic surgical training by the attainment of a 'satisfactory' standard of knowledge and clinical skills. In essence, the standard of performance expected is that of an experienced, well-motivated and able senior house officer (SHO) who has completed a 2 year rotation through a series of approved basic surgical training posts. I provide a broad overview of the regulations for the English College examination appropriate from September 2002. Changes in format and sequence will apply to those taking the clinical section for the first time after May 2002. You must study those for your preferred College as early as possible.

What of the philosophy that lies behind the MRCS? The aims of the examination can be expressed succinctly by stating that it aims to be fair and thorough. 'Fair' means that we shall examine to a consistent standard, explicitly stated as clearly as possible in the examination syllabus and also in the curriculum. Curriculum (Latin *currere* = to run) defines the whole breadth of knowledge and skills to be acquired during training; the syllabus (Greek *sittuba* = book label; programme, abstract) sets out the segments that will be assessed by the examination. Great care is taken in all modern examinations to achieve consistency. The expertise required to achieve this is substantial and is reflected by the infrastructure necessary to support the examination and subsequently in the cost of the examination which, surprisingly, runs at a loss! Fair also means that all candidates will be treated in similar manner without bias of any kind.

'Thoroughness' is the other, as yet unachieved, ambition of examinations. Ideally, examinations test all areas of knowledge and skill outlined in the curriculum. The aim of basic surgical training is to train and educate aspiring young surgeons to a level of 'competence' across a range of skills. Clearly, an examination set outside the workplace cannot assess all of these competencies. Operating skill, attitude and values must be assessed in the workplace. Factual knowledge, ability to examine a patient properly and communicate effectively can be tested reliably in an artificial setting. Overall, the examination sets a demanding agenda of quality and development for the examiners.

The MRCS examination is the main hurdle for aspiring young surgeons and, during the 5 years since its introduction, it has come to be accepted as a well-conducted, fair and thorough examination. Basic science is emphasized to create an adequate foundation of core scientific knowledge.

Key points

- **The MRCS examination aims to be a fair and thorough series of assessments.**
- **It will continue to develop to fulfil the demands of training and available reliable methods of assessment.**

Requirements (Table 49.1)

1. You must have completed a minimum of 24 months of training in approved posts. Type 1 posts provide general experience, Type 2 provide specialist experience and training. Details are available from the examinations

Table 49.1   Timetable and eligibility for the sections of the MRCS (England)

Section	When held	Where held	Criteria for eligibility
Papers	March and September	London and regional centres	Any time after enrolment
Viva	June and December	Royal College of Surgeons, London	A pass in MCQ papers 20 months in approved posts
Communication skills	June and December	Royal College of Surgeons, London	A pass in MCQ papers 20 months in approved posts
Clinical examination	January and July	Regional centres	22 months in approved posts A pass in MCQ papers A pass in the viva section

departments of the respective Royal Colleges and their web sites.

2. You must have satisfactorily completed an approved course in basic surgical skills.

3. You may sit the multiple choice question (MCQ) papers at any time after enrolling with the College. You may attempt it an unlimited number of times. Once you pass the MCQs you may take the viva after a minimum period of 20 months in recognized training posts.

4. Once you have taken the viva for the first time you must pass this plus the clinical examination within 2 years.

5. You must attain a pass in all sections of the examination.

6. The MRCS itself will not be awarded until the full 24 months of training have been completed.

Advice

1. Prepare by taking every opportunity to examine patients thoroughly and confidently (see Ch. 3). Use your clinical time wisely, assiduously acquire new skills, take every opportunity to practise what you have learned and be totally committed to your craft.

2. Plan your training to mirror the philosophy of the examination. Choose your training post carefully to acquire clinical experience. Choose a committed trainer in preference to a prestigious one.

3. If possible, work with friends and colleagues at the same stage, as it is difficult to work in isolation. It may be convenient to meet up once a week or in the evenings. Ask your senior colleagues to monitor you, question you, advise you, criticize you and encourge you.

4. You will benefit from the Advanced Trauma Life Support (ATLS) and Care of the Critically Ill Surgical Patient (CCrISP) courses if possible. Progress through to the clinical examination will only be allowed if the viva is passed, but the communication skills section may be retaken separately if failed and will not hold up progress to the clinicals.

5. On the day of each examination, you will have been asked to present yourself at a time and a place. Note this carefully, together with any documents that are required. Arrive on time; do not fail to allow for heavy traffic or bus and train delays. Examiners try to be helpful but the margin for error is extremely slim and if you miss your appointment slot you may be deferred.

6. If you fail any section, the examiners will have made notes in order to provide some feedback should you fail the whole examination. You can obtain this information through the Examinations Department on request. It is intended to help you direct your learning towards a more successful outcome at your next attempt.

ASSESSMENTS, STANDARDS AND MARKING

1. *Formative* assessments are designed to aid you and your trainer. They may involve tests or assessments conducted by your trainer; your performance is then used to help you and your trainer decide on the requirements for future training. In other words, they help to 'form' subsequent teaching.

2. *Summative* assessments are designed to confirm that a prescribed standard of skill, knowledge and/or competence has been achieved. The driving test is an example. Understand that the MRCS falls firmly into the summative category.

3. A single isolated examination at the end of a substantial period of training is considered unsatisfactory, as it is unlikely to provide the necessary range of assessments. More importantly, it is unlikely to stimulate you to acquire skills and knowledge systematically during training.

4. A single 'exit' examination also suffers from the drawback that it gives you no indication of your progress until the end of the course. This is unhelpful and wastes energy and resources.

5. The MRCS examination addresses this by providing a series of assessments during, as well as at the end of, basic surgical training. These will be further refined and developed as surgical training evolves in the UK, and worldwide, within a society that is increasingly prescriptive and regulated.

6. The curriculum for basic surgical training in the UK is being, and will be, revised, as will the pattern and assessment of training. The end of training will soon be marked by the award of a certificate of completion of basic surgical training (CCBST) but the MRCS examination will remain the most important assessment to be met and overcome by you.

7. The pass mark must be set at a fair and appropriate level, and maintained at a constant level from one examination to the next. When constructing the question papers (which incidentally are marked by optical scanning), a series of standard setting exercises is conducted to agree a cut-off point between pass and fail, under the direction of an expert. The time-consuming and demanding Angof technique combines the views of a substantial group of surgeons. Such methods are now a prerequisite for conducting professional examinations. A panel of external advisors was established initially and continues to direct the appropriate technical measures for setting and maintaining standards.

8. You may wish to know the principles of marking methods. An aggregate of marks is used to measure performance in an MCQ paper or objective structured clinical examination (OSCE). A check list system is impractical and inefficient for complex tasks such as clinical examinations: examiners must make judgements. To ensure consistency, new examiners undergo training. Existing examiners undergo refresher training and regular appraisal of their performance during *each* examination. Furthermore, each examiner has available a set of established criteria to help form that judgement, and at the end of each interview the examiners mark *independently* before conferring, discussing details and agreeing a final mark. Pass/fail is decided on the combined total of marks across each section, with some small leeway for adjustment for borderline candidates resolved at the daily examiners' meeting.

Key points

- **Do you match the knowledge and standards of a well-motivated, competent, experienced SHO?**
- **Do you understand the difference between summative and formative assessment?**

- **Remember, in the clinical examination you may be able to compensate a substandard performance in one bay with a good performance in another.**

OVERVIEW OF THE EXAMINATION

1. Examiners must make judgements regarding the emphasis on particular areas of the curriculum. This is intended to encourage systematic learning and training so you develop sound insights, knowledge and skills. Throughout your professional life you need a grasp of the scientific base for surgical practice. In response to this, the MCQ papers have been increased to accommodate extra scientific content. Take every opportunity thereafter to refresh this knowledge beyond the examination, or it will decay. Be aware that basic sciences are needed for the Intercollegiate Board examinations sat during higher surgical training.

2. The examination is divided into four sections:

a. Multiple choice questions (MCQs)

b. Viva voce (Latin *vivere* = to live + *vocare* = to call; oral testimony)

c. Communication skills test, which takes place on the same day as the vivas

d. Clinical examination (Greek *kline* = bed; strictly, by the bedside).

The vivas, clinical examinations and communication skills tests are taken towards the end of basic surgical training and pitched at the standard expected of an experienced SHO. Until recently, the clinical examination preceded the vivas. A relatively high failure rate in the vivas was ascribed to the fact that, following clinical success, candidates had only 2 weeks to prepare for the vivas. Clinical examination with bays taking 10 min each was considered too rushed and was expanded. The vivas are largely knowledge based. The clinical examinations are rightly the highest tests of skill, knowledge and decision making.

THE SECTIONS OF THE EXAMINATION

Multiple choice papers

1. There are two papers, each lasting two and a half hours. One is held in the morning, the other during the afternoon. They can be taken together or on separate occasions. The examinations are held twice a year.

2. The papers cover two aspects: 'core' topics – a knowledge of the basic sciences that underpin surgical practice; and 'systems' topics – general surgical practice

itself. Both papers aim to test these two key areas. When the examiners set the papers they place the questions into one of these two categories, or a third 'mixed' category that combines both basic sciences and clinical knowledge.

3. Each paper is divided into two sections. The first comprises 65 questions that are in the multiple true/false format (MTF); the other comprises 60 items that are in the extended matching (EM) format. MTF questions test a very basic level of recall of factual knowledge and the answers are, in effect, a pure memory test. Extended matching questions require you to match one, more or none of a series of options with a series of clinical sketches (vignettes). This format is designed to simulate questions that may be encountered within genuine clinical situations, thereby testing your ability to *apply* knowledge. This is considered to be a better, or more 'valid', assessment (Table 49.2).

Table 49.2   Example of extended matching question

Theme: postoperative complications
Options:
a. Tension pneumothorax
b. Unstable angina
c. Septicaemia
d. Acute massive pulmonary embolism
e. Myocardial infarction

For each of the clinical vignettes described below, select the single most likely postoperative complication from the options listed above. Each option may be used once, more than once or not at all.
1. A man of 75 had emergency surgery for a perforated diverticulum of the sigmoid colon. Twenty-four hours after operation he was peripherally warm, hypotensive (95/40 mmHg), and oliguric. The ECG was within normal limits.
2. A man of 75 had a hip fracture treated by hemiarthroplasty. In the history it was apparent that he had fallen a couple of days before he presented. He received subcutaneous heparin from the time of admission. Six days after operation he became hypotensive (95/75 mmHg) and was blue, cold and clammy, with a high central venous pressure. He had inverted T waves in lead III.
3. A man of 75 had a laparoscopic cholecystectomy. The following day he was noted to be peripherally cold with a tachycardia. He had crackles at the lung bases. The ECG showed Q waves and ST segment elevation in the chest leads.

Answers: 1 – c, 2 – d, 3 – e

---

4. There is no negative marking for this or the extended matching section – marks are not deducted for incorrect answers. However, effective statistical techniques are applied to counteract the effects of overselecting choices. Remember that the papers are marked using optical scanning, so use only pencils of the appropriate grade, which are supplied, together with erasers. Sampling is carried out to check the system for accuracy and the scanner queries uncertain pencil marks; however, be positive with your pencil marks and if you wish to erase a mark, do so thoroughly.

 Key points

- **Carefully read the glossary and instructions set out in the front of the papers.**
- **Read the stems of the questions carefully.**
- **Do not be tempted to 'random guess' the answers.**

Viva voce section

1. This is a test of your ability to apply both pure and applied basic sciences to the practice of surgery. There are three sections, each of which is conducted by at least two examiners:

a. *Applied surgical anatomy and operative surgery.* A specialist takes you through some anatomical questions that may involve photographs, sketches, a model or a cadaver. A colleague at the same table questions you on the surgical application of anatomical knowledge for operations and other practical procedures, and the principles underpinning them. Your logbook may be used as a guide to your experience for the purposes of framing questions.

b. *Clinical pathology and principles of surgery* are examined at another table. One examiner poses questions on knowledge of basic pathology, the other questions you on applied pathology.

c. *Applied physiology and critical care.* At the final table an examiner with a specialist interest explores your knowledge of basic physiology; the surgeon examiner tests your clinical knowledge on critical care or other acute clinical situations, also assessing your understanding of the underlying physiological principles.

2. Questions are constructed to provide a uniform approach. They usually start with a fairly straightforward lead into the subject so as to focus your mind on the topic. Subsequent questions progress to the limits of your knowledge before moving on. You may be taken far beyond the level set for a pass in order to establish that

you have attained an adequate level of knowledge across a range of topics.

3. The examiners are mostly interested in eliciting what you know. They provide as much opportunity as possible for you to display it by covering a range of topics. Questions are framed carefully and it is vitally important that the candidate listens and responds to the question asked rather than obfuscating. Much better to admit that the answer to a question is not known so that the interview can move on to other, hopefully more productive, areas rather than leaving awkward silences or filling the space with irrelevant material.

Key points

- **Listen to the questions and respond to them.**
- **Admit ignorance straightforwardly so that the examiner can move to another subject.**

The clinical examination

1. This tests your ability to examine a patient, elicit the appropriate physical signs, discuss their significance and formulate a plan of management. It is conducted simultaneously at several centres throughout the UK and you are allocated as close as possible to, but not usually at, your own hospital. If you had not taken the clinical examination for the first time by May 2002, the clinical section comprises four bays, in each of which you will spend 15 minutes. The bays contain cases categorized as follows:

> Bay 1 – Superficial swellings and skin
> Bay 2 – Musculoskeletal and neurological conditions
> Bay 3 – Circulatory and lymphatic conditions
> Bay 4 – Trunk (including thorax).

2. You are briefed as a group by the supervising examiner and a member of the examinations department. You are then shown to a holding area where the documentation is checked. Thereafter you are addressed by number to provide anonymity. Following a roll call you are shepherded by examination staff, ready for the bell. When this sounds you are introduced to a pair of examiners who take you to the bay for examination.

3. Since time is limited, be prepared to move through topics and cases fairly rapidly. The examiners are anxious to test the breadth as well as the depth of your knowledge.

Key points

- **Listen closely to the instructions you are given. If you are uncertain, ask for clarification.**

- **Do not 'short cut' the routine of inspection, palpation, percussion and auscultation.**

4. Be prepared to be asked to tell the examiner what you are doing, why, what you find and what it means, as you proceed. Practise doing this beforehand. The clinical problems tend to be straightforward, so concentrate initially on common conditions, not rarities.

5. One examiner takes the lead in directing the examination and the other listens, taking notes.

6. Hand-cleaning facilities are available by the bed or nearby but avoid wasting examination time.

7. A limited number of stations will be based on the Objective Structured Clinical Examinations (OSCE) format. These test your expertise in clinical examination *technique*. This has been introduced because some candidates are defective in the correct technique. The format has not yet been finalized, but it is likely to comprise a station, lasting 3–5 minutes, where you are required to perform a task under observation by the examiners. A typical test is the examination of a joint or another region. A bell rings to finish the interview. The examiners have 2–3 minutes only to mark you independently, confer, and agree a final mark, so leave promptly.

8. You are ushered from the examination. The supervising examiner carries out a short, collective debriefing. You may then leave.

9. You may be given the option of reattending at the end of the day to receive your results. If you are successful, there is a short congratulatory ceremony.

Communication skills

1. This section aims to assess your ability to communicate effectively with a patient or patient's relatives in a typical clinical situation (see Ch. 47). Until the end of 2002 it focuses on the giving of information; for example, informing an anxious relative about the condition of the patient, or providing preoperative information to patients (see Ch. 14). Subsequently it is intended to pilot a test of the candidate's ability to extract information from a patient, analyse it and communicate it to fellow professionals. It should provide little difficulty if you have occupied a busy training post.

2. You may wait in a holding room for a maximum of three-quarters of an hour as your group is directed, singly, into the examination cycle. You enter the reading room to be given a vignette – a short character sketch or word picture – to read for 5 minutes. It outlines a fairly realistic clinical situation in which you, as the SHO, are obliged to interview a relative or patient, assess the situation and communicate appropriately. The vignette defines your task.

3. You are now conducted to the interview room and greeted by the two examiners, who introduce you to the

'patient' or 'relative' by the role-play name. You are now in control of the interview. The examiners observe but do not intervene. The actor stays 'in character' throughout and is instructed and coached to behave in a typical manner in that situation and given an itemized series of 'Points of Concern' to discuss with you. You will find that the atmosphere rapidly ceases to be artificial.

4. After 10 minutes the interview ends, or before this if you are satisfied you have covered the concerns satisfactorily. The examiners then discuss the interview with you.

5. As yet, the format of the new sections is not fixed. Probably you will take an observed history from a simulated patient, followed by a presentation to the examiners. You may be asked to prepare a written communication. The time allotted to testing communication skills is likely to be at least 40 minutes, reflecting the recognition of their importance.

2. At present the examinations conducted by the four Royal Colleges of the UK and Ireland are broadly 'equivalent'. It is hoped that an intercollegiate MRCS can be developed.

3. The curriculum for basic surgical training for the English Royal Colleges is intended to integrate in-training and external assessments, including the MRCS examination. Comprehensive assessments during basic surgical training should encourage those with appropriate aptitudes and commitment, and discourage those without the essential traits.

4. It is likely that a certificate of completion of basic surgical training (CCBST) will be introduced.

5. Modern working practice, for example the European Working Time Directive, discourages long hours of clinical work. The required study will need to be undertaken out of defined working time.

Key points

- **Read the vignette carefully to determine the task you have been set.**
- **Give the simulated patient accurate information and behave in a professionally correct manner.**

FUTURE DEVELOPMENTS

1. The MRCS examination will develop in line with accepted good practice in education and in response to changes in clinical surgery and assessment techniques.

Summary

- Do you appreciate that facts alone are insufficient unless they are organized and produced to the examiners at the right time?
- Have you practised taking a history, examining a patient and interpreting your findings until you are confident in your clinical skills?
- Is the scope of your knowledge broad enough and sufficiently up to date?
- Have you fulfilled all the requirements to sit the examination?

50 The intercollegiate examinations in surgery

R. E. C. Collins

Objectives

- Provide an introduction to the intentions of the examination.
- Display the need to obtain current details of your subspeciality examination.
- Outline the conduct of the examination.

INTRODUCTION

The four Royal Colleges of the British Isles have formed the Intercollegiate Examinations Board. Each of the Specialist Advisory Committees (SAC) in the nine recognized surgical disciplines have produced their own specialty examination. The examination has exposed areas of ignorance in some trainees that are a reflection of suboptimal standards of training. The intention is to create a higher standard of rigorous annual assessment of all trainees, to identify their deficiencies at an earlier stage and take corrective action. Meanwhile, there have been significant changes to basic surgical training. In 2003, the first candidates who have not taken the Primary FRCS or Clinical Surgery in General (CSIG) examinations (which contained a significant element of basic sciences) take the intercollegiate examinations. Inevitably, the intercollegiate examination will evolve to take these changes into account.

A balance will need to be reached between all-round surgical competence and the recognition that surgery is now practised on an increasingly subspecialist basis. In general surgery, for example, candidates may choose to have a significant part of their examination devoted to the subspeciality they intend to pursue. In some subspecialities, such as vascular surgery, pressure exists for an examination purely in that subject. However, this clashes with the need for surgeons to be capable of contributing to an on-call rota for emergencies in the generality of surgery. It is therefore in that aspect of speciality interest that the emphasis is placed in the examination.

This examination is a serious hurdle. Initially it was considered a mere formality but the first candidates had received many years of prolonged intensive training. It demands an understanding of the syllabus, appropriate reading, and capability to respond to questions at consultant level. You need knowledge of and competence in the generality of your speciality subject that fit you to be on emergency call. In addition, you must be fully competent in your subspeciality interest, in which you might be the sole representative in your hospital.

REGULATIONS RELATING TO THE INTERCOLLEGIATE SPECIALTY EXAMINATION

These vary from specialty to specialty and also are regularly updated. You should contact the intercollegiate specialty examinations board for up to date details of the regulations in your subject. The address is:

The Intercollegiate Examinations Board
3 Hill Square
Edinburgh EH8 9DR
Tel: 0131 6629222
Fax: 0131 6629444
Web site: http://www.intercollegiate.org.uk

Some regulations are common to all nine SAC subjects:

1. You must hold a medical qualification recognized for qualification by the General Medical Council or the Medical Council of Ireland and must have been qualified for at least 7 years.

2. You must satisfy the current requirements for entry to an approved higher surgical training programme in Great Britain or Ireland.

3. You must have completed satisfactorily 4 years of higher training in the specialty acceptable to the relevant board:

a. If you are a type I trainee, you are training with a view to being awarded the Certificate of Completion of Specialist Training (CCST) by the Specialist Training Authority of the United Kingdom, the Certificate of

Specialist Doctor (CSD) or Specialist Registration with the Medical Council of Ireland. You must have enrolled with the relevant SAC and completed the above 4 years of training within a programme approved by them. You need to have satisfactory fourth year clinical assessment form(s) covering this year of training, and the appropriate declaration form signed by the Programme Director.

b. If you are a type II trainee, you are not eligible for the CCST. You need to be registered with the relevant SAC and must have spent at least one of the above 4 years in a training programme in Great Britain or Ireland approved by the relevant SAC. This mandatory clinical year must offer experience equating to fourth year level within the specialist registrar grade and you must obtain written confirmation of this from your trainer. You require a satisfactory fourth year clinical assessment form(s) covering this year of training and the appropriate declaration form signed by the Programme Director. Any other training posts completed in Great Britain and Ireland must be approved by the relevant SAC in order to count towards the examination. If you wish training acquired outside Great Britain and Ireland to be taken into consideration, you need to present supporting documentation at the time of registration with the SAC.

Key points

- **If you are a type II trainee you are not be eligible for the award of a CCST.**
- **Passing the examination does not automatically entitle you to enter type I training.**

4. From 1 January 2003 you will be limited to three attempts at the examination, after which you must seek specific counselling, retraining where necessary, and written support from the Postgraduate Dean and Programme Director in order to resit again. Attempts prior to January 2003 will not be counted.

THE FORMAT OF THE EXAMINATION

1. The format and style of the examinations differ from specialty to specialty. Although anxieties have been expressed about lack of consistency in such an approach, it is apparent that the nature of the different specialties, and particularly the clinical material involved, varies from subject to subject. Thus in orthopaedics the value of a clinical examination with long cases is considered very important. You need to be able to talk to an individual patient and outline the lifestyle problems and relevant

clinical signs. You must then decide upon an appropriate course of management pertinent to that patient. In urology, on the other hand, there is very limited scope for spending much time on clinical examination so there is an understandable natural reluctance to expose patients and candidates to the evaluation of multiple rectal examinations. The technical skills required of a neurosurgeon clearly differ from those of a general surgeon with an interest in hepatobiliary disease. In my judgement, it is not only appropriate that there is a difference in examination format between the subjects but that such differences are actually essential.

2. Examiners are very concerned to maintain consistent standards. You can be confident of having an examination and subject content of equal standard to the other candidates. This has produced much debate within the examinations boards; it is now common practice for all of the questions in oral examinations to be structured and to conform to a set pattern. A perceived problem in the clinical arena is the difficulty of arranging for large numbers of candidates to see a large number of similar patients. In practice, the clinical examination, particularly of short cases, closely mirrors the procedure in an outpatient clinic, where we encounter the vagaries of life and variances of clinical presentation. The examination tests your ability to deal with whatever problem presents.

3. Recognize that the examination is not an interrogation on surgical esoterica (Greek *esoterikos – eso* = within; revealed to an elect few), but a standard of international authority. However, we all encounter some rare conditions and you must demonstrate your ability to tackle an unusual problem sensibly. In many of the specialist subjects, particularly general surgery, the field and syllabus are quite colossal. It is almost impossible to go through the day of an examination without coming across a subject where one's knowledge or experience is insufficient. You must not be unsettled. This is a fact of life in consultant practice. The examination is carefully designed to balance areas of difficulty with areas of outstanding competence or experience.

Key points

- **Recognize that as a surgeon you must expect to encounter unfamiliar problems.**
- **As a surgeon you must display common sense in difficult circumstances.**

To varying degrees, therefore, each of the examinations is composed of essentially two parts: oral examinations with two examiners, usually lasting half an hour; and clinical examinations with two examiners, again lasting half an hour. Some of the subjects also have written examinations that are usually multiple choice.

4. In all of the oral and clinical tests, examiners are instructed to treat you as if you are a consultant colleague asked to see an interesting or unusual case. There is room for debate, and you will be questioned on management strategies, but the examination should never become rude or aggressive. Almost without exception the examiners go out of their way to make you feel at ease within the understandable constraints of the circumstances.

5. If, however, you feel you have had an unfair or difficult experience in any part of the examination, speak to the chairman of the examination board, or one of the individuals who help organize the examination. You should settle any matter of discontent immediately, between parts of the examination. You can then start the next part in a calm and collected frame of mind, and not carry over any frustrations or anxieties that might otherwise threaten your subsequent performance.

6. Take the minimum baggage into the examination. Briefcases are not permitted. You need little instrumentation for clinical examinations, as it is usually provided. Regard the clinical examination as a demonstration of your routine skills. Do not start with rare tests that you would not normally employ. Concentrate on being thorough, carrying out appropriate examinations, avoiding inappropriate ones.

7. Be prepared to discuss papers from the literature. You may be invited to present some of your own work for discussion, usually of how you performed the studies, how they relate to previous or subsequent work and how, in retrospect, your study could have been improved. You may be asked to comment on a paper, usually taken from a major journal. Do not, on this account, assume it is without fault. The discussion concentrates on the strengths and weaknesses of the paper.

8. Note that statistical method may enter into the format. This is not, though, an examination in statistics but on your understanding and use of simple statistical methodology in the evaluation of scientific work.

9. The emphasis on basic sciences varies, depending on the speciality. Although there is a view that basic science teaching and examination belongs to basic surgical training, you will be expected to apply relevant, and only relevant, basic sciences to your clinical subject. A candidate whose main interest is in upper gastrointestinal/hepatobiliary disease should understand the basic physiology of digestion and pancreatic secretion, but will not be asked the details of the relationships of the thalamus.

THE END OF THE EXAMINATION

1. You either fail or pass. No distinction is made between a bare pass and high marks. However, in some subjects a prize or medal is awarded for outstanding candidates. As a rule you are notified of your result in an envelope at the end of the day's examination. If you have been successful you are usually invited to celebrate with your examiners before departing. If you are unsuccessful you do not discuss with the examiners why you have failed. This is because early experience showed that examiners and failed candidates can become adversarial, prejudicing the atmosphere at subsequent examinations or consultant appointment interviews.

2. If you are unsuccessful, you will, in the following weeks, receive written details from the chairman on your weaknesses, together with advice for the future. If you are unsatisfied with your treatment by the examiners you may appeal. You can obtain details from the Examinations Board in Edinburgh.

Good luck to all those who undertake the examination.

Summary

- Do you know whether or not you are eligible to sit the examination?
- Are you aware of the standard and conduct of the examination?
- Do you recognize that the Colleges owe it to the public to pass only those who demonstrate competence?
- Will you accept that the examiners appreciate the stress involved and will treat you courteously?

Index

Page numbers in **bold** refer to figures or tables.